A. Leblanc · The Cranial Nerves

Springer
*Berlin
Heidelberg
New York
Barcelona
Budapest
Hong Kong
London
Milan
Paris
Tokyo*

André Leblanc

The Cranial Nerves
Anatomy Imaging Vascularisation

Forewords by C. Libersa, G. Cornélis, and P. Lasjaunias

Second enlarged edition
with 293 figures comprising 722 illustrations in all

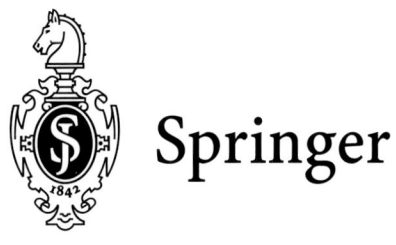 Springer

André Leblanc
Author – Researcher
Service de Radiologie
Centre Hospitalier Régional et Universitaire d'Amiens
F-80030 Amiens, France

Private address:
20, rue Sainte Colombe, F-80800 Aubigny, France

Originally published with the title: *Anatomy and Imaging of the Cranial Nerves*

ISBN 3-540-58702-0 Springer-Verlag Berlin Heidelberg New York

ISBN 3-540-18240-3 1. Auflage Springer-Verlag Berlin Heidelberg New York
ISBN 0-387-18240-3 1st edition Springer-Verlag New York Berlin Heidelberg

Library of Congress Cataloging-in-Publication Data
Leblanc, André, 1934–. [Imagerie anatomique des nerfs crâniens. English] The cranial nerves : anatomy, imaging, vascularisation / André Leblanc ; prefaces by C. Libersa, G. Cornélis, and P. Lasjaunias ; [English translation by David Le Vay]. — 2nd enl. ed. p. cm.
Rev. ed. of: Anatomy and imaging of the cranial nerves / André Leblanc. © 1992.
Includes bibliographical references and index.
ISBN 3-540-58702-0 (alk. paper). — ISBN 0-387-58702-0 (alk. paper)
1. Nerves, Cranial—Magnetic resonance imaging—Atlases. 2. Nerves, Cranial—Tomography—Atlases. I. Leblanc, André, 1934–. Anatomy and imaging of the cranial nerves. II. Title. [DNLM: 1. Cranial Nerves—anatomy & histology—atlases. 2. Magnetic Resonance Imaging—methods—atlases. 3. Tomography, X-Ray Computed—methods—atlases. WL 17 L445i 1995a] RC410.L4413 1995 616.8'7—dc20 DNLM/DLC 95-8410

This work is subject to copyright. All rights are reserved, whether the whole or part of the material is concerned, specifically the rights of translation, reprinting, reuse of illustrations, recitation, broadcasting, reproduction on microfilm or in other way, and storage in data banks. Duplication of this publication or parts thereof is only permitted under the provisions of the German Copyright Law of September 9, 1965, in its current version, and permission for use must always be obtained from Springer-Verlag. Violations are liable for prosecution under the German Copyright Law.

© Springer-Verlag Berlin Heidelberg 1992, 1995
Printed in Germany

The use of general descriptive names, registered names, trademarks, etc. in this publication does not imply, even in the absence of a specific statement, that such names are exempt from the relevant protective laws and regulations and therefore free for general use.
Product liability: The publishers cannot guarantee the accuracy of any information about dosage and application contained in this book. In every individual case the user must check such information by consulting the relevant literature.

Cover illustration: André Leblanc

English translation: Dr David Le Vay, Burwash, East Sussex, England

Typesetting, printing and binding: Graphischer Betrieb K. Triltsch, Würzburg
SPIN 10661141   21/3111 – 5 4 3 – Printed on acid-free paper

Foreword

André Leblanc's book was originally conceived to help in the radiologic location of the orifices at the skull base transmitting the cranial nerves. With the passage of time it has become a true atlas of anatomy, radiology, computed tomography and magnetic resonance imaging, whose final range far exceeds the initial aims.

Having followed the conception of this book from the outset, I am well able to assess the stringency with which this study has been pursued. Based on everyday radiologic practice, André Leblanc has perfected a series of methods allowing very precise visualization of even the smallest orifices of the skull base, using a relatively simple technique and confirming this with clear pathologic evidence.

He has set out, with intense and laudable personal endeavor, to perfect his anatomic knowledge so as to provide even greater precision to the interpretation of the radiographs. It is for this reason that he was induced to collaborate with my laboratory, where he was able to utilize the remarkable studies of my friend and pupil, Professor Jean-Paul Francke. Finally, thanks to the kindness of Professors Cornélis and Doyon, he has enriched his book with computed tomographic sections and magnetic resonance images which add even more importance to this remarkable production.

The final outcome of this long research is the work now completed after so much persistent exertion, and also after so many transient hold-ups that André Leblanc has been able to overcome, thanks to an unwavering faith in the utility of his work.

Thus it is that collected here, for each cranial nerve, will be found its anatomic description, its course and distribution, its radiologic identification in the different regions it traverses, a review of its pathology and the computed tomographic aspects of its relations. All this is clear, precise and profusely illustrated.

Though mainly intended for radiologists and their co-workers, it will also be of the greatest usefulness to students, anatomists and clinicians. André Leblanc's work is a veritable treatise on the cranial nerves, a valuable guide of indisputable didactic importance, and one that merits the esteem that everyone is bound to accord it.

Professor Claude Libersa
Lille Medical Faculty

Foreword

When, in 1980, André Leblanc showed me the first outline of his work, I immediately agreed to collaborate in the performance of the research in computed tomography required to bring it to fruition. I did, indeed, have a good many reasons to welcome André Leblanc's "new method" with enthusiasm. Among these, I stress the fact that I had never had the good fortune to come across a work so rich in detail, one in which willingness to go to the extremes of precision in description was obvious in every line and every diagram. Another reason, as I saw it, lay in the organization of the book: its division into 12 chapters, each corresponding to the study of a single nerve; the actual study of this nerve, itself divided into 3 sections: a precise and profusely illustrated anatomic description, a complete review of the pathology and symptomatology relevant to the nerve in question with a detailed account of the necessary radiologic postulates; and, finally, a description of the computed tomographic images that can be obtained.

A third reason, which also seemed to me one of the most important, was that André Leblanc's "new method" arrived at the very time to coincide with the perfection of the so-called "high-resolution" scanners and of magnetic resonance imaging. In fact, the great advances in scanning technology have allowed us, in the space of a years, to pass from coarse imaging of the brain substance to imaging of very high resolution. Our present scanners produce real anatomic sections of the skull base that are extremely sharp, precise and detailed. It is unfortunate that too few are able to validly interpret them because of inability to keep in mind – and this is perfectly normal – the multitude of details comprised in the thorough study of the cranial nerves and their pathways.

This is why I am convinced that André Leblanc's book, based on his new investigative technique, constitutes a reference work of outstanding value, both for students, who will find there very many diagrams as well as descriptions, and for technicians – whether or not they work with scanners – who can inform themselves effectively and without waste of effort on the views to carry out and the images to obtain. Radiologists themselves can only feel happy to have at hand this genuine working tool, which should allow them to direct procedure effectively and rapidly and to make interpretation of the images obtained less arduous and problematic.

I pay due homage to André Leblanc for having carried through this gigantic work, and I am grateful for the trust he showed in asking me to collaborate with him. I dare to expect that his book will achieve the success it deserves. But, whatever the outcome, I shall always feel very proud to have had the opportunity to add my modest contribution.

Professor Georges Cornélis
St-Luc University Neuroradiology Clinic
Louvain en Woluwe, Brussels

Foreword

This is the second, enlarged edition of André Leblanc's atlas of the cranial nerves. The first edition, published in 1992, was a successful conclusion of long and fastidious work that was carried out with a meticulousness that did credit to its author. André Leblanc's roots are firmly in the French anatomoclinical tradition: he combined dissections, cross-sections, and views of the skull with functional anatomical information on the cranial nerves and with conventional tomography and magnetic resonance imaging. He contributed to the anatomoradiological tradition with this work, a compilation which featured architectural ideas and rigorous selection in terms of both, information and images. In short, he became a model for the French school. He did not seek to make strict correlations, but managed to associate views in the same planes with general views centred on the cranial nerve, thereby combining the three-dimensional, two-dimensional, and schematic aspects. This capacity for linking detailed vision with a general view is rare today and certainly deserves emphasis here: it is modern and at the same time true to our tradition.

The first edition and the posters which accompanied it were a showcase for the French school. André Leblanc's book can now be found all over the world, and his posters hang in the majority of general radiological and neurological departments. The wide recognition is a source of pride for him and for us, and surely an encouragement to read this work in a little more detail. This distribution over international boundaries of the work of a man whom our own system might classify as marginal should prompt reflection on the part of those responsible for the system. Does progress not always have its origins in a marginal phenomenon?

The multidisciplinary character of André Leblanc's approach and the addition of vascularisation in this new edition illustrate the extent to which the anatomical foundations of imaging are an essential accompaniment to the development of therapeutic techniques. Indeed, some years after the creation of groups for neurosurgery of the skull base and the introduction of minimally invasive or endovascular approaches, knowledge of the anatomy of the cranial nerves and their vascularisation has become a source of clinical precision, a series of significant markers, and a surgical challenge. Just a few years ago, skull base syndromes represented obstacles or contraindications to therapy. Today, surgeons' knowledge of the anatomy of the nerves and ability to respect them during treatment are an index of their skill and precision. Functional rehabilitation and immediate reconstruction of these anatomical structures are the aspects most recently focused on.

This second edition is thus a reference not only for clinicians, surgeons, and neuroradiologists but also for anatomists. It represents a successful balance between erudite detail and clinical practice. Working with a book like this is a sheer pleasure: it provides authentic material for teachers, and will be pleasantly easy to use for students or others who have the good fortune to become acquainted with it.

I share the pride of Professor Cornelis in the first edition at having had the opportunity to follow this project from its very beginning and to see the author's persistence rewarded.

Professor Pierre Lasjaunias
UFR Kremlin Bicêtre, Université Paris Sud

Preface and acknowledgments

This work presents a simple and original radiologic technique, thanks to which most of the vulnerable points of the cranial nerves, wherever they may be situated, can be rapidly visualized. The course of each nerve is studied both anatomically, by dissections and macroscopic serial sections, and radiologically.

Naturally, the classical lesions are reviewed. But, over and above the association with the anatomy and computed tomography (CT), the main interest of this book lies in the description of the numerous unpublished lesions at the foramina and orifices of the skull base. These lesions, demonstrated by myself, called for numerous preliminary explorations of the dry bone and anatomic specimens, contrasting with the facility of actual execution. They are valid whatever the morphology and the patient's condition, and take account of possible asymmetries.

The different pathologic affections of the cranial nerves are summarized. In the presence of a given syndrome, they allow precise definition of the zones to be radiographed. By simple angular calculation, and whatever the radiologic material utilized (old or otherwise), it is possible to clearly visualize the suspect zones, easily and rapidly.

Each nerve is studied from its origin right up to its muscle, with its anastomotic, ganglionic and terminal branches, with its intracranial, extracranial and intracanalicular course and path. The canals and orifices transmitting the cranial nerves are visualized precisely in their axes.

It is true that computed tomography and magnetic resonance imaging have become the preferred methods for radiologic exploration of the skull. But while these techniques are more particularly suited to detecting intracranial pathologic processes, the images of the foramina at the skull base often still lack definition.

These images are rarely made along an axis allowing detection of a lesion of small dimensions or a minimal fracture line, as can be done by radiography using the methods described in this work. It is common to obtain films of CT scans showing the foramen ovale, the foramen lacerum, the auditory tube, the jugular foramen, etc.; but it remains rare to see the orifices and courses of the greater and lesser petrosal nerves, superficial and deep, and of their grooves, which run in different directions. The importance of obtaining such films is set out in the book.

Progress in computed tomography and magnetic resonance imaging has made available greater possibilities in multidimensional orientation and reintegration; the new methods are readily applied for our present purposes, but interpretation of the films is all the trickier. This means that the radiologist must be able to refer to very detailed anatomic studies; and in the anatomical field, as in that of imaging, this atlas will be a valuable guide. It is supplemented by numerous sections obtained by the most recent types of magnetic resonance imaging and CT scanning (high definition).

The importance of this book may be illustrated by reference to some of its essential features. It provides valuable teaching material in a field where exploration is difficult. It is a guide for the anatomist, the radiologist, the neurosurgeon, the otorhinolaryngologist, the ophthalmologist and the medical student. It deals with the neuralgias, and with the early diagnosis of neurinomata, fractures and small tumors from the appearance of the earliest clinical signs. The radiographs discussed are easy to perform, whatever the morphology or condition of the patient, and the films are obtainable with a minimum of time and radiation, even with simple equipment. There is a general revival of interest in view of the development of computed tomography and magnetic resonance, whose better spatial resolution allows demonstration of the foramina of the skull base in their axes and of the course of the cranial nerves.

This book summarizes fifteen years of work and research in electroradiology carried out by me with the help of the Anatomy Institute of Lille Medical Faculty, then in neuroradiology [computed tomography (CT)] at the Saint-Luc University Clinic of Brussels, in the Department of Neuroradiology (MRI) of Kremlin Bicêtre Hospital Center in Paris, and finally in the Department of Neuroradiology (MRI) of A. Z. St-Jan in Brugge. I thank particularly my brother René Leblanc and Dr Jean Jacquier who taught me the rudiments of this discipline around 1955 at the Medicosocial Center of Mines at Auchel, so making it possible to produce this work. I also thank the members of the Photographic Department of the Lille Medical Faculty: Messrs Gérard Espouy, Jean-Pierre Delattre, Jacques Delattre, Jules Herman, and Ms. Maryse Caron of the Sud Hospital in Amiens for the production of the greater part of the photographic material in this book and Jean-Jacques Vérité for the reproduction of my drawings and anatomic diagrams, as well as Mr and Ms Deraison (polygraphique, Amiens) for the preparation of most of the photoengravings. I wish to express my warmest thanks to Dr David Le Vay who undertook the difficult task of translating the book into the English language.

Finally, I am deeply indebted to Professor P. Lasjaunias, thanks to whom my book could at long last – even though I did not believe in it – appear, for the possibility to use his angiographic views enhancing this new edition.

A. Leblanc

The author would like to thank Professor J.P. Francke for carrying out all the dissections and serial macroscopic sections in color intended for this book.

This second edition is further enhanced by numerous recent MRI views and additionally by angiographic views of the craniofacial arteries.

Participants

Alejandro Berenstein
Professor of Radiology and Neurosurgeon
New York University and
Bellevue Medical Center
New York

Jan W. Casselman
Doctor of Neuroradiology and
Head and Neck Radiology
A. Z. St-Jan Brugge
Ruddershove, Belgium

Georges Cornélis
Professor of Neuroradiology
Catholic University of Louvain
Saint Luc University Clinic
Brussels

Dominique Doyon
Professor of Radiology
University Hospital Center
Kremlin Bicêtre
Université Paris Sud

Jean-Pierre Dumortier
Department of Neuroradiology
Saint Luc University Clinic
Brussels

Jean-Paul Francke
Professor of Anatomy and
Organogenesis
Faculty of Medicine
Université Lille II

Philippe Halimi
Professor of Radiology
Hospital Center Boucicaut
Paris

Pierre Lasjaunias
Professor of Anatomy
University Hospital Center
Kremlin Bicêtre
Université Paris Sud

Claude Libersa
Professor of Anatomy and
Organogenesis
Faculty of Medicine
Université Lille II

Jean-Claude Libersa
Professor of Dental Pathology and
Therapeutics
Université Lille II

Natacha Belly Touge
Radiologist
Hospital Center Laënnec
Paris

List of contents

Foreword (Professor Claude Libersa) V
Foreword (Professor Georges Cornélis) VI
Foreword (Professor Pierre Lasjaunias) VII
Preface and acknowledgments VIII
Participants IX

Olfactory nerves (I) 1
Optic nerve (II) 17
Oculomotor nerve (III) 33
Trochlear nerve (IV) 47
Trigeminal nerve (V) 59
Abducent nerve (VI) 155
Facial nerve (VII) 171
Vestibulocochlear nerve (VIII) 211
Glossopharyngeal nerve (IX) 227
Vagus nerve (X) 241
Accessory nerve (XI) 251
Hypoglossal nerve (XII) 259
The twelve pairs of cranial nerves 273
Vascular relations: Craniofacial arteries
   (Professor Pierre Lasjaunias) 275
Bibliography 293
Index 295

Olfactory nerves (I)

Anatomy (course – terminals – collaterals) 3
Imaging (regions examined) 3
Pathology 3
Cribriform plate of ethmoid
    Anatomy and imaging (examination) 6
    Frontal view (CT) 7
    Sagittal view (CT) 8
    Axial view (CT) 10
Olfactory tracts
    Anatomy and imaging (examination) 12
    Computed tomography (CT) and magnetic
    resonance imaging (MRI) 13
       Cingulate gyrus
          Sagittal and frontal views (MRI) 14
       Longitudinal striae, dentate gyrus
          Sagittal view 15
    Magnetic resonance imaging (MRI)
       Hippocampal uncus
          Sagittal view 16

Vascular relations:
Olfactory branch of the anterior cerebral artery .. 276, 277

The olfactory nerves arise from neurosensory cells situated in the olfactory mucous membrane.
The apparent origin of the olfactory fibers occurs at the olfactory mucous membrane (nasal cavity, superior nasal concha).
The true origin of the constituent nerve fibers is located at each olfactory patch, where each nerve fiber separates from the base of the olfactory cell.

Olfactory nerves (I)

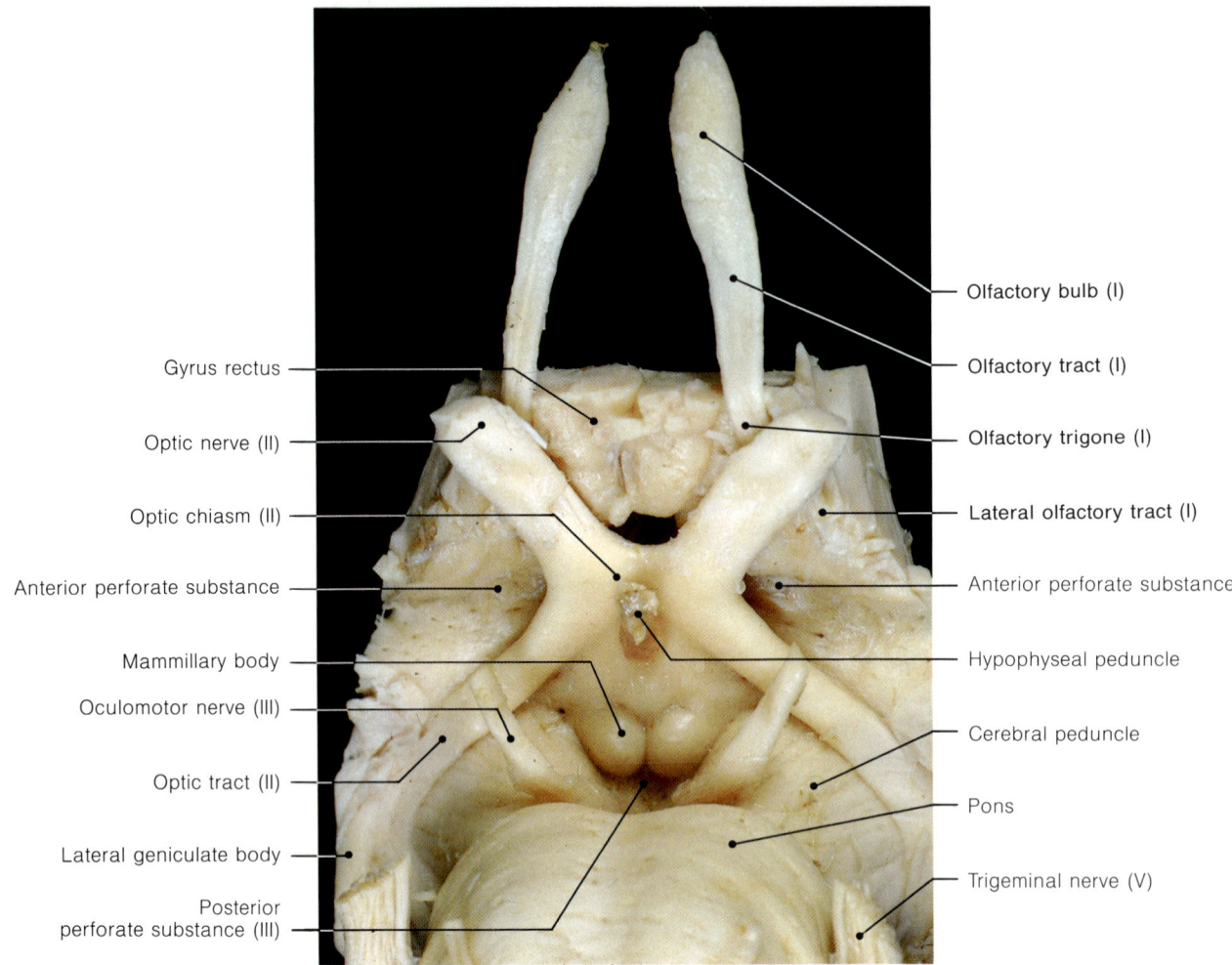

Fig. 1.1. Inferior view of olfactory bulbs

Anatomy

COURSE – TERMINALS – COLLATERALS

Origin (yellow patch, olfactory mucosa)

Fibers of olfactory nerves, olfactory bulb

Lateral, intermediate, medial olfactory tracts
Olfactory pathways:

– cingulate gyrus (corpus callosum),
– longitudinal striae,
– dentate gyrus,
– fasciolar gyrus,
– parahippocampal gyrus and uncus

Accessory olfactory cavities (paranasal sinuses)

Imaging

REGIONS EXAMINED

Imaging of the nasal cavity (superior nasal concha, nasal septum, lateral and medial walls)

Imaging of foramina of cribriform plates of ethmoid

Study of the cingulate sulcus (corpus callosum) with the parahippocampal gyrus, uncus, olfactory bulbs and olfactory tracts

Imaging of the frontal sinuses, maxillary sinuses, sphenoidal sinuses, ethmoidal cells and meatuses of the nasal cavity

Pathology

– Hyposmia, anosmia, hyperosmia, parosmia,
– Paget's disease (osteitis deformans),
– meningiomata of the ethmoid, lesser wing of sphenoid, olfactory sulcus,
– craniopharyngiomata of middle fossa,
– frontal tumors,
– tumors of third ventricle and hypophysis,
– tumors of corpus callosum,
– agenesis of septum pellucidum,
– fractures of the anterior cranial fossa and the ethmoid, involving the foramina of the cribriform plate,
– posttraumatic epistaxis with rhinorrhea; ethmoiditis.

Topography

Origin of olfactory nerves (I)
- Yellow patch, olfactory mucosa (superior nasal concha)

Olfactory bulb, tract, fibers of olfactory nerves
- Cribriform plate of ethmoid

Olfactory pathways
- Cingulate gyrus
- Sulcus of corpus callosum
- Longitudinal striae
- Dentate gyrus
- Hippocampal uncus

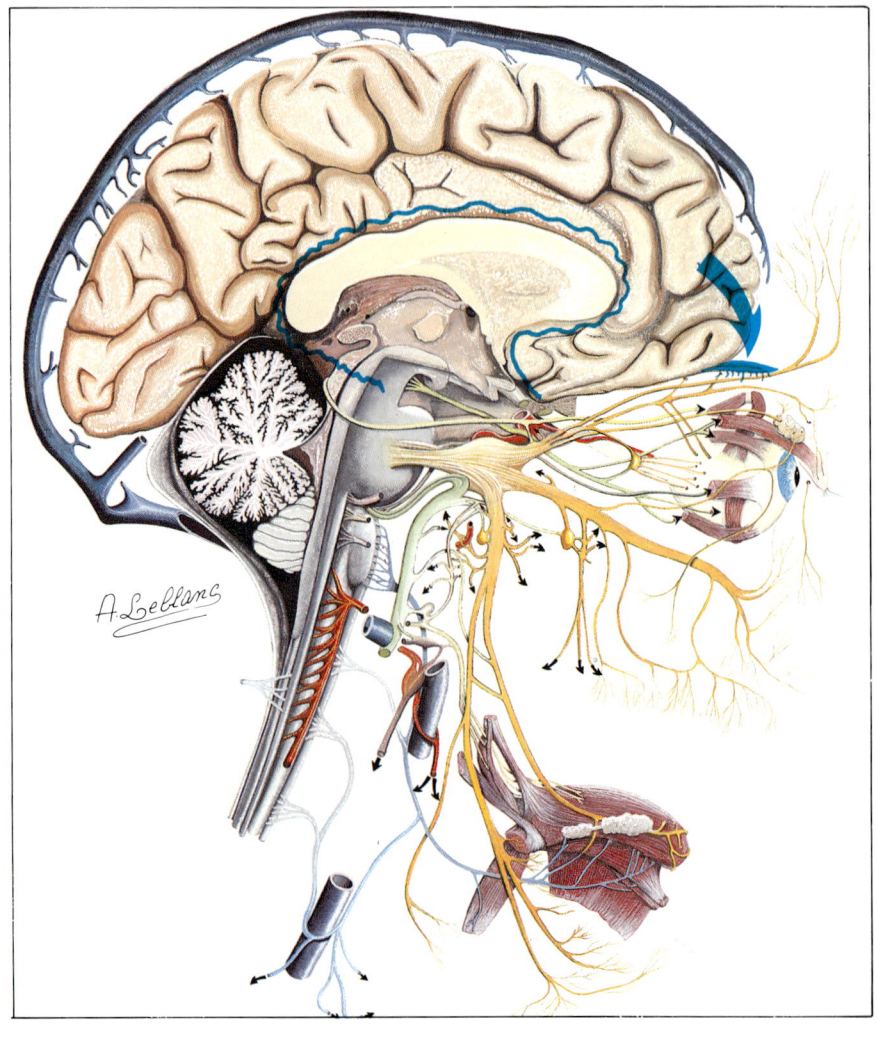

Fig. 1.2

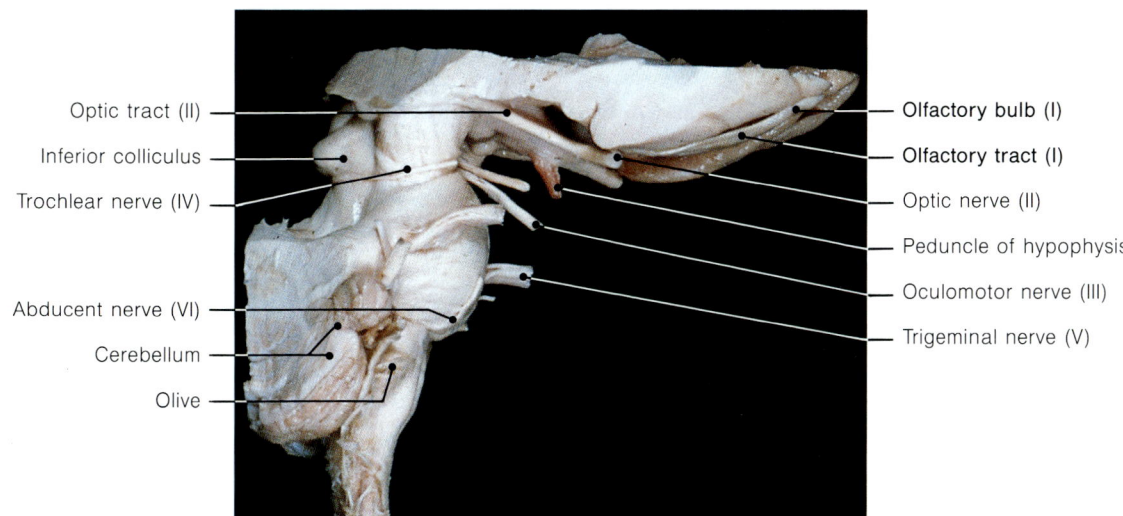

Fig. 1.3a. Sagittal view of olfactory bulbs

Cribriform plate of ethmoid

Anatomy

The olfactory nerves arise from nerve cells situated outside the neuraxis. These cells are in the *olfactory mucosa* clothing the *upper part of the medial and lateral walls of the nasal cavity,* extending from the cribriform plate of the ethmoid (Fig. 1.6b) to a plane tangential to the *superior nasal concha*. In their totality these cells form a ganglion as extensive as a spinal ganglion. Their domain ends at the surface of the olfactory mucosa in some very fine short hairs (Fig. 1.6b, c). The cylindraxial prolongation becomes a nerve fiber of the olfactory nerves. Travelling beneath the olfactory mucosa, the *fibers* of the olfactory nerve are applied to the bony wall and excavate very fine grooves (Fig. 1.6a), before they reach the *foramina* of the cribriform plate (Fig. 1.6a, b). In their submucosal course, the nerve fibers join together to form increasingly larger branches which are united by a certain number of anastomoses to give this submucosal part of the olfactory nerves a plexiform arrangement.

The average number of *medial branches* of the olfactory nerves derived from the nasal septum is twelve to sixteen (Fig. 1.6c). The *lateral branches* arising from the lateral wall of the nasal cavity are rather more numerous: twelve to twenty (Fig. 1.6b). Each olfactory fiber (ensheathed by the pia mater) accesses the anterior cranial fossa by the foramina of the cribriform plate of the ethmoid and terminates at the inferior aspect of the olfactory bulb, which it penetrates.

Olfactory bulb, cribriform plate (I)

Magnetic resonance imaging (MRI)

FRONTAL VIEW

Imaging

Injuries are a common cause of hyposmia or anosmia. Depending on the case, there may be:

- a skull injury, particularly occipital, even without detectable fracture but with avulsion of the olfactory nerves, which are sheared off at the cribriform plate during the impact;
- a fracture of the anterior cranial fossa involving the cribriform plate of the ethmoid (rhinorrhea), so damaging the olfactory nerves that traverse it.

Compression of the olfactory tracts may be the cause of anosmia or hyposmia. This may be due to either:

- a bony lesion of the skull base secondary to a neoplastic process or to Paget's disease (osteitis deformans),
- or an intracranial tumor, the commonest causes being tumors developing in the anterior cranial fossa: frontal tumors, meningiomata of the lesser wing of the sphenoid or of the ethmoid.

EXAMINATION

- Study of the maxillary, frontal and sphenoidal sinuses and ethmoidal cells,
- clarification studies, radiologic and tomographic, of the middle and anterior cranial fossae and of the wings of the sphenoid in profile and high frontal view (projection of the lesser wings of the sphenoid into the orbits),
- clarification study of the cribriform plates of the ethmoid in sagittal views: a strictly lateral radiograph and one in "false profile",
- computed tomographic (CT) study of the cribriform plate of the ethmoid in frontal, sagittal and axial views (Fig. 1.4b, c; 1.5a–c; 1.7).

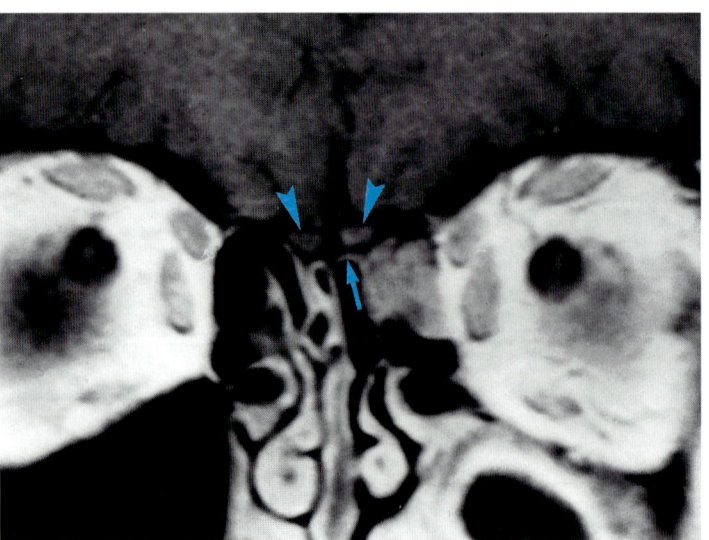

Fig. 1.3b. Magnetic resonance imaging (MRI), frontal view of cribriform plate (*arrow*) and olfactory bulb (I) (*arrowheads*). (MRI: Dr. J.W. Casselman, A.Z. St-Jan, Brugge)

Olfactory nerves (I)   7

TECHNIQUE (FRONTAL VIEW)

Frontal tomography or computed tomography (CT):

- The subject is in dorsal decubitus, the head strictly face-forward, the beam centered at the supraorbital margins making an angle of 0° to 5° in relation to the orbito-meatal plane (OM);
- the first plane of section is situated at 1.5 cm from the skin of the frontal region; the sections are made extending from this plane to 3 cm of depth (Fig. 1.4a).

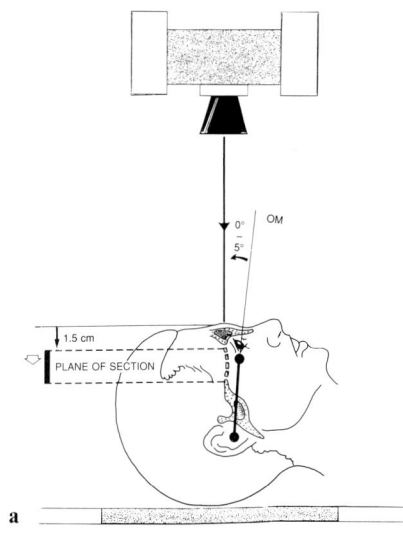

Fig. 1.4. a Reference diagram for imaging of the cribriform plate of the ethmoid; **b** frontal computed tomographic (CT) section; **c** radiograph of an anatomic section at the level of the cribriform plate

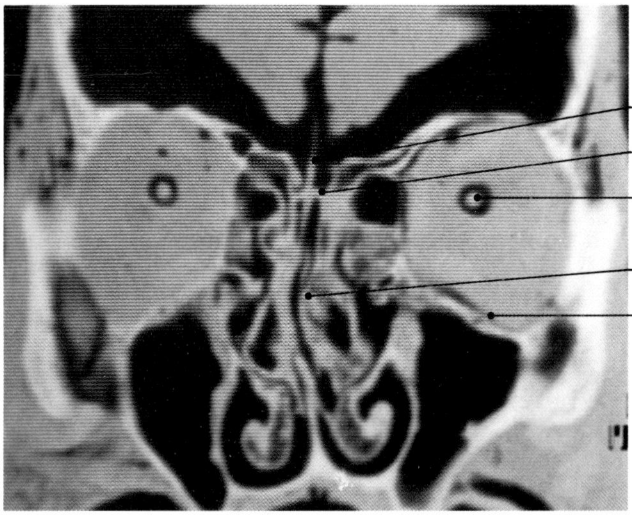

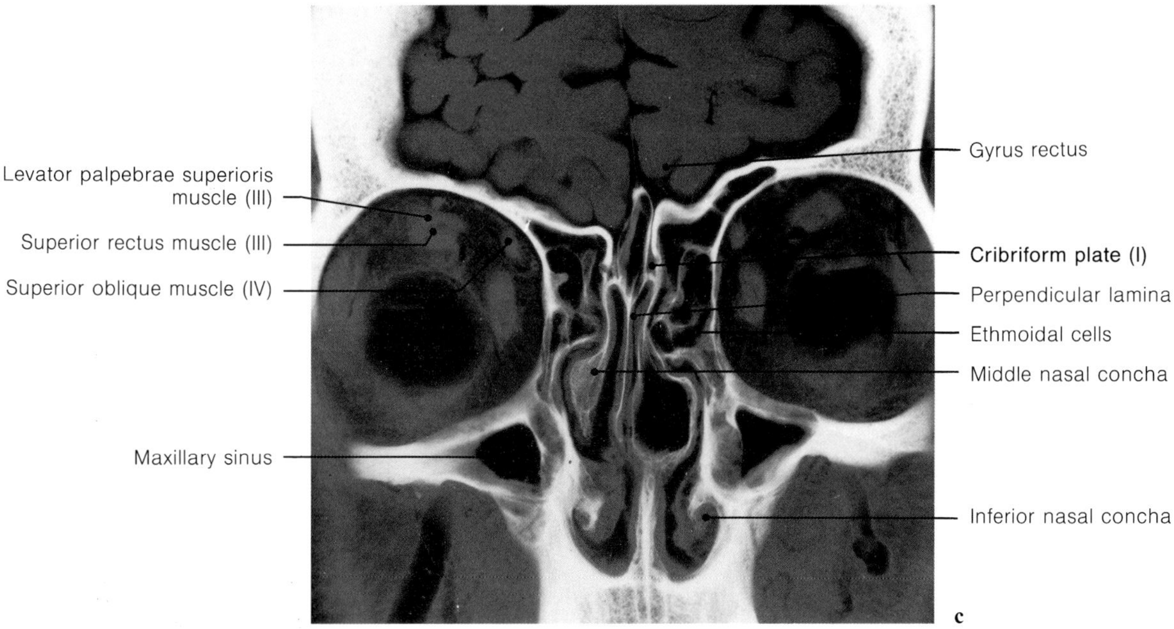

TECHNIQUE (SAGITTAL VIEW)

Sagittal computed tomographic (CT) or tomographic study:

- The subject is in the prone position, the head strictly in profile. Bags of flour are placed in front of the facial massif so as to obtain good homogeneity of the region to be examined;
- the centering point is situated above the lateral angle of the eye;
- the sections are made in like fashion on the two sides, starting from the median sagittal plane and extending for 1 cm outward, remembering to lateralize the films (Fig. 1.5).

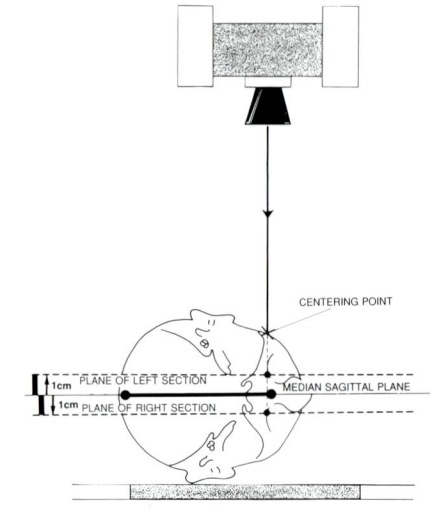

Fig. 1.5. Reference diagram for sagittal study of cribriform plate

Fig. 1.5 a–c. Diagram (**a**) and computed tomography (CT) (**b, c**) of cribriform plate of ethmoid

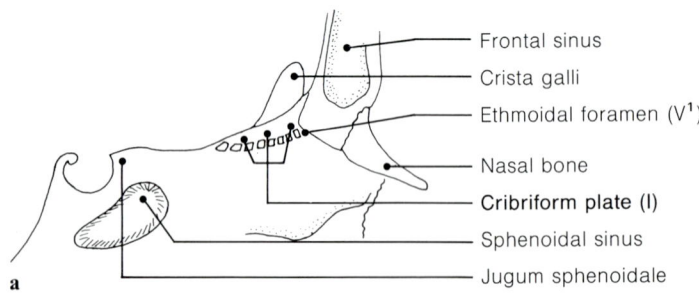

— Frontal sinus
— Crista galli
— Ethmoidal foramen (V^1)
— Nasal bone
— **Cribriform plate (I)**
— Sphenoidal sinus
— Jugum sphenoidale

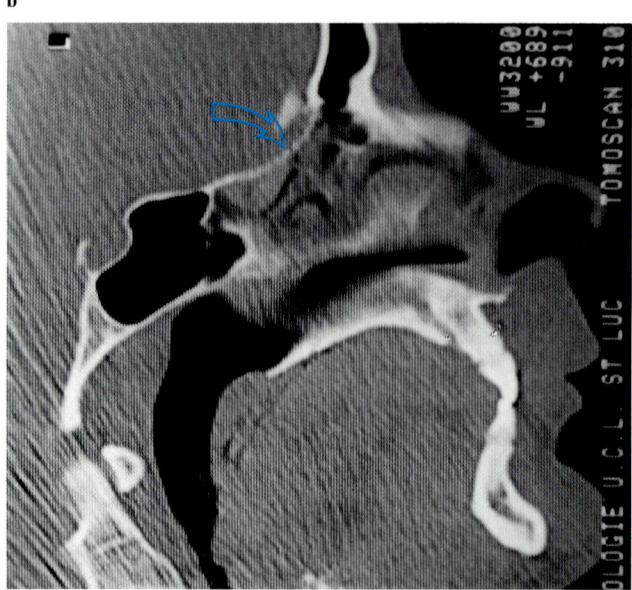
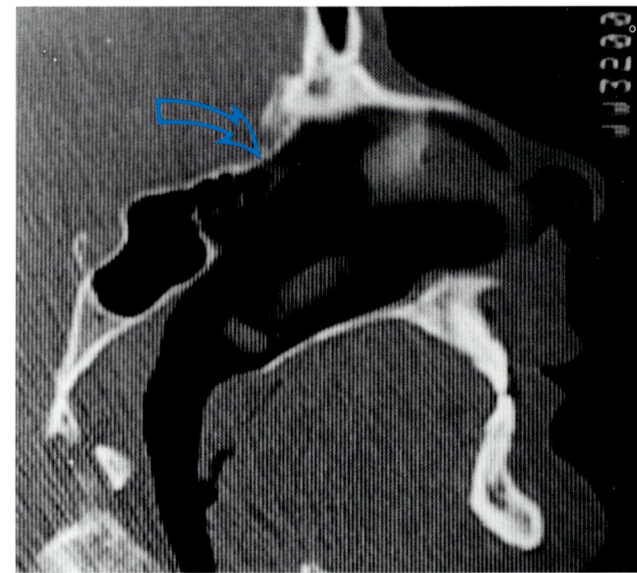

Olfactory nerves (I)

Fig. 1.6a–c. Section of dried specimen (**a**) at nasal cavity showing sulci for olfactory nerves; diagrams of nerves on lateral (**b**) and medial wall (**c**) of nasal cavity

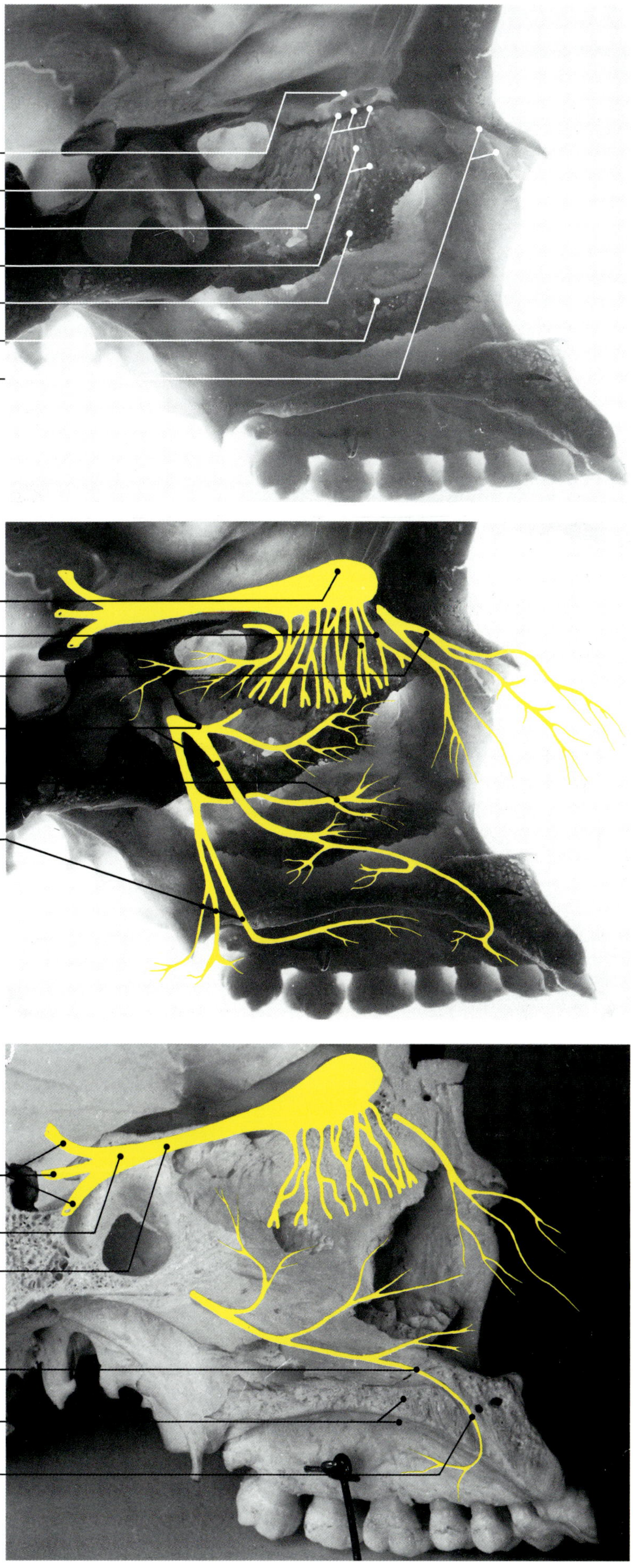

Sulcus for anterior ethmoidal nerve (V^1)
Cribriform plate (I)
Superior nasal concha
Sulci for fibers of olfactory nerves (I)
Middle nasal concha
Inferior nasal concha
Sulcus for nerve to levator labii superioris muscle

a

Olfactory bulb (I)
Fibers of olfactory nerves (I)
Nerve to levator labii superioris muscle (V^1)
Superior nasal nerves, nasopalatine nerve (V^2 – VII – IX)
Postero-inferior nasal branches
Greater palatine, lesser palatine and accessory palatine nerves

b

Lateral, medial, intermediate olfactory tracts (I)
Olfactory trigone (I)
Olfactory tract (I)

Nasopalatine nerve
Hard palate
Incisive canal

c

TECHNIQUE (AXIAL VIEW)

Axial tomographic and computed tomographic (CT) studies:

- The subject is in dorsal decubitus, with the back elevated on cushions and the head turned in the Hirtz position, with the orbitomeatal plane (OM) making an angle of 0° to 8° to the horizontal (Fig. 1.7);
- centering is at the midline 3 cm from the mental symphysis;
- the planes of section are made from 1 cm below the supraorbital margin, every 3 mm towards the infraorbital margin (Fig. 1.7). A series of 4 films should be obtained.

CENTERING POINT
OM
0°
8°
SUPRAORBITAL MARGIN
PLANE OF SECTION
CRIBIFORM PLATE OF ETHMOID
a

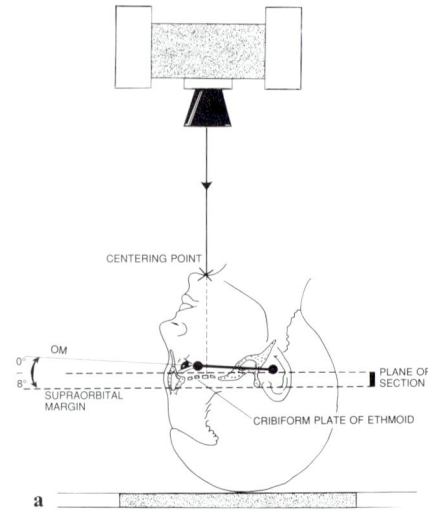

Fig. 1.7. **a** Centering diagram for axial imaging of cribriform plate; **b–d** axial tomographic section of cribriform plate of ethmoid; **e** axial magnetic resonance imaging (MRI) of olfactory bulbs (I) (*arrows*). (MRI: Dr. J.W. Casselman, A.Z. St-Jan, Brugge)

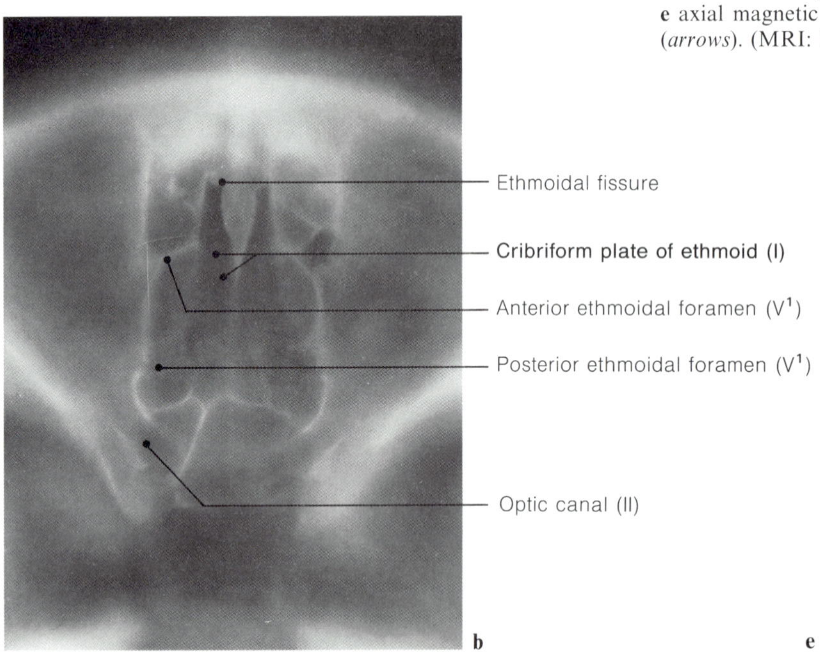

Ethmoidal fissure
Cribriform plate of ethmoid (I)
Anterior ethmoidal foramen (V¹)
Posterior ethmoidal foramen (V¹)
Optic canal (II)
b

Olfactory bulb (I)

Magnetic resonance imaging (MRI)

AXIAL VIEW

e

c

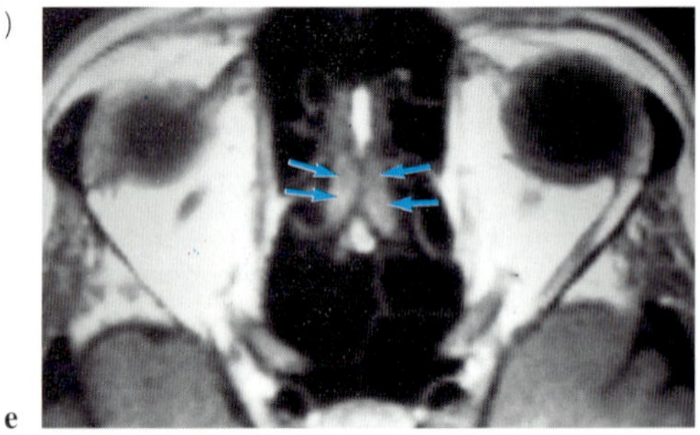

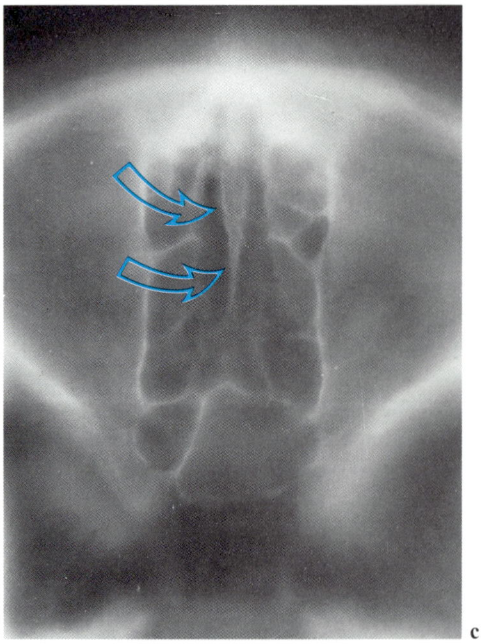

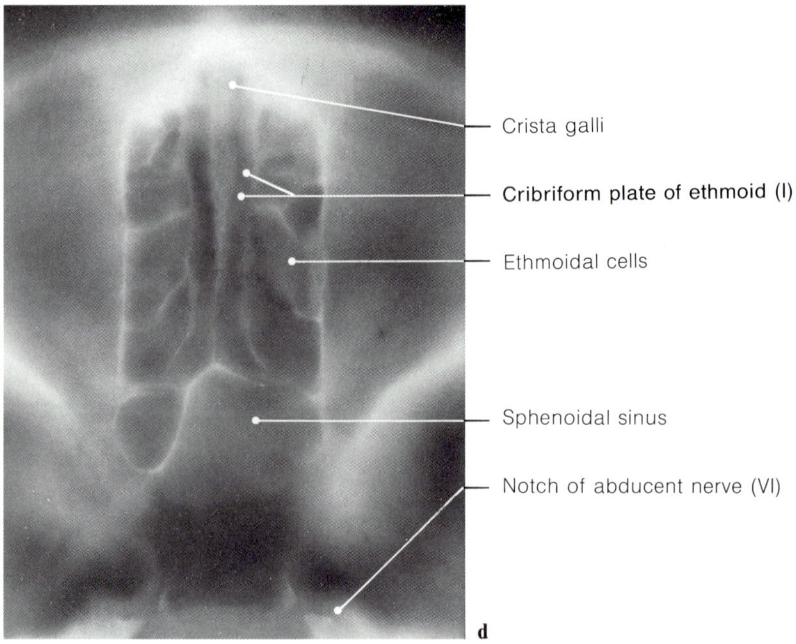

Crista galli
Cribriform plate of ethmoid (I)
Ethmoidal cells
Sphenoidal sinus
Notch of abducent nerve (VI)
d

Olfactory nerves (I)

Fig. 1.8. a Endocranial view of cribriform plate of ethmoid; **b** diagram of inferior view of cerebral hemispheres showing relations of olfactory bulbs, olfactory tracts (or roots) and tracts of Lancisi (or longitudinal striae); **c** superior anatomic view of olfactory bulbs

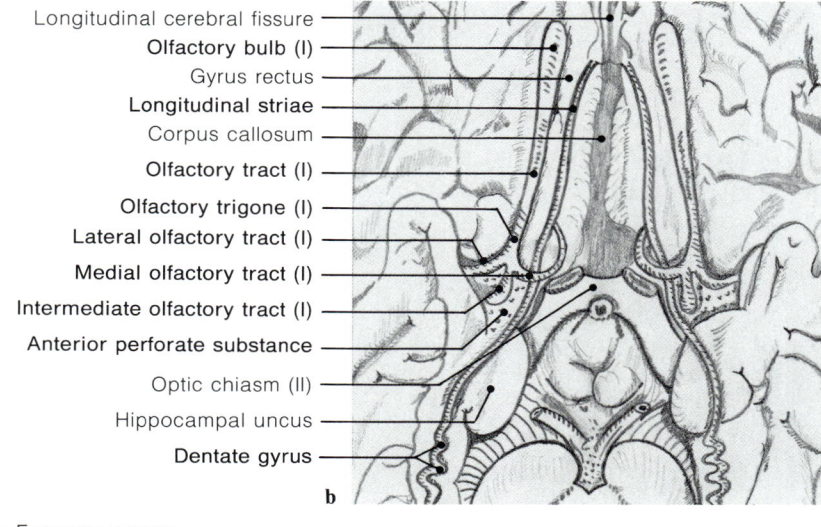
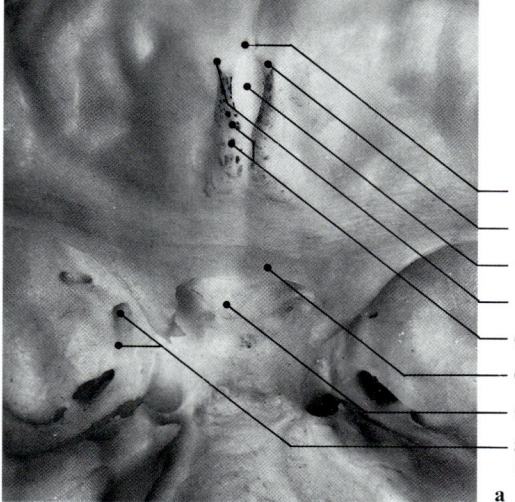

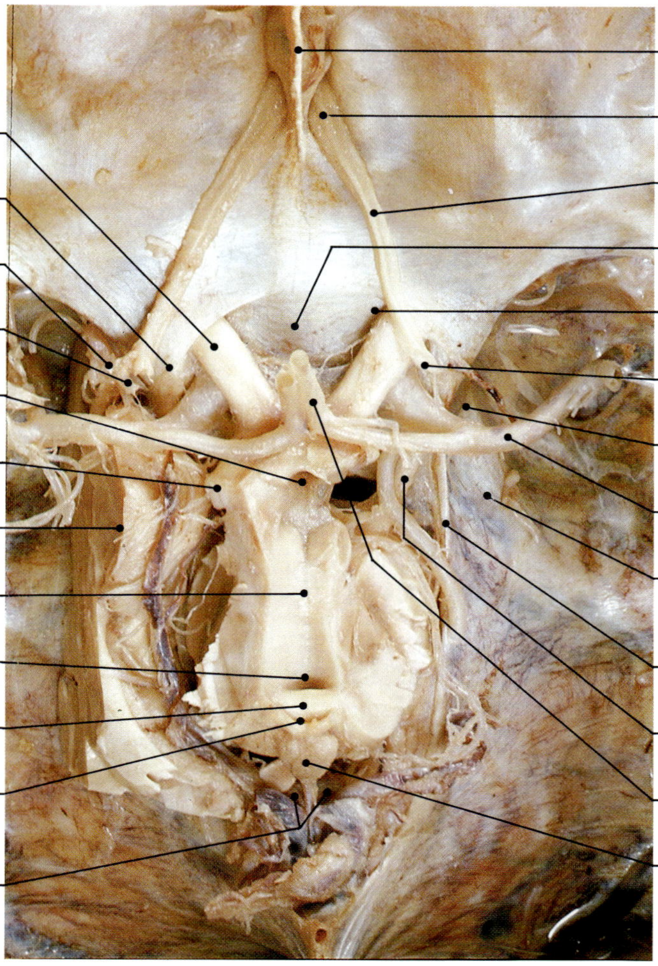

Olfactory pathways, olfactory bulb (its roots), limbic gyrus, hippocampal uncus

Anatomy

The olfactory structures are situated on the orbital aspect of the frontal lobe and constitute the olfactory peduncle; its anterior bulge is known as the olfactory bulb.

Olfactory bulb: Symmetrically paired, this is an expansion of the cerebral hemisphere and therefore forms part of the central nervous system; the peduncle terminates opposite the anterior perforate substance as the olfactory trigone (Fig. 1.3; 1.6 b; 1.8 b, c)

The latter divides into three striae (or roots):

- The *lateral stria* travels outwards and leads to the bend of the 5th temporal gyrus or hippocampal uncus, where it is distributed to two prominences, the gyrus ambiens and the semilunar gyrus (Fig. 1.8 b).
- The *medial stria* curves upwards and medially to reach the subcallosal and precommissural septal regions, close to the rostrum and genu of the corpus callosum (Fig. 1.2; 1.8 b, c; 1.11 a).
- The *intermediate stria* ends at the anterior perforate substance, giving rise to a slight elevation known as the olfactory tubercle (Fig. 1.8 b).

Imaging

Compression of the olfactory pathways may also be caused by tumors developing in the middle cranial fossa, especially by those situated in the midline such as hypophyseal tumors, tumors of the third ventricle, tumors of the corpus callosum and craniopharyngiomata. They may also be damaged in agenesis of the corpus callosum.

Examination

– Imaging by magnetic resonance (MRI) or computed tomography (CT) of the olfactory pathways visualizing the olfactory junction, the sulcus of the corpus callosum, the cingulate gyrus and third ventricle, with demonstration of the olfactory bulbs (Fig. 1.9 b–e; 1.10 a; 1.11 a).

Temporal lesions, particularly those of the hippocampal uncus, may also be evidenced by olfactory symptoms, such as hyposmia and especially olfactory hallucinations. When of recent occurrence, the possibility of a temporal tumor must be suspected, but a vascular lesion and a craniocerebral injury may also be responsible; however, when they are of long standing, the most likely explanation is obstetric injury.

– Sagittal magnetic resonance imaging of the temporal region for the hippocampal uncus (Fig. 1.12 a, b).

Computed tomography (CT) and magnetic resonance imaging (MRI)

Fig. 1.9. a Frontal computed tomography section (CT) of bulb; **b, c** horizontal sections of bulbs, olfactory trigones and sulci of olfactory striae up to hippocampal unci; **d, e** sagittal sections at the level of olfactory bulbs (anatomic specimens); **f** magnetic resonance imaging (MRI) frontal view of olfactory tract (I) (*arrow*); **g** MRI sagittal view of olfactory bulb (I) (*arrow*)

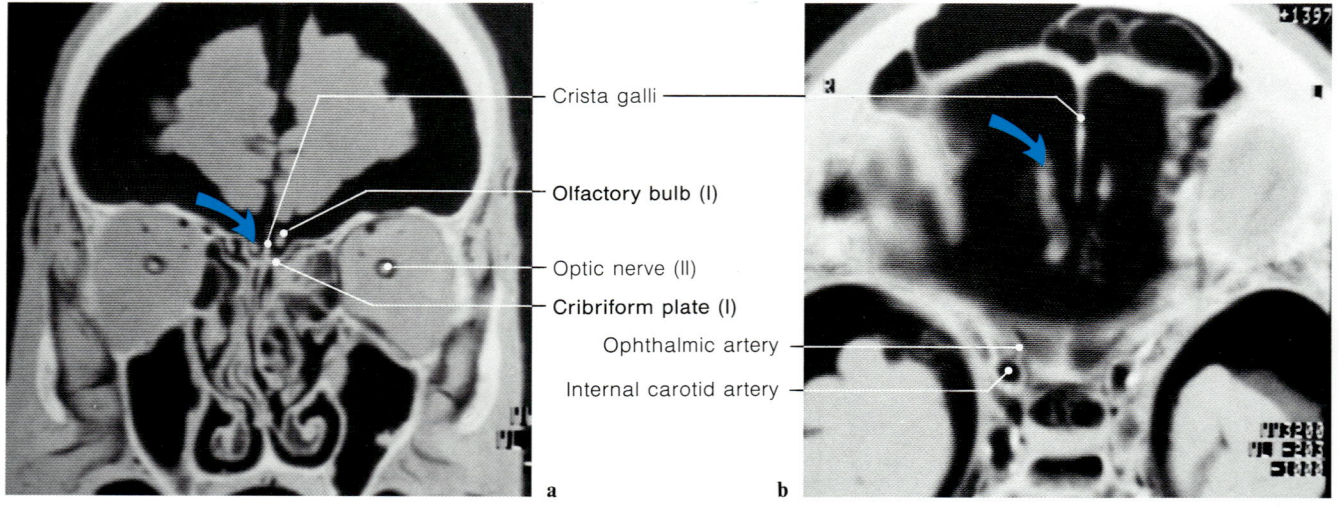

Olfactory nerves (I) 13

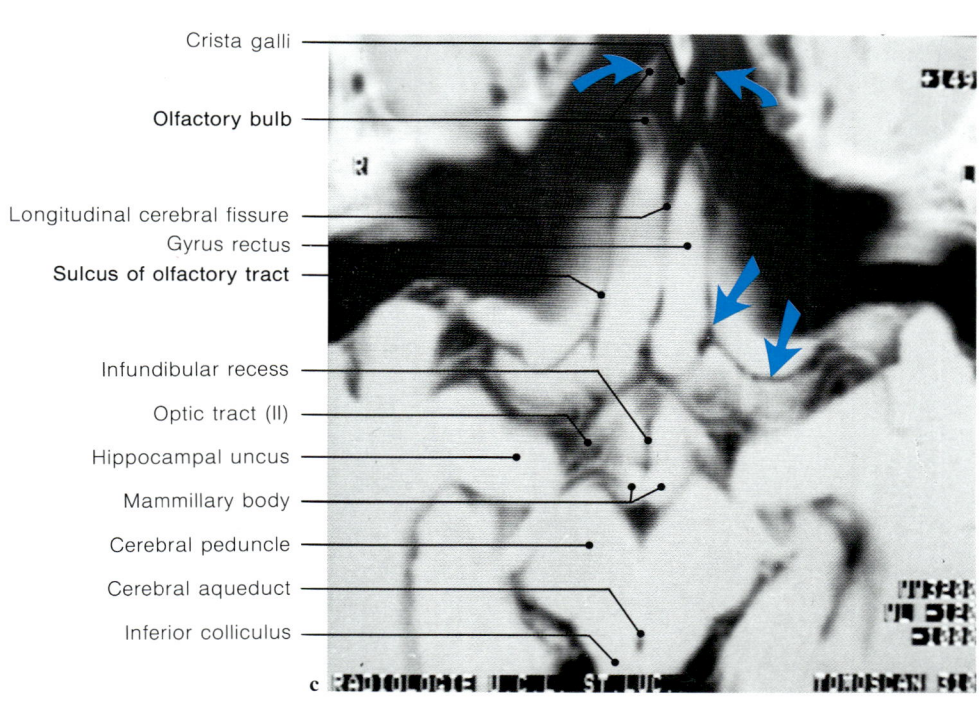

Crista galli
Olfactory bulb

Longitudinal cerebral fissure
Gyrus rectus
Sulcus of olfactory tract

Infundibular recess
Optic tract (II)
Hippocampal uncus
Mammillary body
Cerebral peduncle
Cerebral aqueduct
Inferior colliculus

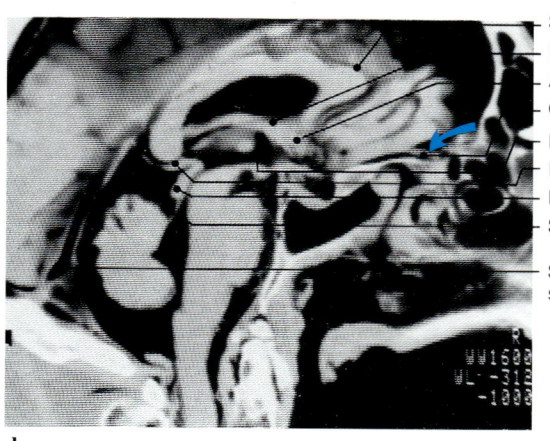
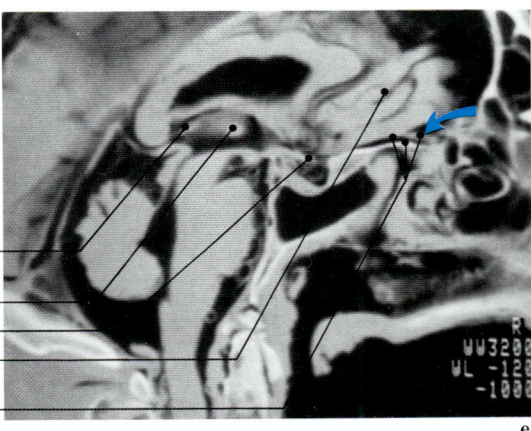

Sulcus (corpus callosum)
Fornix
Anterior commissure
Olfactory bulb (I)
Interventricular foramen
Pineal body
Inferior colliculus
Superior medullary velum
Straight sinus
Tenia thalami
Interthalamic adhesion
Optic chiasm (II)
Cingulate sulcus
Olfactory bulb, cribriform plate (I)

d   e

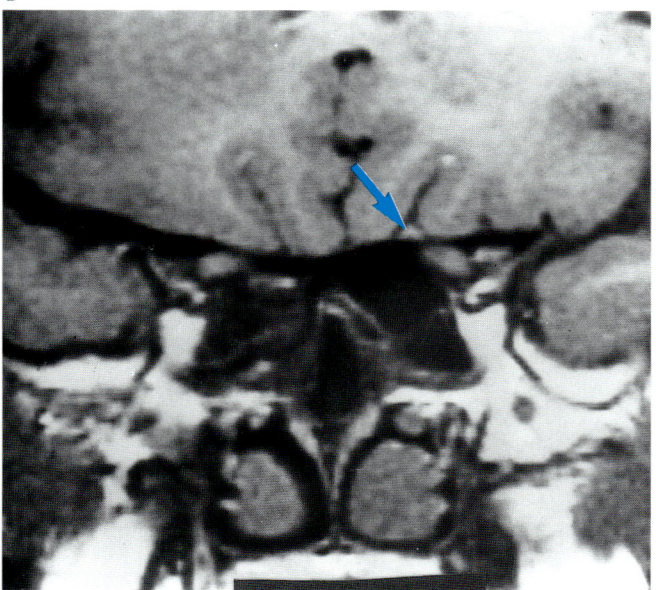
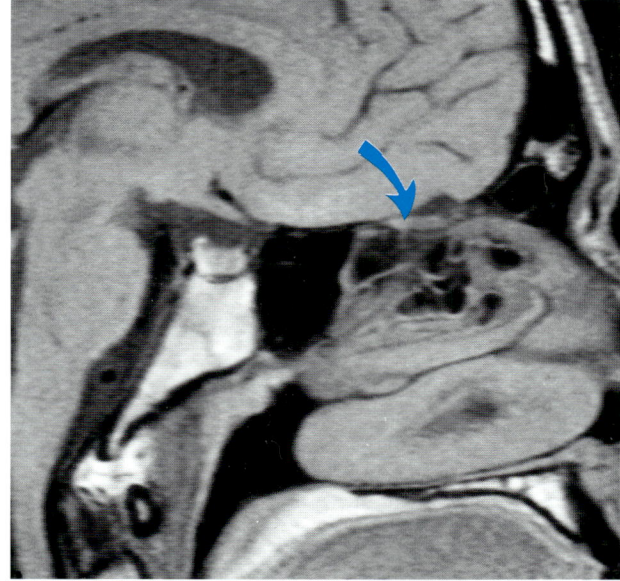

f g

14 Olfactory nerves (I)

CINGULATE GYRUS
Sagittal and frontal views

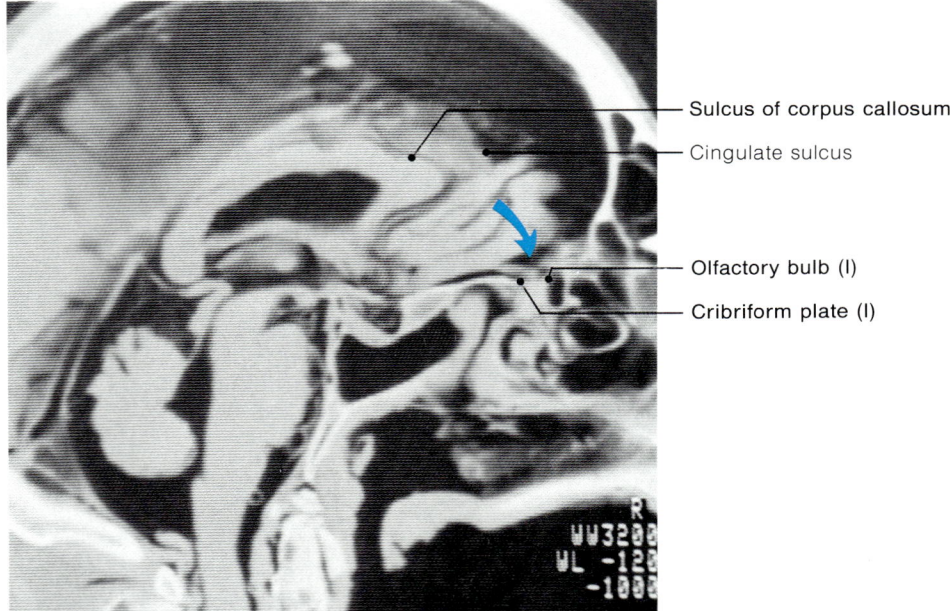

Fig. 1.10a, b. Sagittal computed tomography (CT) (**a**) and diagram (**b**) for cingulate gyri and olfactory pathways

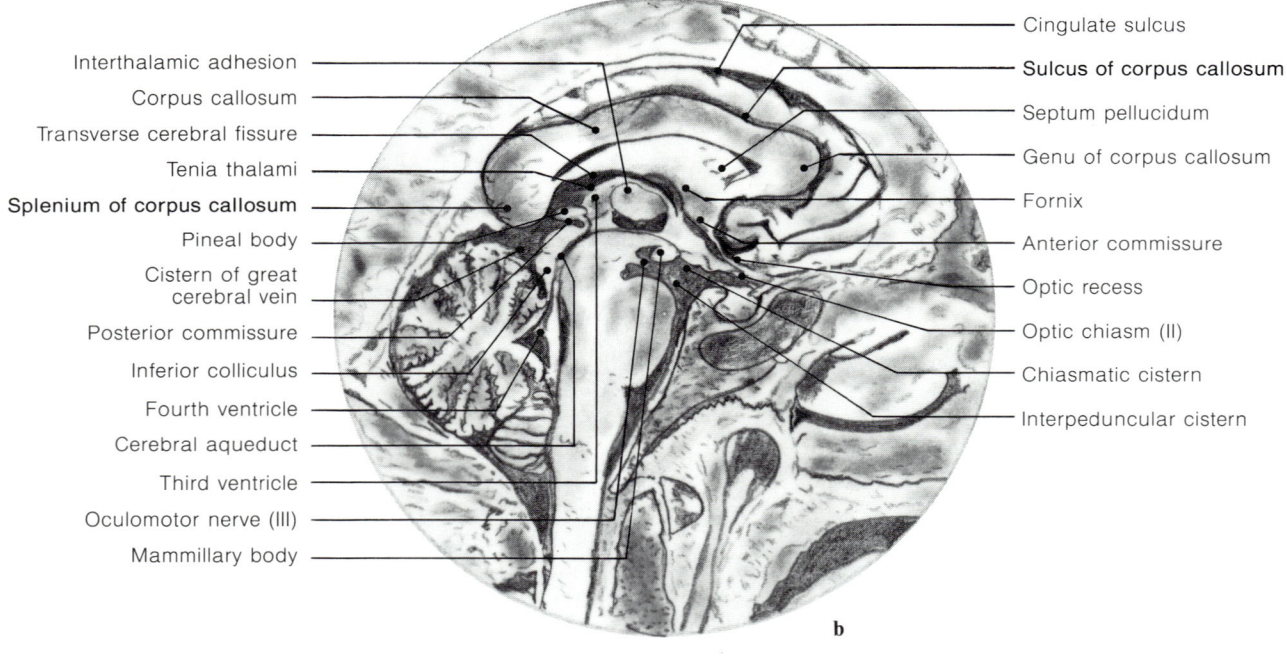

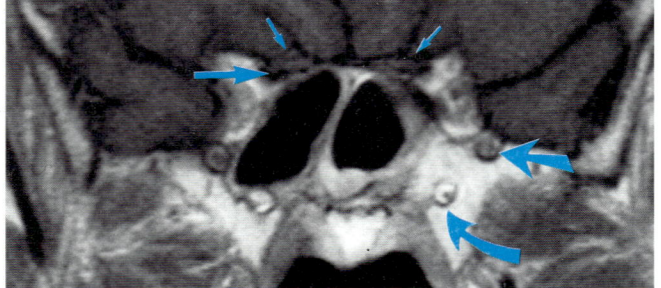

Fig. 1.10c. Frontal magnetic resonance imaging (MRI) of olfactory tract (*small arrow*); optic nerve (*straight arrow on left*); maxillary nerve (*straight arrow on right*); pterygoid nerve (*curved arrow*). (MRI: Dr. J.W. Casselman, A.Z. St-Jan, Brugge)

Longitudinal striae, dentate gyrus

Sagittal view

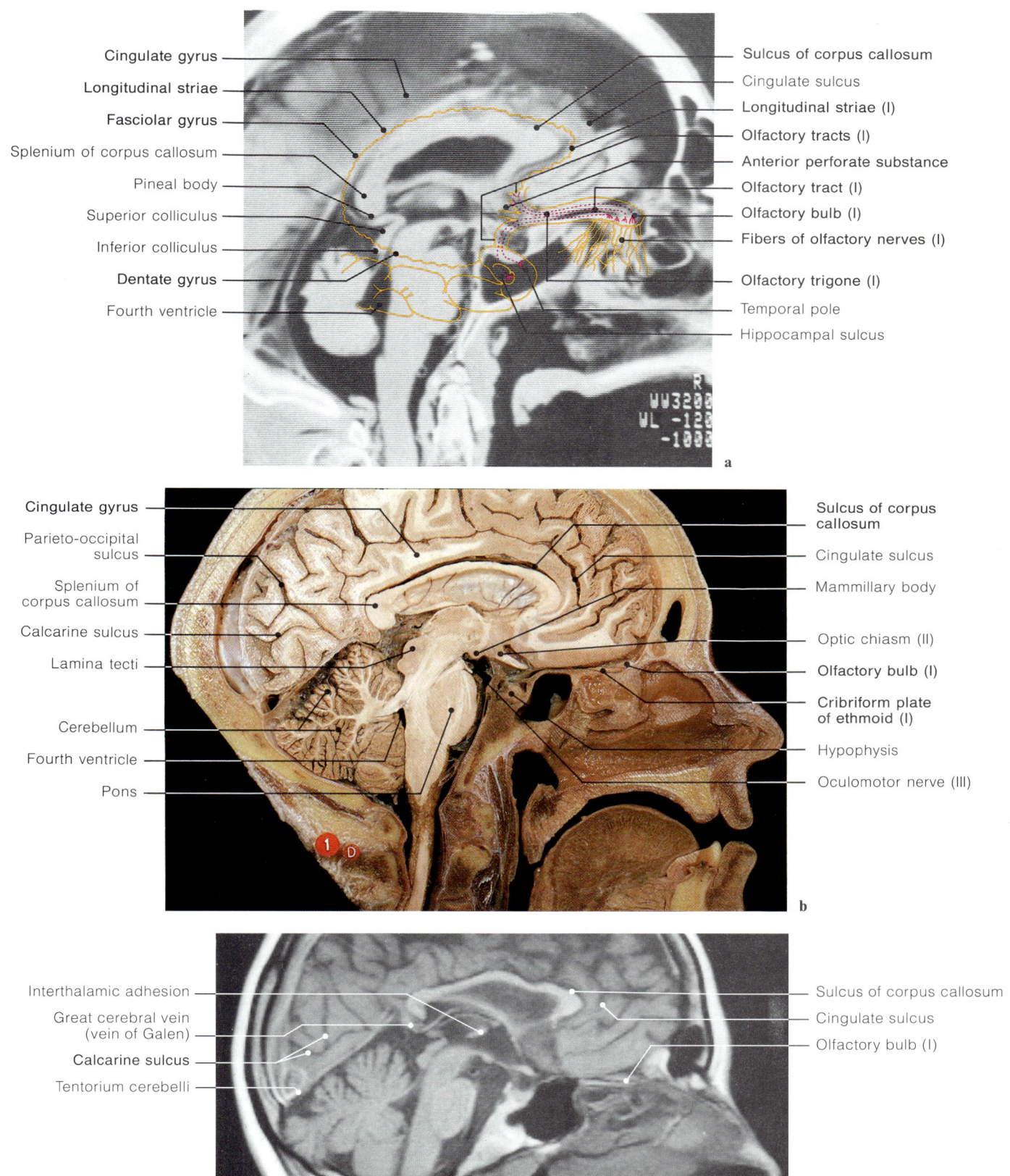

Fig. 1.11. a, b Cisternal computed tomography (CT): sagittal diagram and anatomic section of olfactory pathways; **c** sagittal magnetic resonance imaging (MRI) of olfactory bulb (I)

Magnetic resonance imaging (MRI)

HIPPOCAMPAL UNCUS

Sagittal view

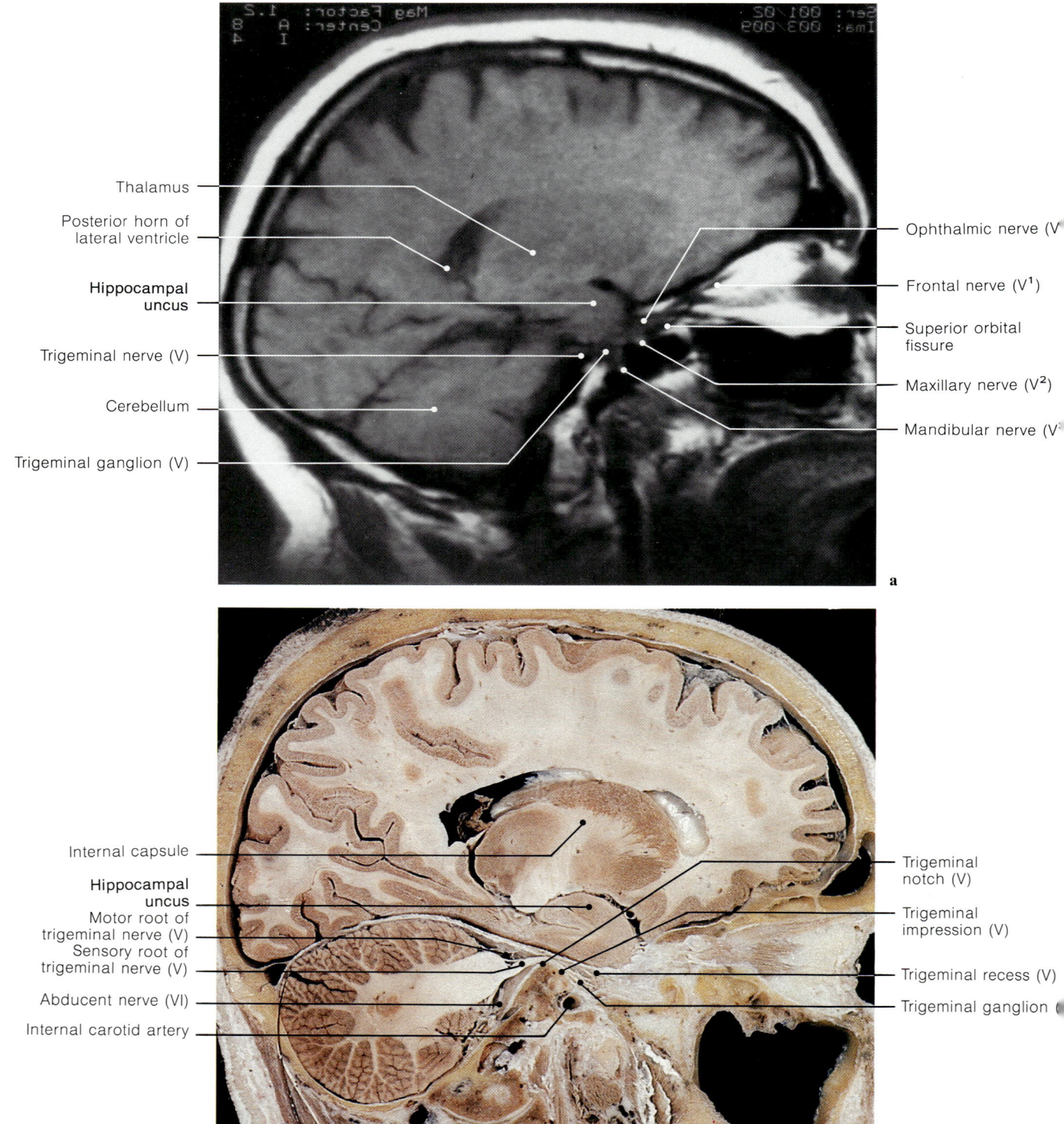

Fig. 1.12a, b. Sagittal magnetic resonance imaging (a) and sagittal anatomic section (b) at level of hippocampal uncus

Optic nerve (II)

Anatomy (course – terminals – collaterals) 19
Imaging (regions examined) 19
Pathology 19
Optic canal
    Anatomy and imaging (examination) 21
    Oblique view (CT) 22
    Axial view (CT) 23
Optic pathways
    Magnetic resonance imaging (MRI) and
    computed tomography (CT) 24
Chiasmatic cistern, optic chiasm, optic tracts, optic pathways
    Anatomy and imaging (examination) 25
    Chiasmatic cistern
        Sagittal view (CT, MRI) 26
        Frontal view (CT) 28
    Optic pathways, optic chiasm, optic tracts
        Oblique sagittal and axial views (MRI) 29
    Optic pathways
        Axial views (MRI) 30
        Diagram and magnetic resonance imaging
        (MRI) 31
Lateral geniculate body, pulvinar, calcarine sulcus
    Axial and sagittal views (MRI) 32

Vascular relations:
Ophthalmic artery, anterior ciliary arteries 278

The optic nerve is formed by numerous nerve fibers arising from the cells of the retina. These converge towards the optic disk, traverse the sclera and choroid, and emerge from the eyeball to form a bulky rounded cord, the optic nerve.

The optic nerve traverses the orbital cavity, enters the optic canal and ends at the optic chiasm, where the nerve fibers partially cross over to form the optic tracts. These tracts terminate in the lateral geniculate body, from which arise the optic radiations; these travel towards the occipital lobe and divide into different fibers that wind round the lateral ventricle to reach the calcarine sulcus.

Optic nerve (II)

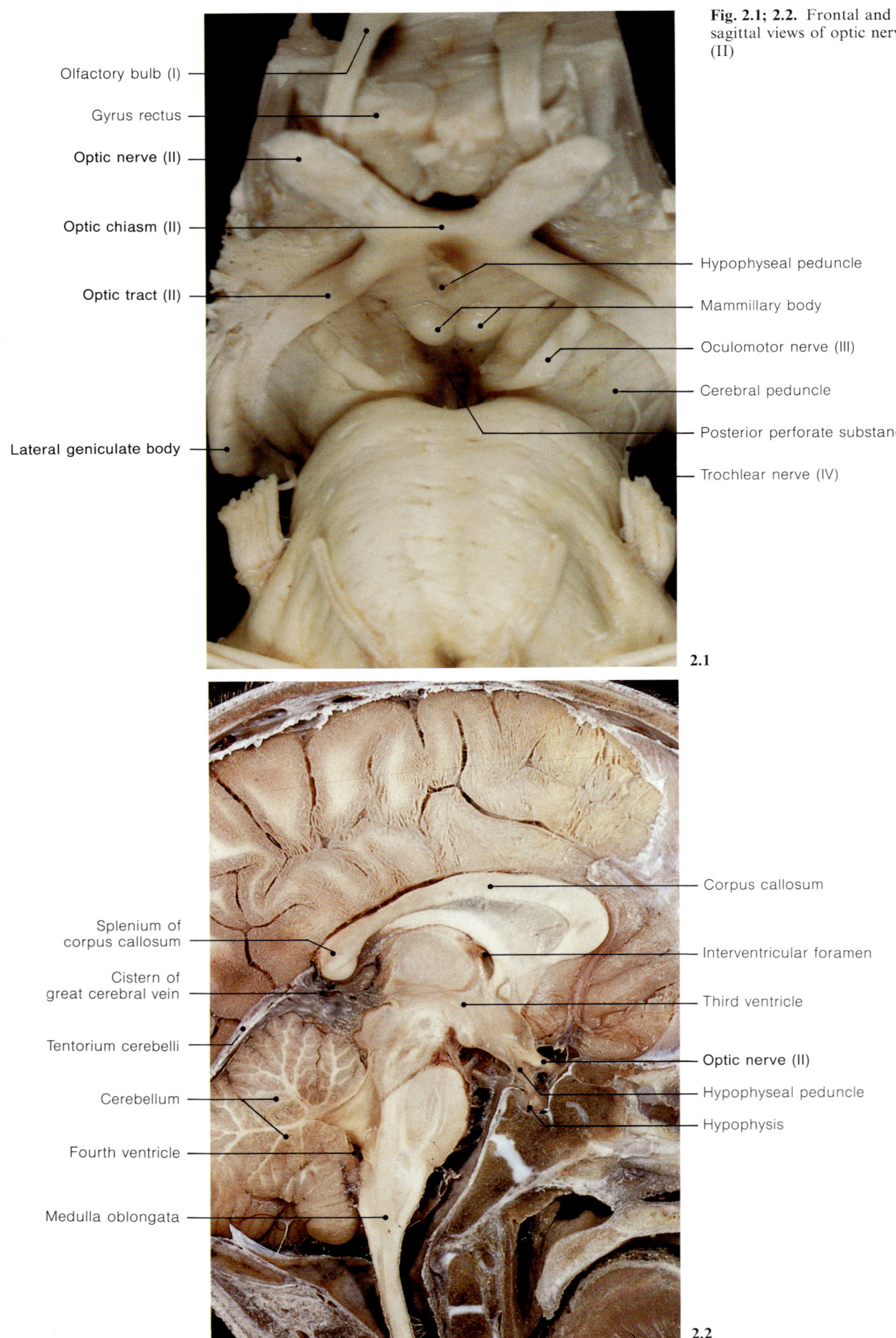

Fig. 2.1; 2.2. Frontal and sagittal views of optic nerve (II)

Anatomy

COURSE – TERMINALS – COLLATERALS

Origin and intracranial course

Optic pathways:
– chiasm, optic tracts
– lateral geniculate body, pulvinar

Cerebral cortex (occipital lobe), calcarine sulcus

Imaging

REGIONS EXAMINED

Examination of orbital cavity and optic canal

Imaging of third ventricle, interpeduncular and chiasmatic cisterns

Imaging of occipitotemporal junction (posterior and inferior horns) with demonstration of calcarine sulcus

Pathology

- Hypophyseal tumors (compression of chiasm),
- tumors of third ventricle (compression of optic nerves and chiasm),
- meningiomata of lesser wing of sphenoid (ophthalmoplegia),
- neurinoma of optic canal,
- Crouzon's disease,
- orbital apex syndrome (or Rollet's syndrome),
- fracture of optic canal or anterior clinoid process,
- major aneurysm of internal carotid artery,
- ventricular tumors at occipitotemporal junction (optic radiations).

Topography

Optic canal

Chiasm and optic tracts

Optic pathways
– Lateral geniculate body, pulvinar, calcarine sulcus

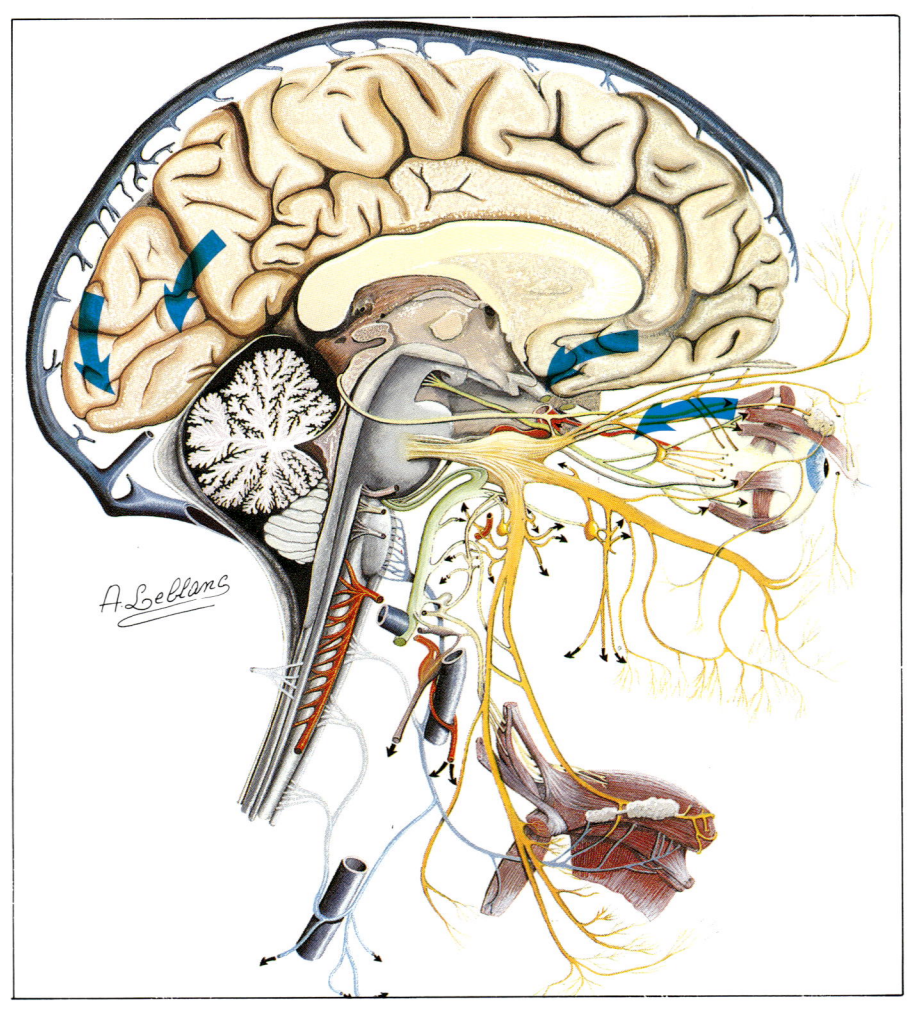

Fig. 2.3

Optic canal

Anatomy

The **optic pathways** ensure transmission of the visual impulses, which, after arising from the retina, arrive at the perceptive centers of the occipital lobe (Fig. 2.12a).
The retina is the organ of visual perception and is formed of a series of superimposed layers:

1) the sensory cells,
2) the internal granular layer,
3) the layer of ganglion cells whose axons converge towards the disk to form the optic nerve.

The **optic nerve,** paired and symmetrical, emerges from the eyeball near its posterior pole (Fig. 2.5b; 2.12a), then traverses the orbital cavity and optic canal, accompanied by the ophthalmic artery. The optic nerve then becomes intracranial and travels to the anterolateral angle of the chiasm, where it terminates (Fig. 2.5c; 2.10a, c; 2.11b; 2.12a).

The **optic chiasm,** situated above the sella turcica, receives the optic nerves and gives off the optic tracts at its posterolateral angles.

Imaging

CLINICAL FEATURES

– Posttraumatic diminution of visual acuity,
– progressive affection of extrinsic ocular motility, beginning with the lateral rectus muscle (VI) and spreading to the muscles supplied by III and, later, the superior oblique muscle (IV), severe headaches with type V^1 and sometimes V^2 trigeminal neuralgia, finally unilateral exophthalmos with homolateral blindness.

POSSIBLE CAUSES

– Fracture of optic canal (hematoma),
– aneurysm of internal carotid artery in the cavernous sinus,
– meningioma of lesser wing of sphenoid,
– Crouzon's disease.

EXAMINATION

– Comparative imaging study of optic canal in oblique anteroposterior view,
– tomographic study of optic canals and anterior clinoid processes in symmetric oblique and axial views (Fig. 2.4a, b, f; 2.5b),
– axial, sagittal and frontal computed tomographic (CT) studies of optic nerves and canals and cavernous sinuses (Fig. 2.6a–f; 2.10a, b)

TECHNIQUE (OBLIQUE ANTEROPOSTERIOR VIEW)

– The subject is in dorsal decubitus, with the head turned to the side opposite to that to be examined by 40° to 45° in relation to the median sagittal plane (Fig. 2.4b);
– the head is deflected in such a way that the guide-beam makes an angle of 35° in relation to the orbitomeatal plane (OM), open downwards (Fig. 2.4a). The centering point is located at the inferolateral angle of the orbit (Fig. 2.4c, d). This study must be performed comparatively.

Optic canal

Imaging

TECHNIQUE (OBLIQUE VIEW)

Important remarks

Study of the optic canal in dorsal decubitus is preferable to study in the prone position, both for the comfort of the patient in whom injury has fractured the facial massif and also if any structural abnormality exists: malformations, asymmetries, nasal or mandibular prominences; this position allows adjustment of the centering, so that the optic canal may be properly studied in its axis.

For good diagnostic procedure, the optic canal must be centered exactly in its axis and projected in the inferolateral quadrant of the orbit, and it must appear perfectly round (Fig. 2.4c, d).

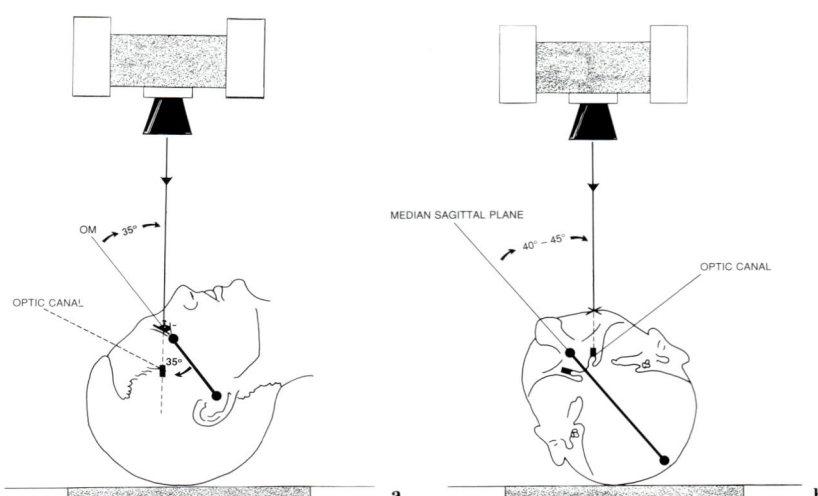

Fig. 2.4a, b. Centering diagrams for study of optic canal

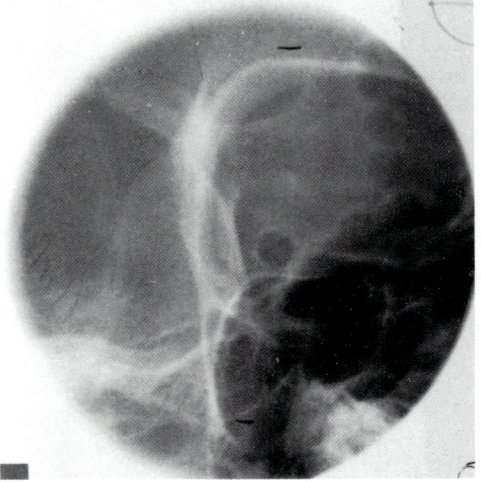

Fig. 2.4c. Imaging of optic canal in antero-posterior view

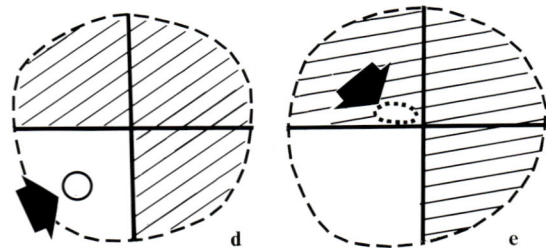

Fig. 2.4. d Good projection of optic canal; **e** poor projection of optic canal

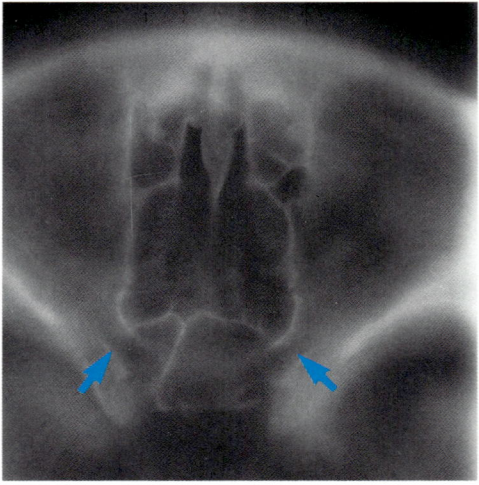

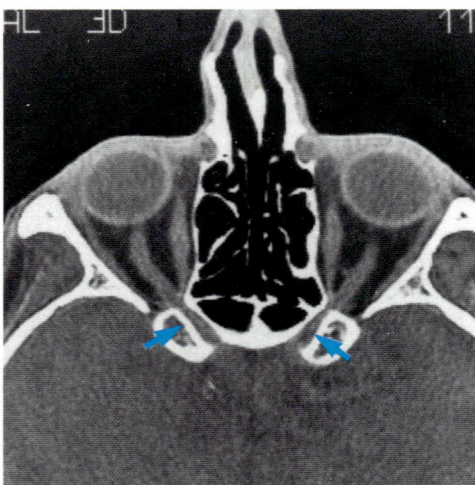

Fig. 2.4. f Conventional axial tomography of optic canals; **g** axial computed tomography (CT) of optic canals and nerves (II)

Optic canal

Computed tomography (CT)

AXIAL VIEW

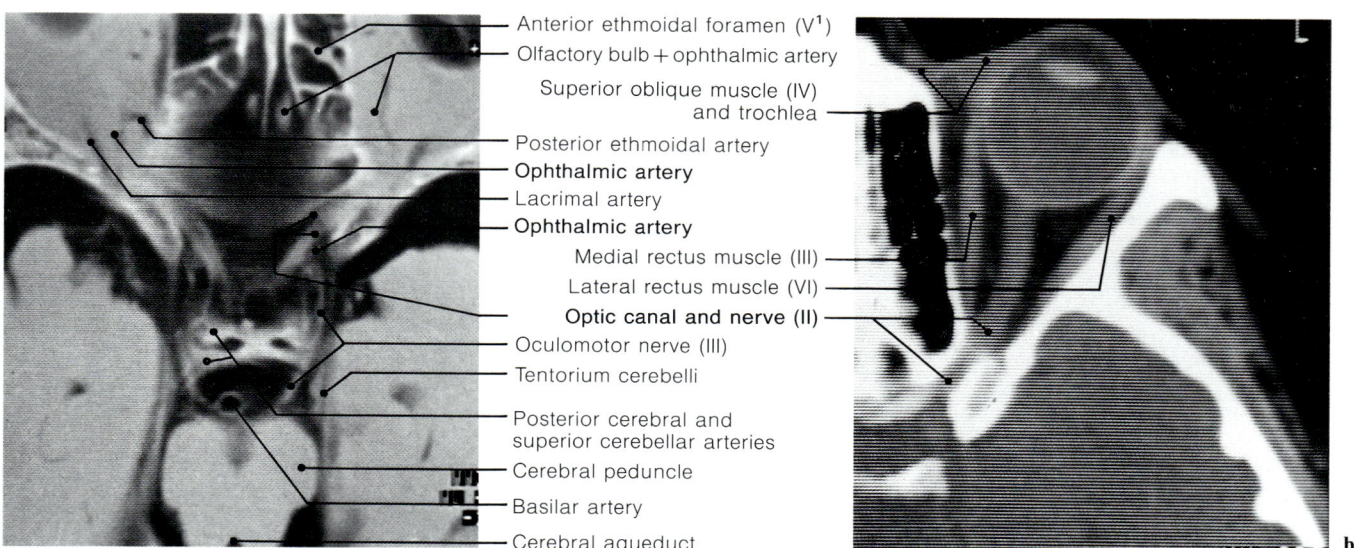

Fig. 2.5. a, b Axial computed tomographic (CT) sections of optic nerves and canals; c superior anatomic view of intracranial portion of optic nerves and relations of optic chiasm to third ventricle

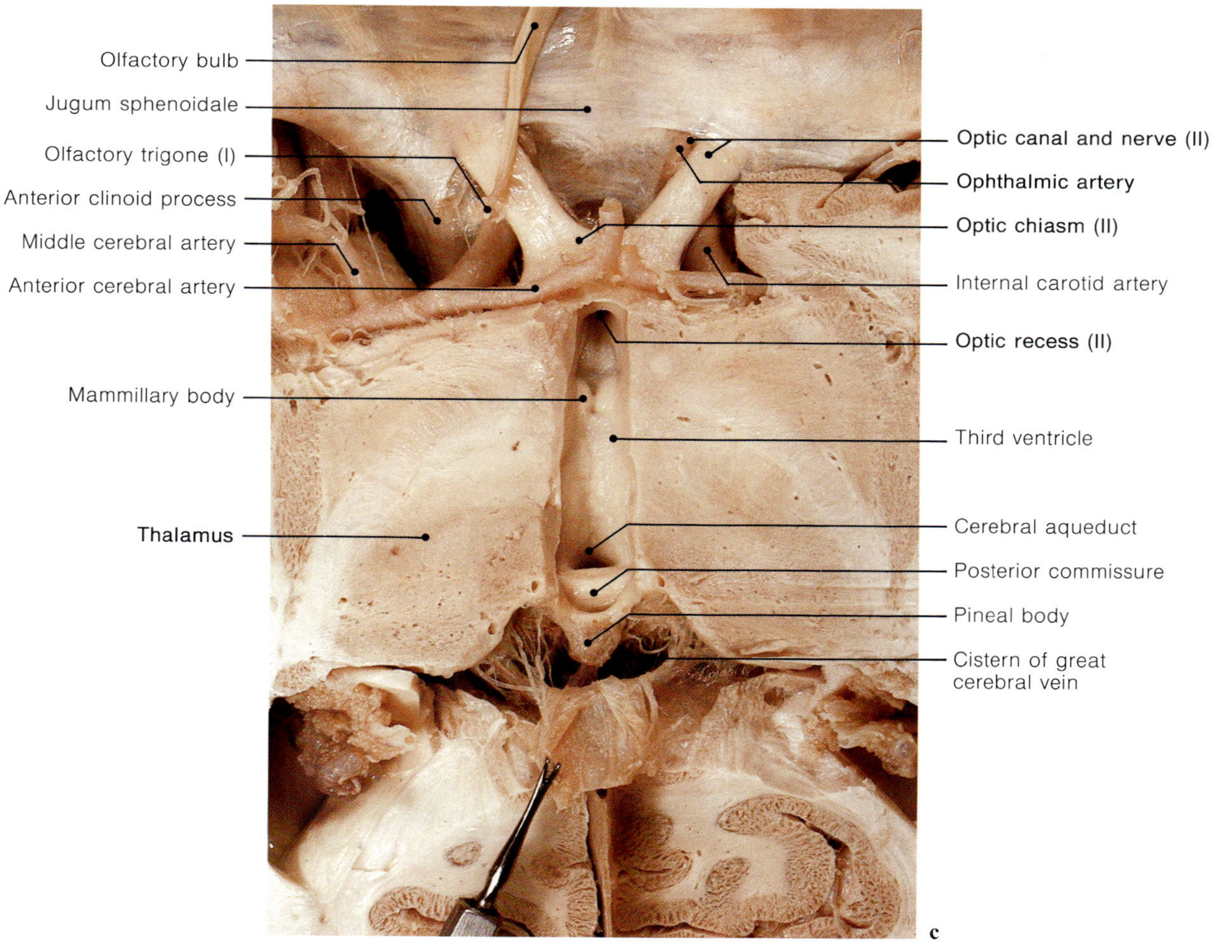

Optic pathways

Magnetic resonance imaging (MRI) and computed tomography (CT)

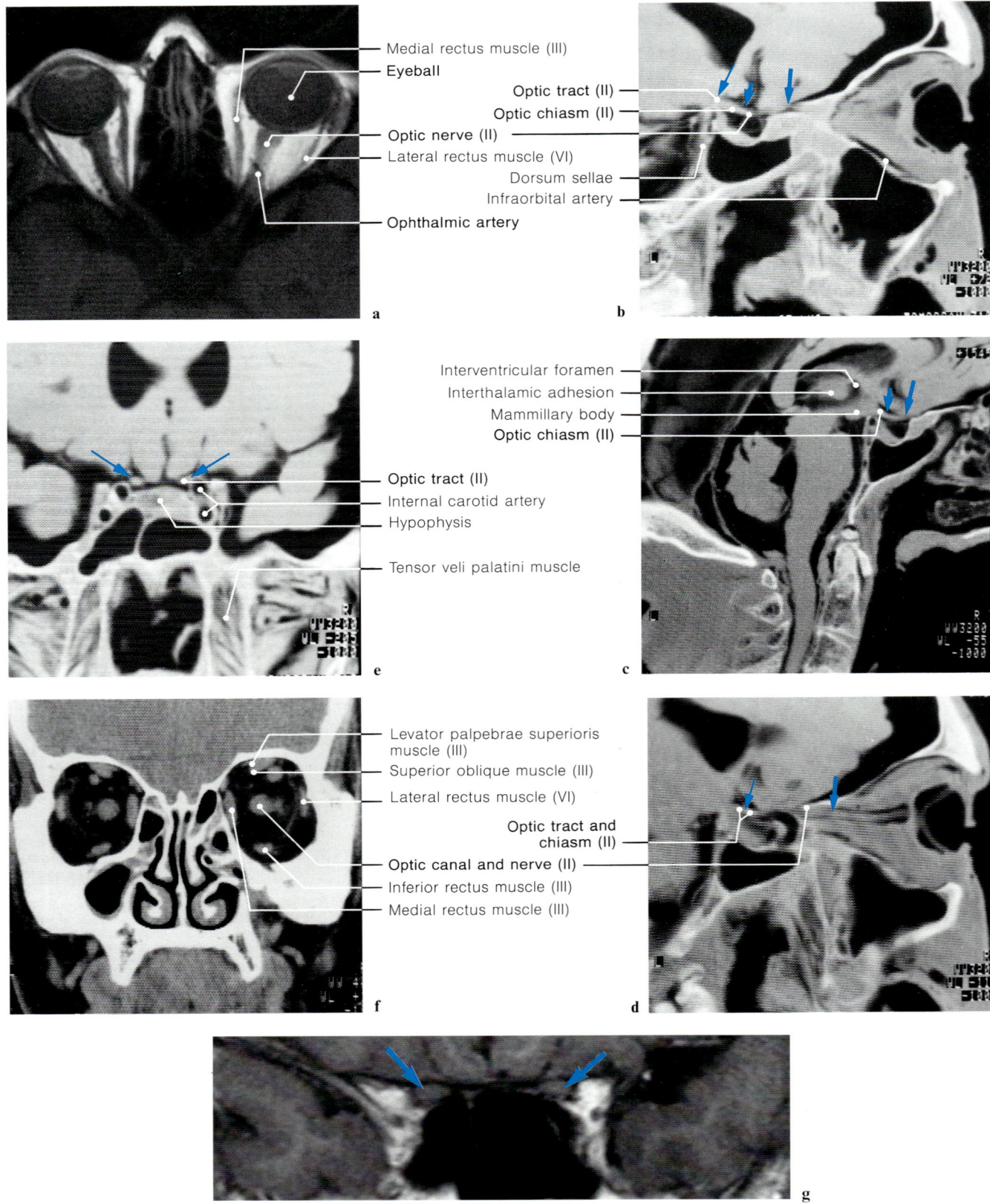

Fig. 2.6a–g. Axial (**a**), sagittal (**b–d**) and frontal (**e, f**) sections of optic pathways by magnetic resonance imaging (MRI) and computed tomography (CT), visualizing optic nerve, chiasm and tract; frontal MRI (**g**) of optic nerves (II) (*arrows*)

Chiasmatic cistern, optic chiasm, optic tracts, optic pathways

Anatomy

Each *optic tract* is formed by the temporal bundle derived from the retina of the same side, the nasal bundle derived from the retina of the opposite side and by macular fibers derived from both retinae.
The optic tracts terminate in the lateral geniculate body (Fig. 2.12a, b and MRI Fig. 2.13a, b), where the nerve fibers are relayed.
The optic radiations arise in the *lateral geniculate body* (Fig. 2.12a) and travel towards the occipital lobe where they divide into two groups of fibers:

- an anterior bundle which courses round the *inferior horn of the lateral ventricle* to terminate in the *lower lip of the calcarine sulcus* (Fig. 2.11a; 2.13a),
- a posterior bundle which courses round the *posterior horn of the lateral ventricle* to terminate in the *upper lip of the calcarine sulcus*.

Thus, the *cortical visual center* is formed by the two lips of the calcarine sulcus at the medial aspect of the occipital lobe.

Fig. 2.6h–k. Frontal, sagittal and axial magnetic resonance imaging (MRI) views showing successively the optic nerves, optic chiasm, optic tract, lateral geniculate body, and calcarine sulcus (II). (MRI: Dr. J.W. Casselman, A.Z. St-Jan, Brugge)

Imaging

CLINICAL FEATURES

- Headaches, vertigo, visual disorder with lessened acuity and decreased visual field.

POSSIBLE CAUSES

- Hypophyseal tumors compressing the chiasm,
- tumors of the third ventricle involving the chiasmatic region or the lateral geniculate body,
- pinealoma, ventricular tumors at the collateral trigone expanding towards the cerebral cortex (calcarine sulcus),
- parietal syndrome: visual field defect associated with involvement of the fibers reaching the upper lip of the calcarine sulcus,
- temporal syndrome: lower lip of calcarine sulcus.

EXAMINATION

- Magnetic resonance imaging (MRI) and computed tomography (CT) of the chiasmatic and interpeduncular cisterns in sagittal views (Fig. 2.7a–c), frontal views (Fig. 2.9a, b; 2.6e) and axial views (Fig. 2.5a; 2.6a) to visualize the optic chiasm, nerve and tract (Fig. 2.6a–f).

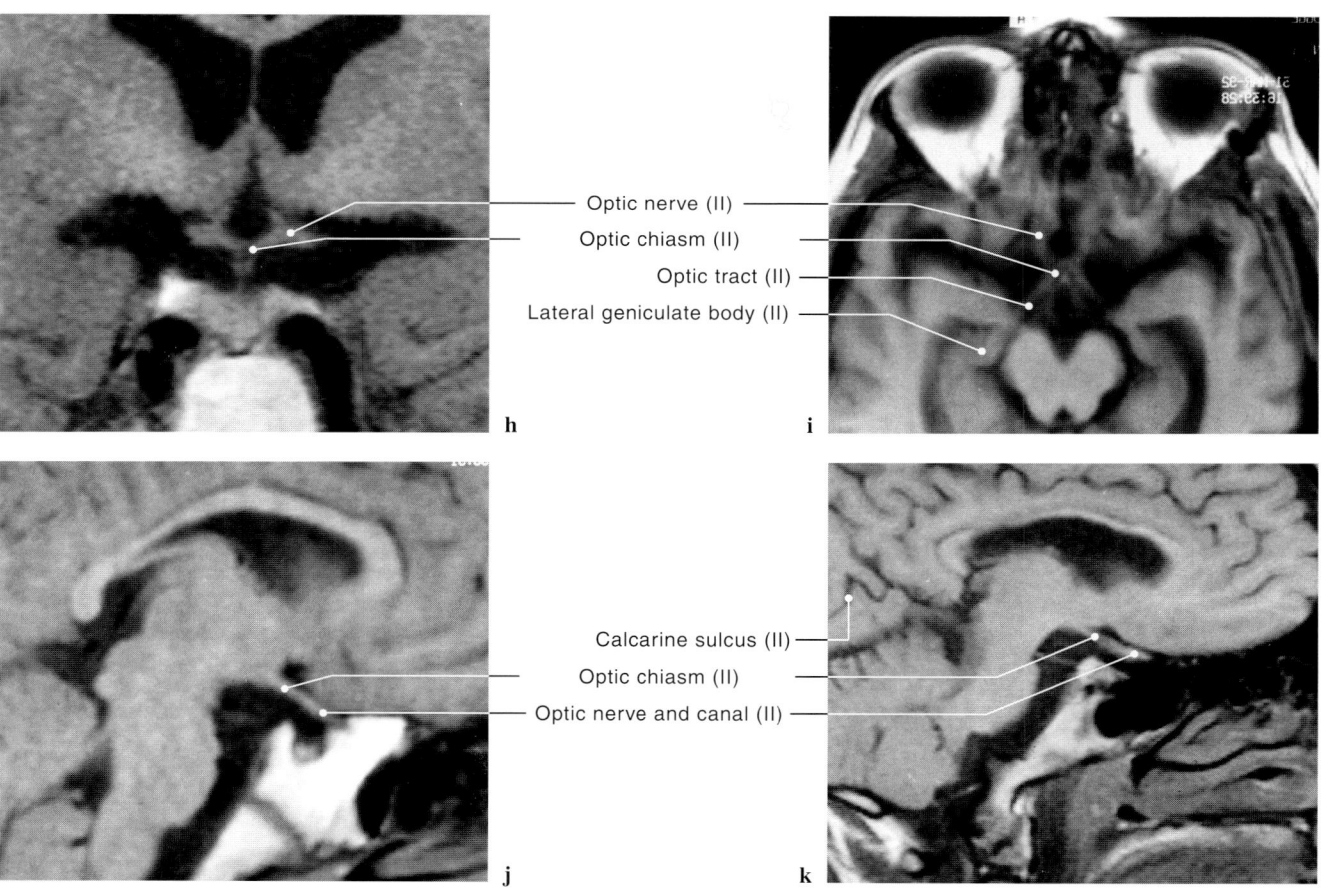

Chiasmatic cistern

Magnetic resonance imaging (MRI) and computed tomography (CT)

SAGITTAL VIEW

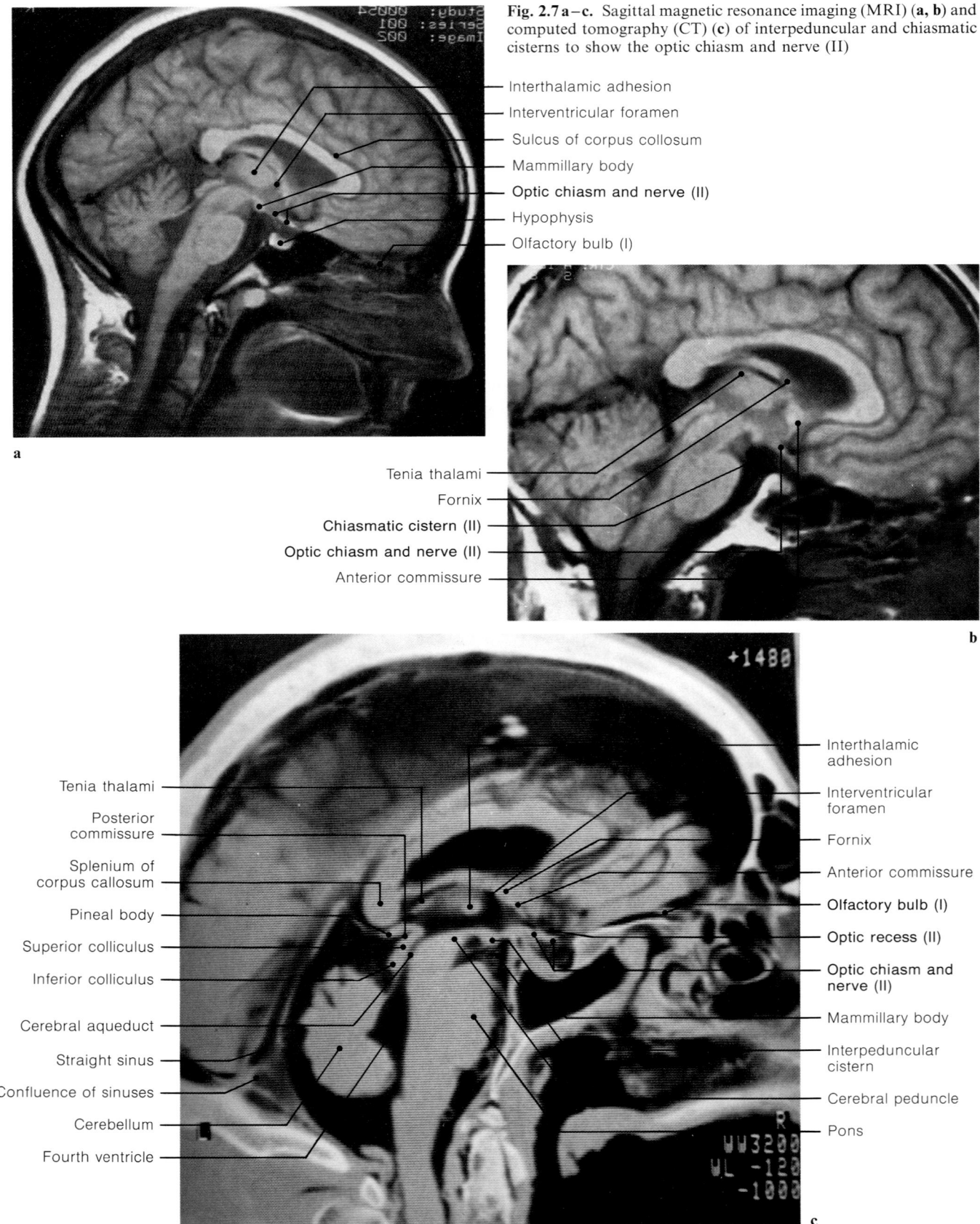

Fig. 2.7 a–c. Sagittal magnetic resonance imaging (MRI) (**a, b**) and computed tomography (CT) (**c**) of interpeduncular and chiasmatic cisterns to show the optic chiasm and nerve (II)

Optic nerve (II) 27

Fig. 2.8 a, b. Sagittal anatomic sections at the level of the optic chiasm (II)

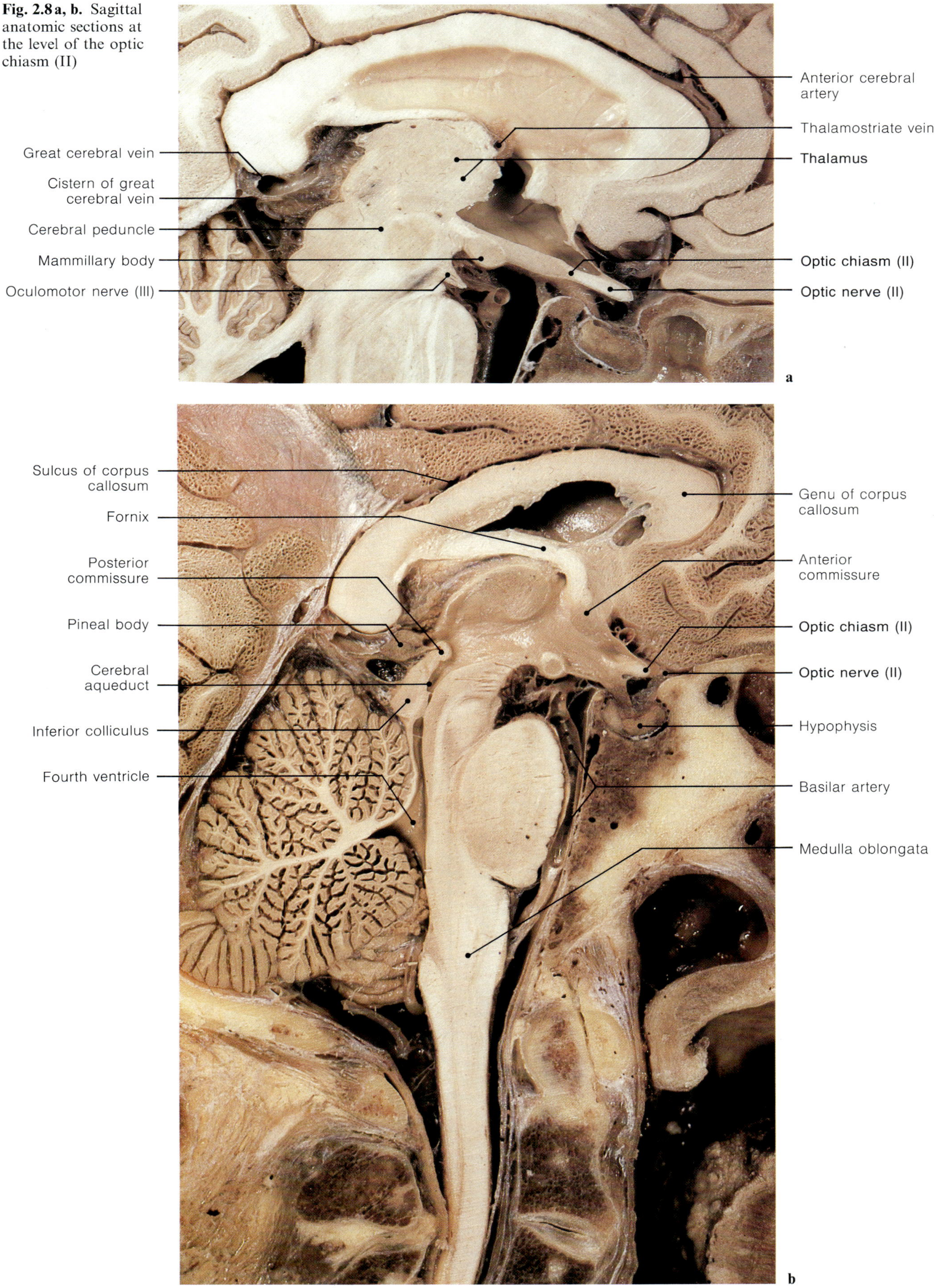

Great cerebral vein
Cistern of great cerebral vein
Cerebral peduncle
Mammillary body
Oculomotor nerve (III)

Anterior cerebral artery
Thalamostriate vein
Thalamus
Optic chiasm (II)
Optic nerve (II)

Sulcus of corpus callosum
Fornix
Posterior commissure
Pineal body
Cerebral aqueduct
Inferior colliculus
Fourth ventricle

Genu of corpus callosum
Anterior commissure
Optic chiasm (II)
Optic nerve (II)
Hypophysis
Basilar artery
Medulla oblongata

Chiasmatic cistern

Computed tomography (CT)

FRONTAL VIEW

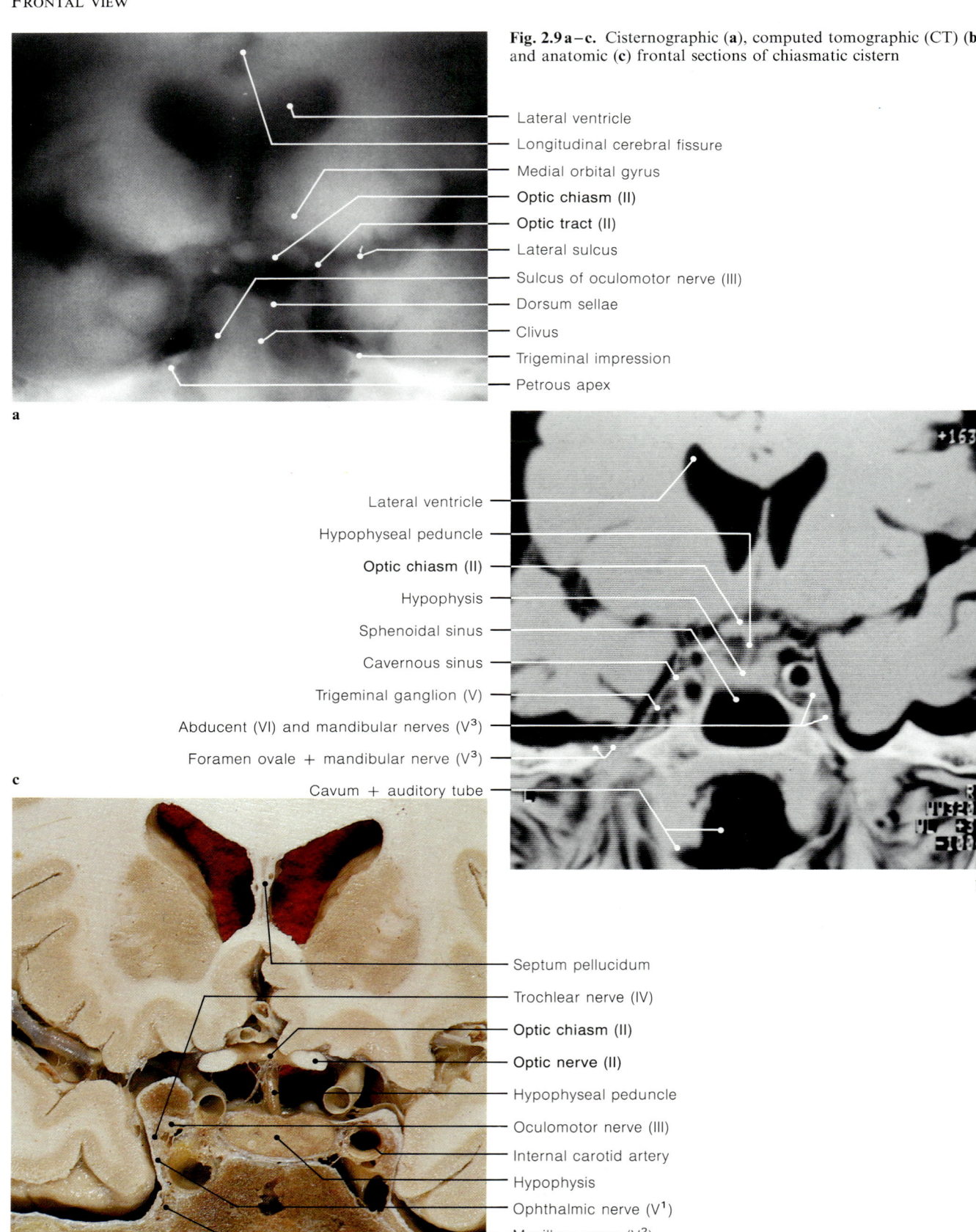

Fig. 2.9a–c. Cisternographic (a), computed tomographic (CT) (b) and anatomic (c) frontal sections of chiasmatic cistern

Optic pathways, optic chiasm, optic tracts (See vascular relations, p. 278)

Magnetic resonance imaging (MRI)

OBLIQUE SAGITTAL, AXIAL VIEWS

Fig. 2.10a. Orientation diagram for "oblique sagittal" magnetic resonance imaging (MRI) of right optic nerve, chiasm and left optic tract

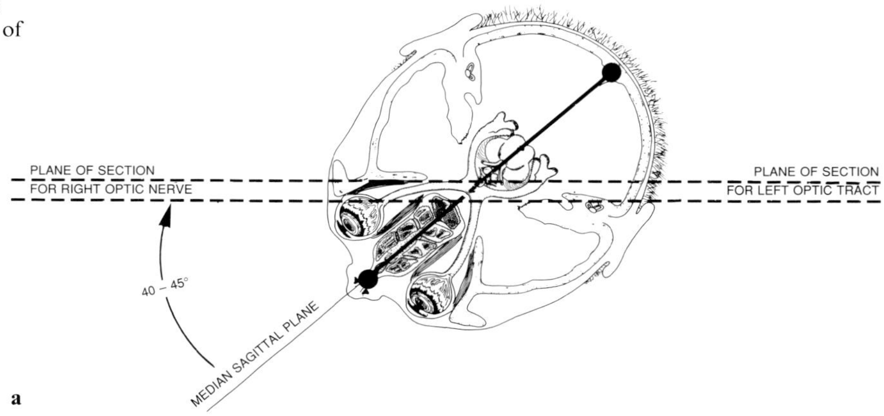

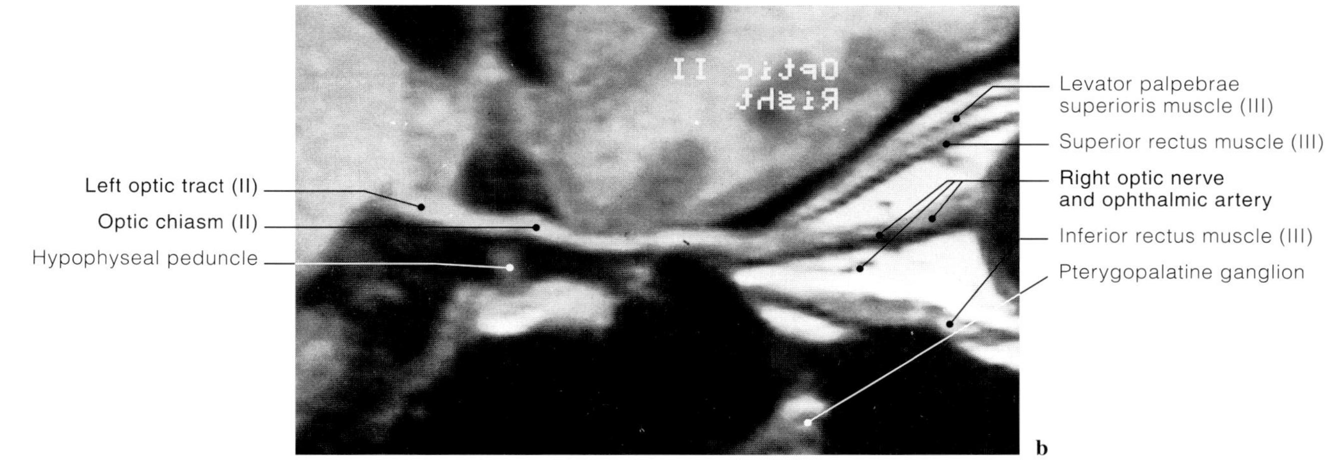

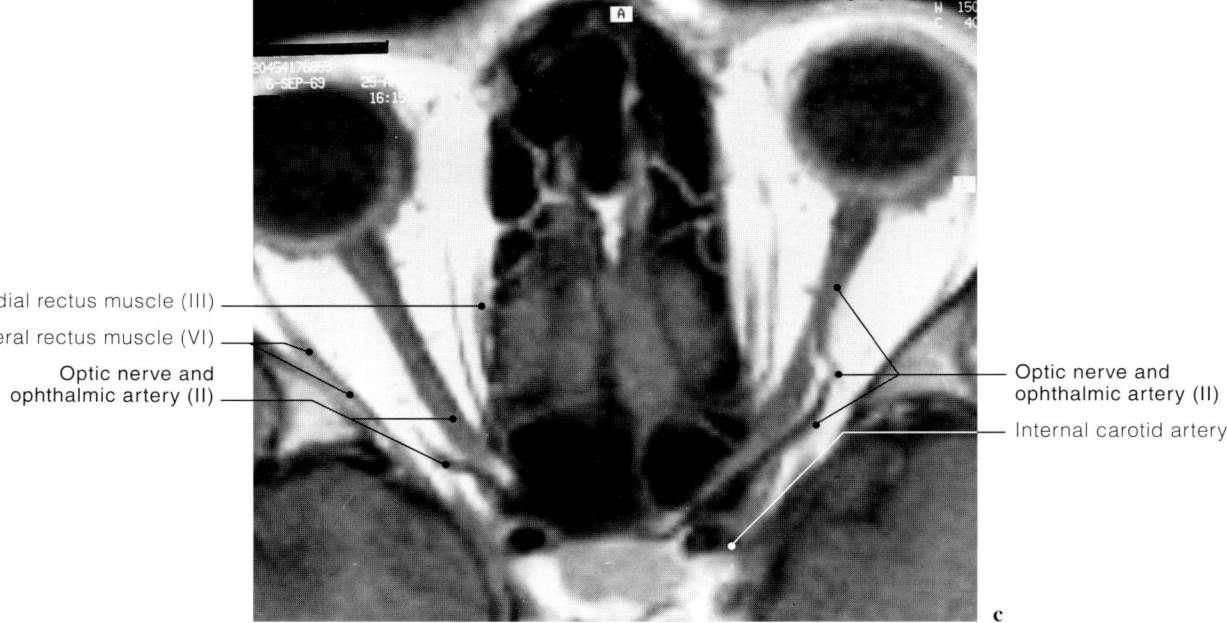

Fig. 2.10b, c. Oblique sagittal magnetic resonance imaging (MRI) section of right optic nerve, chiasm and left optic tract. **c** Axial and symmetric MRI of optic nerves (II). (MRI: Dr. J.W. Casselman, A.Z. St-Jan, Brugge)

Optic pathways

Magnetic resonance imaging (MRI)

AXIAL VIEWS

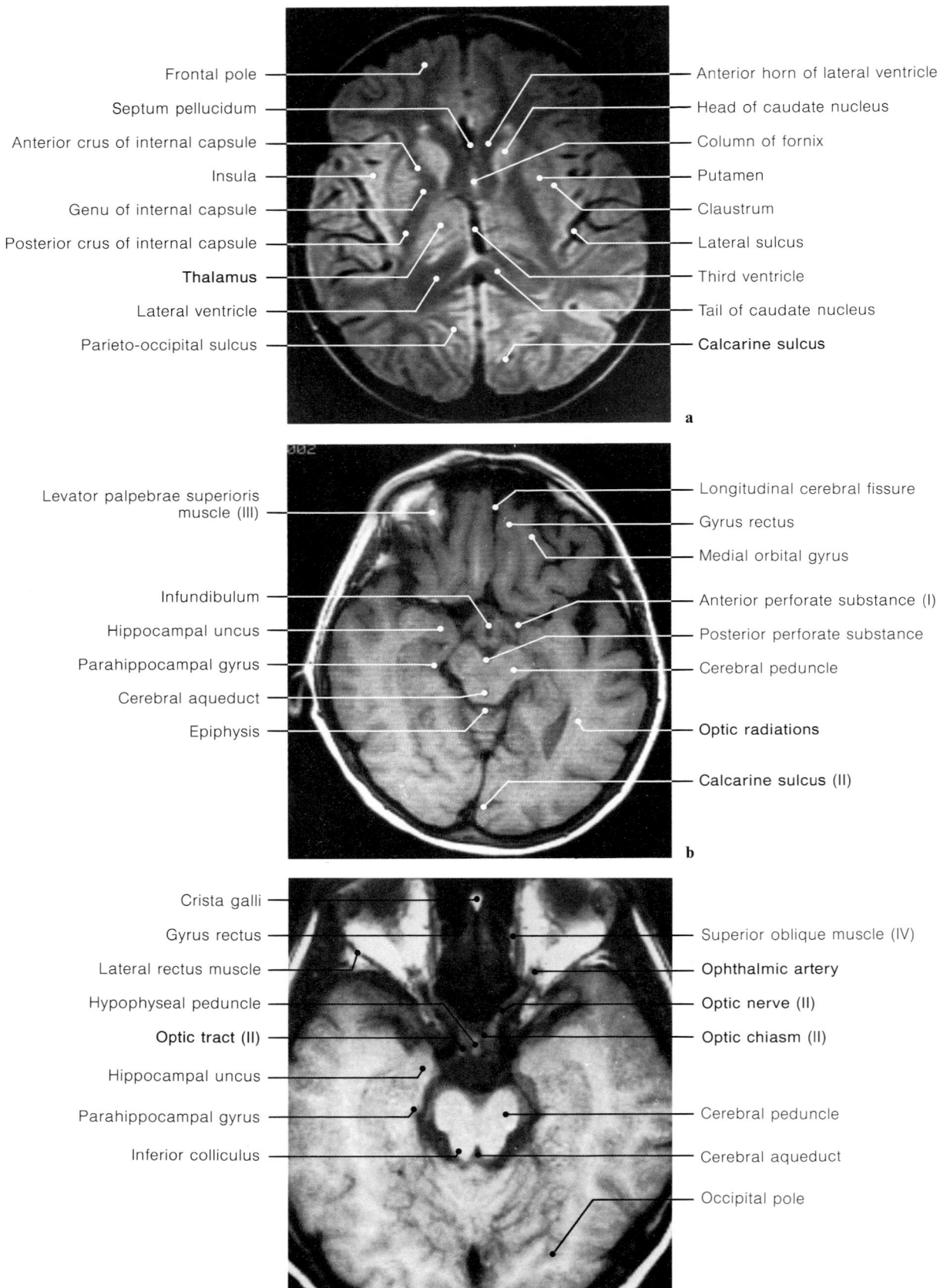

Fig. 2.11 a–c. Magnetic resonance imaging: sections at level of cerebral hemispheres passing through the frontal and occipital poles to show the central gray nuclei and the optic pathways

Optic pathways

Fig. 2.12 a, b. Horizontal diagram (**a**) and magnetic resonance imaging (MRI) (**b**) showing courses and relations of optic pathways

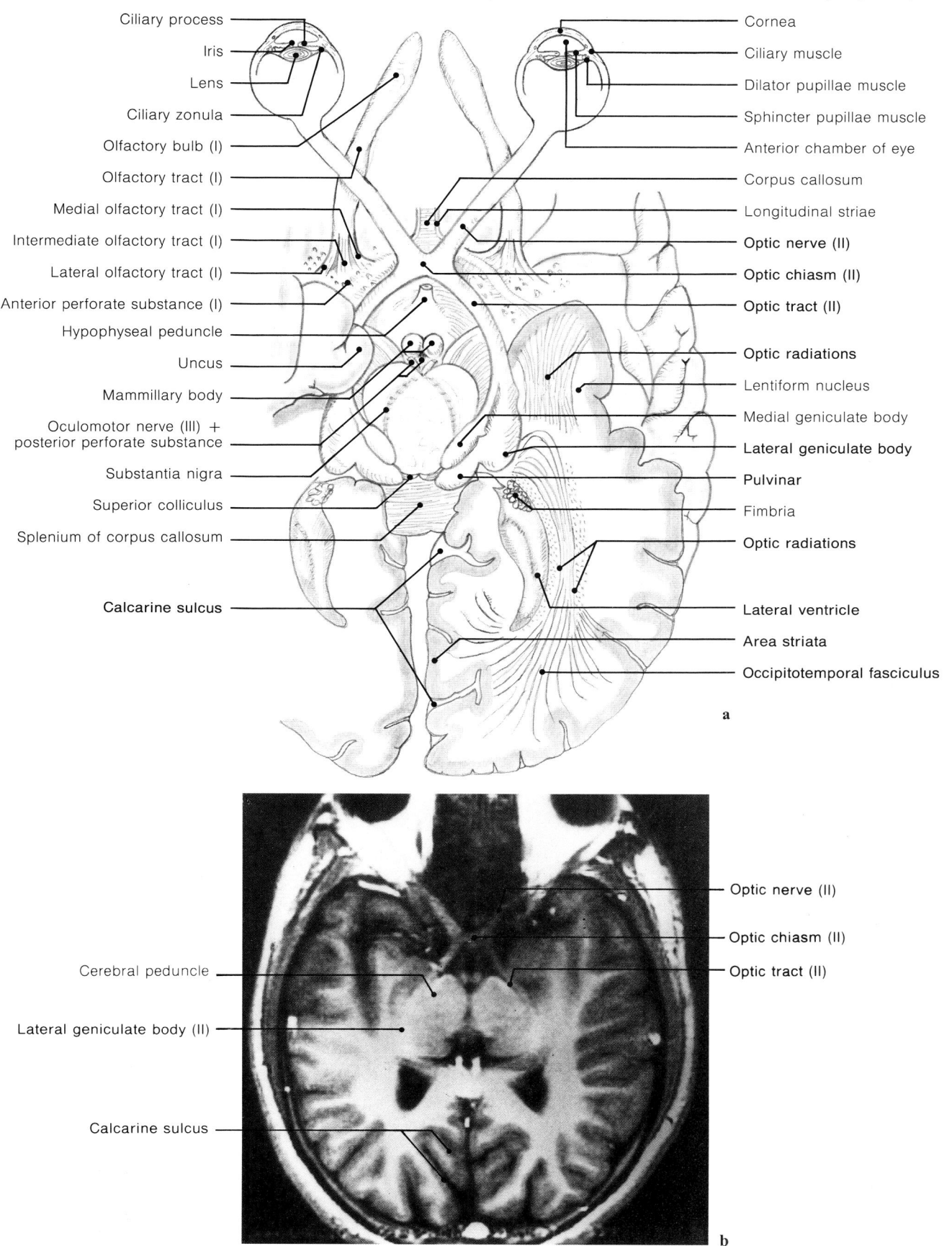

Lateral geniculate body, pulvinar, calcarine sulcus

Magnetic resonance imaging (MRI)

Axial and sagittal views

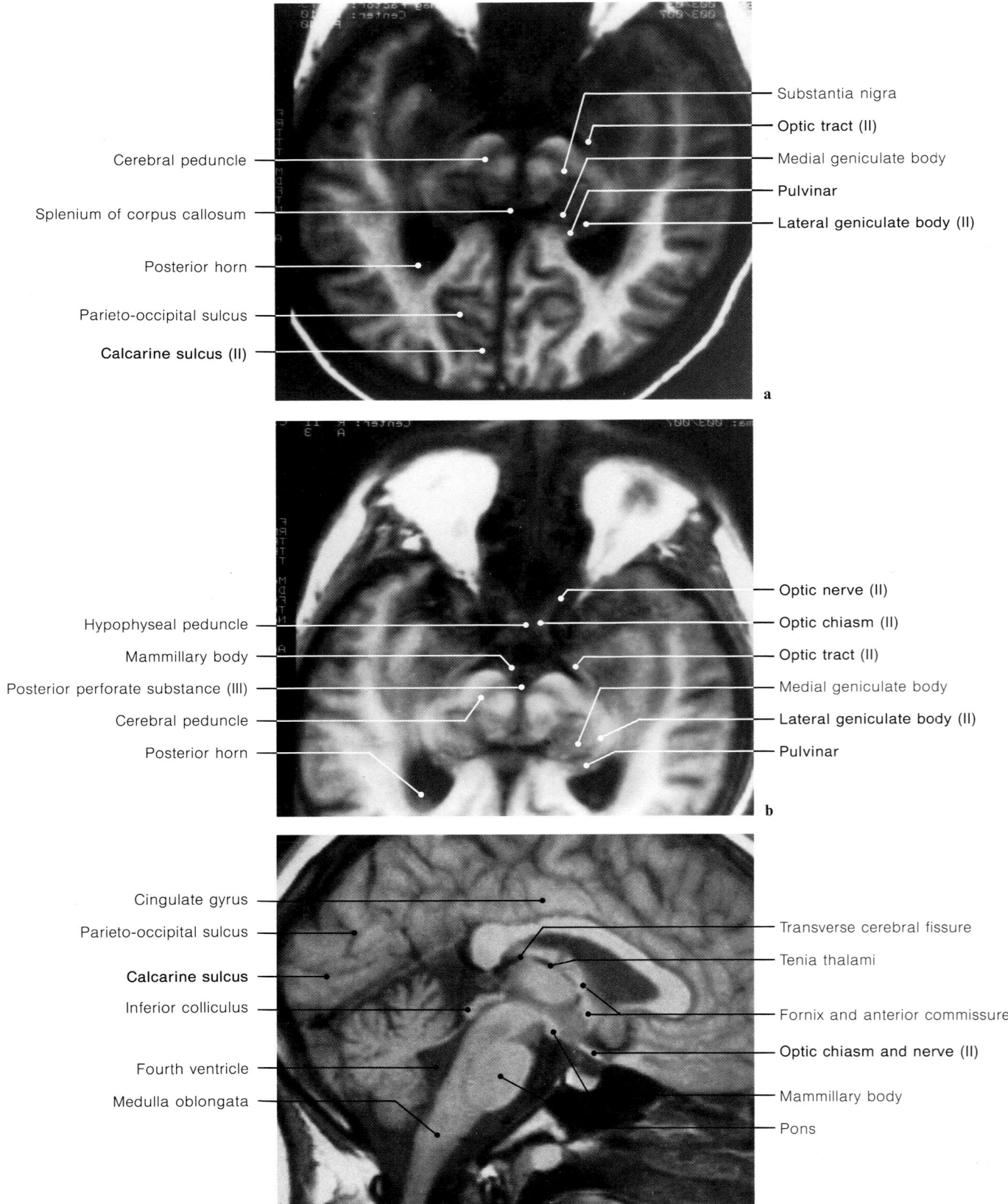

Fig. 2.13a–c. Axial magnetic resonance imaging (MRI) (a, b) of brain-stem, geniculate bodies, pulvinar, floor of third ventricle, hypophyseal peduncle and mammillary bodies; sagittal image (c) for calcarine sulcus

Oculomotor nerve (III)

Anatomy (course – terminals – collaterals) 35
Imaging (regions examined) 35
Pathology 35
Apparent origin of oculomotor nerve, cerebral
peduncle, interpeduncular cistern
    Anatomy and imaging (examination) 38
Interpeduncular cistern
    Sagittal view (MRI) 39
    Axial view (CT, MRI) 40
Course, vascular relations of oculomotor nerve
    Axial views (MRI, CT), anatomic views 41
Course, sulcus of oculomotor nerve, cavernous sinus,
superior orbital fissure
    Anatomy and imaging (examination) 42
Dorsum sellae (CT) 42
Sulcus of oculomotor nerve, superior orbital fissure
    Axial views (MRI) 43
Extrinsic ocular movements
    Anatomy and imaging 44
    Frontal and sagittal views (CT) 44
Ocular muscles
    Frontal and axial views (CT) 45
Intrinsic ocular movements
    Anatomy and diagram 46

Vascular relations:
Posterior cerebral and superior cerebellar
    arteries 37, 39–41, 43, 48
Cavernous sinus
    Venous drainage at the skull base 167, 290
    Inferolateral trunk 276, 277

The oculomotor nerve is a motor nerve. It supplies the levator palpebrae superioris muscle and most of the oculomotor muscles except the lateral rectus (VI) and superior oblique (IV); also, via its parasympathetic fibers, the annular part of the ciliary muscle and the pupillary sphincter muscle.
Paralysis may severely affect eye movements, involving both extrinsic and intrinsic ocular motility.

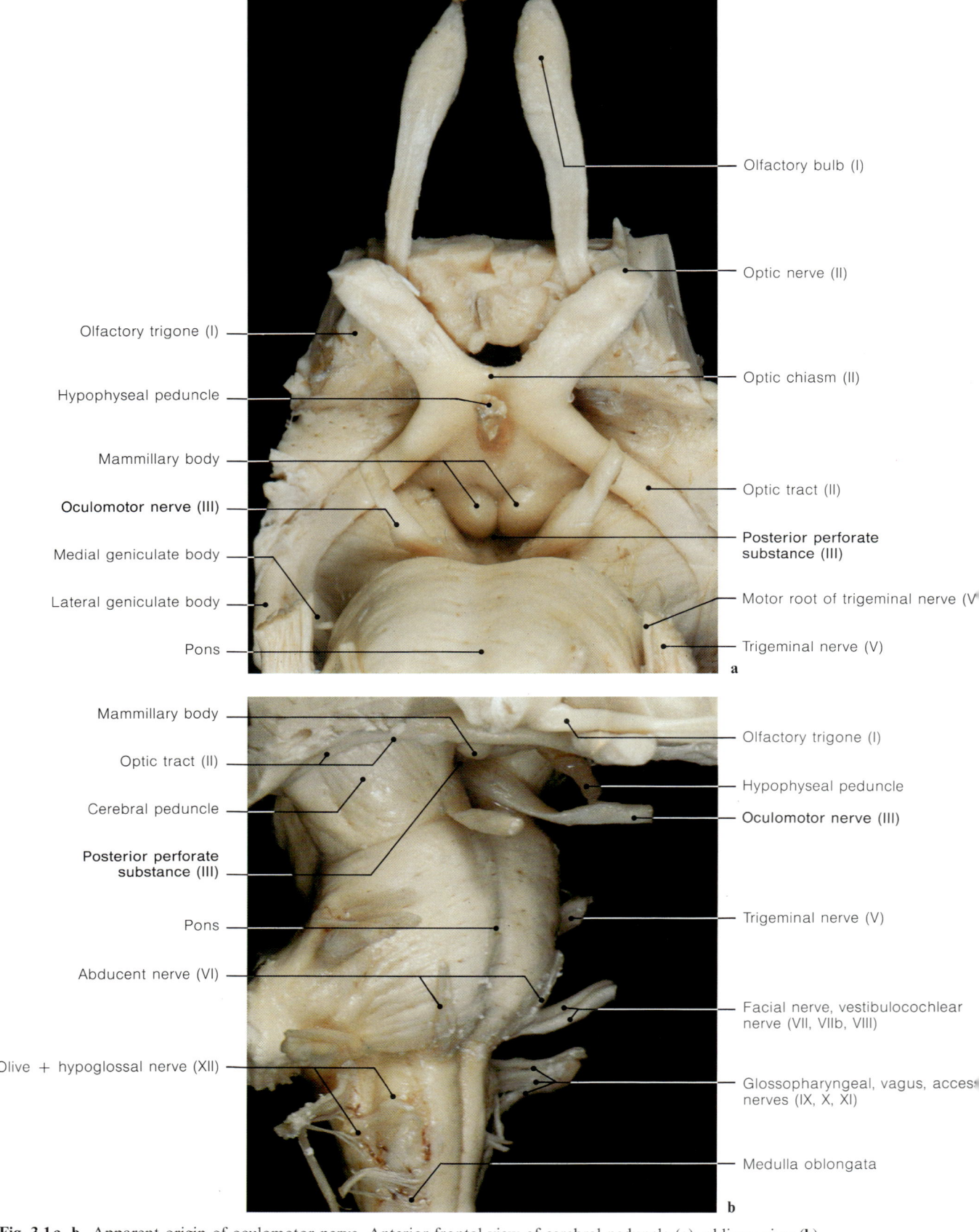

Fig. 3.1 a, b. Apparent origin of oculomotor nerve. Anterior frontal view of cerebral peduncle (a); oblique view (b)

Anatomy

COURSE – TERMINALS – COLLATERALS

Apparent origin and intracranial course

Sulcus of oculomotor nerve

Cavernous sinuses

Superior and inferior branches (terminal)

Medial rectus, inferior oblique, superior rectus, inferior rectus, and levator palpebrae superioris muscles

Imaging

REGIONS EXAMINED

Exploration of cerebral peduncles (posterior perforate substance)
Imaging of interpeduncular and chiasmatic cisterns

Sulcus of dorsum sellae, with computed tomographic and tomographic studies in lower frontal view

Imaging of cavernous sinuses

Study of superior orbital fissure

Orbital imaging for musculo-aponeurotic cone of eye

Pathology

- Syndrome of cerebral peduncle (Weber's syndrome),
- syndrome of lateral wall of cavernous sinus (Foix's syndrome),
- syndrome of superior orbital fissure (Rochon-Duvigneaud's syndrome),
- syndrome of orbital apex (Rollet's syndrome),
- syndrome of petrosphenoidal junction (Garcin's syndrome) affecting cranial nerves II, IV and VI,
- osteitis of petrous apex (Gradenigo's syndrome),
- aneurysm of internal carotid artery,
- agenesis of corpus callosum,
- hypophyseal tumor,
- trigeminal neuralgia (V^1),
- fracture of lesser wing of sphenoid,
- fracture of sphenoidal sinus (medial wall of cavernous sinus).

Oculomotor nerve (III)

Topography

Apparent origin of oculomotor nerve (III)
- Cerebral peduncle
- Posterior perforate substance
- Interpeduncular cistern

Course
- Sulcus of oculomotor nerve
- Cavernous sinus
- Superior orbital fissure

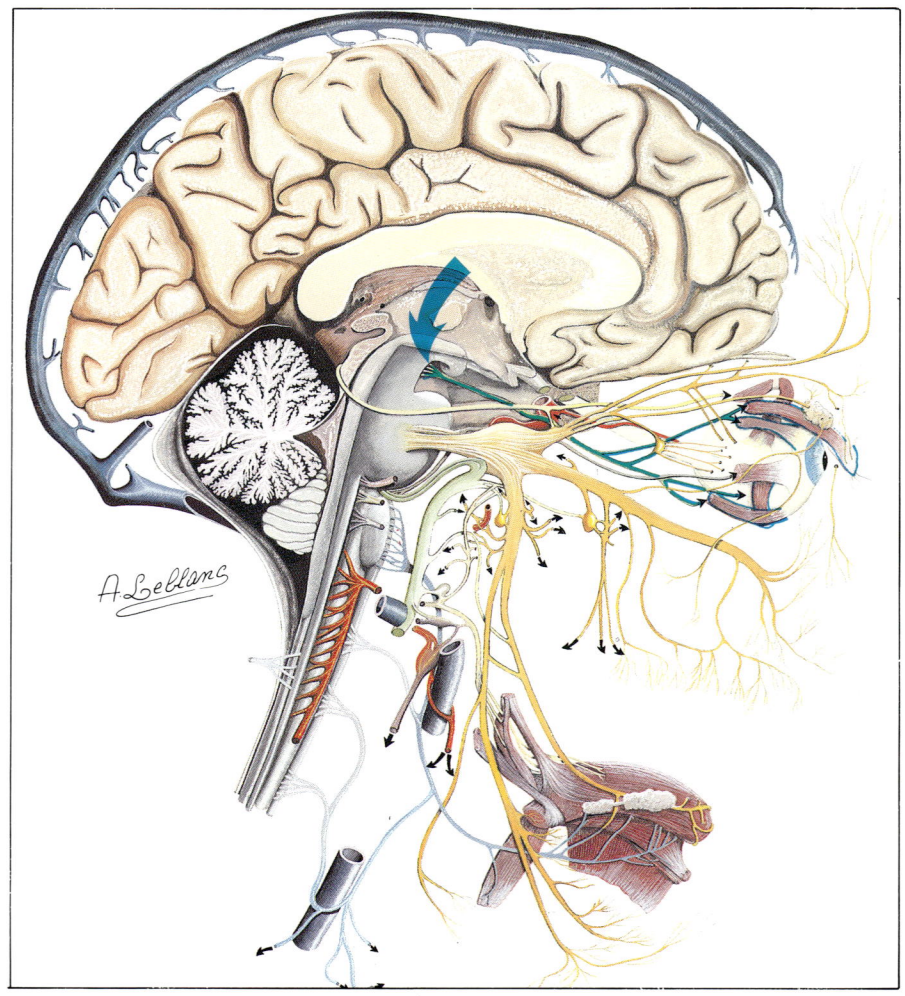

Fig. 3.2

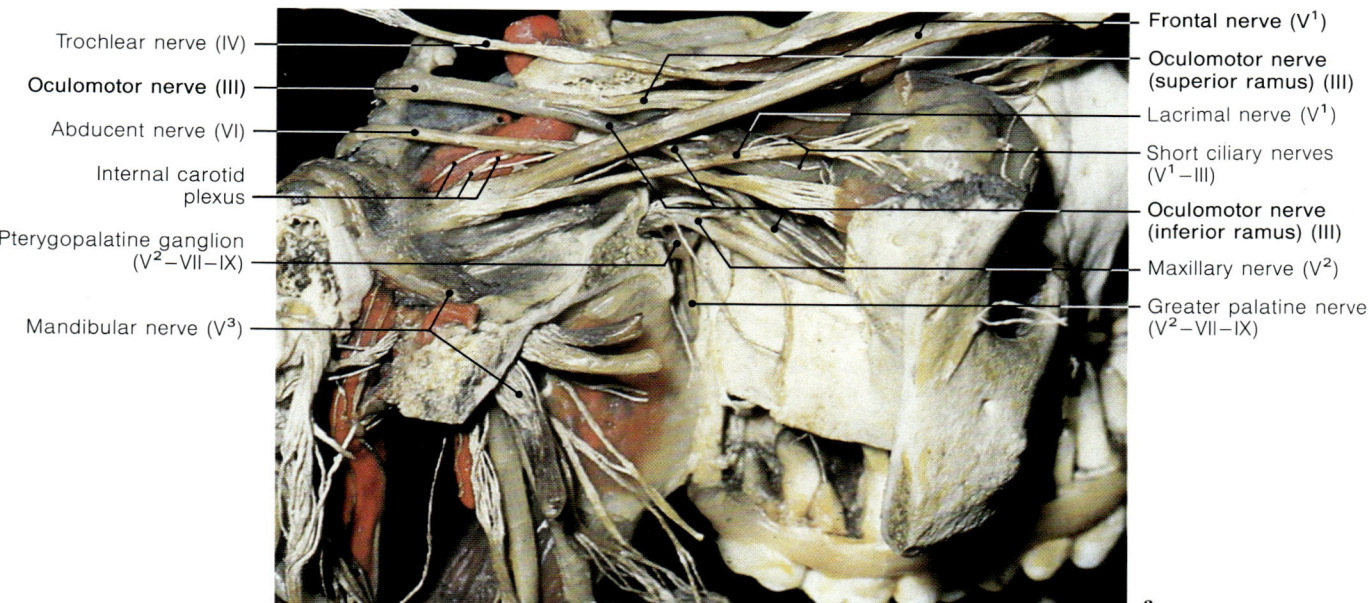

Fig. 3.3a. Sagittal section of anatomic specimen showing oculomotor nerve (III)

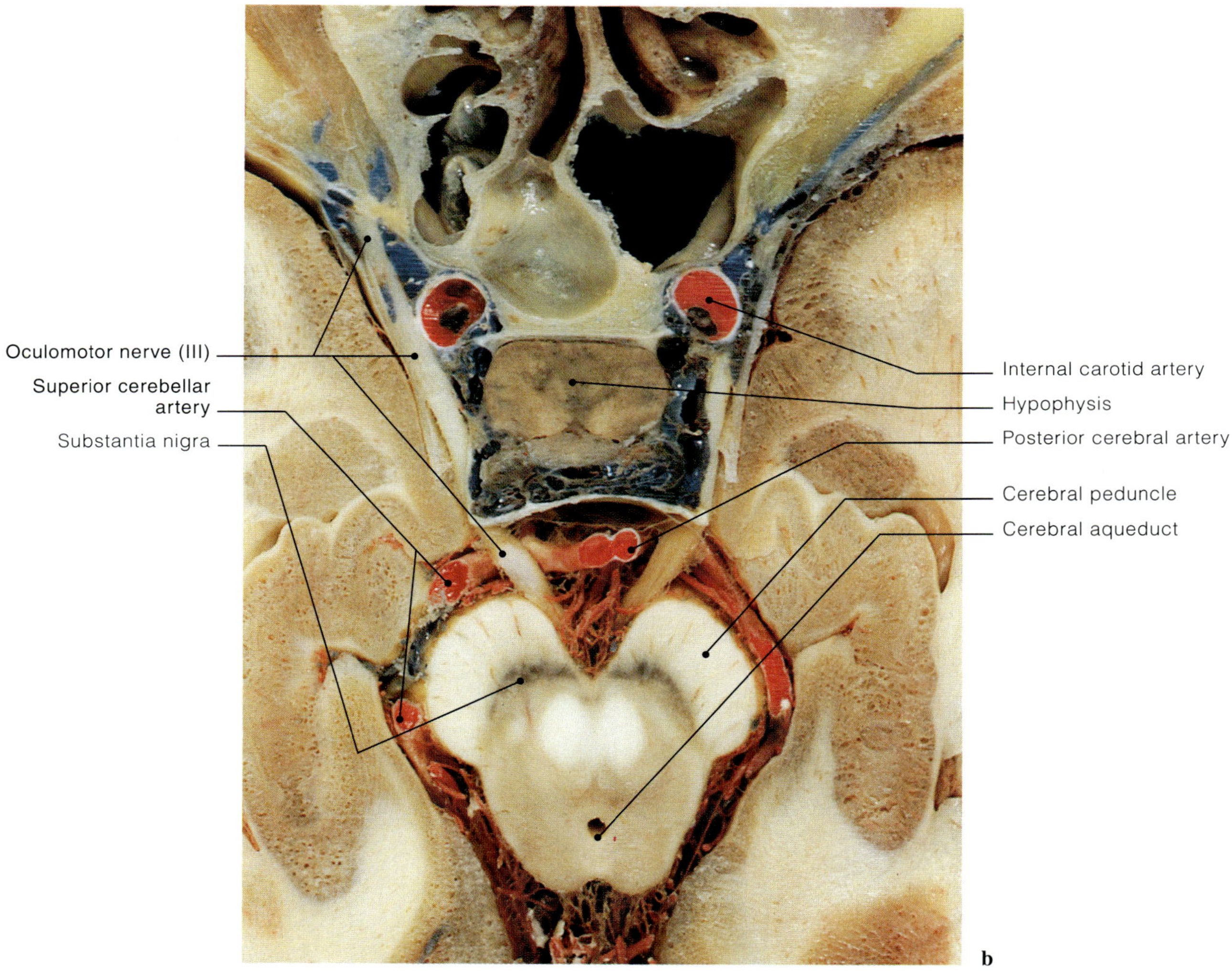

Fig. 3.3b. Axial anatomic section of cerebral peduncle showing vascular relations of oculomotor nerves (III). (Anatomic section: Pr. J. P. Francke, Faculty of Medicine, Lille)

Apparent origin of oculomotor nerve, cerebral peduncle, interpeduncular cistern

Anatomy

The symmetrically paired oculomotor nerve (III) arises in the cerebral peduncles and travels to the orbital cavity, where it terminates.

True origin

- Its **nuclei of origin** are situated at the superior colliculus in front of and lateral to the cerebral aqueduct under cover of the cerebral peduncles. They consist of several cell-groups:
- the symmetrically paired **lateral nuclei,** which provide the innervation of the extrinsic ocular muscles (superior, inferior and medial rectus; levator palpebrae superioris; inferior oblique),
- the symmetrically paired **parasympathetic nuclei,** situated above, medial to and in front of the preceding nuclei. They provide the innervation of the intrinsic ocular muscles (Fig. 3.12),
- the **nuclei of the oculomotor nerve** emit fibers destined for all the ocular muscles except the superior oblique and lateral rectus. All the fibers come together in slender root strands which are grouped shortly after in the mainstem of the oculomotor nerve.

Apparent origin

This is situated at the anterior aspect of the brain-stem, at the medial border of the base of the cerebral peduncle (Fig. 3.12).

Interpeduncular cistern

Magnetic resonance imaging (MRI)

SAGITTAL VIEW

Imaging

CLINICAL FEATURES

- Direct paralysis of oculomotor nerve (III), complete or partial,
- homolateral paralysis of oculomotor nerve with involuntary movements of opposite side.

POSSIBLE CAUSES

- Weber's syndrome (syndrome of cerebral peduncle),
- syndrome of Benedikt or Claude (inferior syndromes of red nucleus (cerebral peduncle)),
- hypophyseal adenoma,
- agenesis of corpus callosum (possible compression of III and posterior cerebral and superior cerebellar arteries).

EXAMINATION

- Magnetic resonance imaging (MRI) or computed tomography (CT) of interpeduncular cistern to show apparent origin of oculomotor nerve (III) in sagittal, frontal and axial views (Fig. 3.4a–c; 3.5a–c).

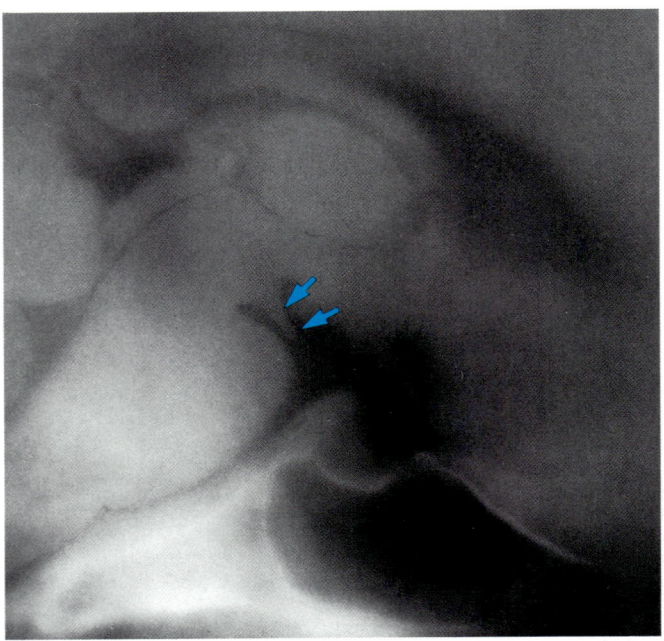
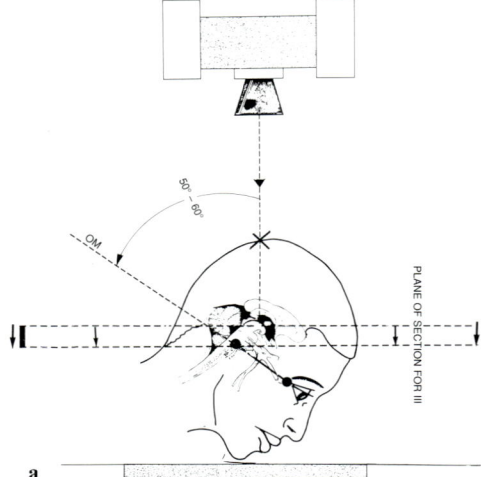

Fig. 3.4a–f. Reference diagram (**a**) for conventional study of interpeduncular cistern; tomography (**b**); sagittal magnetic resonance imaging (**c, e, f**) and sagittal anatomic view (**d**) to show oculomotor nerve (III)

b

Oculomotor nerve (III) 39

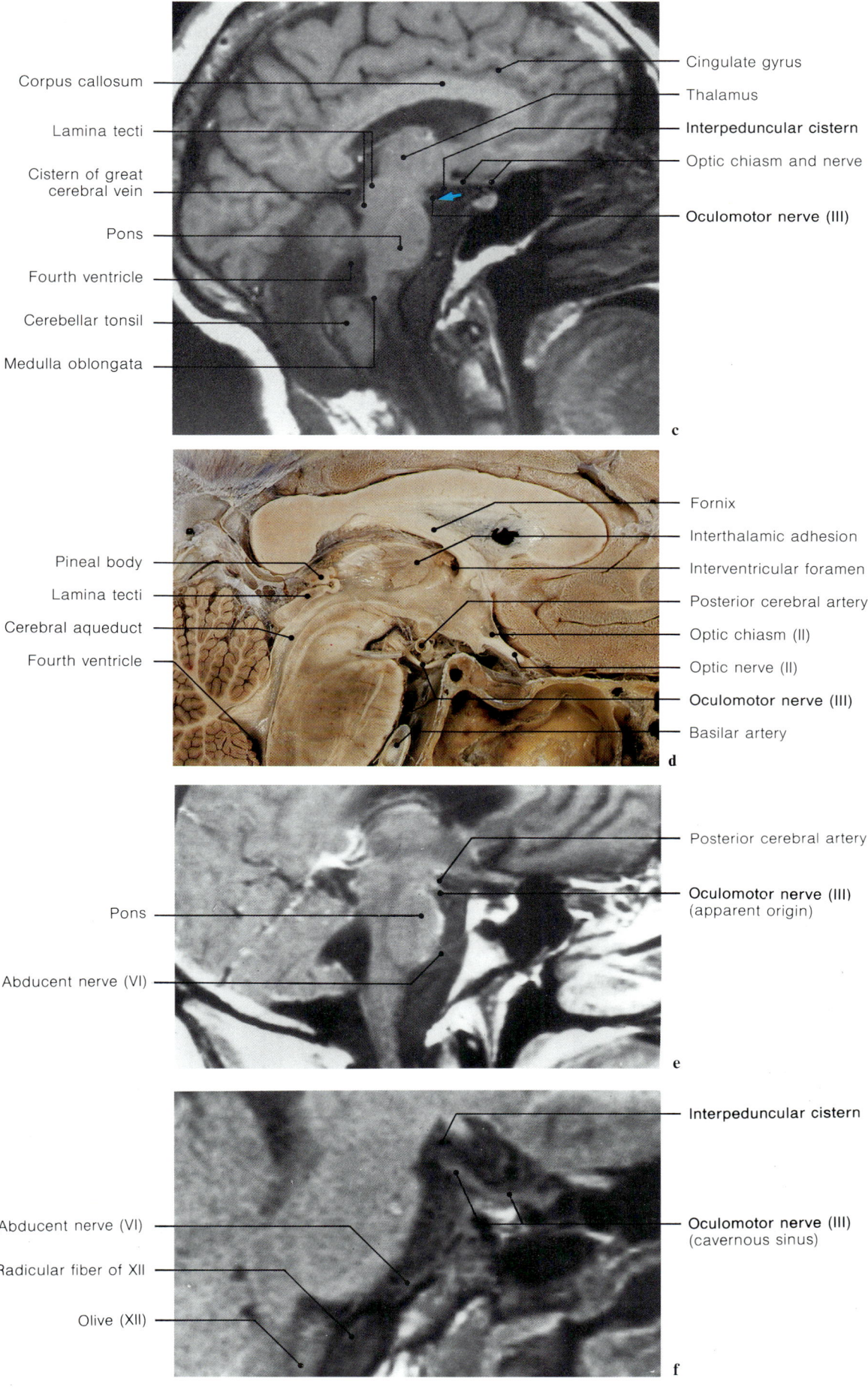

Interpeduncular cistern

Computed tomography (CT) and magnetic resonance imaging (MRI)

AXIAL VIEW

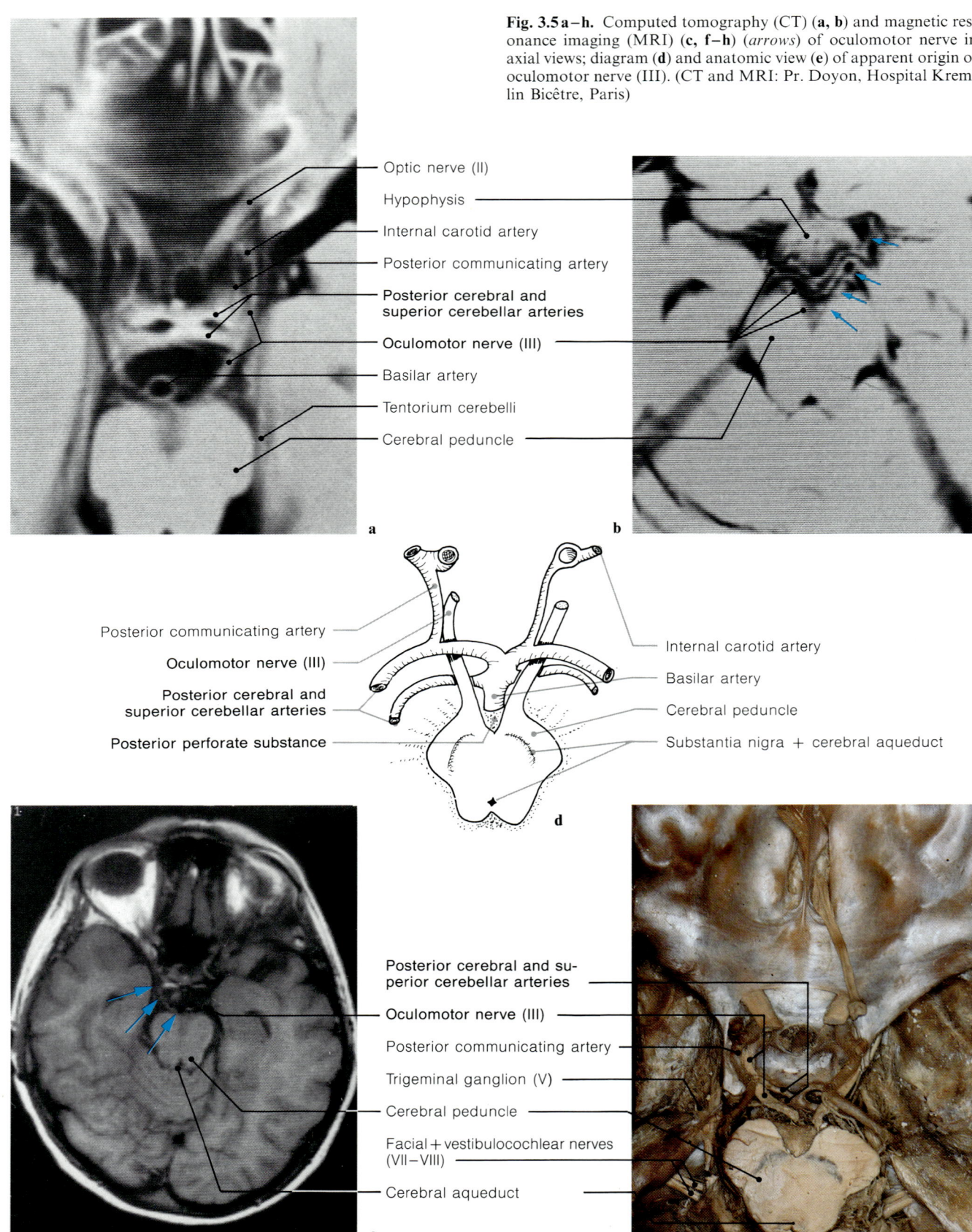

Fig. 3.5 a–h. Computed tomography (CT) (**a**, **b**) and magnetic resonance imaging (MRI) (**c**, **f–h**) (*arrows*) of oculomotor nerve in axial views; diagram (**d**) and anatomic view (**e**) of apparent origin of oculomotor nerve (III). (CT and MRI: Pr. Doyon, Hospital Kremlin Bicêtre, Paris)

Oculomotor nerve (III) 41

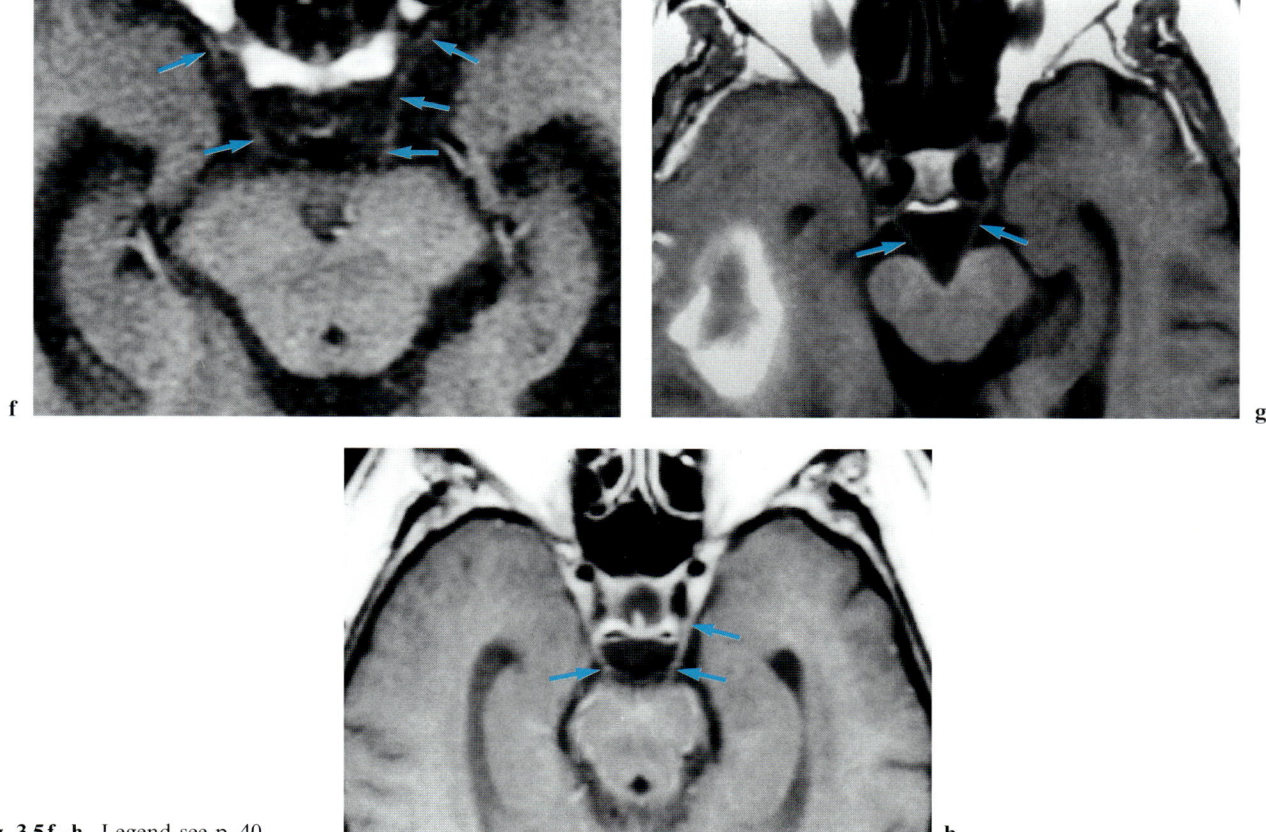

Fig. 3.5f–h. Legend see p. 40

Fig. 3.6. Dissection of brain-stem showing vascular relations of oculomotor nerves

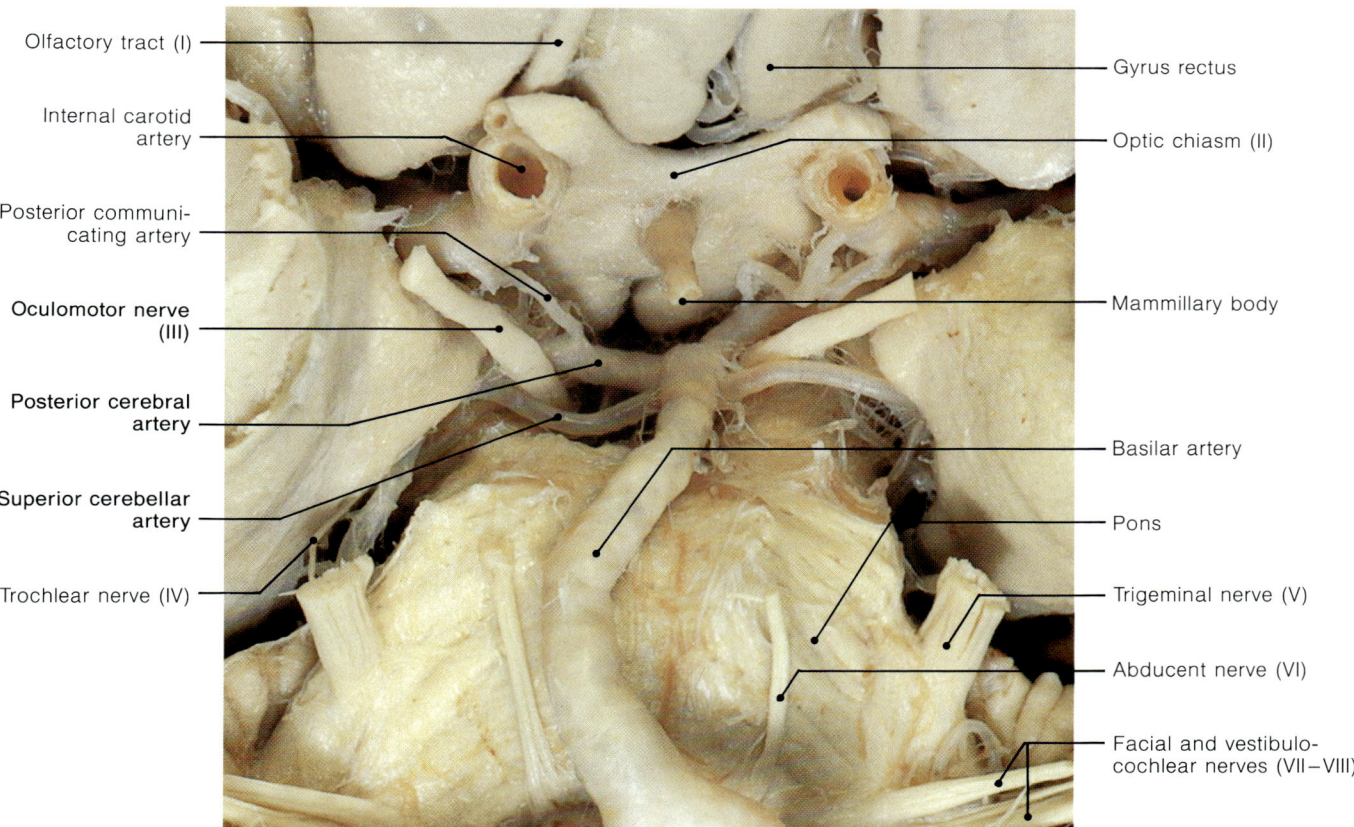

Course, sulcus of oculomotor nerve (dorsum sellae), cavernous sinus, superior orbital fissure

Anatomy

Intracranial course

After leaving the cerebral peduncle and the posterior perforate substance, the oculomotor nerve (III) passes between the superior cerebellar and posterior cerebral arteries (Fig. 3.5a, b, d, e; 3.6c), travels forwards, glides under the posterior clinoid process, making a more or less marked sulcus on the lateral margin of the dorsum sellae (Fig. 3.6b; 3.7a, b; 3.8a) and then penetrates the superolateral wall of the cavernous sinus (Fig. 6.10).

When it arrives at the medial portion of the superior orbital fissure, it divides into two terminal branches as it passes into the ciliary zonula, a superior and an inferior branch (Fig. 3.2; 3.3).

Imaging

Clinical features

- Trigeminal neuralgia involving III,
- paralysis of cranial nerves III, IV and VI with involvement of ophthalmic (V^1) and maxillary (V^2) branches of trigeminal nerve,
- total extrinsic and intrinsic ophthalmoplegia due to involvement of cranial nerves III, IV and VI.

Possible causes

- Osteitis of petrous apex (neuralgia of V and paralysis of VI, Gradenigo's syndrome),
- Foix's syndrome (lateral wall of cavernous sinus),
- aneurysm of internal carotid artery (cavernous sinus),
- Garcin's syndrome, involvement of cranial nerves II, IV, V and VI (petrosphenoidal junction),
- sarcoma of skull base,
- Rollet's syndrome (orbital apex),
- Rochon-Duvigneaud's syndrome (superior orbital fissure), fractures.

Examination

- Tomographic or computed tomographic (CT) study of the dorsum sellae for the sulcus of III, using the lower frontal view of Worms and Bretton (with modifications), with projection of the dorsum sellae into the foramen magnum (Fig. 3.7b),
- axial and frontal CT studies of the cavernous sinuses (Fig. 4.7; 6.10),
- computed tomographic (CT) or ordinary tomographic studies of the superior orbital fissure using symmetric frontal and unilateral oblique views, and also "discontinuous scanning"

For performance of these views of the superior orbital fissure, see the study of the ophthalmic nerve (V^1; trigeminal nerve).

Sulcus of oculomotor nerve (dorsum sellae)

Fig. 3.7a, b. Tomography (a) and anatomic transoccipital view (b) of dorsum sellae to show sulcus of oculomotor nerve (III)

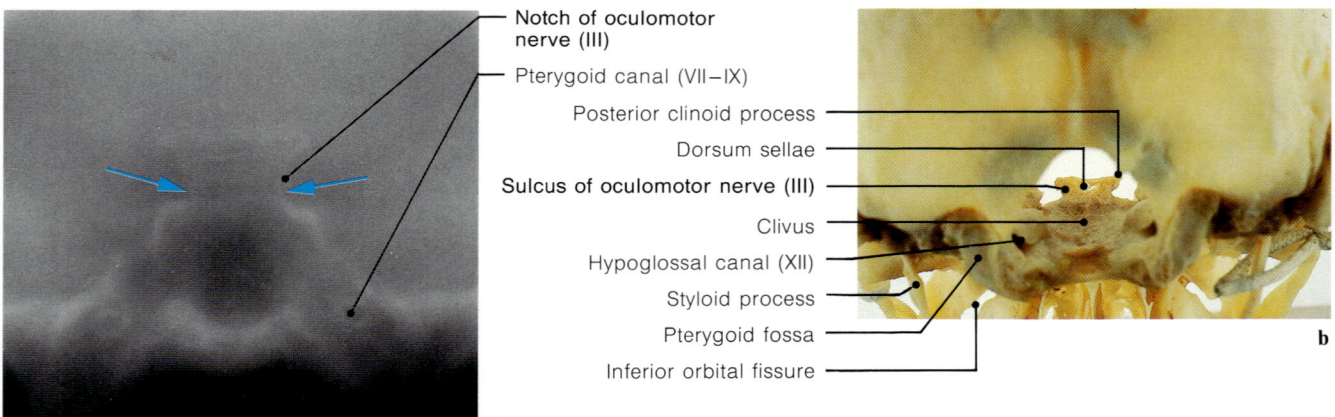

Sulcus of oculomotor nerve, superior orbital fissure

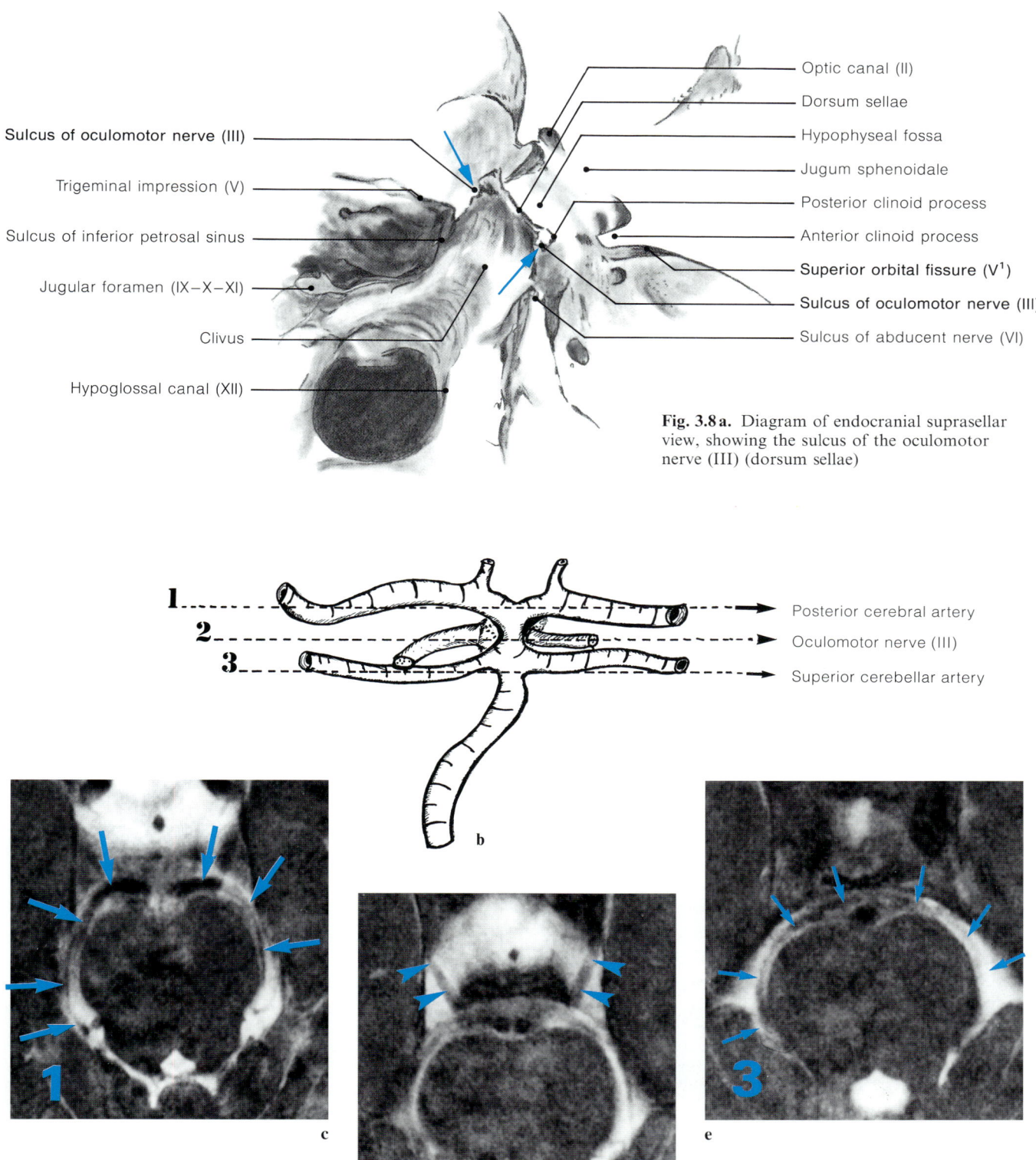

Fig. 3.8 a. Diagram of endocranial suprasellar view, showing the sulcus of the oculomotor nerve (III) (dorsum sellae)

Fig. 3.8 b–e. Axial magnetic resonance imaging (MRI) and diagram visualizing successively the oculomotor nerve (III) and its vascular relationship: *1*, posterior cerebral artery (*arrows*); *2*, oculomotor nerve (*arrowheads*); *3*, superior cerebellar artery (*small arrows*). (MRI: Dr. J.W. Casselman, A.Z. St-Jan, Brugge)

Extrinsic ocular movements of the oculomotor nerve (innervation of all ocular muscles except superior oblique (IV) and lateral rectus (VI))

Anatomy

Terminal branches

The **superior ramus** of the oculomotor nerve (III) courses round the optic nerve and supplies the superior rectus and levator palpebrae superioris muscles (Fig. 3.3; 3.9).
The shorter and larger **inferior ramus** divides into three other branches:

- the branch to the inferior rectus muscle,
- the branch to the medial rectus muscle,
- the branch to the inferior oblique muscle (Fig. 3.9).

From this last branch there arises above and behind a short slender communicating branch to the ciliary ganglion (V^1 – III) which supplies the sphincter pupillae muscle and the annular portion of the ciliary muscle via the short ciliary nerves (Fig. 3.9; 3.12). It also contributes to the parasympathetic innervation (see intrinsic ocular movements).

Computed tomography (CT)

FRONTAL AND SAGITTAL VIEWS

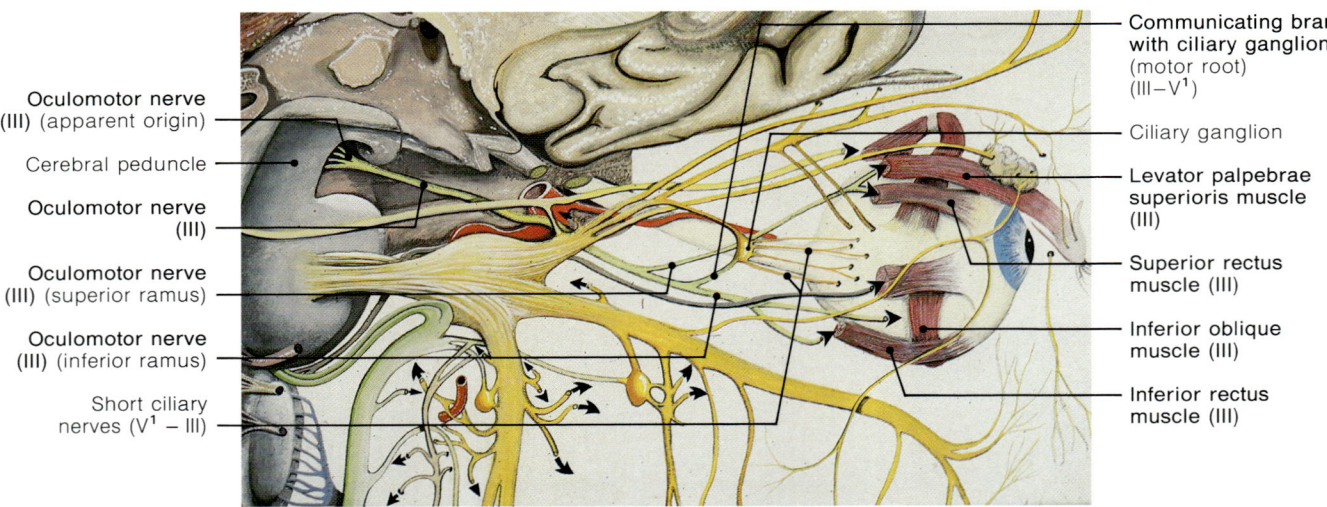

Fig. 3.9. Diagram of course and relations of oculomotor nerve (III)

Fig. 3.9 a, b. Frontal (a) and sagittal (b) computed tomographic (CT) sections of ocular muscles

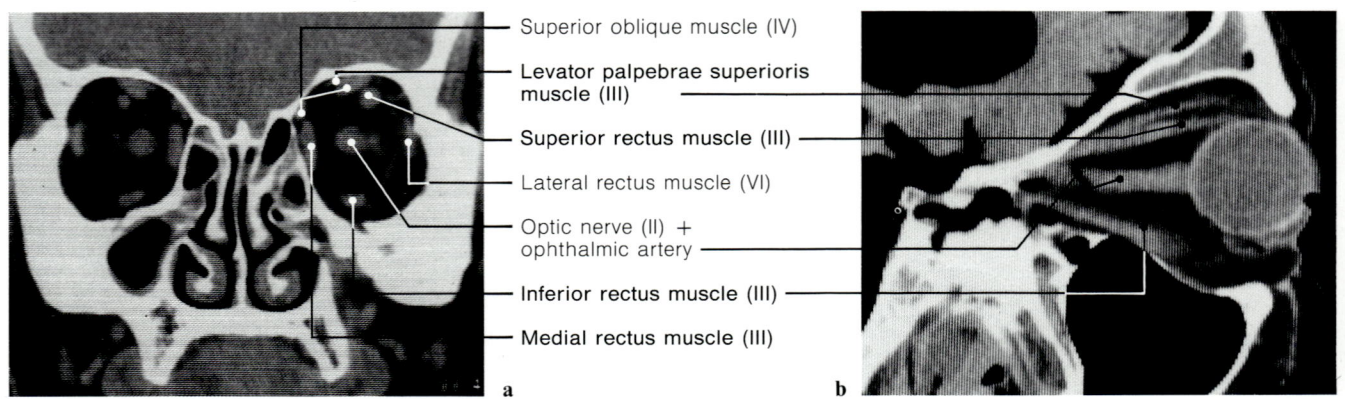

Ocular muscles

Computed tomography (CT)

FRONTAL AND AXIAL VIEWS

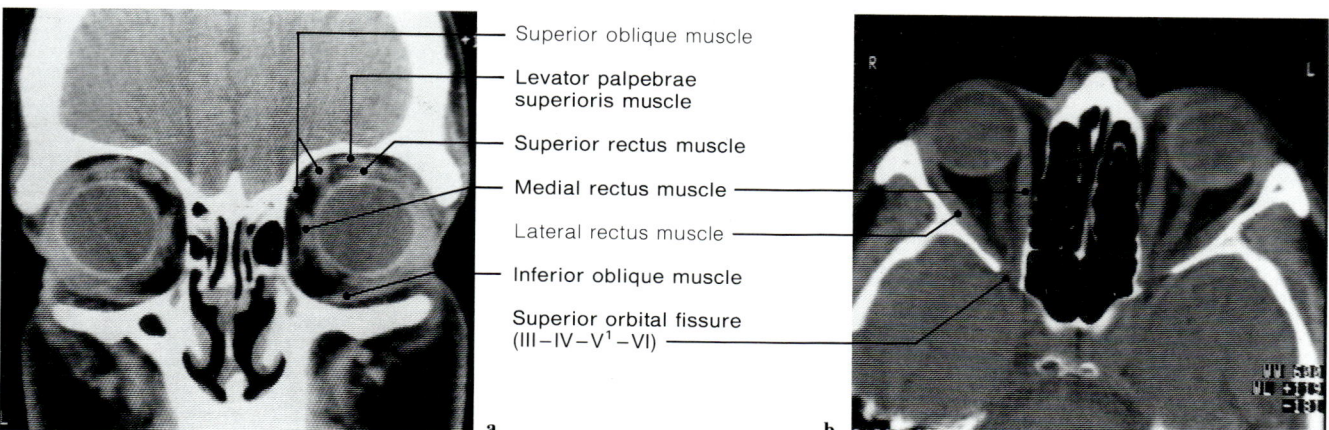

Fig. 3.10a, b. Frontal (**a**) and axial (**b**) computed tomography (CT) of ocular muscles

Fig. 3.10c, d. Axial computed tomography of levator palpebrae superioris muscles (**d**) and of superior rectus muscles (**c**)

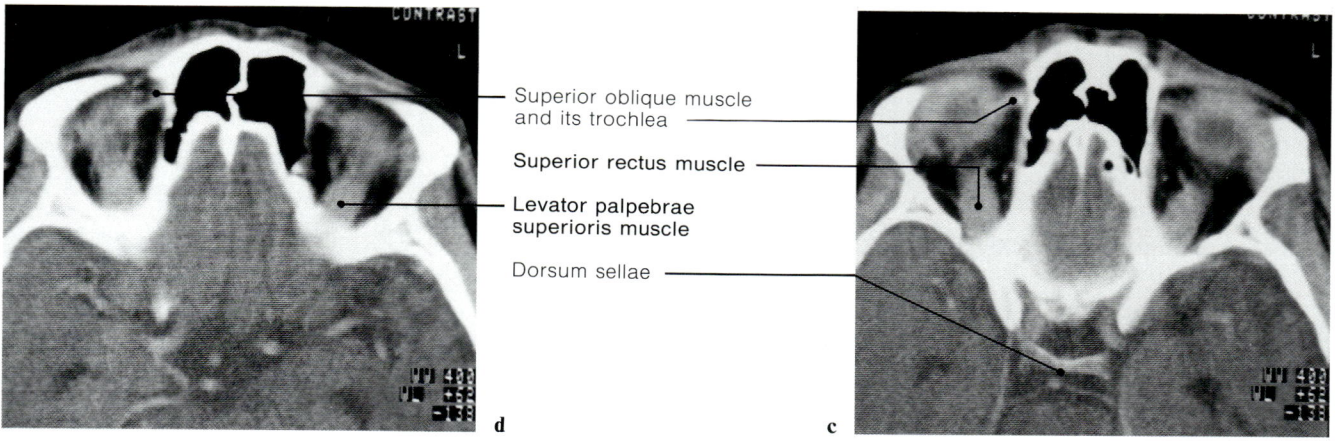

Fig. 3.11. Superior view of orbital cavity showing the levator palpebrae superioris muscle

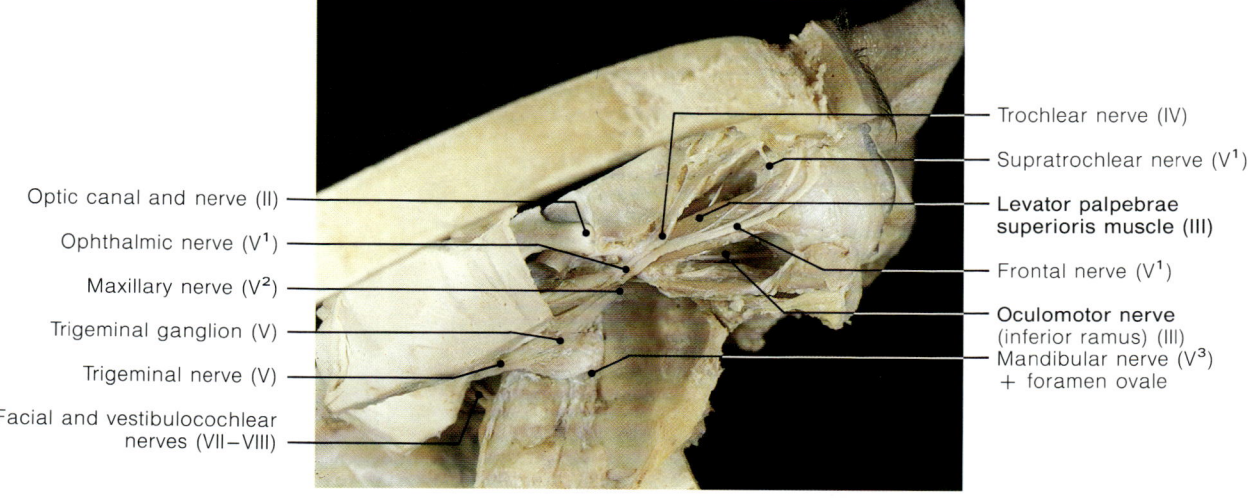

Intrinsic ocular movements (III–V^1)
(innervation of sphincter and dilator pupillae muscles)

Anatomy

The nasociliary nerve (V^1–III) gives off several branches, the first of which is the communicating branch with the ciliary ganglion, from which the short ciliary nerves arise (Fig. 3.9; 3.12).

The short ciliary nerves number 7 to 16 on average and are applied to the lateral aspect of the optic nerve. They perforate the sclera around the optic nerve and supply the cornea, the choroid, the iris, the ciliary body and the sclera.

They innervate the sphincter pupillae muscle and derive from the parasympathetic component of the oculomotor nerve (III), which arises from the Edinger-Westphal nucleus situated in the cerebral peduncle (Fig. 3.12).

They give off the pupillary sphincter tracts, which follow the course of the oculomotor nerve and the nerve to the inferior oblique muscle to reach the ciliary ganglion via its (short) oculomotor root (Fig. 3.9; 3.12).

The sphincter pupillae allows accommodation in near vision.

The nasociliary nerve gives off two other branches, the long ciliary nerves which innervate the dilator pupillae muscle. The pupillary dilator paths derive from the cervical sympathetic chain and proceed successively via the pericarotid plexus, the cavernous plexus, the ophthalmic nerve, the nasociliary nerve and the long ciliary nerves to reach the dilator pupillae muscle (Fig. 3.12).

This muscle allows accommodation in distant vision.

Intrinsic ocular movement includes pupillary movements and movements of accommodation.

Fig. 3.12. Diagram showing intrinsic ocular motility. — — — parasympathetic innervation: sphincter pupillae; - - - sympathetic innervation: dilator pupillae

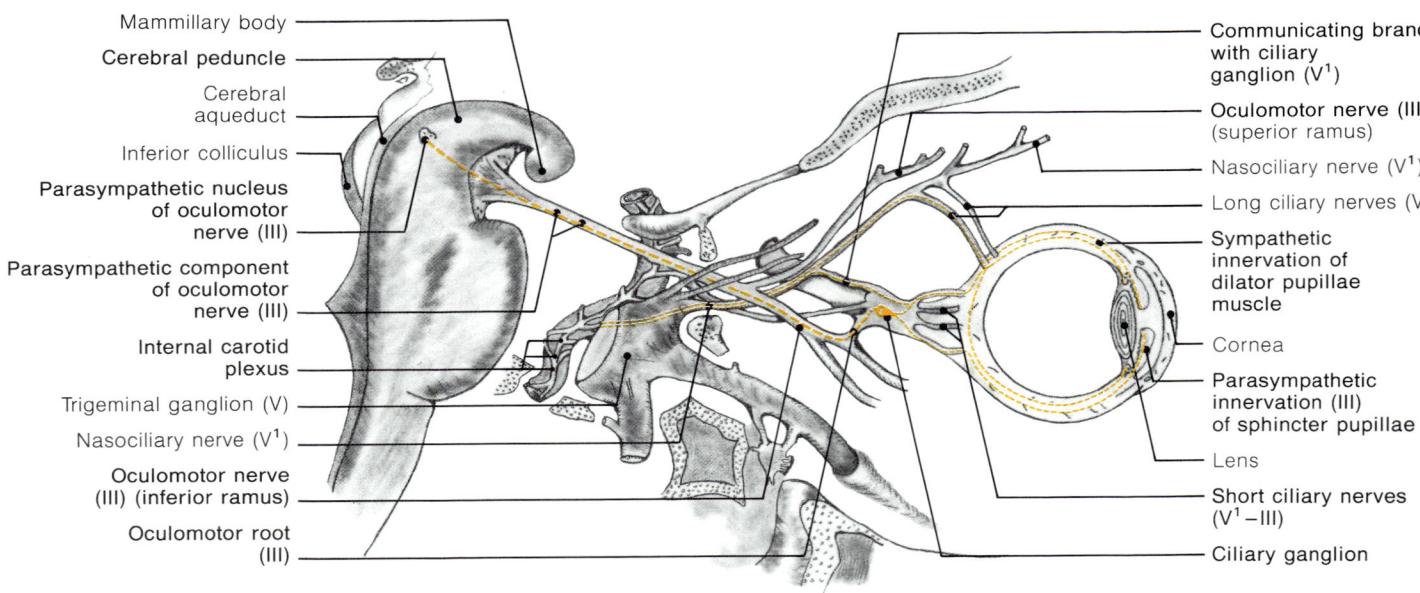

Trochlear nerve (IV)

Anatomy (course – terminals – collaterals) 49
Imaging (regions examined) 49
Pathology 49
Apparent origin of trochlear nerve, inferior colliculus,
cistern of great cerebral vein
    Axial views (MRI) 51
    Anatomy and imaging (examination) 51
Cistern of great cerebral vein
    Sagittal view (MRI) 52
Brain-stem
    Anatomic view and sagittal section 53
Intracavernous course of trochlear nerve
    Axial and sagittal views (MRI, CT) 54
Superior orbital fissure, reflexion pulley (trochlea)
of superior oblique muscle
    Imaging 55
Course of trochlear nerve
    Horizontal, axial and sagittal views (MRI, CT) 56
    Anatomic dissections of oculomotor nerves 57
    Axial view (MRI) and sagittal diagram 58

Vascular relations:
Cavernous sinus
    Venous drainage at the skull base 167, 290
    Marginal tentorial artery 276, 277
    Inferolateral trunk 276, 277

The trochlear nerve is the most slender of the cranial nerves. It is a motor nerve and supplies only the superior oblique muscle.

Its nucleus of origin is situated in the tegmentum of the mesencephalon at the level of the inferior colliculi, below the nucleus of the oculomotor nerve and behind the medial longitudinal fascicle, which it indents.

The radicular fibers pass dorsally, intersect behind the cerebral aqueduct with those of the opposite side, and emerge at the dorsal aspect of each side of the frenulum of the superior medullary velum, beneath the inferior colliculi.

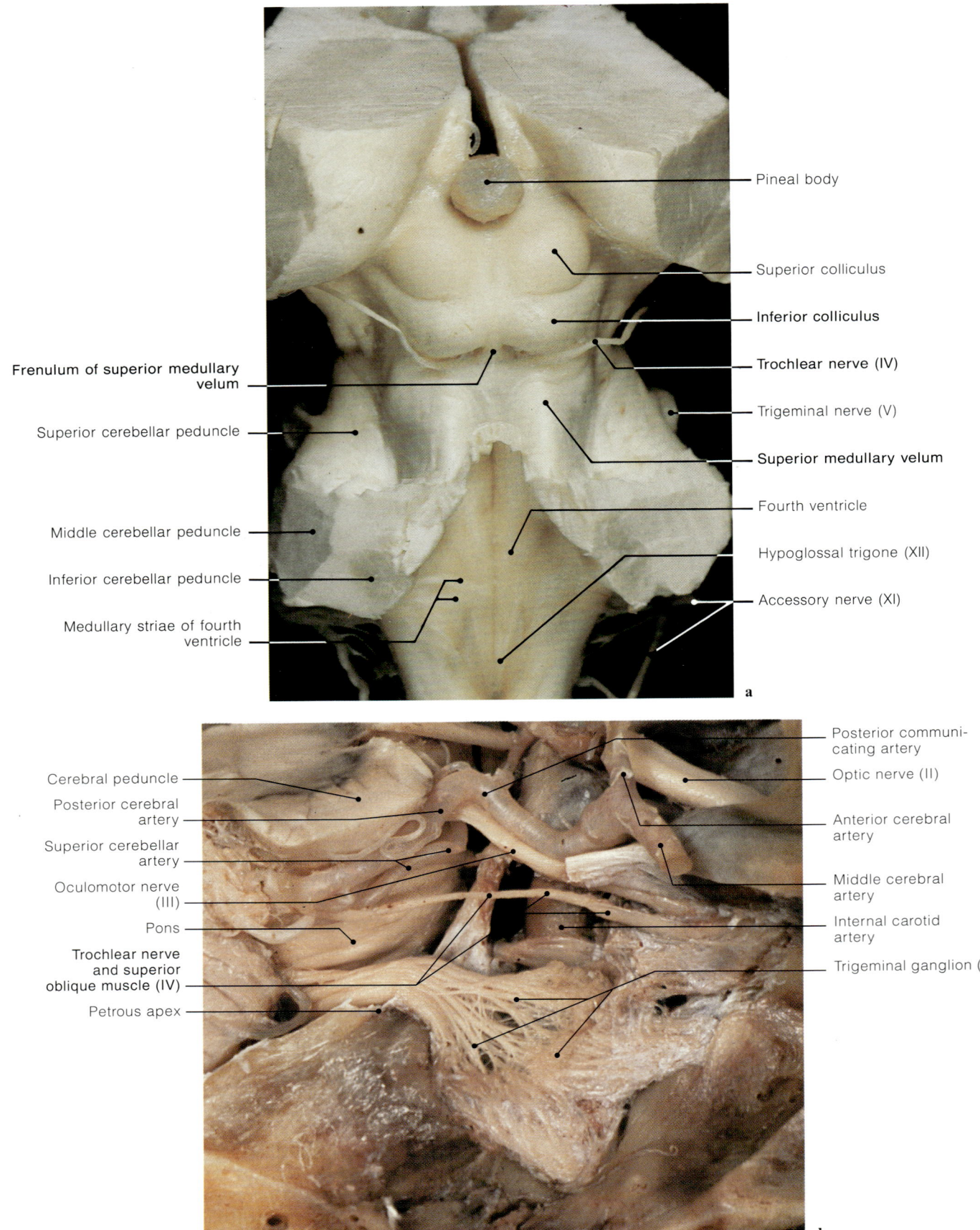

Fig. 4.1. a Apparent origins of trochlear nerves (IV) at the posterior aspect of cerebral peduncle; b sagittal dissection showing the course of the trochlear nerve up to the superior oblique muscle (IV). (Anatomic dissection: Pr. J.P. Francke, Faculty of Medicine, Lille)

Anatomy

COURSE – TERMINALS – COLLATERALS

Apparent origin and intracranial course

Intracavernous and orbital course

Reflexion pulley (or trochlea) of superior oblique muscle

Imaging

REGIONS EXAMINED

Imaging of third ventricle of the cerebral aqueduct and of the cistern of the great cerebral vein, demonstrating the inferior colliculus and the frenulum of the superior medullary velum

Examination of cavernous sinuses and superior orbital fissures

Imaging of medial supraorbital wall of orbit and ocular muscles

Pathology

- Pinealoma,
- petrosphenoidal junction syndrome (Garcin's syndrome),
- syndrome of lateral wall of cavernous sinus (Foix's syndrome),
- syndrome of superior orbital fissure (Rochon-Duvigneaud's syndrome),
- syndrome of orbital apex (Rollet's syndrome),
- syndrome of cerebral peduncle (Weber's syndrome),
- tumors and sarcomata of skull base,
- osteitis deformans (Paget's disease),
- cavernous sinus thrombosis,
- superior cerebellar artery thrombosis or syndrome,
- aneurysm of internal carotid artery,
- meningitides, diabetes,
- fractures of the superior orbital wall (trochlea: pulley of superior oblique muscle),
- tumor of fourth ventricle.

Trochlear nerve (IV)

Topography

Apparent origin of trochlear nerve (IV)
- Inferior colliculus
- Cistern of great cerebral vein

Intracavernous course
- Cavernous sinus

Superior orbital fissure
- Reflexion pulley (trochlea) of superior oblique muscle

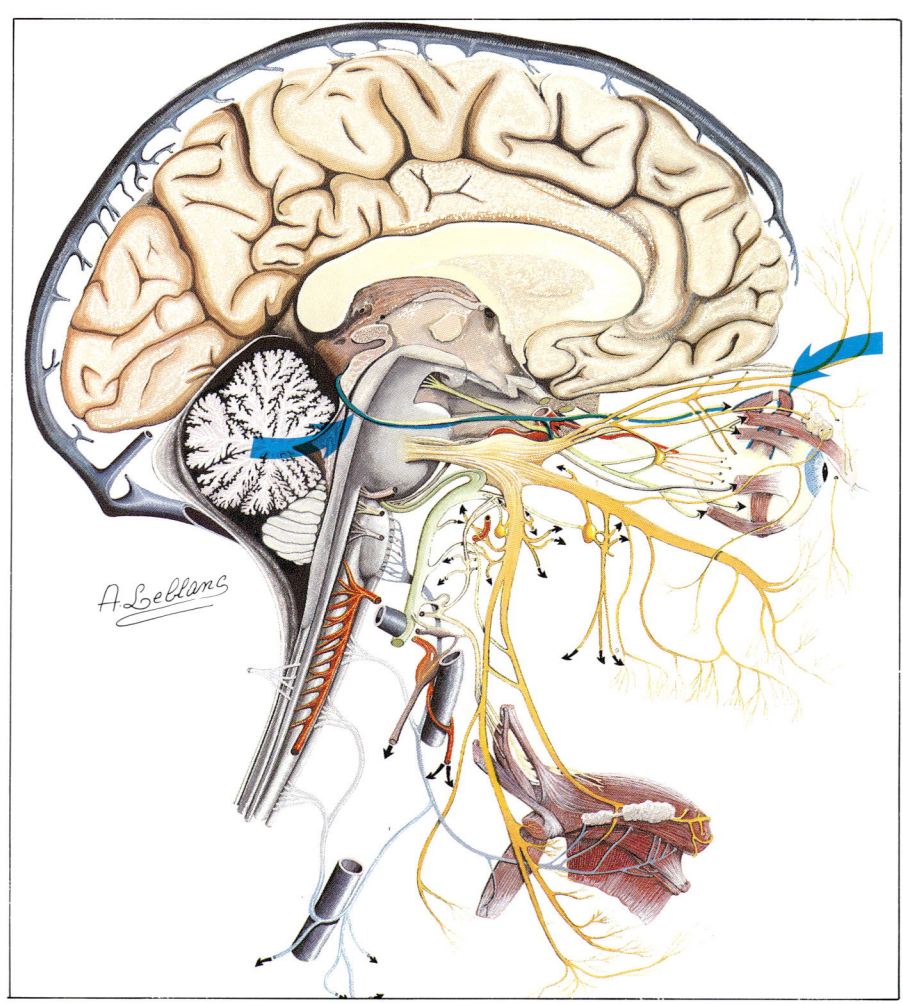

Fig. 4.2

Apparent origin of trochlear nerve, inferior colliculus, cistern of great cerebral vein

Anatomy

After having emerged from the dorsal aspect of the neuraxis, at either side of the frenulum of the superior medullary velum and beneath the inferior colliculus, the trunk of the trochlear nerve travels in the subarachnoid space.

Initially, it is situated in the posterior cranial fossa and courses round the lateral aspect of the cerebral peduncles (Fig. 4.1; 4.2; 4.6; 4.13a, b) skirting the free edge of the tentorium cerebelli. It joins then the upper part of the cavernous sinus at the level of its posterolateral angle. It passes lateral to III, then crosses it and comes to lie above it.

The trochlear nerve anastomoses with the ophthalmic nerve (V^1) before the superior orbital fissure (Fig. 4.11).

It traverses the superior orbital fissure, passing lateral to the common tendinous ring, and joins the orbital cavity.

It glides obliquely forward and inward to reach the superior oblique muscle (Fig. 4.2; 4.9; 4.11; 4.12).

Trochlear nerve (IV)

Magnetic resonance imaging (MRI)

AXIAL VIEWS

Imaging

CLINICAL FEATURES

– Paralysis of the trochlear nerve may occur during oculomotor disorders of varying complexity, it is difficult to demonstrate and specialist diagnosis depends on supplementary techniques.

POSSIBLE CAUSES

– Pinealoma, downward spread,
– thrombosis of superior cerebellar artery,
– tumor of fourth ventricle,
– tumor of cistern of great cerebral vein.

EXAMINATION

– Magnetic resonance imaging (MRI) and computed tomography (CT) of the cistern of the great cerebral vein, demonstrating the inferior colliculus and frenulum of the superior medullary velum to show the apparent origin of the trochlear nerve (IV) in frontal, sagittal and axial views (Fig. 4.4a, b; 4.10b, e, f; 4.13a).

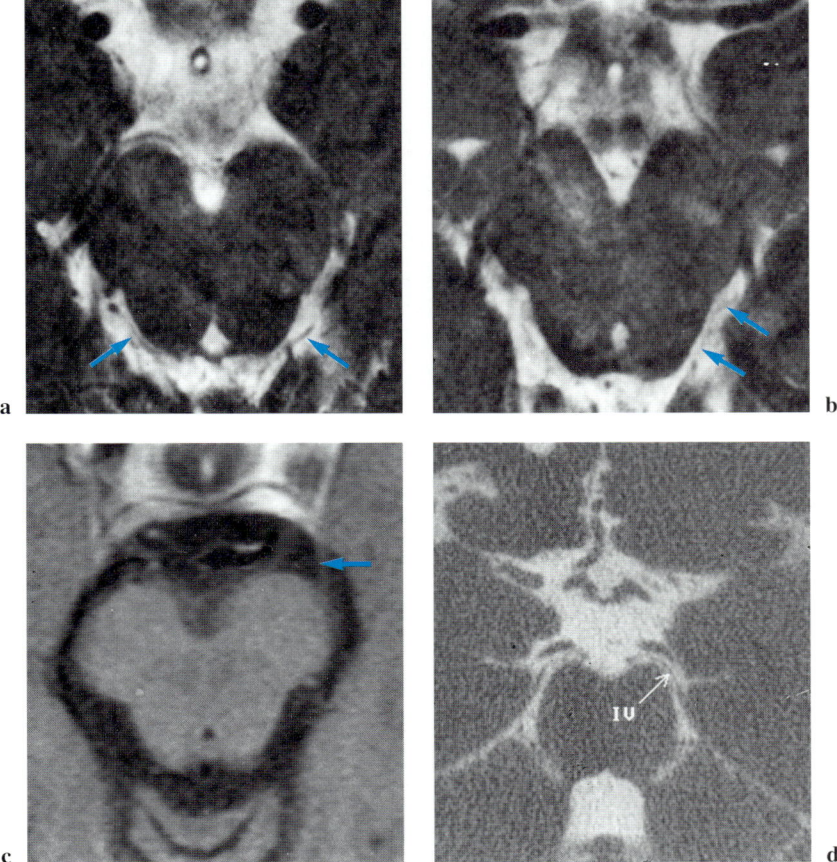

Fig. 4.3a–d. Axial magnetic resonance imaging (MRI) and computed tomography (CT) demonstrating in succession the course of the trochlear nerve (IV) from its origin to its circumpeduncular path (*arrows*). (CT: Pr. Doyon, Hospital Kremlin Bicêtre, Paris; MRI: Dr. J.W. Casselman, A.Z. St-Jan, Brugge)

Cistern of great cerebral vein
Magnetic resonance imaging (MRI)
SAGITTAL VIEW

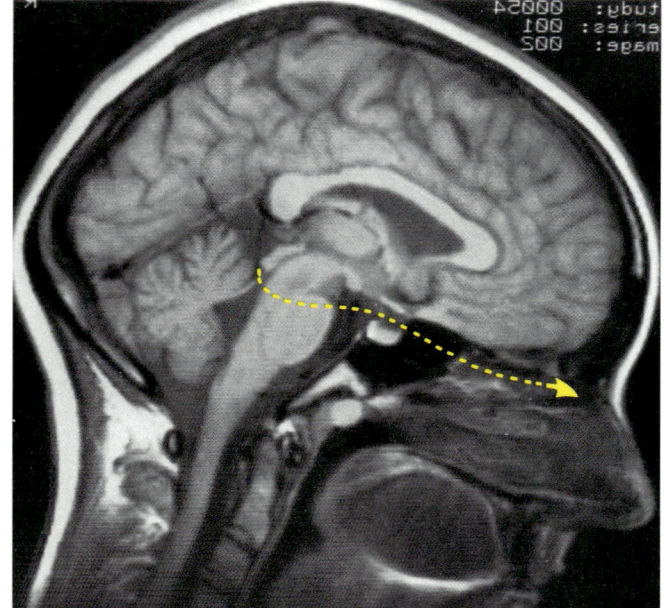

Fig. 4.4a–c. Sagittal magnetic resonance imaging of cistern of great cerebral vein, demonstrating the inferior and superior colliculi as well as the frenulum of the superior medullary velum. Dotted and arrowed: course of trochlear nerve (IV). (MRI: Pr. Doyon, Hospital Kremlin Bicêtre, Paris)

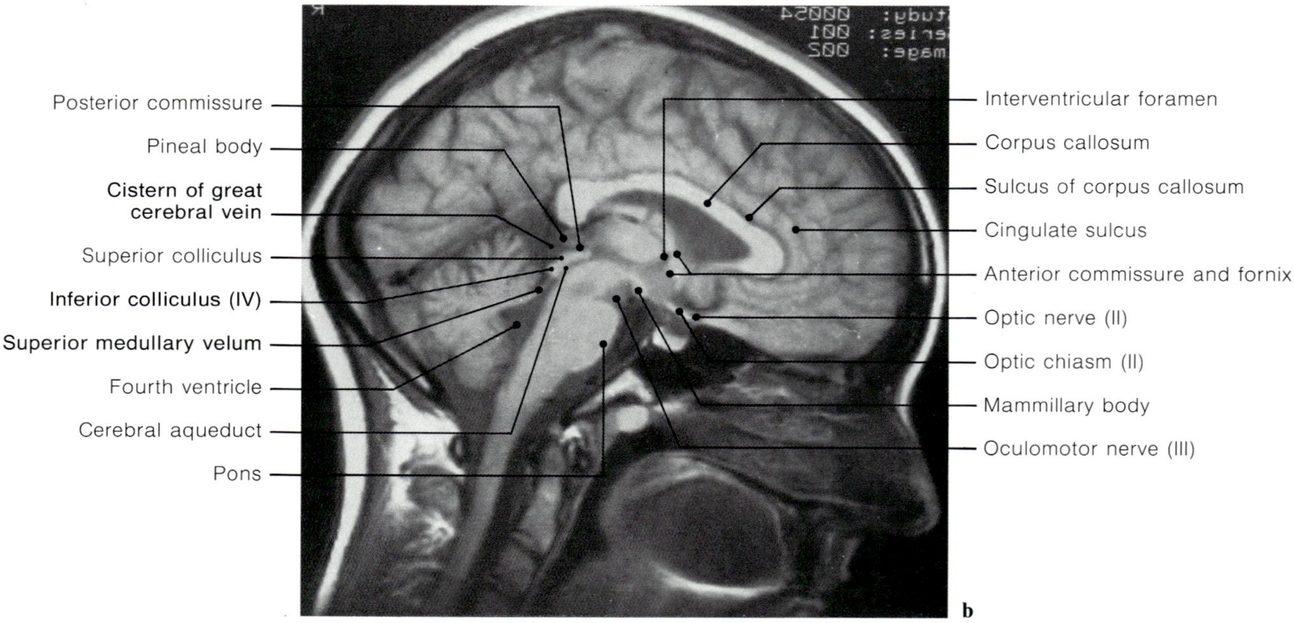

- Posterior commissure
- Pineal body
- Cistern of great cerebral vein
- Superior colliculus
- Inferior colliculus (IV)
- Superior medullary velum
- Fourth ventricle
- Cerebral aqueduct
- Pons

- Interventricular foramen
- Corpus callosum
- Sulcus of corpus callosum
- Cingulate sulcus
- Anterior commissure and fornix
- Optic nerve (II)
- Optic chiasm (II)
- Mammillary body
- Oculomotor nerve (III)

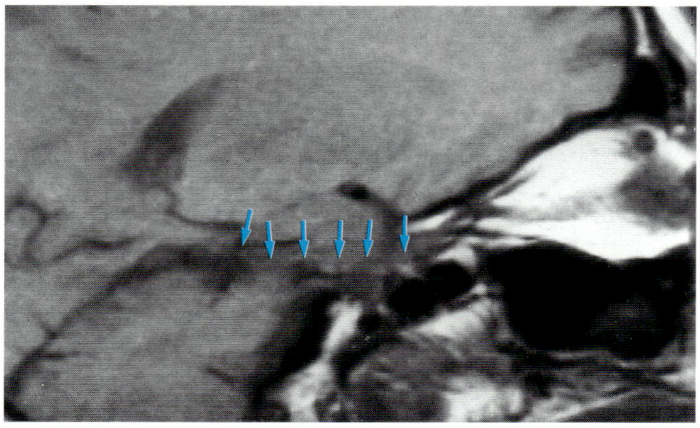

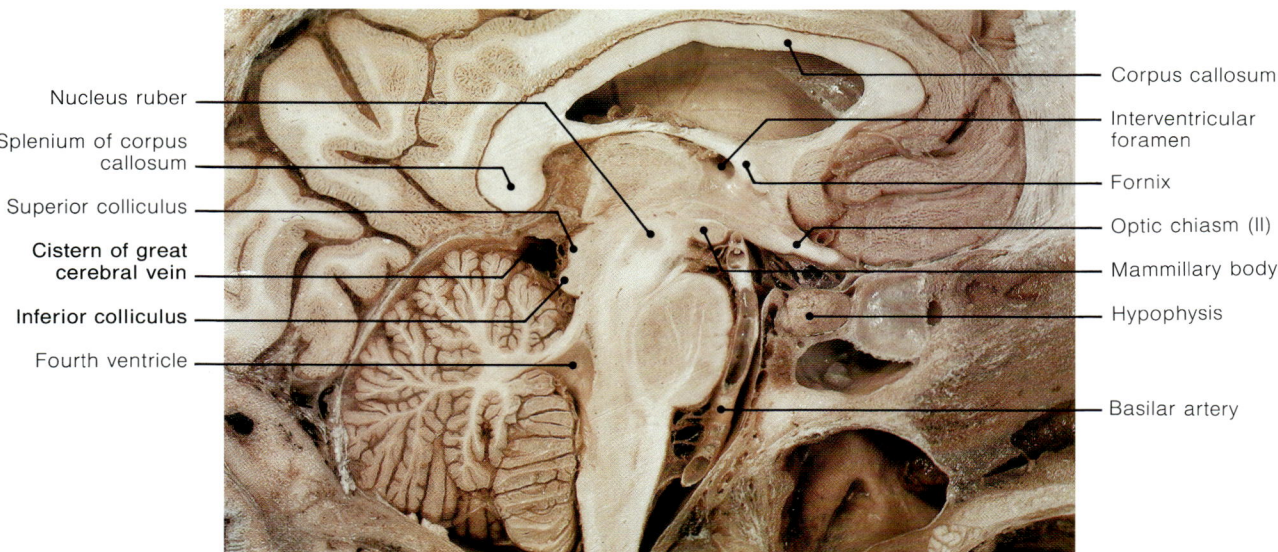

Fig. 4.5. Sagittal anatomic section of brain-stem

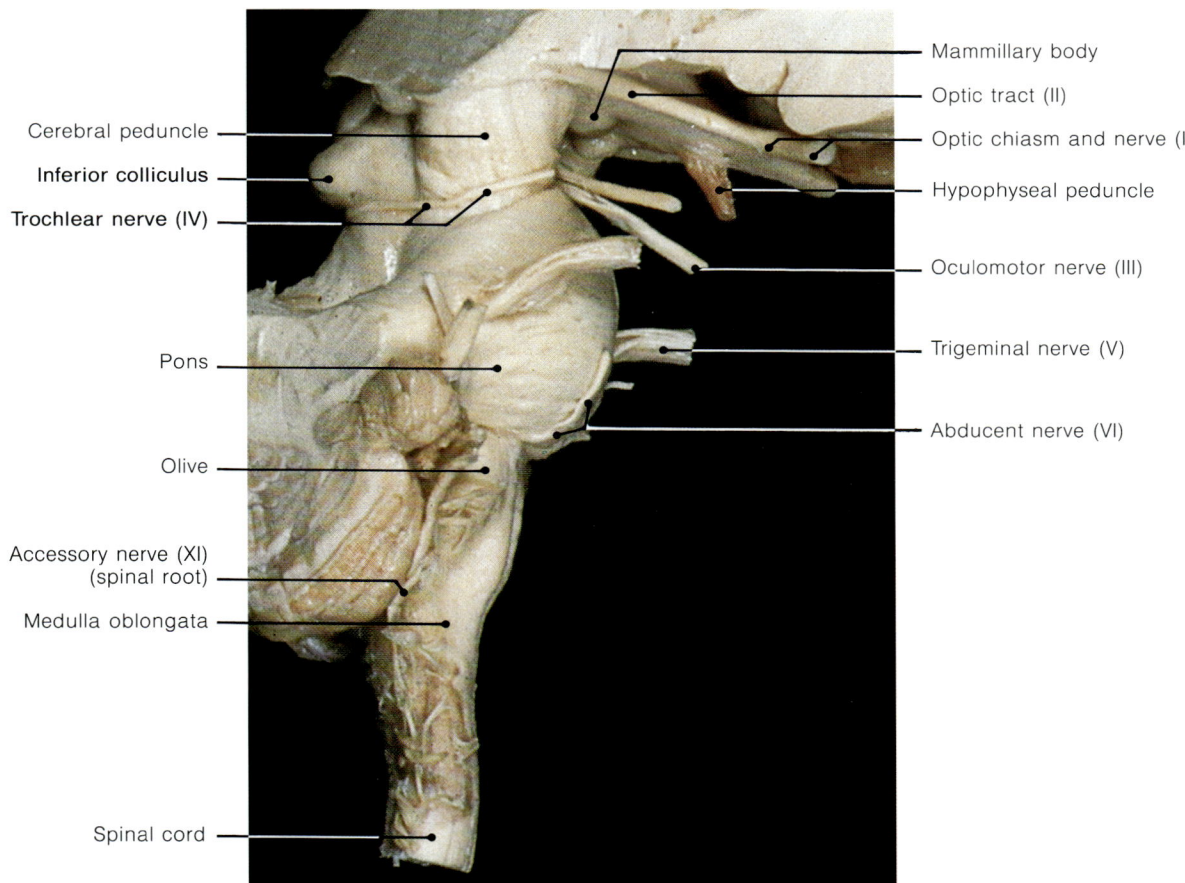

Fig. 4.6. Anatomic view of brain-stem showing the right trochlear nerve (IV) in its circumpeduncular course

Intracavernous course of trochlear nerve

Magnetic resonance imaging (MRI) and computed tomography (CT)

CLINICAL FEATURES

– Paralysis of the trochlear nerve together with the IIIrd and IVth cranial nerves, as well as involvement of the ophthalmic (V^1) and maxillary (V^2) branches of the trigeminal nerve (trigeminal neuralgia, types V^1-V^2)

POSSIBLE CAUSES

– Syndrome of Jacob or Foix (lateral wall of cavernous sinus, possibly associated with an aneurysm of the internal carotid artery),
– hypophyseal tumors,
– tumors or fractures of sphenoidal sinus,
– cavernous sinus thrombosis.

EXAMINATION

– Study of cavernous sinus in frontal, sagittal and axial views (Fig. 4.7; 6.9; 6.10).

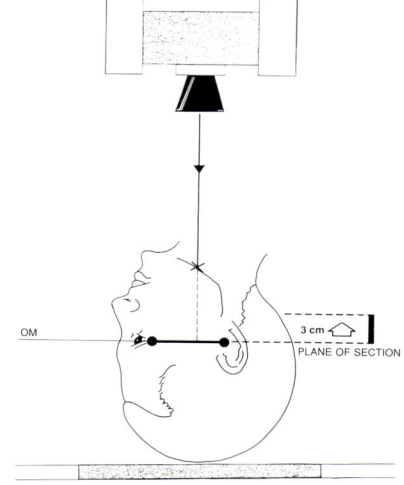

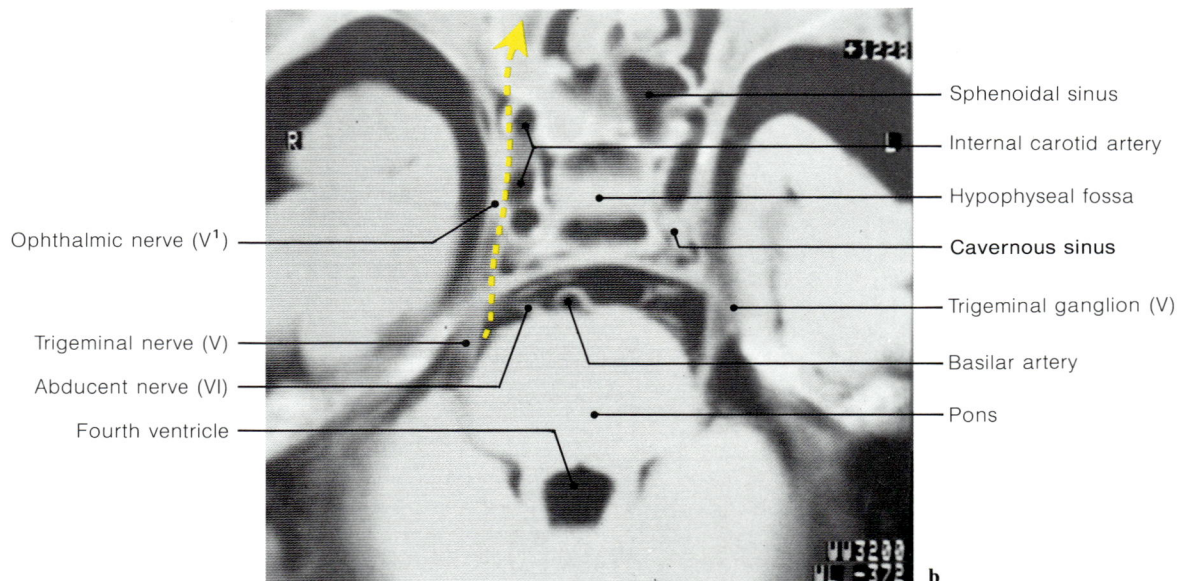

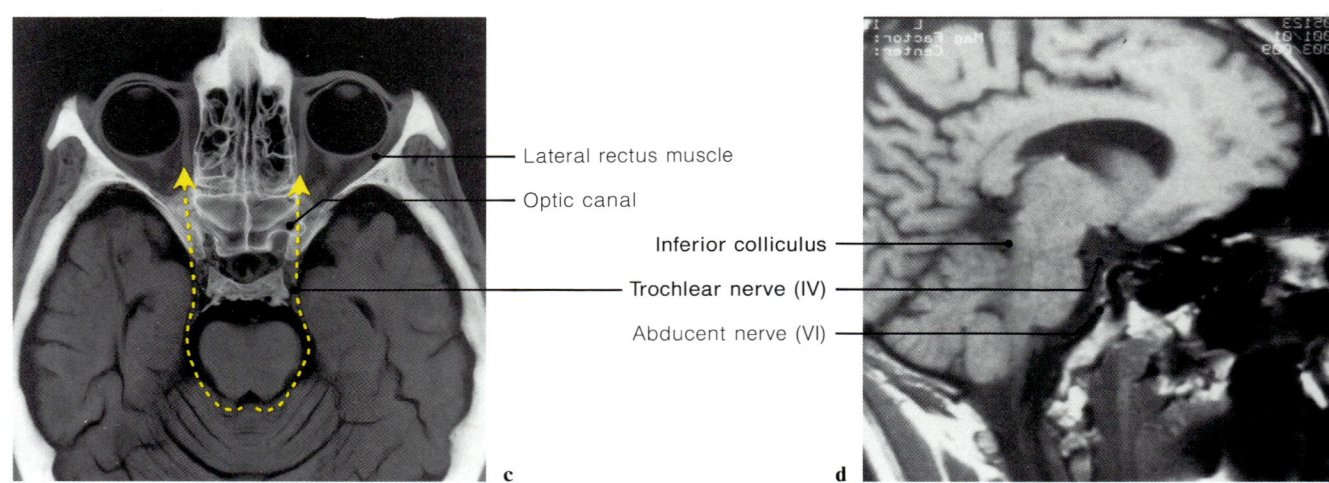

Fig. 4.7a–d. Centering diagram for imaging of cavernous sinuses (**a**); axial computed tomography (**b, c**) and sagittal magnetic resonance imaging (**d**) for the trochlear nerve (IV)

Superior orbital fissure, reflexion pulley (trochlea) of superior oblique muscle

Imaging

CLINICAL FEATURES

– Paralysis of cranial nerves III, IV and VI and involvement of ophthalmic branch (V^1) with evidence of anesthesia of the root of the nose, upper eyelid, forehead and cornea with abolition of corneal reflex, accompanied by complete ophthalmoplegia, but with preservation of vision,
– the same clinical picture, but with amblyopia, involvement of the optic nerve, optic atrophy and homolateral blindness.

POSSIBLE CAUSES

– Syndrome of superior orbital fissure (Rochon-Duvigneaud's syndrome),
– meningioma of lesser wing of sphenoid,
– aneurysm of internal carotid artery,
– syndrome of petrosphenoidal junction (Garcin's syndrome).

EXAMINATION

– Imaging of superior orbital fissure.

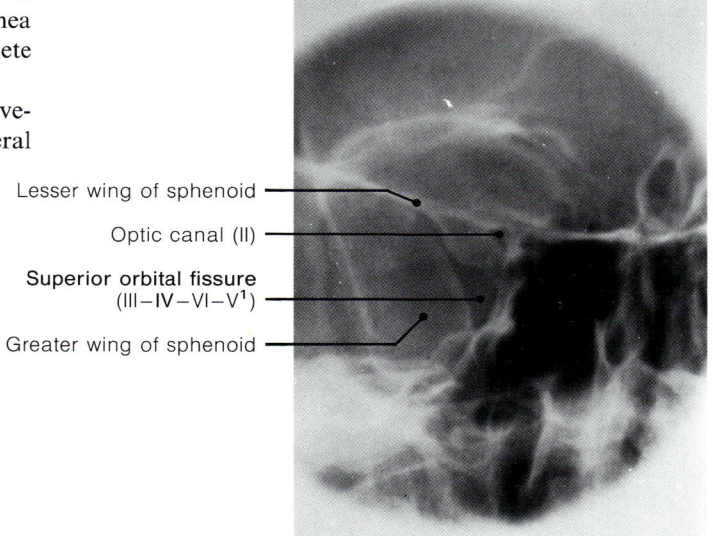

Fig. 4.8. Imaging of superior orbital fissure in unilateral view

Trochlea (reflexion pulley of superior oblique muscle)

The attachments of the reflexion pulley of the superior oblique muscle may be damaged in head injury, when there is suspicion of a fracture of the orbit or, more precisely, of the superomedial orbital margin, or in a case of orbital tumor or of Paget's disease. Such damage produces mechanical dysfunction of this pulley.

Note: It is important to note that the disorder resulting from mechanical trouble with the pulley of the superior oblique muscle is the same as that resulting from paralysis of the trochlear nerve (IV).

Views required

– After having visualized the orbital walls, it is necessary to study the nerve by means of computed tomographic (CT) sections or magnetic resonance imaging (MRI) in several different views (p. 56) to show its origin and its circumpeduncular course to the superior oblique muscle.
– As the trochlear nerve (IV) is very slender, it is difficult to demonstrate. Initially, it must be located along the free margin of the tentorium cerebelli, then at the upper part of the cavernous sinus in the region of its posterolateral angle, then in its passage lateral to III, and subsequent positioning above and finally superomedial to and alongside the ophthalmic nerve (Fig. 4.7; 6.8 d; 6.10; 6.14 a, b).

Fig. 4.9. Diagram of superior oblique muscle and of its reflexion pulley

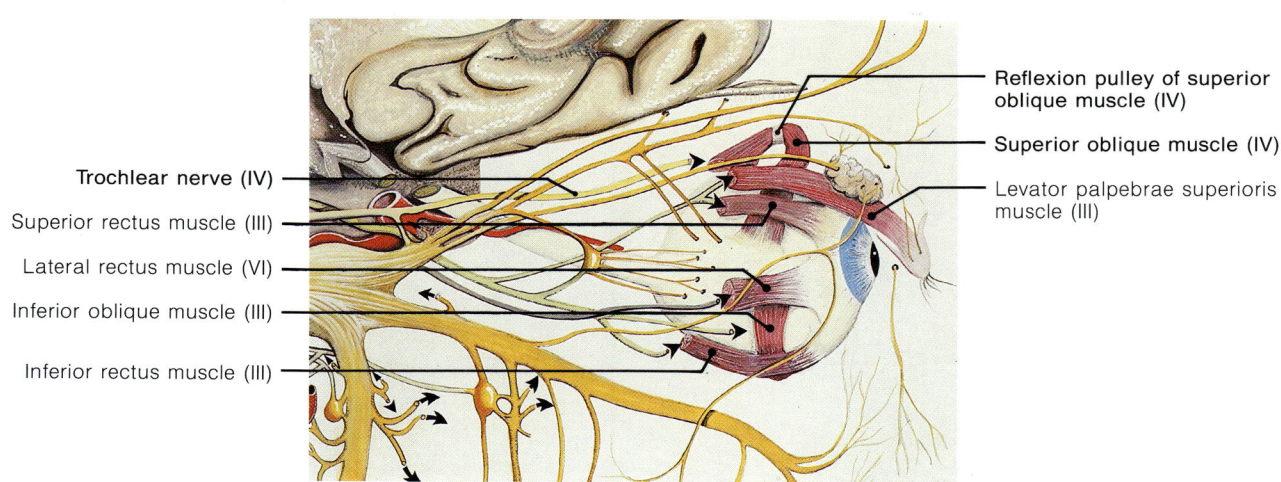

56 Trochlear nerve (IV)

Course of trochlear nerve

Computed tomography (CT) and magnetic resonance imaging (MRI)

HORIZONTAL, AXIAL AND SAGITTAL VIEWS

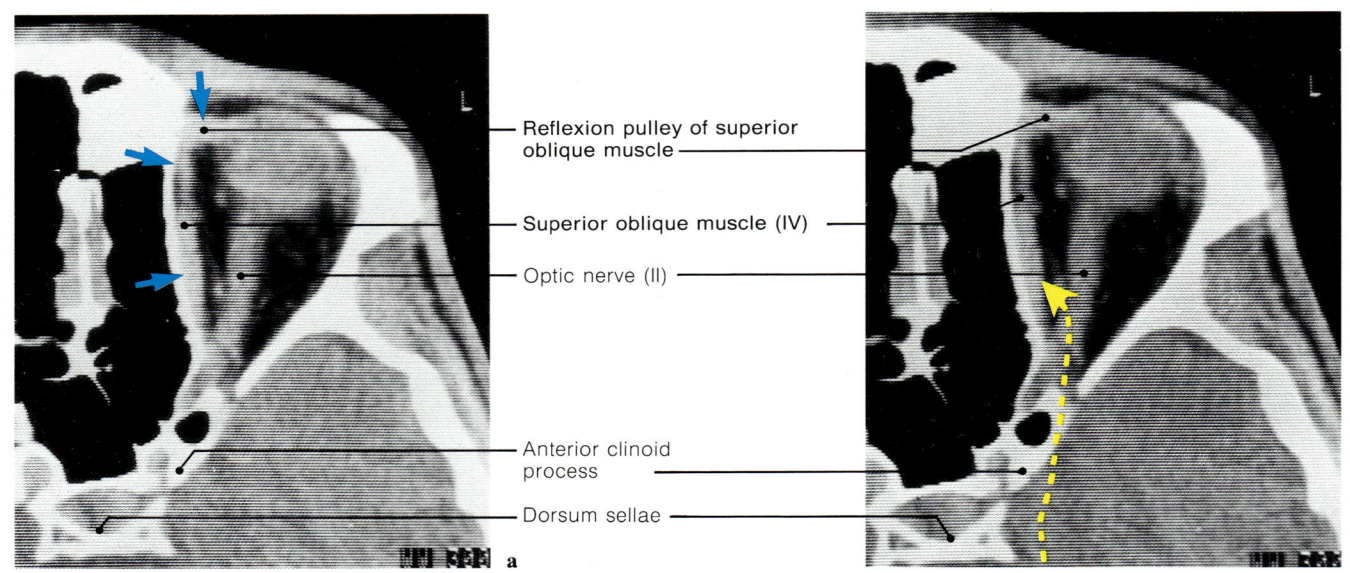

Fig. 4.10 a–c. Horizontal sections of the superior oblique muscle and its reflexion pulley

Fig. 4.10 d. MRI axial section of cerebral peduncles; dotted: circumpeduncular course of trochlear nerve (IV)

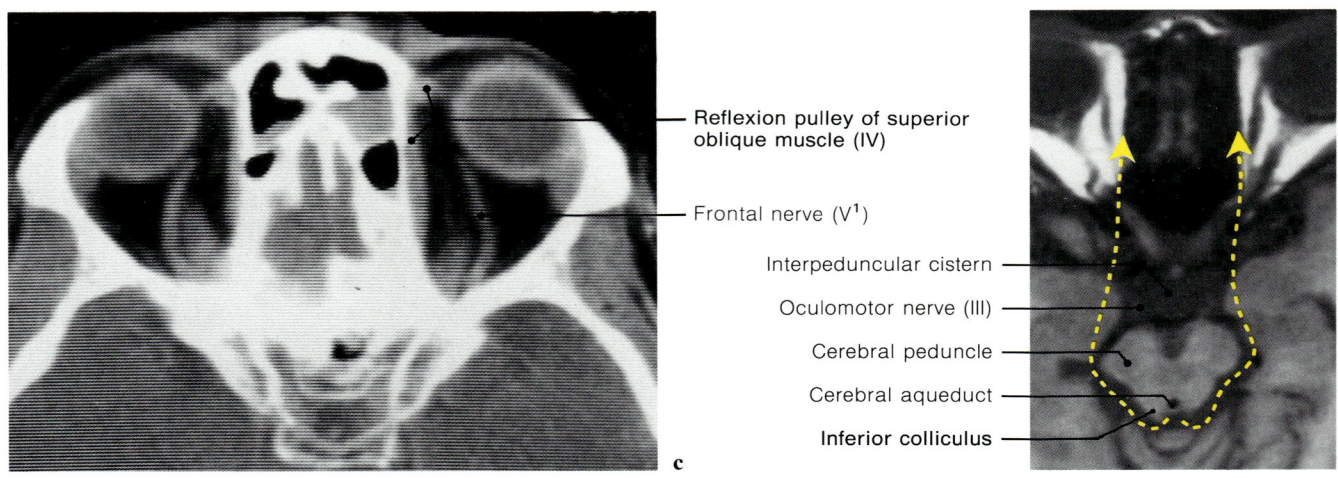

Fig. 4.10 e. Section passing through the lamina tecti in Vatters' view; arrow: origin of trochlear nerve (IV)

Fig. 4.10 f. Median sagittal section; dotted: course of trochlear nerve (IV)

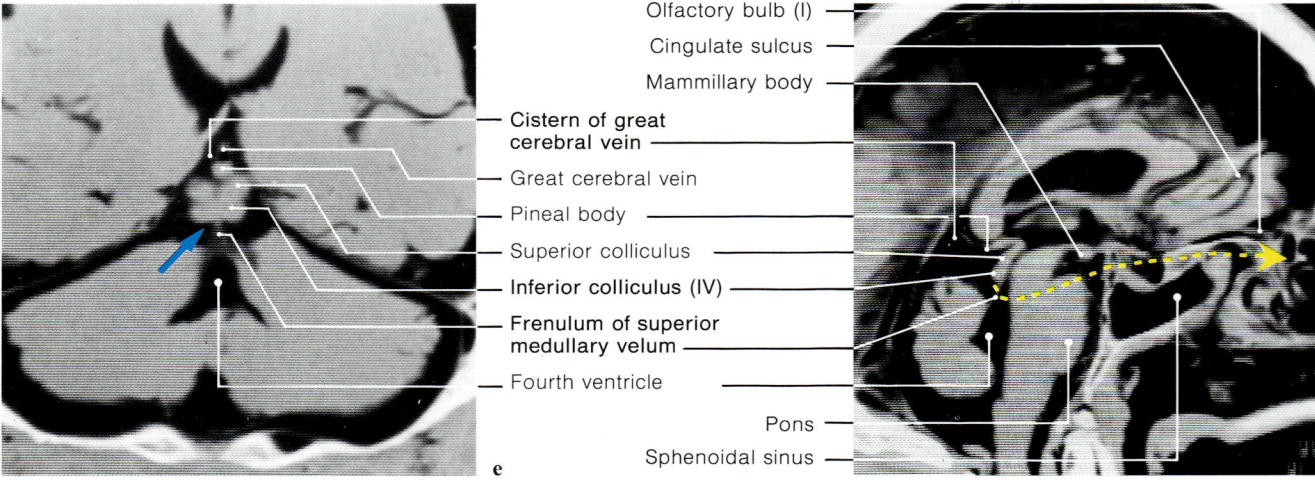

Course of trochlear nerve

Anatomic dissections of oculomotor nerves

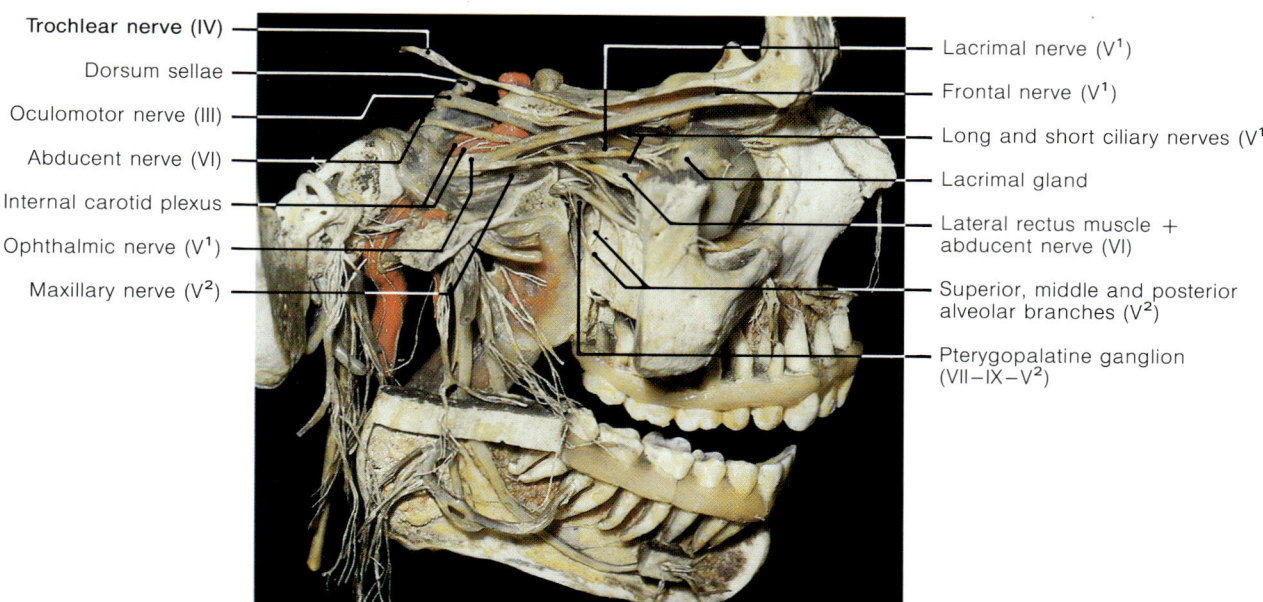

Fig. 4.11. Lateral view showing course of trochlear nerve up to the reflexion pulley of the superior oblique muscle

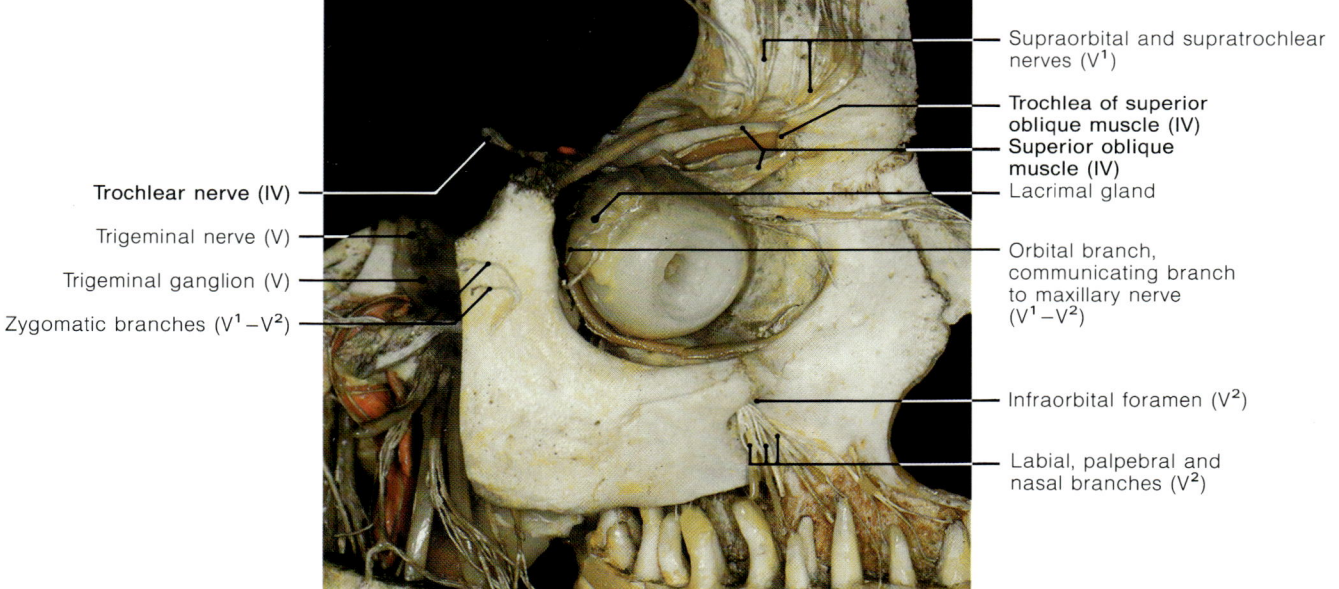

Fig. 4.12. Intraorbital view showing the trochlear nerve, the superior oblique muscle and its reflexion pulley

Course of trochlear nerve

Magnetic resonance imaging (MRI)

AXIAL VIEW AND SAGITTAL DIAGRAM

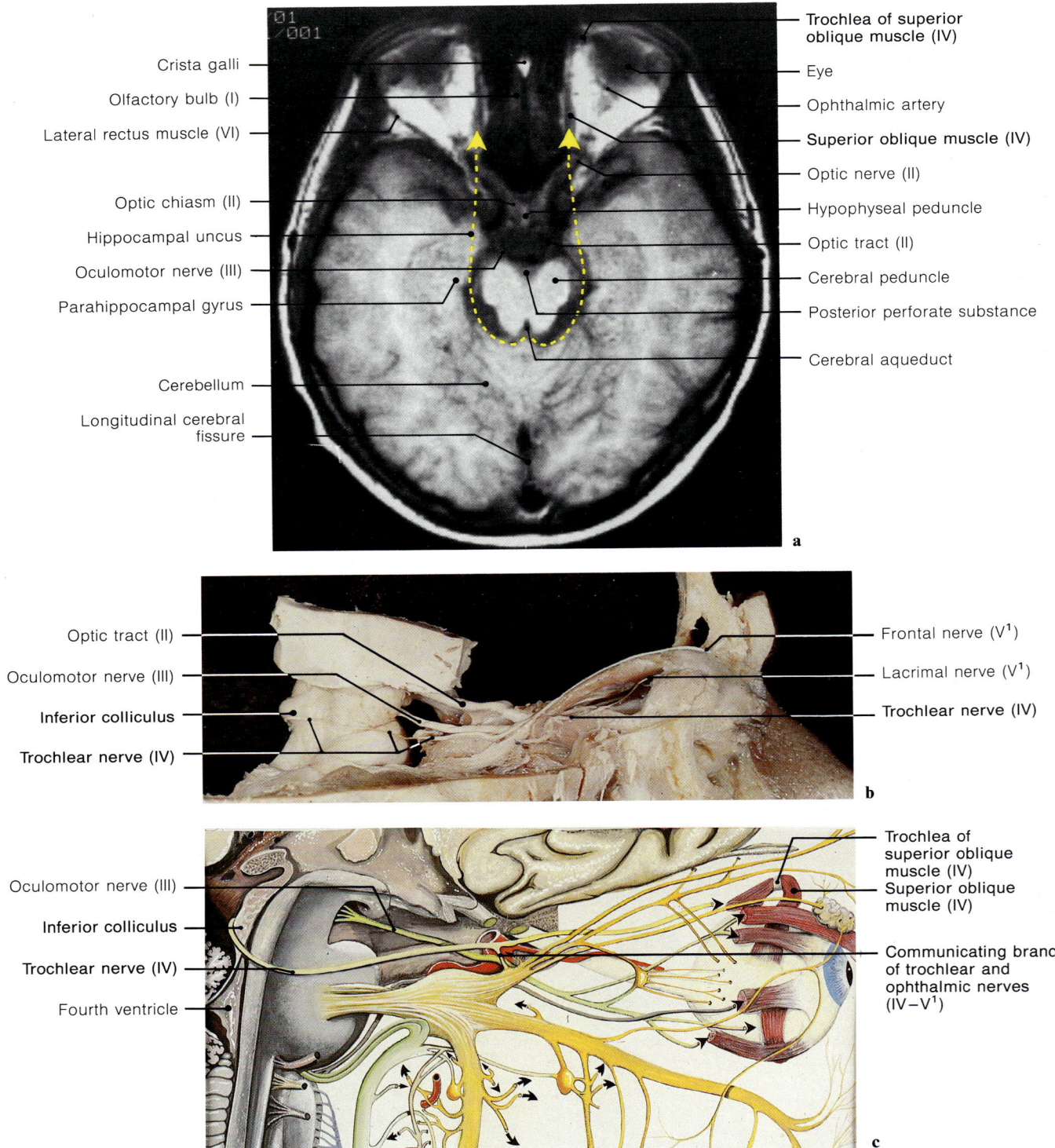

Fig. 4.13a–c. Axial magnetic resonance imaging (**a**), anatomic view (**b**) and diagram (**c**), both sagittal, showing the course of the trochlear nerve from its apparent origin up to the superior oblique muscle (IV)

Trigeminal nerve (V)

Apparent origin of trigeminal nerve 60
Trigeminal ganglion 69
Ophthalmic nerve (V¹) 81
Maxillary nerve (V²) 95
Mandibular nerve (V³) 135
Terminal branches, sensory territories (diagrams) 153

Apparent origin of trigeminal nerve (V)
Diagram of trigeminal nerve 61
Anatomy (course – terminals – collaterals) 63
Imaging (regions examined) 63
Pathology 63
Pons, cistern of cerebellopontine angle
    Anatomy and imaging (examination) 64
    Axial views (MRI, CT) 64
    Sagittal view (MRI, CT) 65
    Frontal and axial views (CT) 66
    Anatomic section and MRI (horizontal view) 67
Axes of foramina of trigeminal nerve 68

Vascular relations:
Cavernous sinus 167, 290
Internal carotid arteries (meningohypophysial) 276
    Inferolateral trunk 276, 277
Trigeminal artery 291

The trigeminal nerve is the largest of the cranial nerves. It emerges from the anterior aspect of the pons by two roots:

– a sensory root gathering sensation from the facial coverings and cavities and from the teeth,
– a motor root supplying the masticator muscles.

The trigeminal ganglion is situated on the course of the sensory root.

It terminates in three nerves:

– the ophthalmic nerve (V¹),
– the maxillary nerve (V²),
– the mandibular nerve (V³).

Trigeminal nerve (V)

Apparent origin

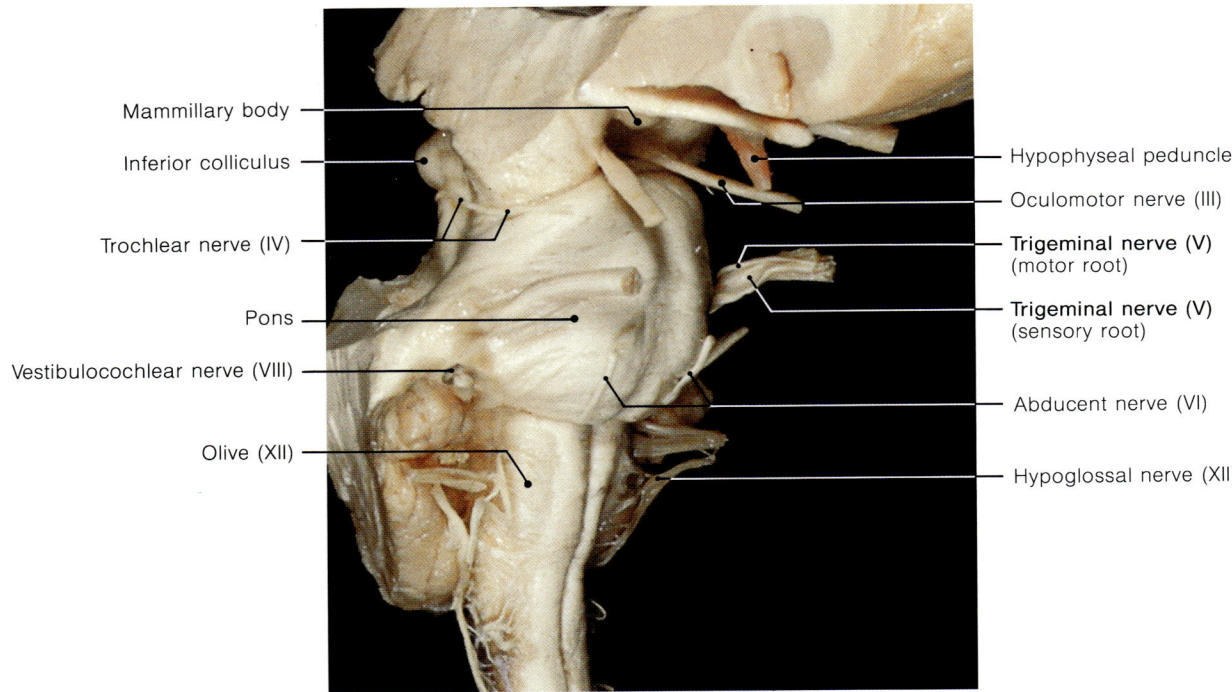

Fig. 5.1. Oblique view of brain-stem to show apparent origin of trigeminal nerve (V)

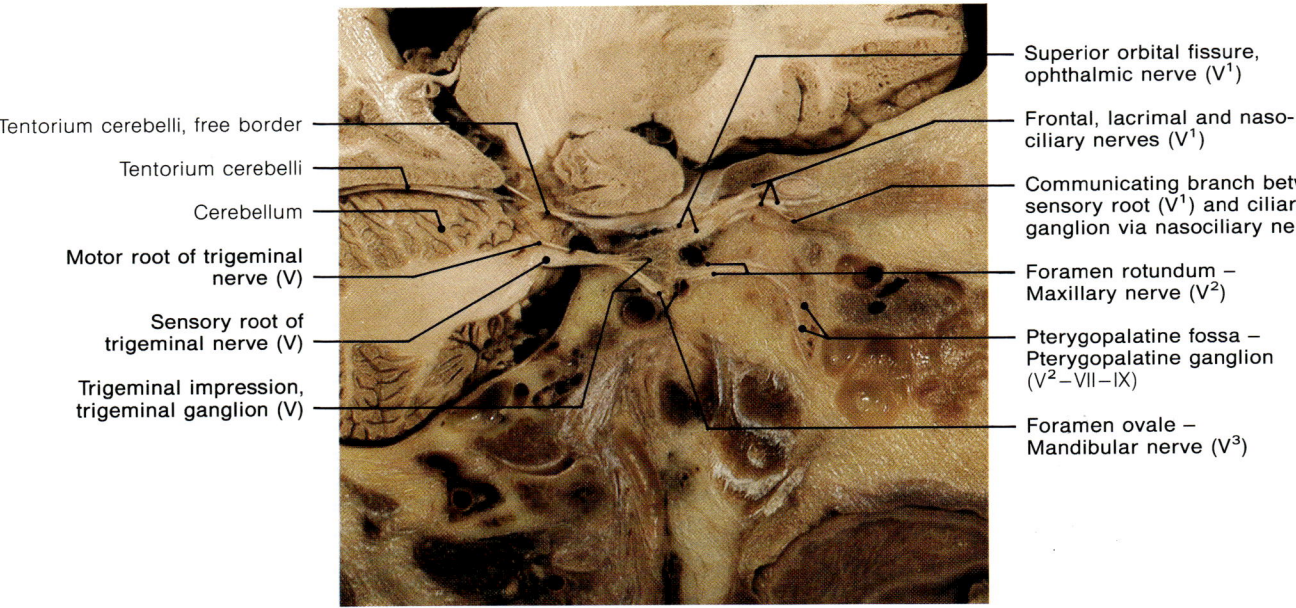

Fig. 5.2. Sagittal anatomic section of trigeminal nerve (V) and of its foramina

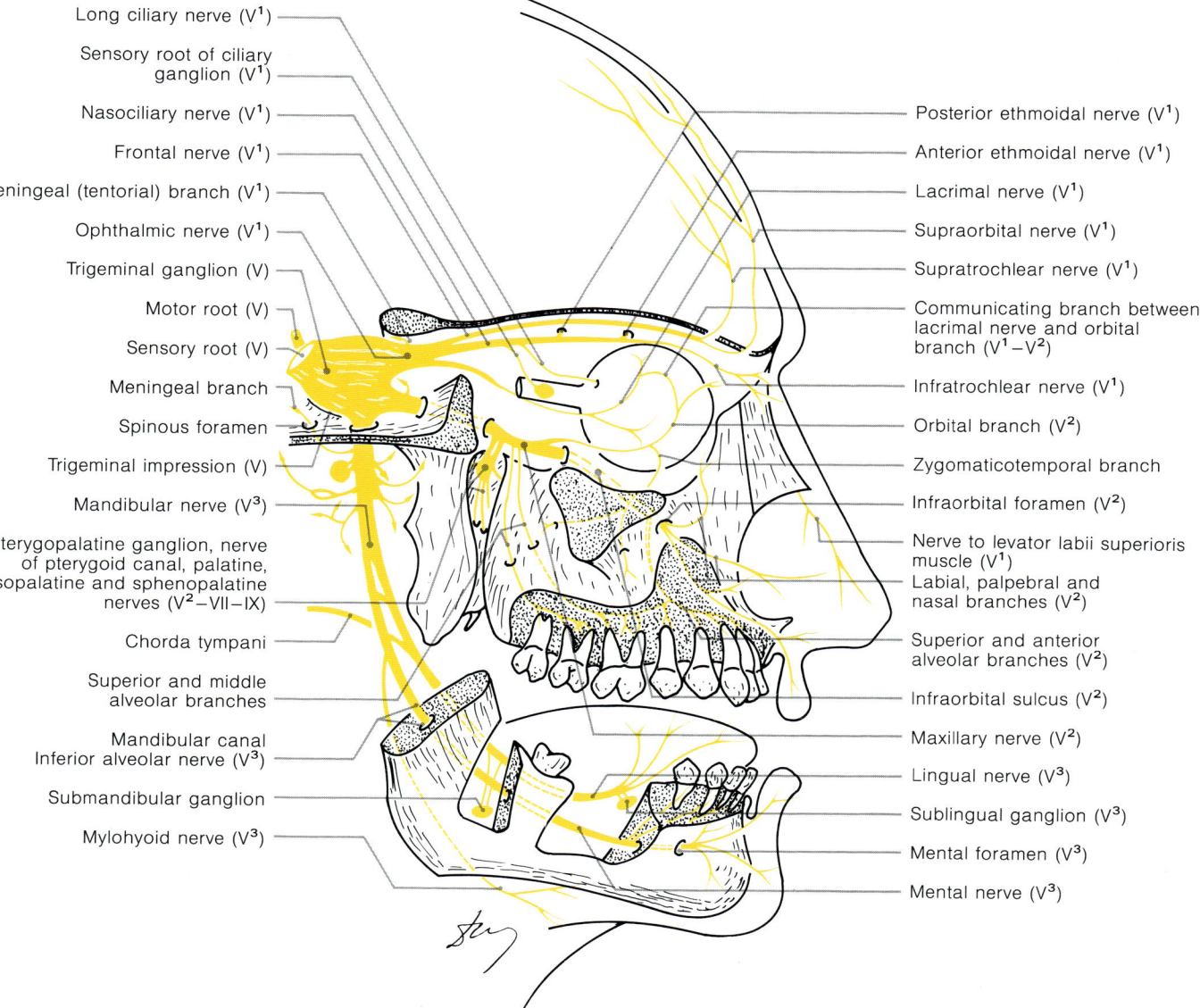

Fig. 5.3. Diagram of trigeminal nerve (V) [Prof. Claude Libersa]

Topography

Apparent origin of trigeminal nerve (V)
- Pons
- Cistern of cerebellopontine angle

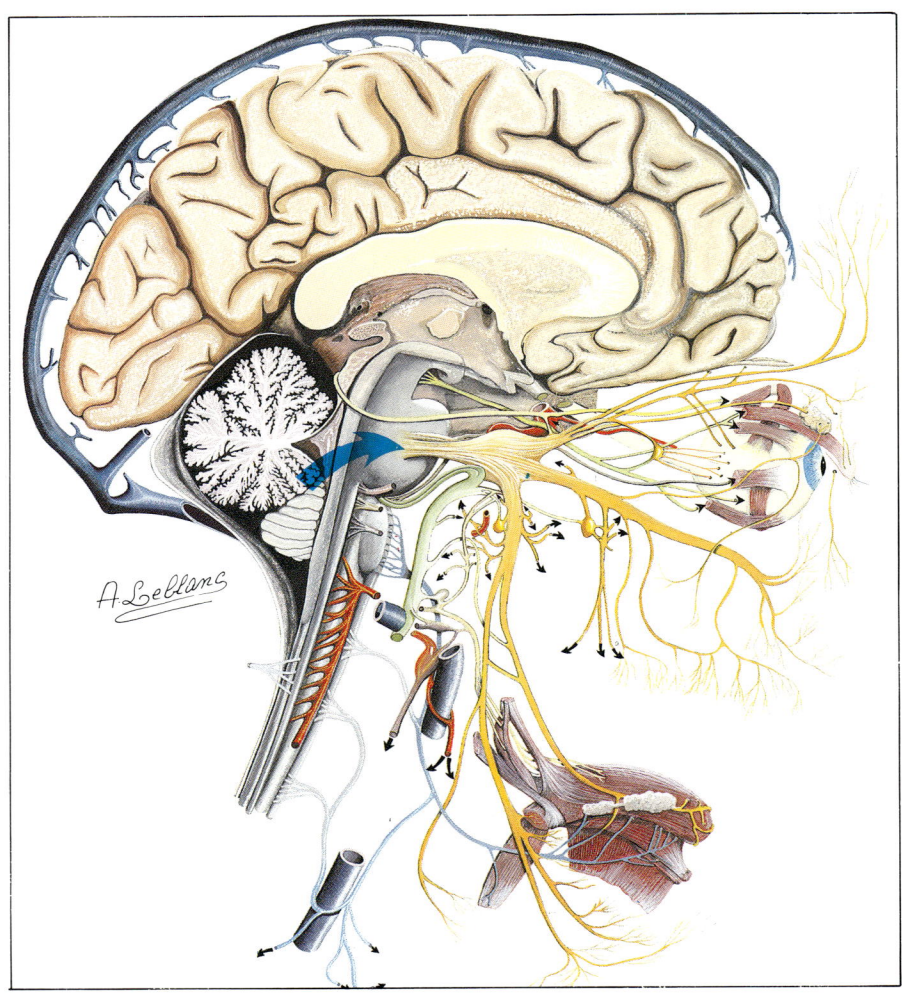

Fig. 5.4

Anatomy

COURSE – TERMINALS – COLLATERALS

Apparent origin
Axes of foramina

Trigeminal ganglion (V)

Ophthalmic nerve (V^1)
(frontal, lacrimal and nasociliary nerves)

Anterior and posterior ethmoidal nerves and nasal branches
(of anterior ethmoidal nerve)

Maxillary nerve (V^2)
(labial, palpebral and nasal branches)

Pterygopalatine ganglion
Greater, lesser and accessory palatine nerves

Mandibular nerve (V^3)

Inferior alveolar and mental nerves, mental branches (V^3)

Imaging

REGIONS EXAMINED

Examination of pons and cistern of cerebellopontine angle

Study of trigeminal impression

Imaging of superior orbital fissure

Imaging of anterior and posterior ethmoidal foramina, ethmoidal foramen and slit

Study of foramen rotundum, inferior orbital fissure, infraorbital sulcus and foramen

Pterygopalatine fossa, greater and lesser palatine foramina, incisive canal

Study of foramen ovale

Examination of mandibular canal and mental foramen

Pathology

- Neurinoma of V,
- extracanalicular acoustic neurinoma (VII, VIIb, VIII) with deficit of V,
- tumor of cerebellopontine angle,
- syndrome of cerebellopontine angle (V, VI, VII, VIII),
- tumor of fourth ventricle.

Apparent origin of trigeminal nerve (pons, cistern of cerebellopontine angle)

Anatomy

This is a sensorimotor nerve. It emerges from the lateral region of the pons by two roots: one sensory, the other motor (Fig. 5.1–3).

INTRACRANIAL COURSE AND RELATIONS

The sensory fibers arise from the trigeminal ganglion. The motor fibers merely traverse the ganglion.
The sensory root is virtually round adjacent to the pons, but becomes progressively flattened laterally and medially as it expands to form a ganglionic swelling: the trigeminal ganglion.
The motor root is much smaller than the sensory root. It is situated anterior and medial to the sensory root, near its upper border, passes beneath it and then arrives at the trigeminal recess (Fig. 5.2; 5.9; 5.18a).
Subsequently, it passes obliquely to reach the inferomedial aspect of the sensory root of the mandibular nerve. It then joins the foramen ovale.

Imaging

EXAMINATION

– Magnetic resonance imaging (MRI) or computed tomography (CT) of the cerebellopontine angle for the apparent origin of the trigeminal nerve (V) in sagittal, frontal and axial views (Fig. 5.6a; 5.7; 5.8).

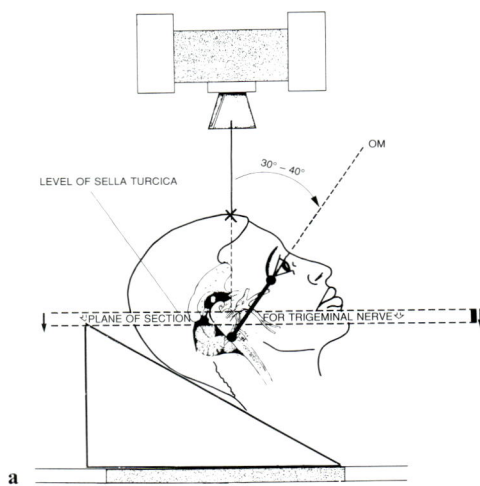

Fig. 5.5a. Centering and reference diagram for (conventional) cisternography of the cerebellopontine angle to show the apparent origin of the trigeminal nerve (V)

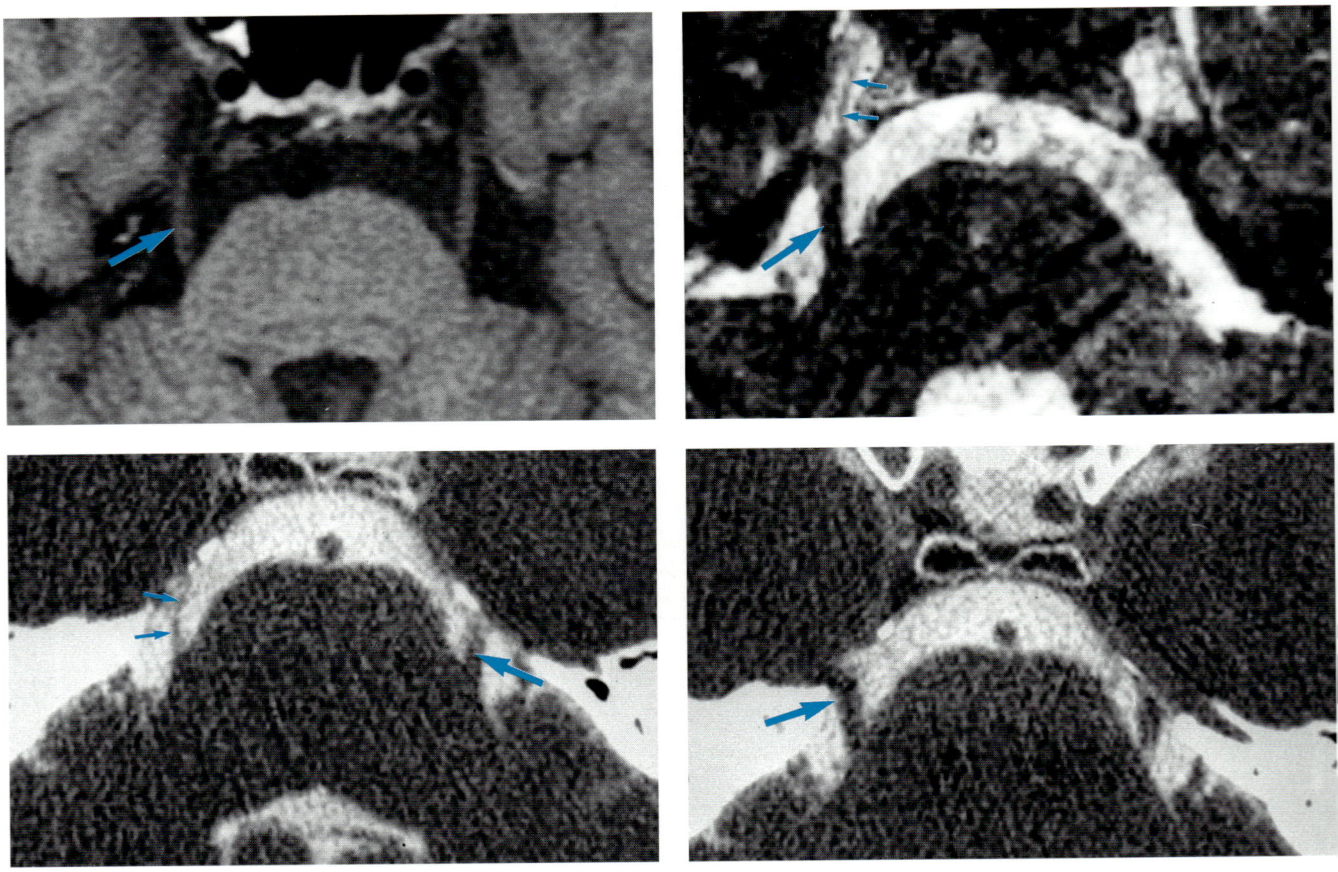

Fig. 5.5b–e. Axial magnetic resonance imaging (MRI) (**b, c**) and computed tomography (CT) (**d, e**) of trigeminal nerve (V), sensory root (*arrows*), motor root (*small, double arrows*). (CT: Pr. Doyon, Hospital Kremlin Bicêtre, Paris)

Apparent origin 65

Cerebellopontine angle

Magnetic resonance imaging (MRI) and computed tomography (CT)

SAGITTAL VIEW

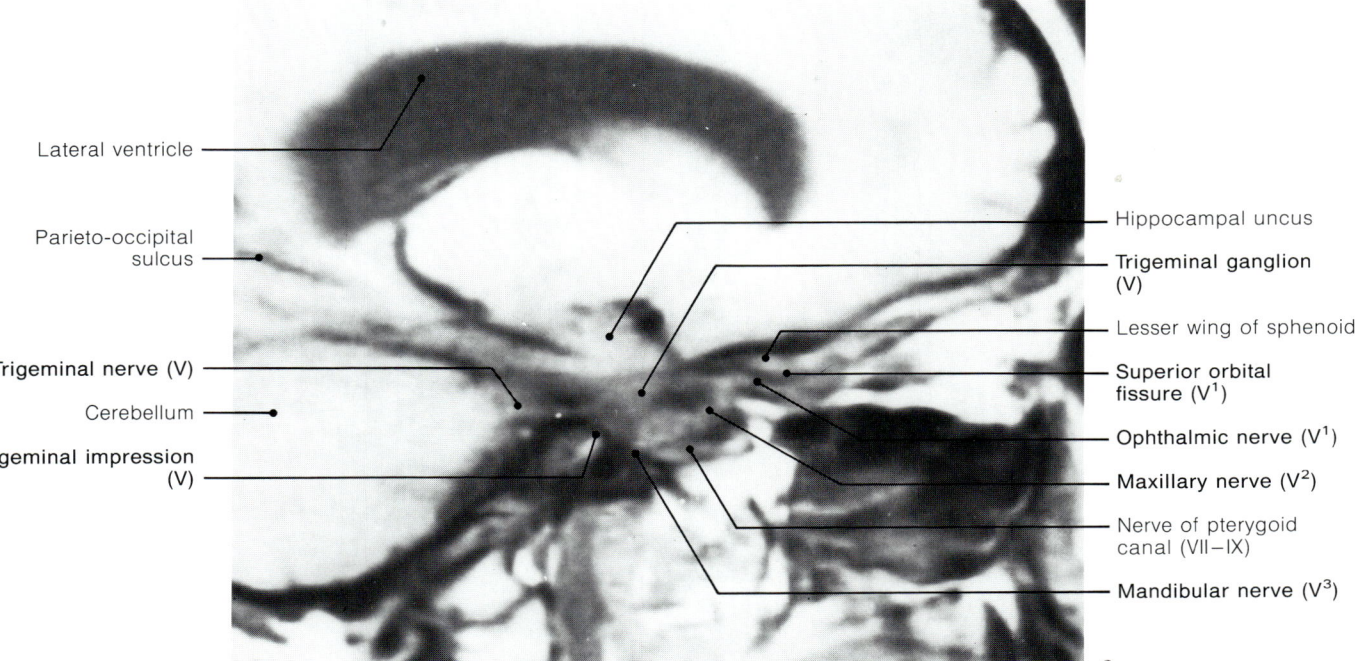

Fig. 5.6 a. (refer to the anatomic section of Fig. 5.2)

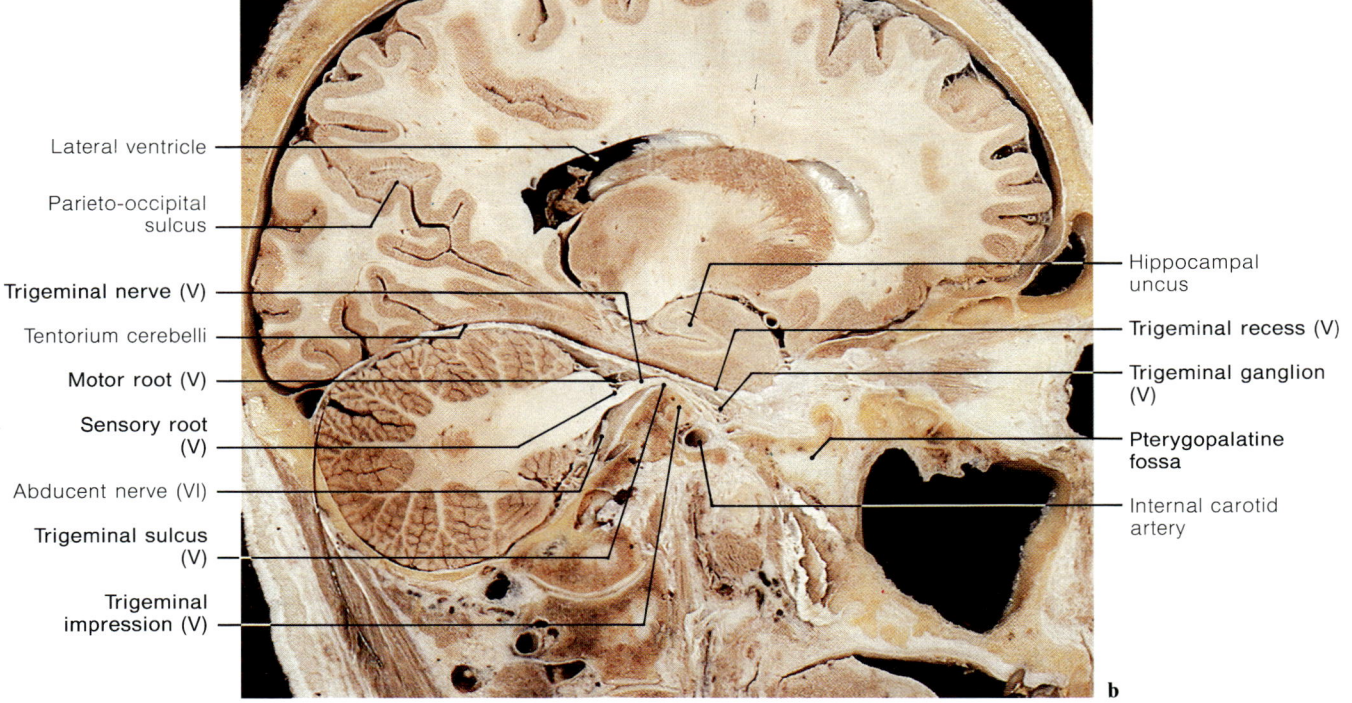

Fig. 5.6 a, b. Sagittal magnetic resonance imaging (**a**) and anatomic section (**b**) at the level of the apparent origin of the trigeminal nerve and its collaterals

Cerebellopontine angle

Computed tomography (CT) and magnetic resonance imaging (MRI)

FRONTAL AND AXIAL VIEWS

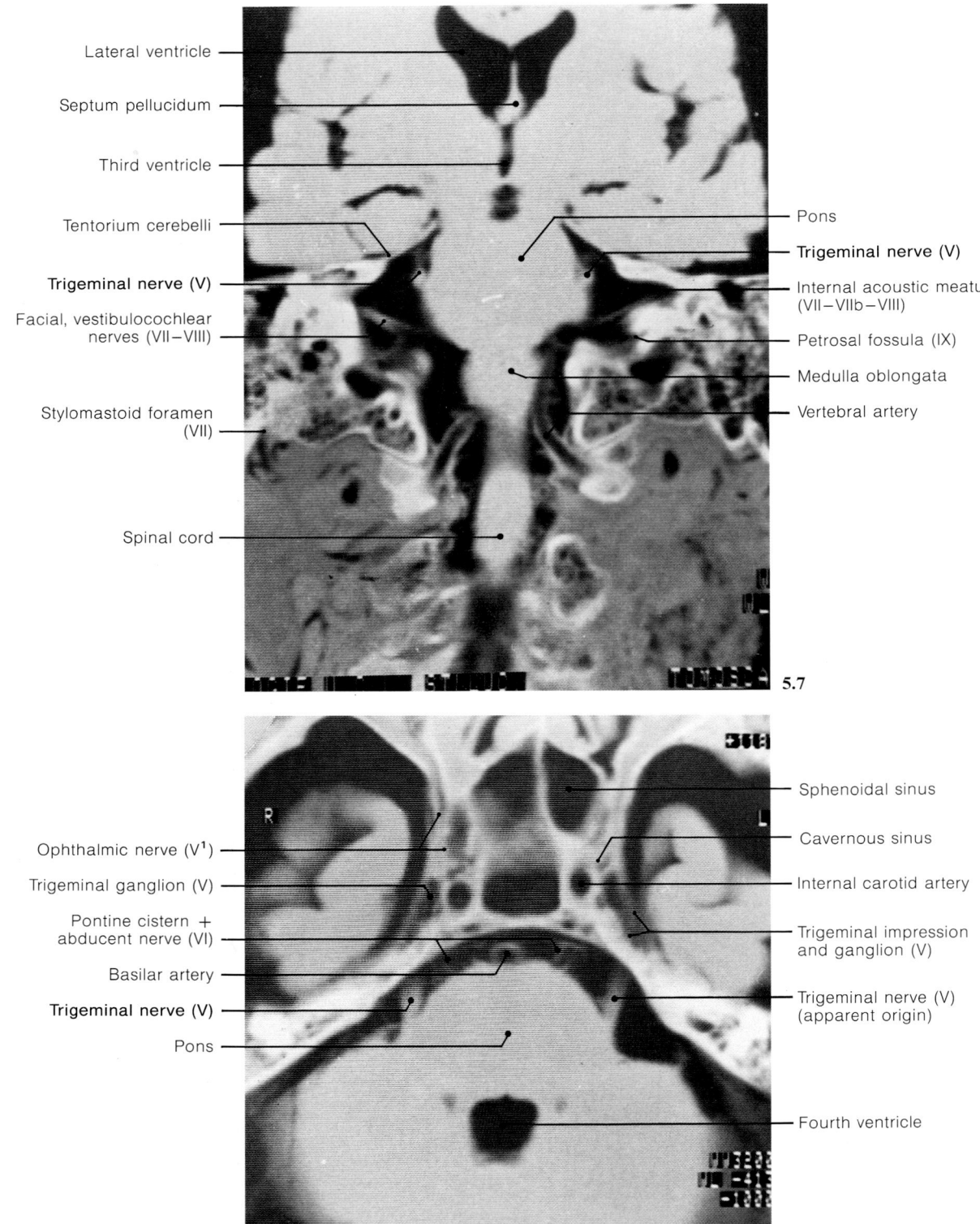

Fig. 5.7; 5.8. Frontal and axial computed tomographic (CT) sections at the apparent origins of the trigeminal nerves

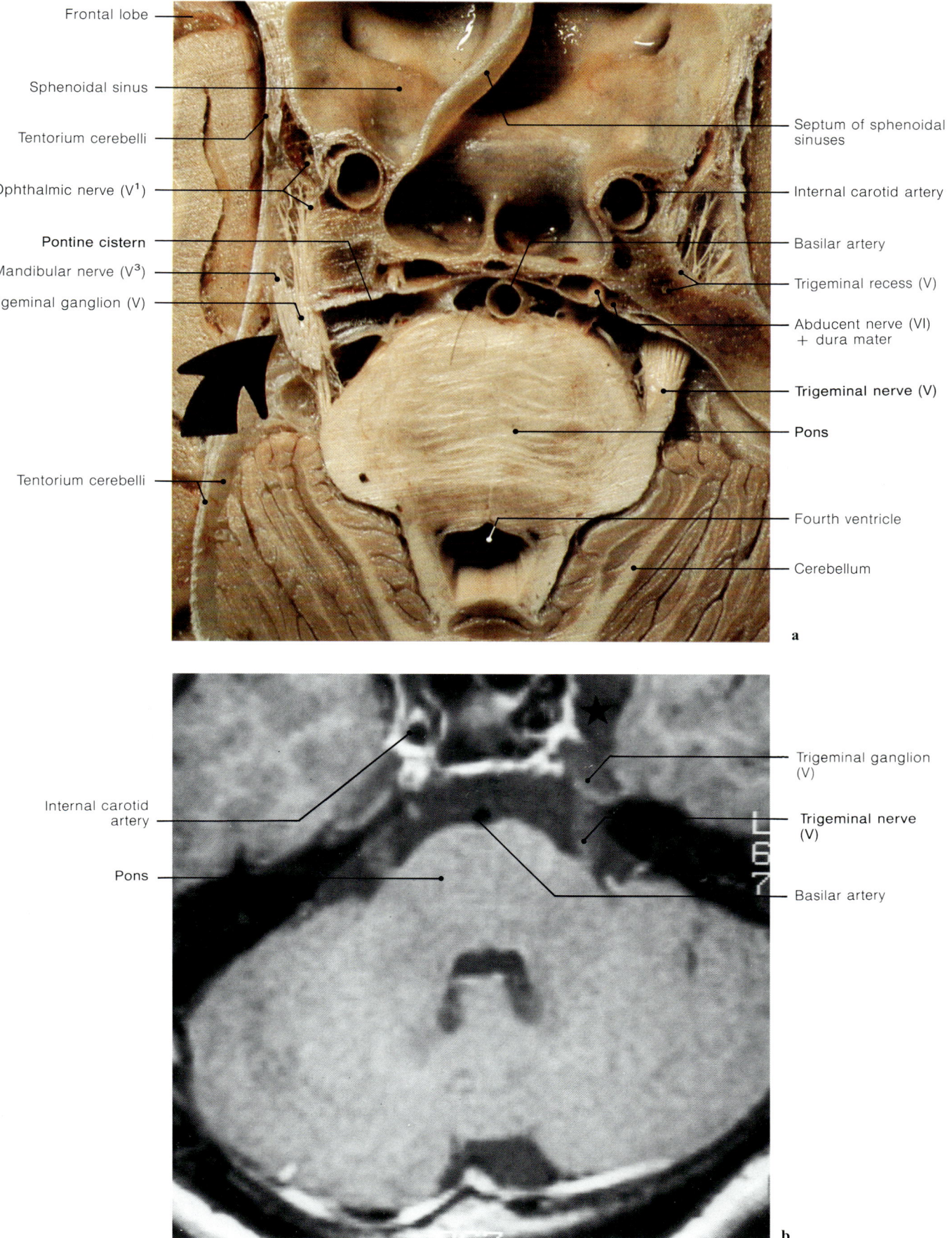

Fig. 5.9a, b. Horizontal anatomic section and MRI view of pons at the level of the apparent origins of the trigeminal nerves (V). (Anatomical section: Pr. J.P. Francke, Faculty of Medicine, Lille)

Axes of foramina of trigeminal nerve

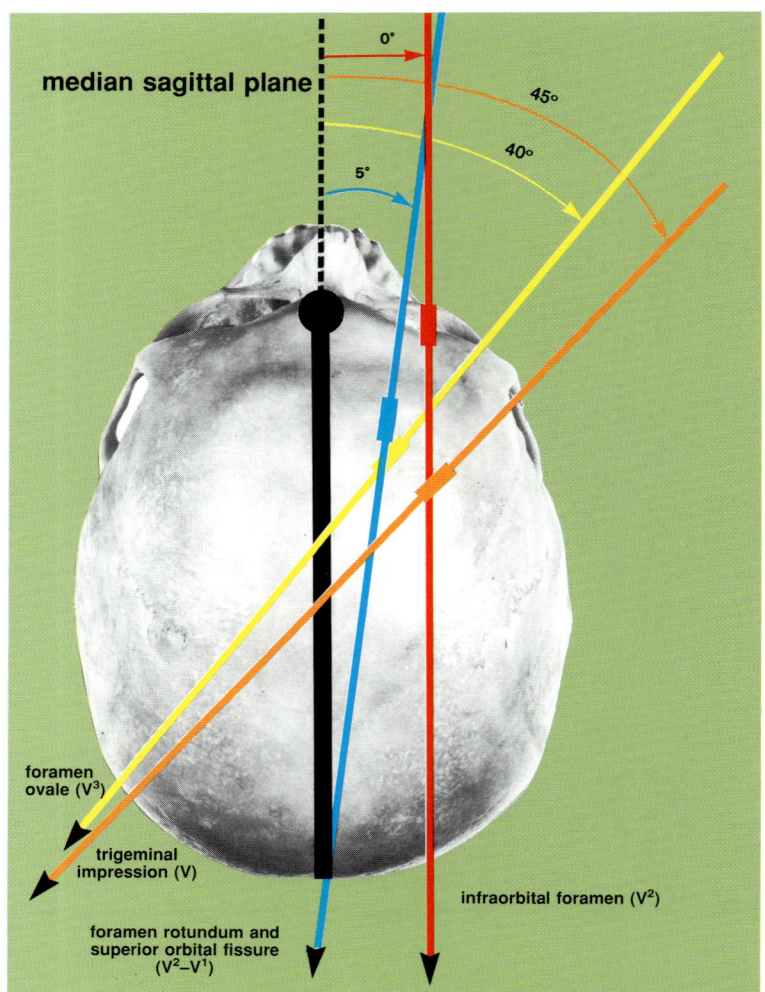

Fig. 5.10 a, b. Angles of study of the course of the trigeminal nerve and its collaterals in relation to the median sagittal plane (**a**) and the orbitomeatal plane (OM) (**b**)

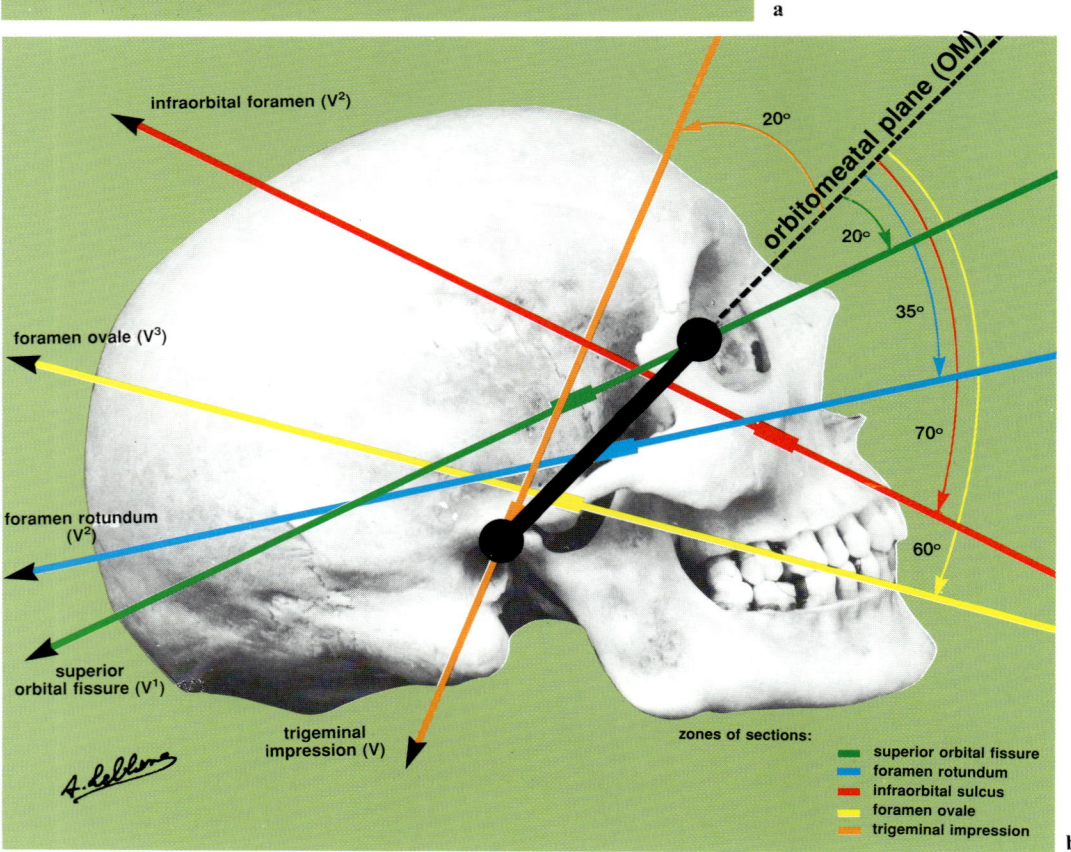

Trigeminal nerve (V)

Trigeminal ganglion (V)
Trigeminal impression (trigeminal ganglion V)
Pathology 70
Anatomy and imaging (examination) 72
    Axial views (MRI) 72
    Frontal (radiology) and axial views (CT) 73
    Oblique view (radiology) 74
    Axial view (MRI) 74
    Discontinuous scanning (radiology) 75
    Frontal views (MRI) 75
    Oblique view (CT) 76
    Sagittal view (radiology) 78

Trigeminal notch
    Anatomy (sagittal view) 80

Vascular relations:
Cavernous sinus 167, 290
Internal carotid arteries (meningohypophysial) 276
    Inferolateral trunk 276, 277
Trigeminal artery 291

Topography

Trigeminal ganglion (V)
- Trigeminal impression

Pathology

- Trigeminal neuralgia,
- osteitis, fractures of the petrous bone,
- osteitis of the petrous apex, neuralgia of V and paralysis of VI (Gradenigo's syndrome),
- syndrome with sensorimotor involvement of V (Raeder's syndrome),
- neurinoma of V,
- aneurysm of internal carotid artery (carotid siphon) extending posteriorly.

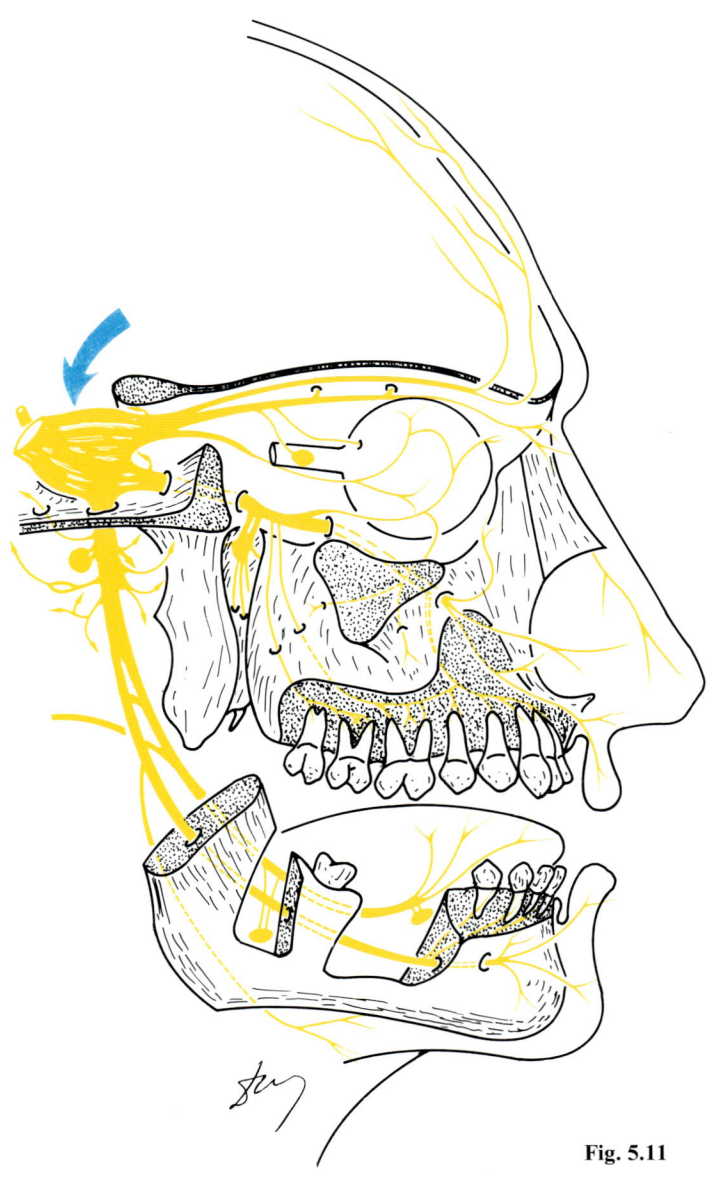

Fig. 5.11

Trigeminal ganglion: Trigeminal impression

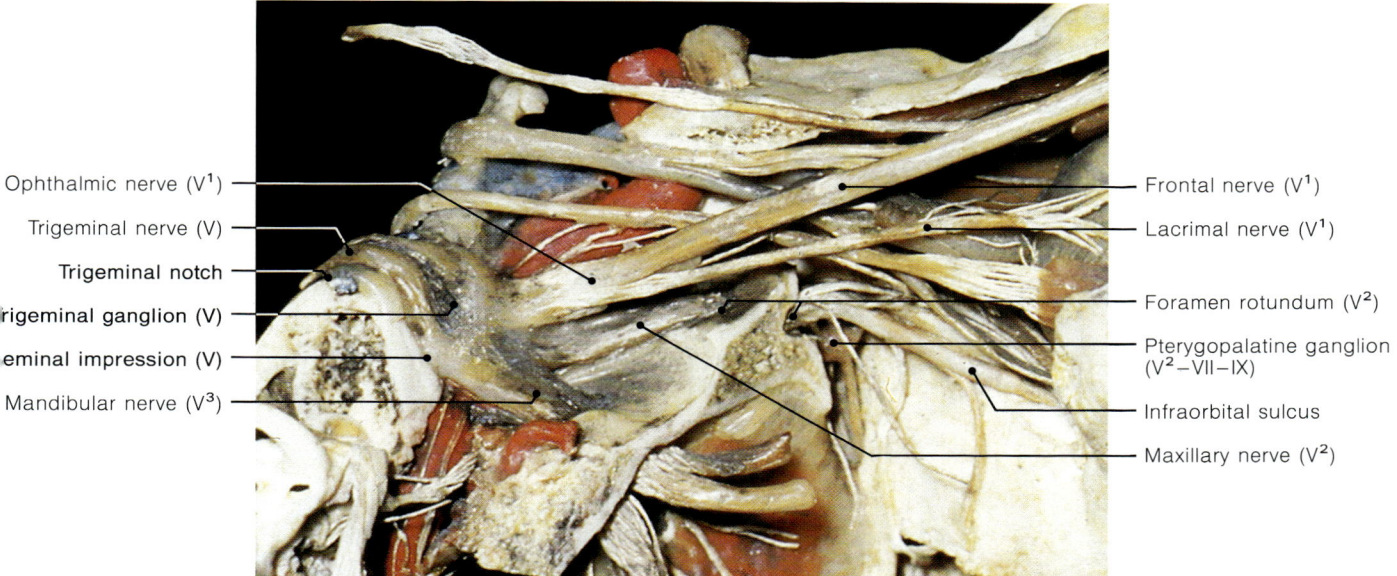

Fig. 5.12a. Anatomic dissection showing the trigeminal ganglion and its impression

Trigeminal ganglion: Trigeminal impression (See vascular relations, p. 291)

Anatomy

The trigeminal (or Gasserian) ganglion is situated in a compartment known as the trigeminal recess (Fig. 5.2; 5.9). Semilunar in shape and flattened, the trigeminal ganglion is a mass of nerve tissue lying on the anterosuperior aspect of the petrous bone, near its apex, in a depression of varying depth: the trigeminal impression (Fig. 5.2; 5.21; 5.22). The foramina of the canals of the greater and lesser petrosal nerves can be seen between the trigeminal impression and the arcuate eminence (Fig. 7.6; 7.22; 7.31 a).

The trigeminal ganglion gives off three main branches:

- the ophthalmic nerve (V^1), which travels to the superior orbital fissure (Fig. 5.11; 5.12),
- the maxillary nerve (V^2), entering the foramen rotundum, the infraorbital sulcus and the infraorbital foramen (Fig. 5.11; 5.12; 5.20),
- the mandibular nerve (V^3), traversing the foramen ovale (Fig. 5.11; 5.12; 5.18a, b).

Imaging

EXAMINATION

- Imaging of the trigeminal impressions in intraorbital projection and in symmetric distinguishing view (Fig. 5.13a),
- study in oblique unilateral intraorbital view (Fig. 5.14a, b),
- exploration of the impression by "discontinuous scanning" in unilateral intraorbital view (Fig. 5.15),
- tomographic study in unilateral view, in the axis of the petrous bone (Fig. 5.17)
- computed tomographic study (CT) or magnetic resonance imaging (MRI) of the trigeminal impression and of the trigeminal ganglion (Fig. 5.13c; 5.29a).

TECHNIQUE

Study in symmetric intraorbital projection:

- The subject is in dorsal decubitus, the head facing strictly forward;
- the beam is centered at the level of the supraorbital margins, and makes an angle of 5° to 10° in relation to the orbitomeatal plane (OM), inclined towards the forehead (Fig. 5.13a).

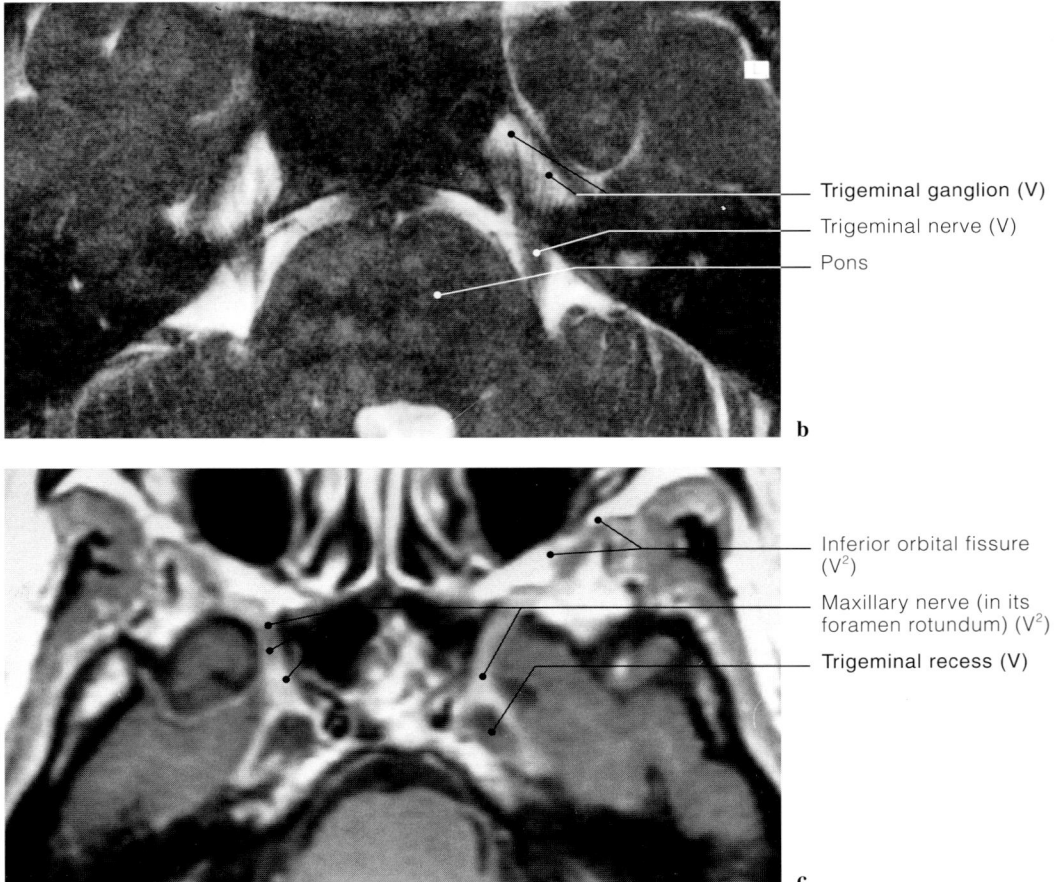

Fig. 5.12b, c. Axial magnetic resonance imaging (MRI) of trigeminal nerve, trigeminal ganglion (**b**) and trigeminal recess with the maxillary nerve (V^2) (**c**)

Trigeminal ganglion: Trigeminal impression

Computed tomography (CT) and radiography

FRONTAL AND AXIAL VIEWS

Fig. 5.13a. Centering diagram for symmetric study of trigeminal impressions and ganglia in intraorbital projection

5 – 10°
OM
LEVEL OF
TRIGEMINAL IMPRESSION

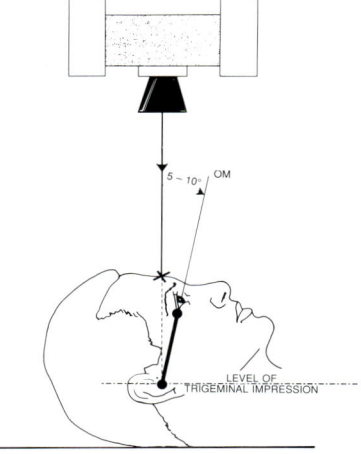

Fig. 5.13b, c. Intraorbital view (**b**) and axial computed tomography (CT) (**c**) of trigeminal impressions and ganglia (for MRI centering, see Fig. 5.28)

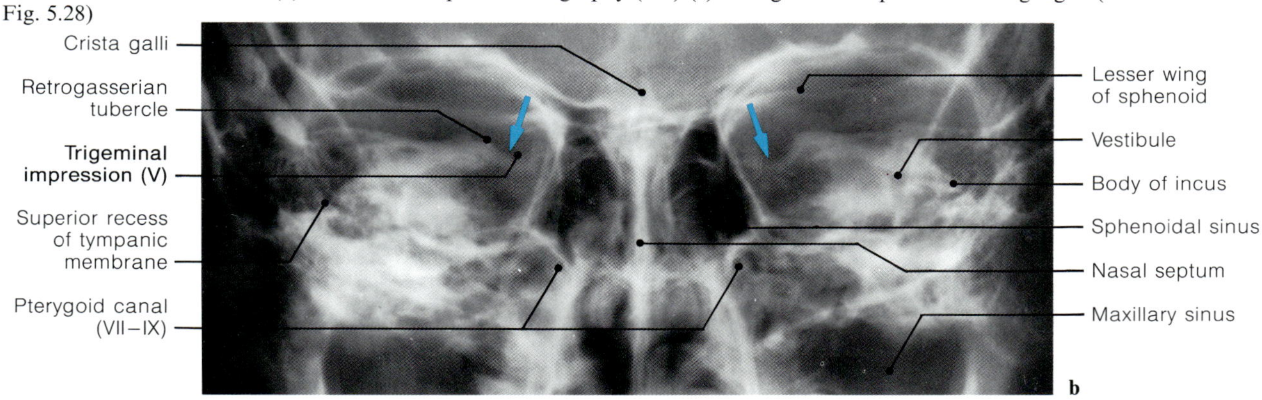

Crista galli
Retrogasserian tubercle
Trigeminal impression (V)
Superior recess of tympanic membrane
Pterygoid canal (VII–IX)
Lesser wing of sphenoid
Vestibule
Body of incus
Sphenoidal sinus
Nasal septum
Maxillary sinus

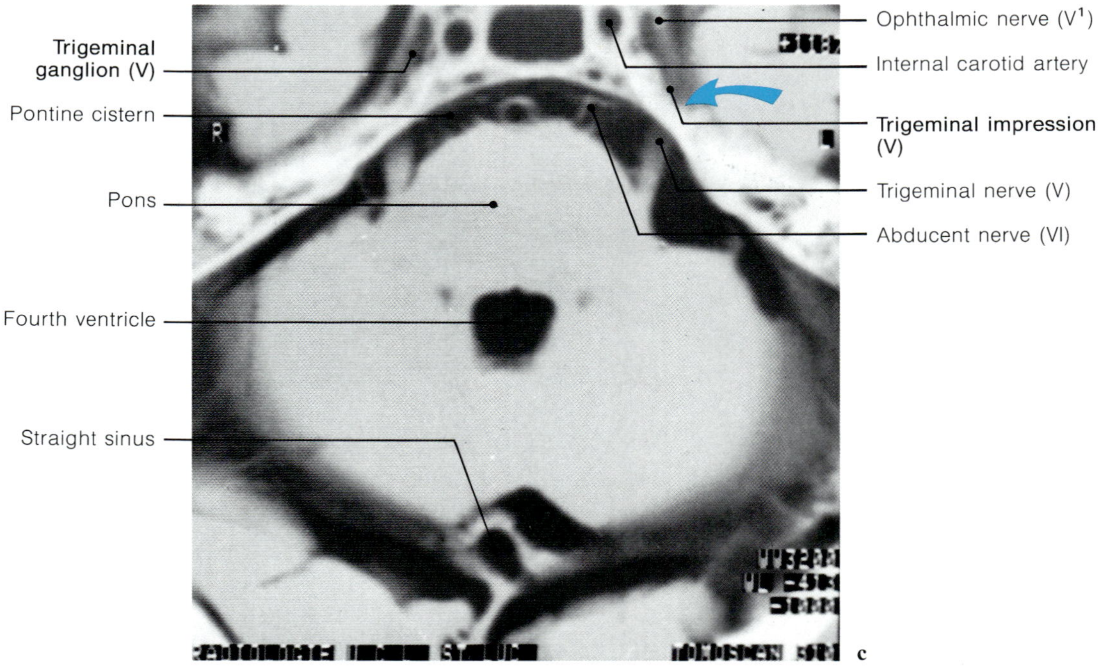

b

Trigeminal ganglion (V)
Pontine cistern
Pons
Fourth ventricle
Straight sinus
Ophthalmic nerve (V^1)
Internal carotid artery
Trigeminal impression (V)
Trigeminal nerve (V)
Abducent nerve (VI)
R

c

Trigeminal ganglion: Trigeminal impression and trigeminal recess (V)

Imaging

TECHNIQUE (OBLIQUE VIEW)

Study of trigeminal impression in oblique unilateral intraorbital view:

- The subject is in dorsal decubitus with the head inclined by 5° to 7° towards the side to be examined (Fig. 5.14a);
- the beam is centered at the supraorbital margin and makes an angle of 5° to 10° with the orbitomeatal plane (OM) inclined upwards (Fig. 5.14b).

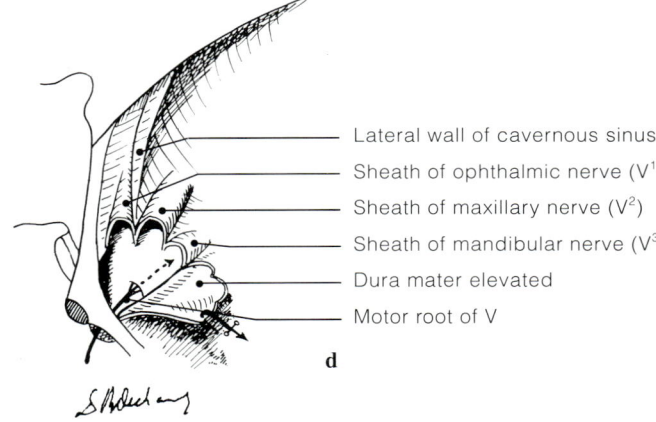

Fig. 5.14d. Diagram of dural compartment containing the triangular plexus, trigeminal ganglion (V) and its three efferent branches (V^1, V^2, V^3)

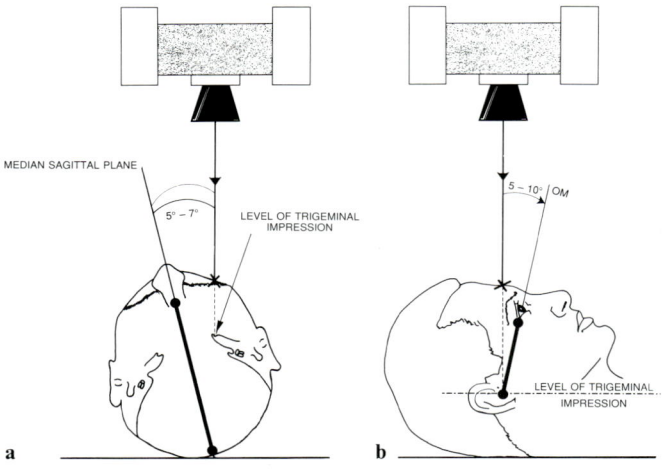

Fig. 5.14a, b. Centering diagrams for oblique unilateral study of the trigeminal impression (V)

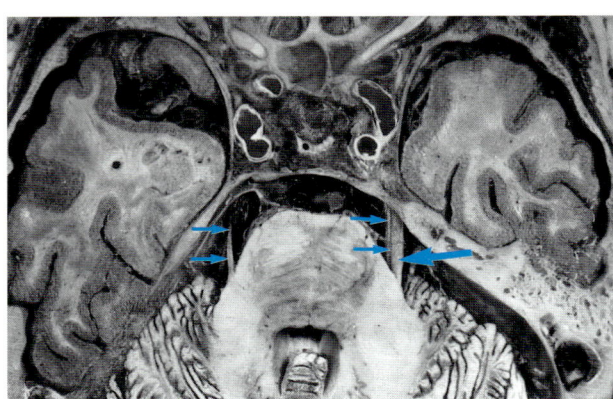

Fig. 5.14e. Axial anatomic section at the level of the trigeminal nerves (V): sensory root (*large arrow*), motor root (*small arrows*)

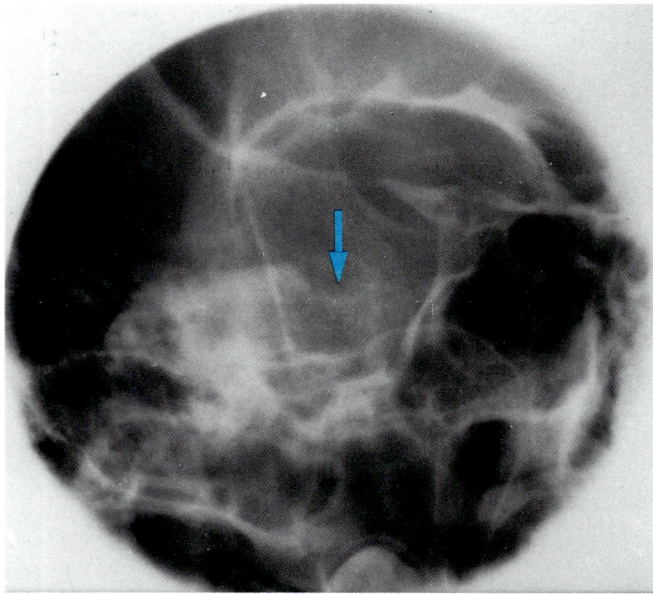

Fig. 5.14c. Radiograph of trigeminal impression (V)

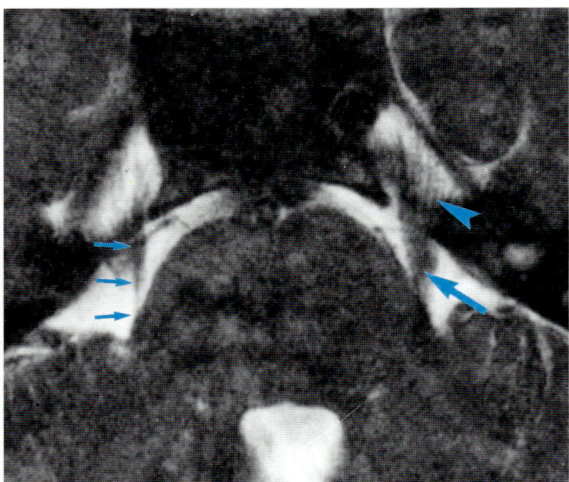

Fig. 5.14f. Axial magnetic resonance imaging (MRI) of trigeminal nerve (V) (*large arrow*), sensory root (*small arrows*) and trigeminal ganglion (V) (*arrowhead*)

Technique (discontinuous scanning)

This technique is identical with that previously described (Fig. 5.14). Only the angle of the tube is varied, the patient's head remaining in the same position. After having taken the film of the trigeminal impression in its axis (Fig. 5.14c), the tube is angled by about 5° in relation to the centering point and 4 films are taken in succession during rotation of the tube (Fig. 5.15).

Note: By means of this technique, this series provides perfect definition of the entire trigeminal impression and retro-gasserian tubercle or colliculus, as well as of the trigeminal notch and the sulcus of the abducent nerve (VI).
If, however, the equipment does not permit rotational movement of the tube, it is always possible to incline the head very slightly (by about 5° of rotation before taking each film).

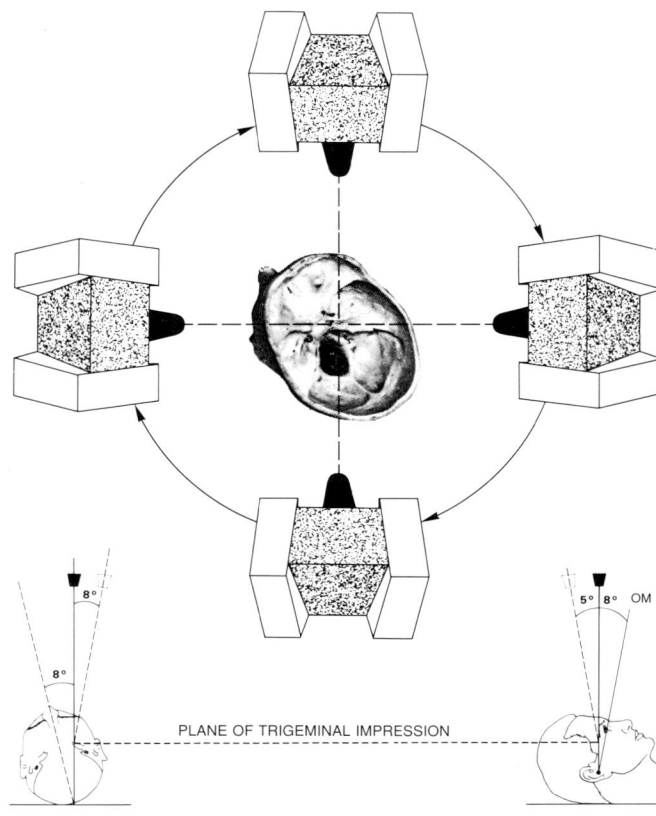

Fig. 5.15. Centering diagram for study of trigeminal impression by "discontinuous scanning"

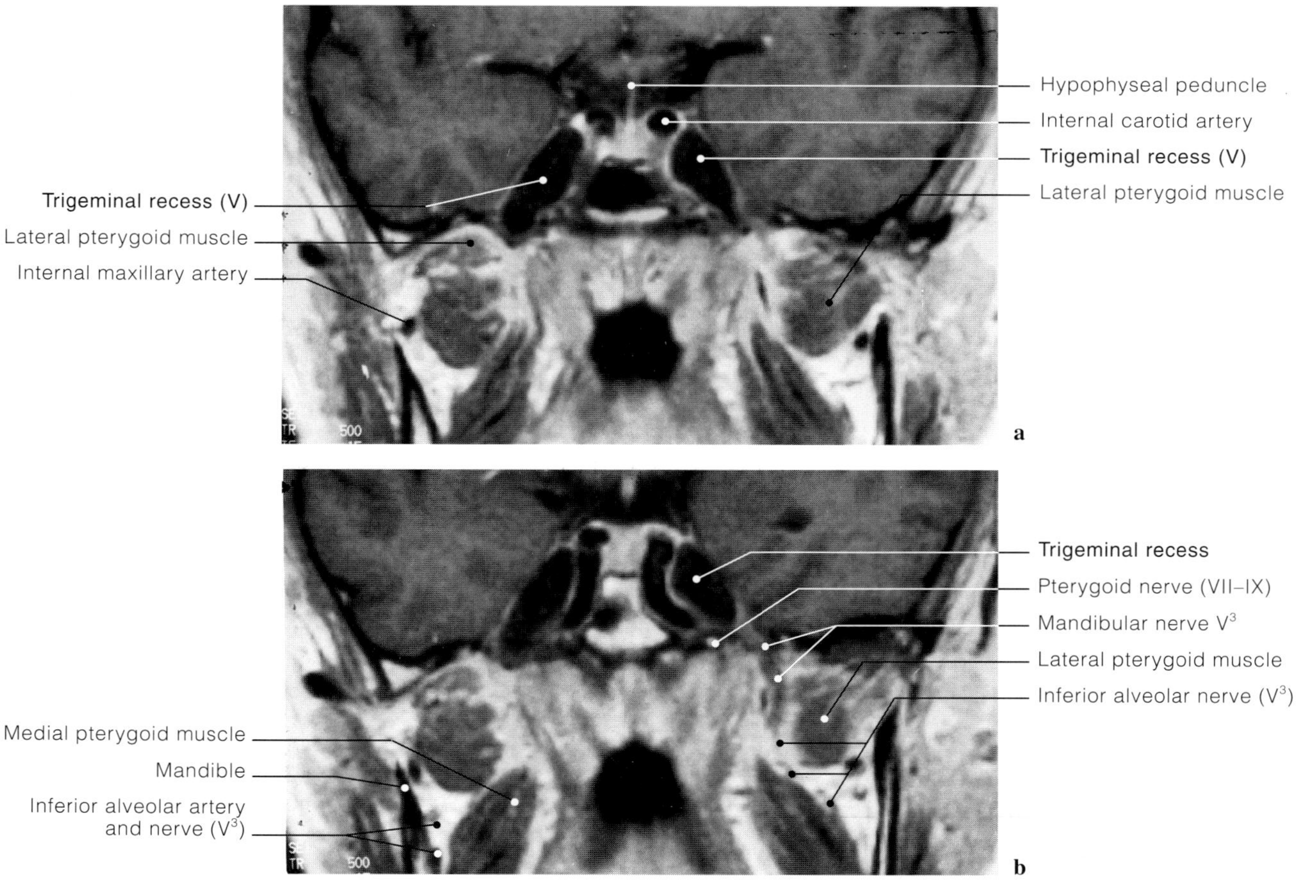

Fig. 5.16 a, b. Frontal magnetic resonance imaging (MRI) at level of trigeminal recess (V). (MRI: Dr. J.W. Casselman, A.Z. St-Jan, Brugge)

Trigeminal ganglion: Trigeminal impression

Imaging

TECHNIQUE (OBLIQUE VIEW IN LONG AXIS)

Oblique unilateral tomography of trigeminal impression in its long axis:

– The subject is in dorsal decubitus, the head turned by 45° to 50° away from the side to be radiographed so as to display the trigeminal impression properly (Fig. 5.17a);
– the incident beam makes an angle of 20° open upwards in relation to the orbitomeatal plane (OM) (Fig. 5.17b);
– the centering point is situated at the superolateral angle of the eye at the level of the external acoustic meatus;
– the tomographic plane is fixed at the level of the internal acoustic meatus (Fig. 5.17b).

The sections are made downward from this plane.

Fig. 5.17. a, b Centering diagrams for imaging of trigeminal impression in unilateral oblique view; **c** tomography and **d** diagram of impression (V)

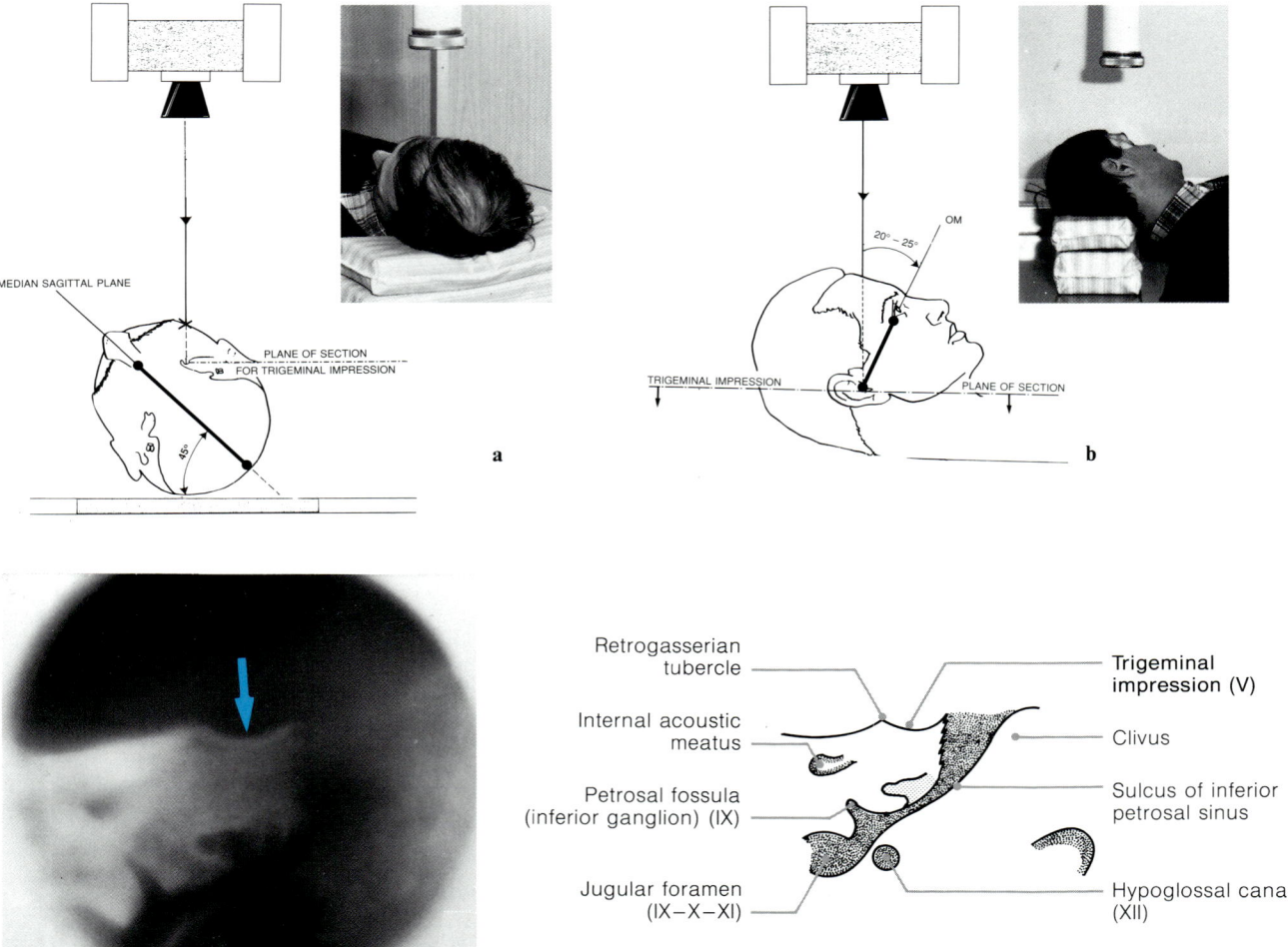

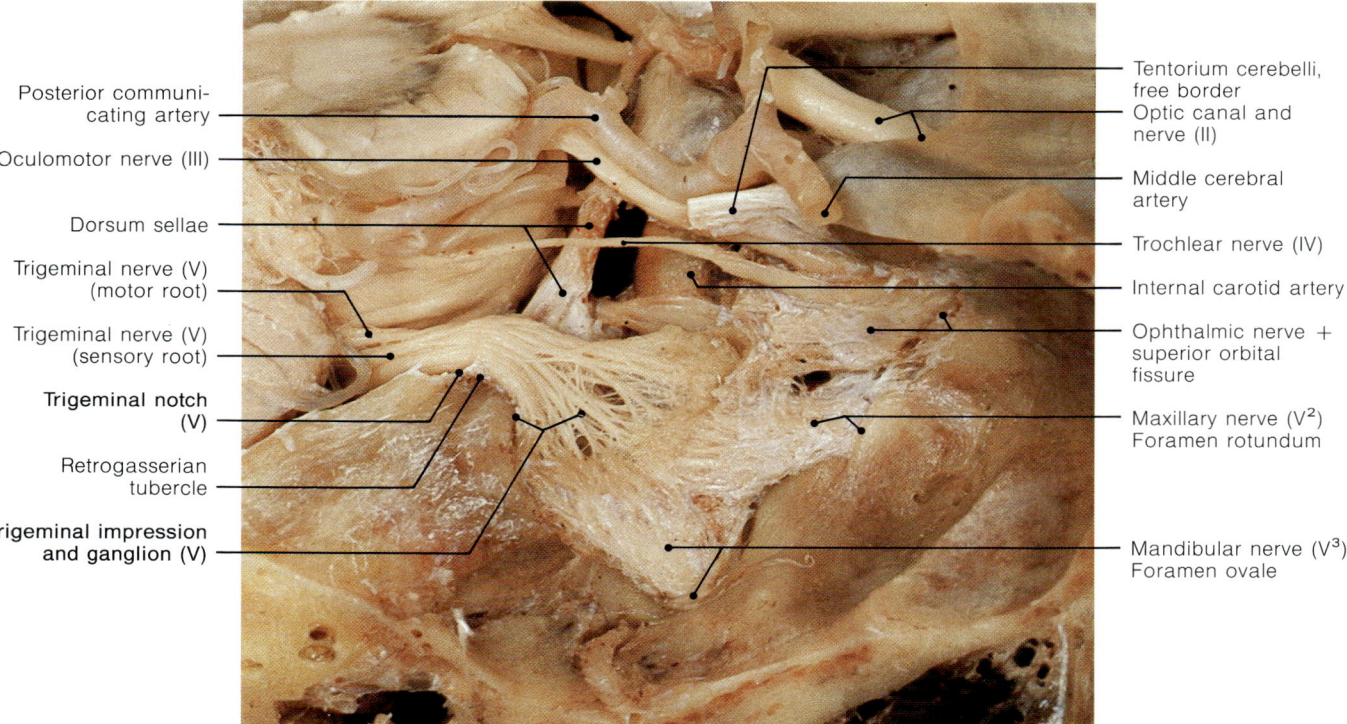

Fig. 5.18a. Dissection of the right trigeminal ganglion and its relations after resection of the temporal lobe, removal of the dura mater and opening of the cavernous sinus

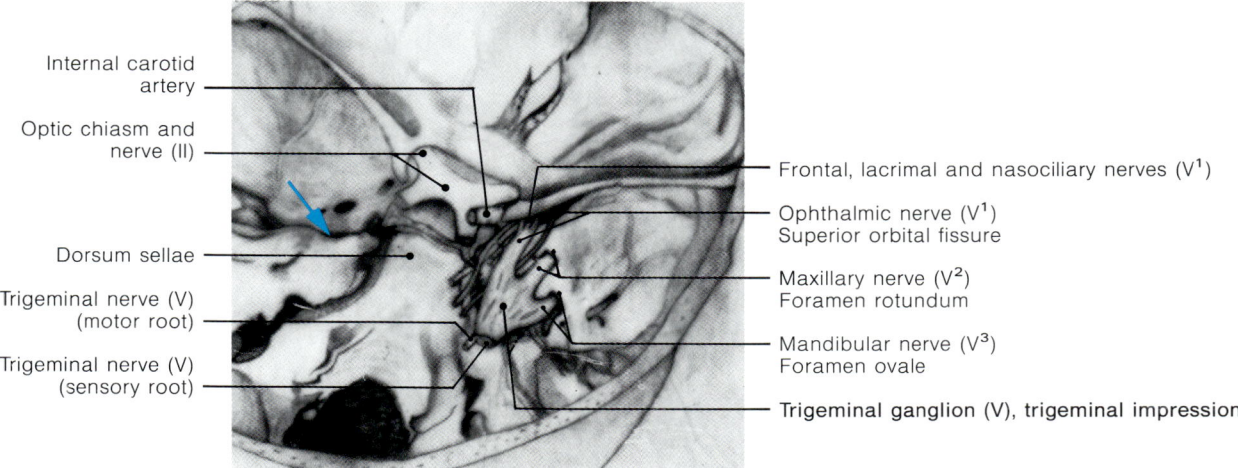

Fig. 5.18b. Diagram of ganglion and its collaterals, right superolateral view

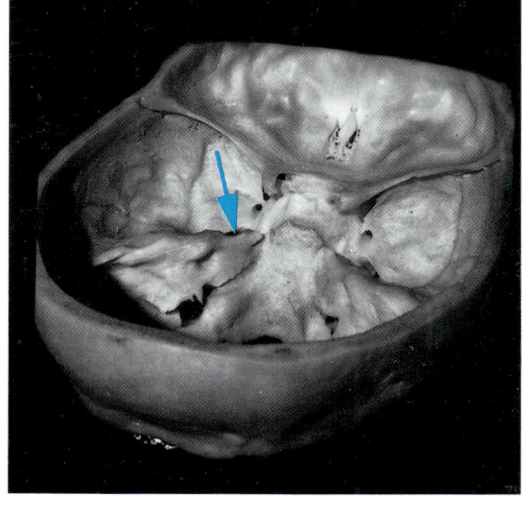

Fig. 5.18c. Dried bone showing trigeminal impressions (V)

Trigeminal ganglion: Trigeminal impression

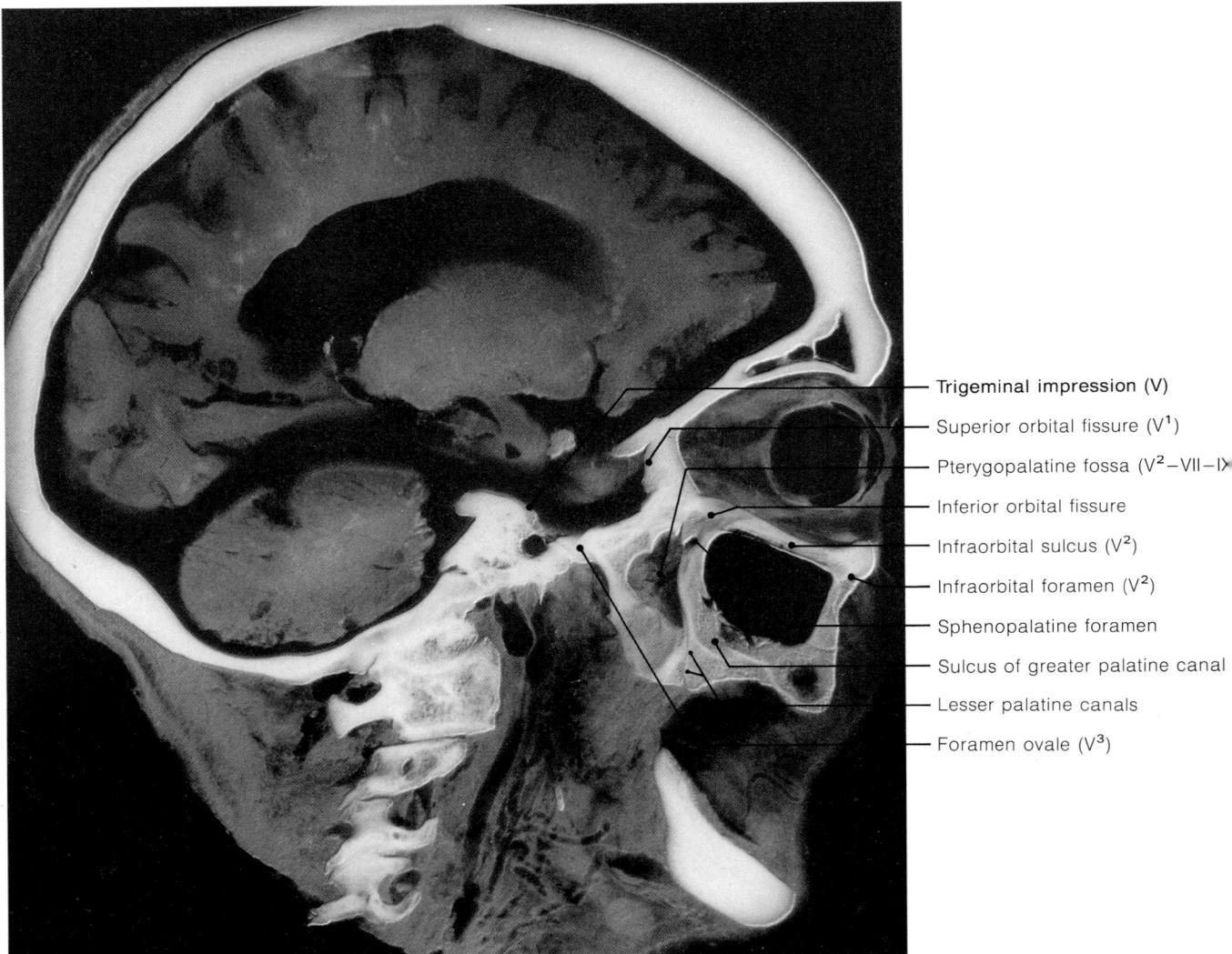

Fig. 5.19. Radiograph of a sagittal anatomic section at the level of the foramina of the trigeminal nerve and its collaterals

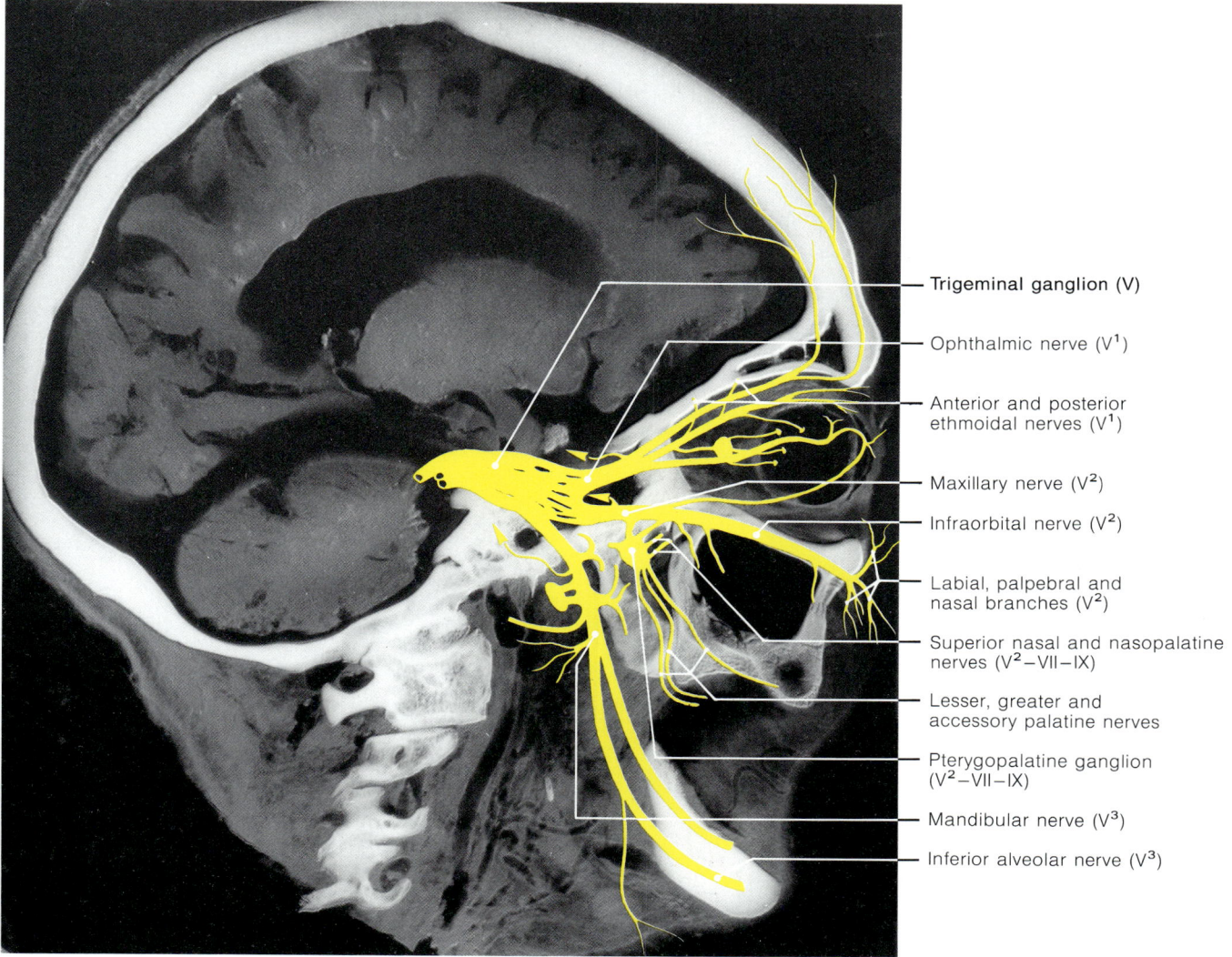

Fig. 5.20. Superimposition of diagram of trigeminal nerve and its collaterals

Trigeminal impression and notch

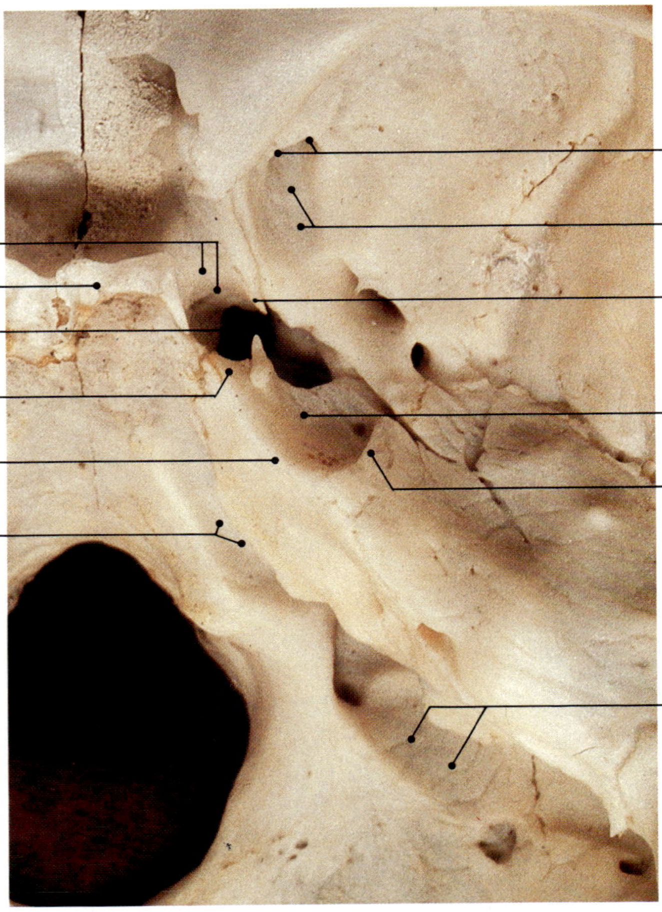

Fig. 5.21. Trigeminal impression

Fig. 5.22. Trigeminal notch, right sagittal view

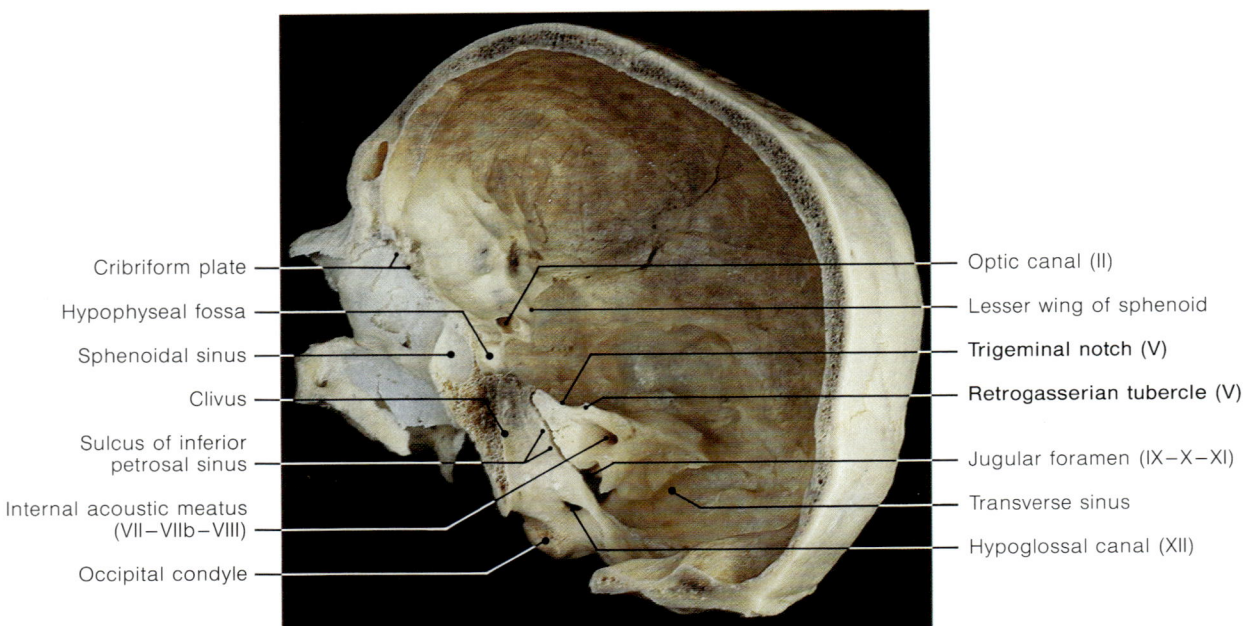

Trigeminal nerve (V)

Ophthalmic nerve (V¹)
Cavernous sinus and superior orbital fissure
Pathology 82
Anatomy and imaging (examination) 84
    Axial view (MRI) 84
Superior orbital fissure
    Oblique view (radiology) 85
    Discontinuous scanning (radiology) 86
    Axial view (MRI) 86
    Axial view (CT) 87

Anterior and posterior ethmoidal nerves
Pathology 88
Anatomy and imaging (examination) 89
Anterior and posterior ethmoidal foramina
    Axial view (radiology) 90
    Diagram of nerves 91
Courses, foramina and sulci
    Anatomic views 93
Vascular relations
    Diagrams 94

Vascular relations:
Anterior and posterior ethmoidal arteries 94, 278
Cavernous sinus
    Venous drainage at the skull base 167, 290
    Inferolateral trunk 276
    Superior ophthalmic vein 276, 277

Topography

Ophthalmic nerve (V^1)
- Superior orbital fissure

Pathology

Cavernous sinus:
- Syndrome of lateral wall of cavernous sinus (Foix's syndrome),
- aneurysm of carotid siphon.

Superior orbital fissure:
- Syndrome of superior orbital fissure (Rochon-Duvigneaud's syndrome),
- meningioma of lesser wing of sphenoid,
- aneurysm of internal carotid artery,
- trigeminal neuralgia (type V^1),
- fractures of lesser wing of sphenoid,
- orbital apex syndrome (Rollet's syndrome),
- syndrome of petrosphenoidal junction (Garcin's syndrome).

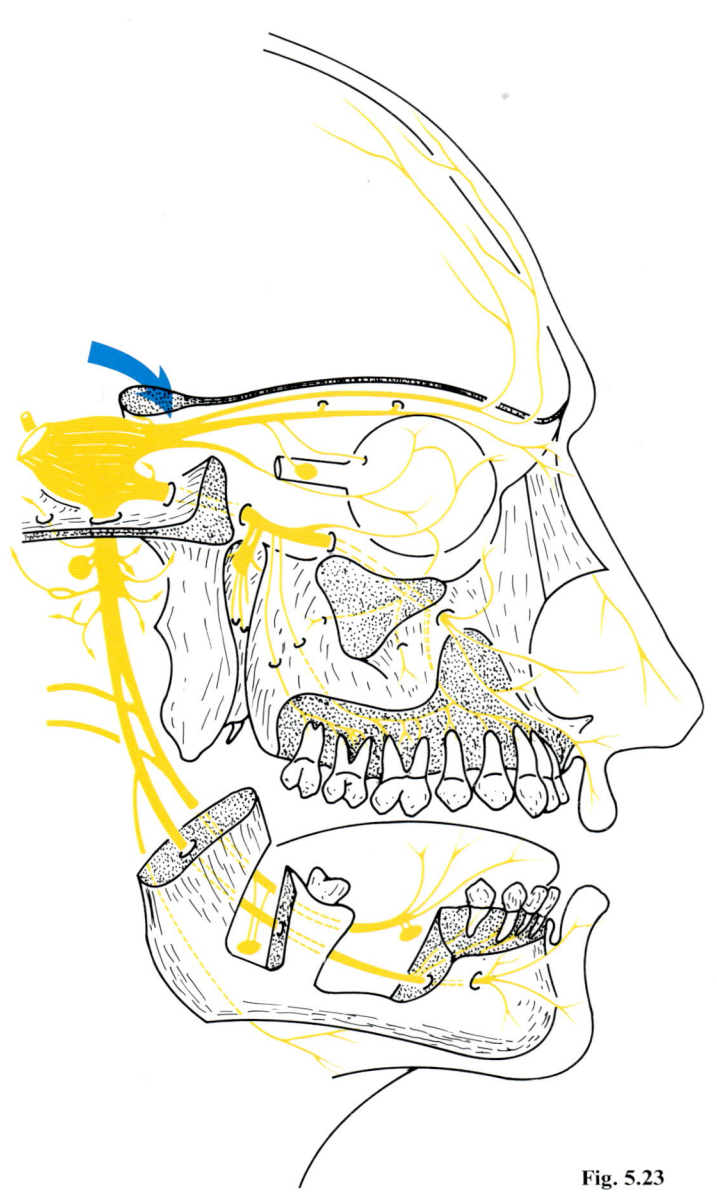

Fig. 5.23

Ophthalmic nerve (V¹): Superior orbital fissure

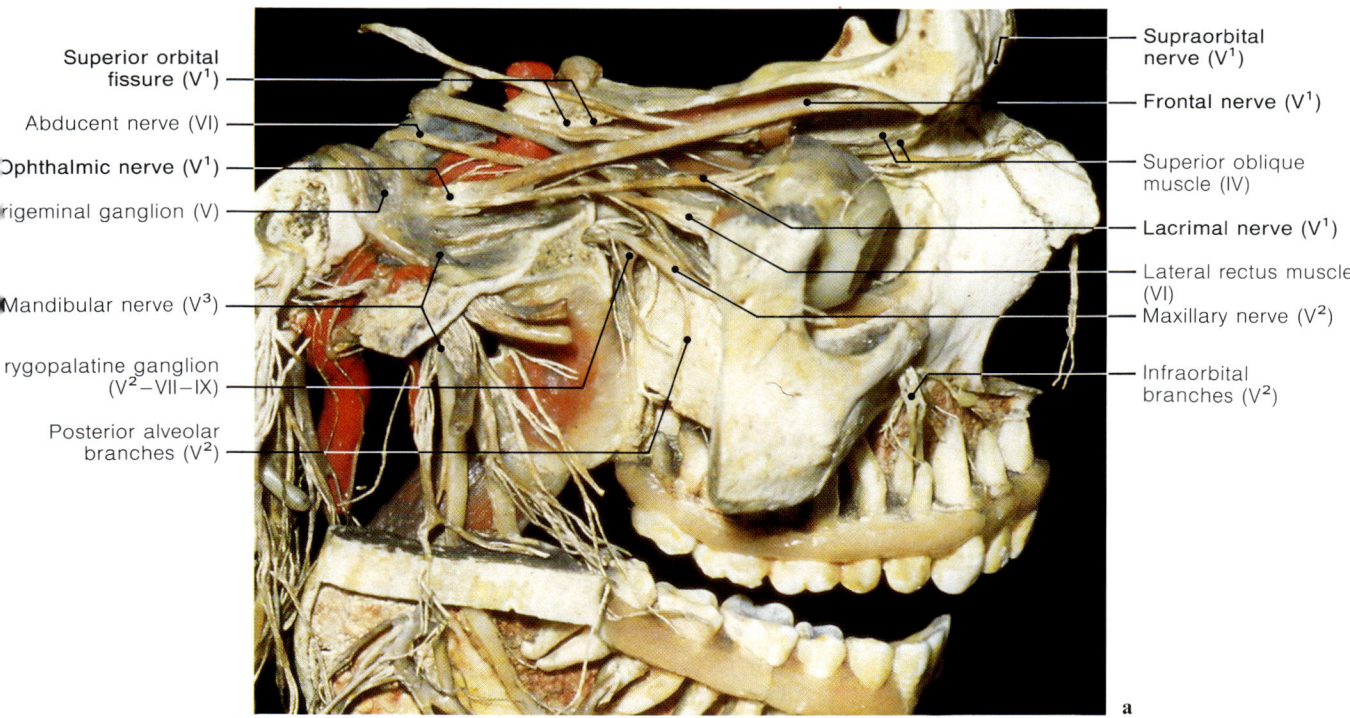

Fig. 5.24a. Anatomic dissection showing the ophthalmic nerve (V¹) in the superior orbital fissure

Fig. 5.24b. Magnetic resonance imaging (MRI) sagittal view of trigeminal nerve showing the ophthalmic nerve in the superior orbital fissure. (MRI: Pr. Doyon, Hospital Kremlin Bicêtre, Paris)

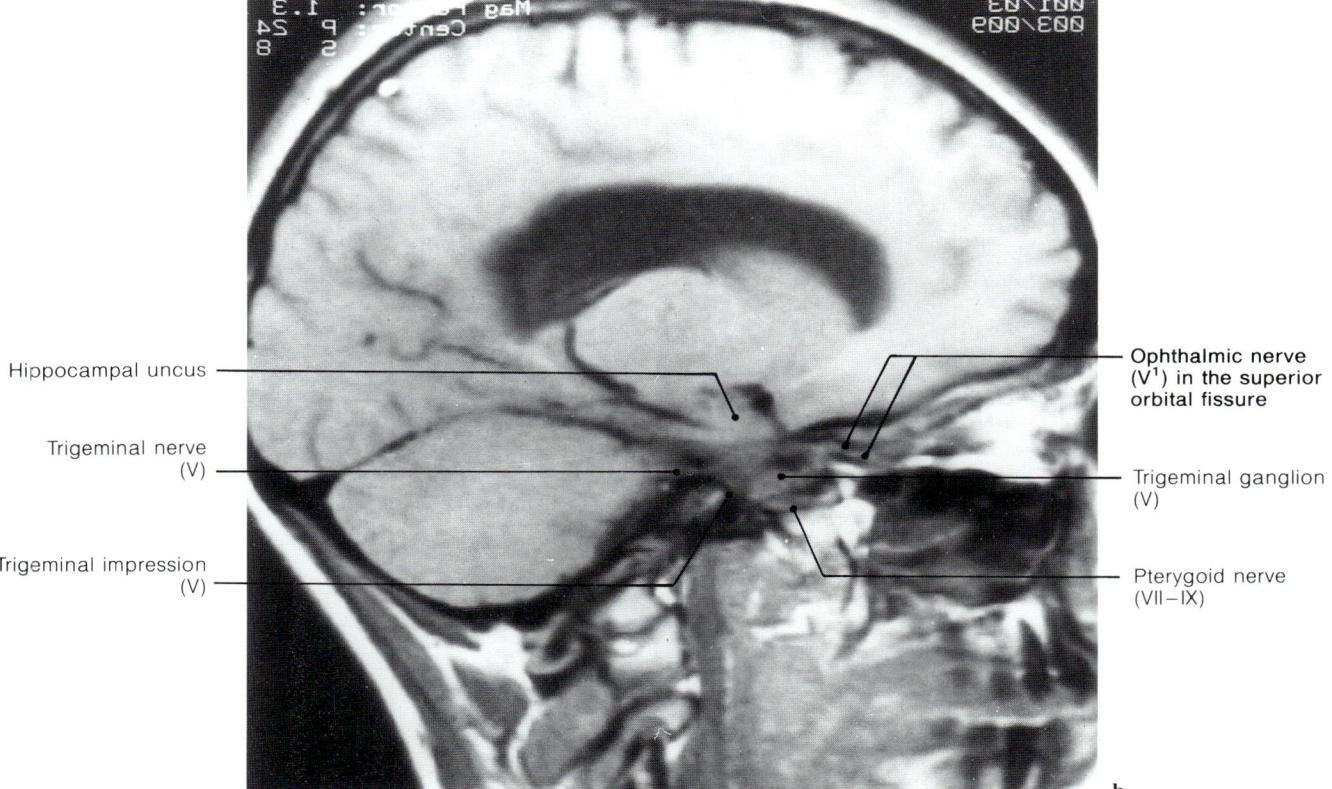

Ophthalmic nerve (V¹): Superior orbital fissure

(MRI sagittal view of ophthalmic nerve: p. 65)

Anatomy

The ophthalmic nerve (V¹) is sensory. It arises from the anteromedial portion of the trigeminal ganglion, passes in a medial direction and receives the anastomotic branch of the trochlear nerve (IV) (Fig. 5.4).
It divides into three branches just before entering the superior orbital fissure:

– the frontal nerve,
– the lacrimal nerve,
– the nasociliary nerve.

The frontal nerve traverses the narrow lateral portion of the orbital fissure, medial to the lacrimal nerve and lateral to the common tendinous ring and the trochlear nerve (IV).
It travels from behind forwards between the orbital roof and the levator palpebrae superioris muscle and then divides behind the supraorbital margin into two branches, the supratrochlear nerve and the supraorbital nerve (Fig. 5.3; 5.34 a).
These branches are distributed to the skin of the forehead, root of the nose and upper eyelid.
The frontal nerve gives off another branch: a supratrochlear branch which passes above the pulley of the superior oblique muscle to anastomose with the infratrochlear nerve.
The lacrimal nerve sometimes anastomoses posteriorly with the trochlear nerve (IV), and sometimes anteriorly with the orbital branch of the maxillary nerve, whence originate the lacrimal branches and then the zygomatic nerve (Fig. 5.3; 5.45 a, b).
The lacrimal nerve traverses the superior orbital fissure lateral to the frontal nerve. It passes forward and outward and branches in the lacrimal gland and in the outer part of the upper eyelid.

The nasociliary nerve enters the orbit via the widest part of the superior orbital fissure and traverses the common tendinous ring (of Zinn).

Imaging

The superior orbital fissure separates the lesser wing of the sphenoid from the anterior edge of the greater wing, both of which form the posterior orbital wall (Fig. 5.25 c).

EXAMINATION

– Symmetric study of the superior orbital fissures in a high frontal distinguishing view,
– radiologic study in unilateral oblique view, beam perpendicular,
– unilateral radiograph of the superior orbital fissure in a "discontinuous scanning"

IMAGING TECHNIQUE

Radiographic study of the superior orbital fissure in an oblique unilateral intraorbital view:

– The subject is in dorsal decubitus, the head turned 5° to 8° in relation to the median sagittal plane, away from the side to be examined (Fig. 5.25 b);
– the beam makes an angle of 25° with the orbitomeatal plane (OM) (Fig. 5.25 a);
– the centering point is situated at the center of the orbit.

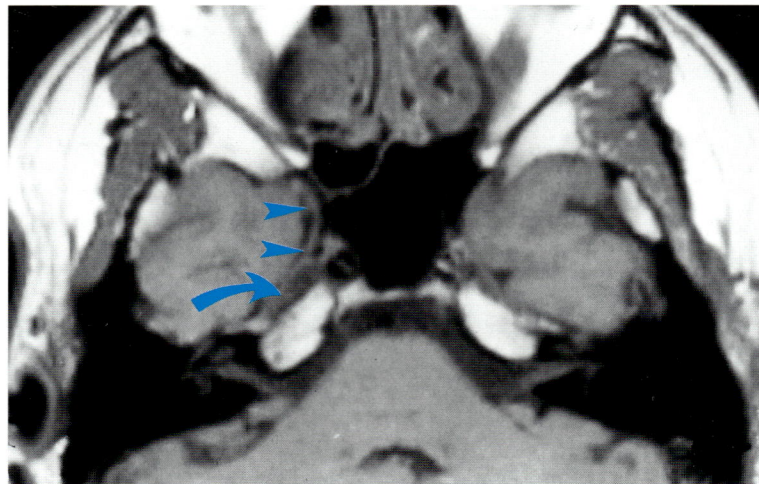

Fig. 5.24 c. Axial MRI imaging of trigeminal ganglion (V) (*curved arrow*) and ophthalmic nerve (V¹) (*arrowheads*)

Ophthalmic nerve (V¹): Superior orbital fissure

Imaging

TECHNIQUE (OBLIQUE VIEW)

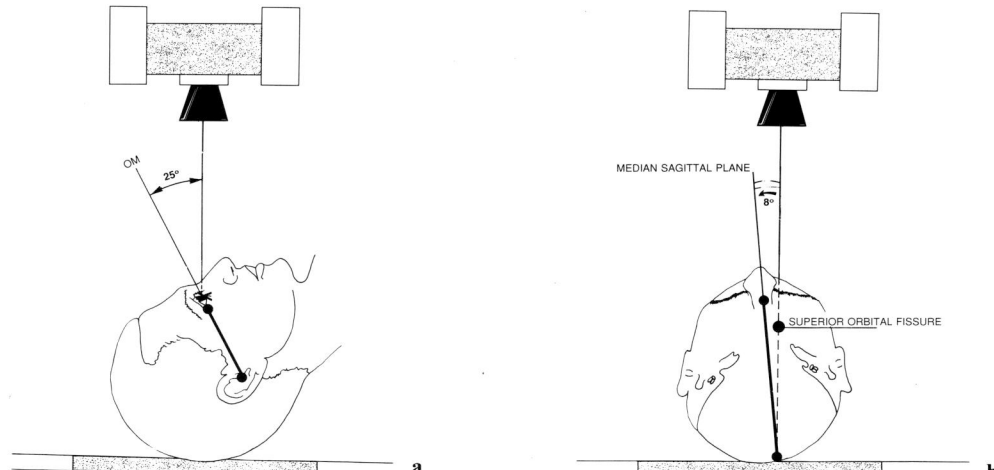

Fig. 5.25 a, b. Centering diagrams for imaging of the superior orbital fissure in unilateral oblique intraorbital view

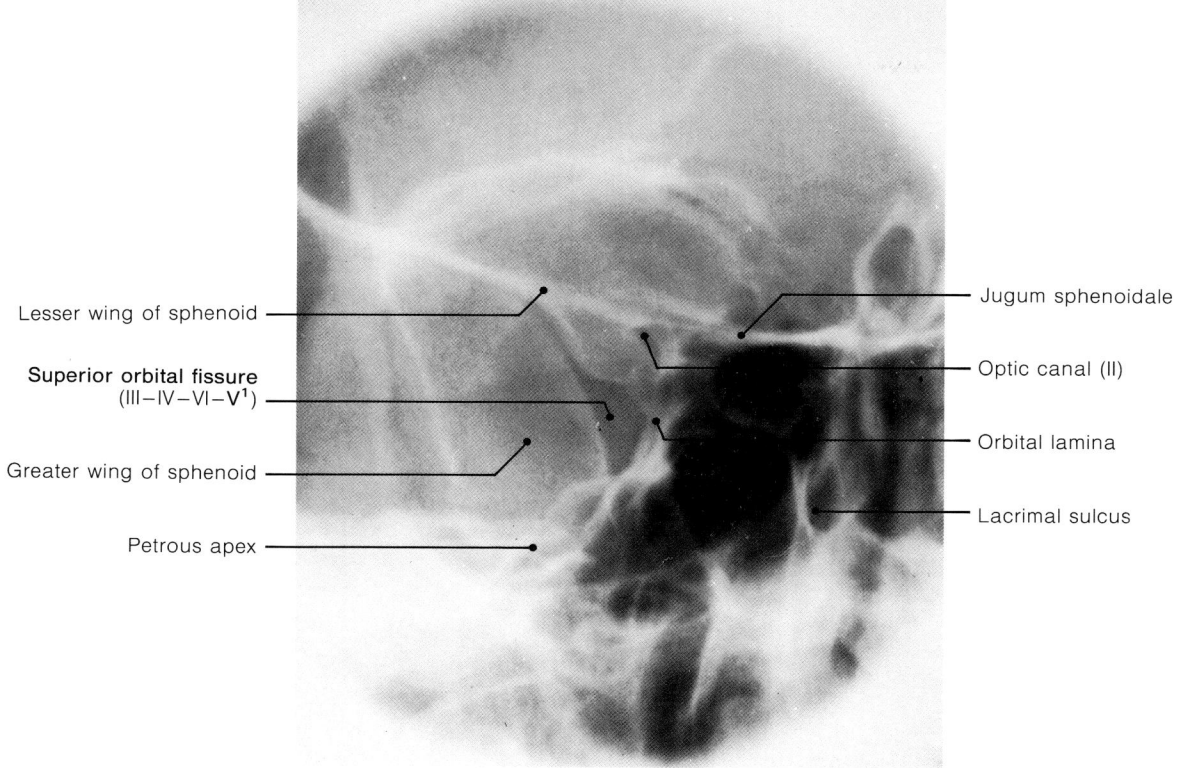

Fig. 5.25 c. Unilateral radiograph of superior orbital fissure

Note: In these conventional radiographs, and even with tomographic sections, the margins and walls of the superior orbital fissure are not registered on the same plane. They are, in fact, fine and irregular and therefore it is necessary to supplement this study by films with "discontinuous scanning".

Ophthalmic nerve (V¹): Superior orbital fissure

Imaging

TECHNIQUE (DISCONTINUOUS SCANNING)

Study of the superior orbital fissure in oblique unilateral and intraorbital view in "discontinuous scanning":
If the equipment allows circular movement of the tube, it is preferable to supplement the examination where this zone is suspect by films in "discontinuous scanning".
The view is identical with that previously stated (Fig. 5.25a), but the tube must be inclined by 7°.
Four films are then taken in succession during rotation of the tube (Fig. 5.26; 5.27).

Note: This technique of successive films gives good definition of all the margins of the superior orbital fissure (Fig. 5.27).

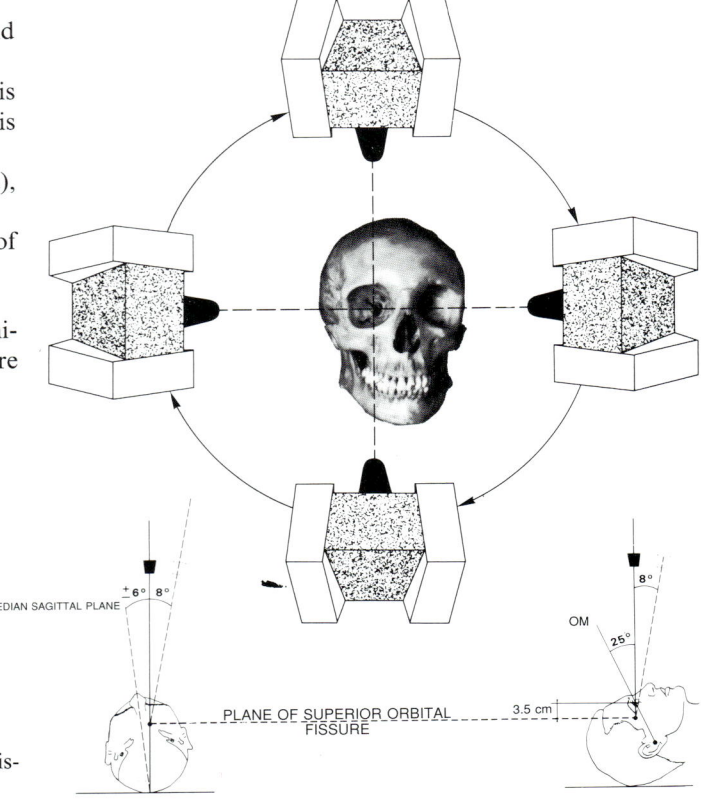

Fig. 5.26. Centering diagram for study of the superior orbital fissure by "discontinuous scanning"

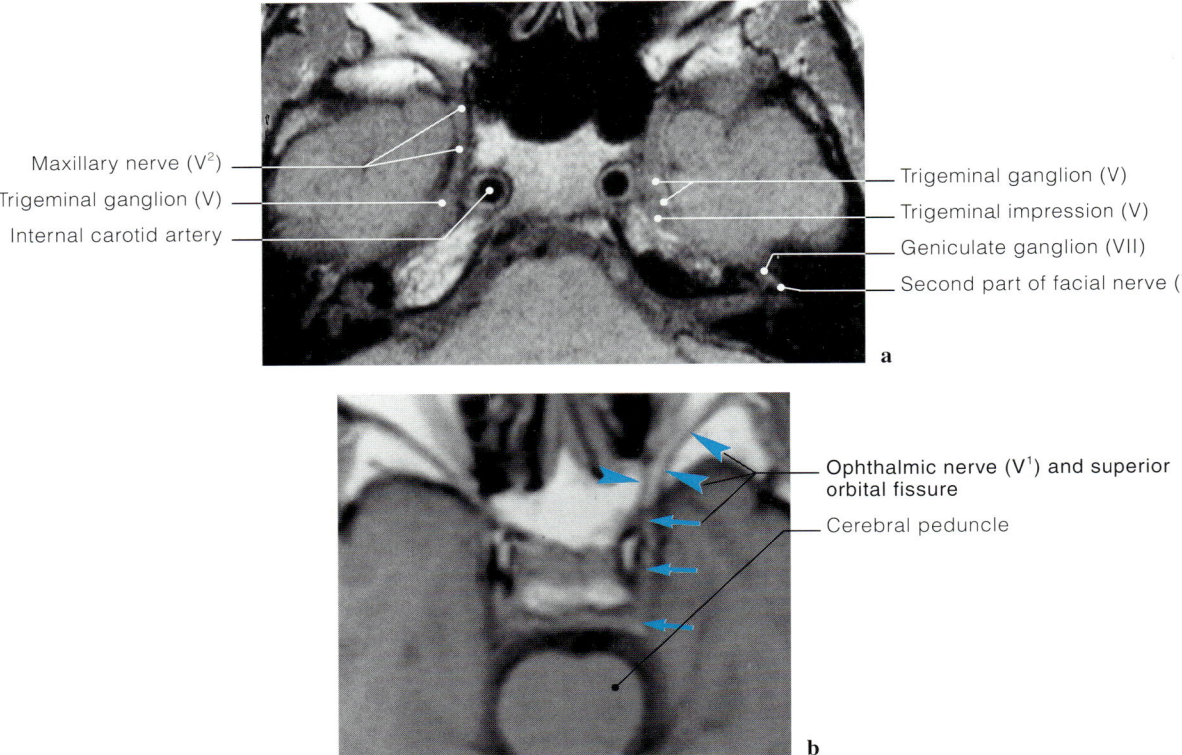

Fig. 5.27 a, b. Axial magnetic resonance imaging (MRI) at level of maxillary nerve (V²) (**a**) and course of ophthalmic nerve (V¹) (**b**) (*arrows*) up to its entry into the superior orbital fissure (*arrowheads*). (MRI: **a** Dr. J.W. Casselman, A.Z. St-Jan, Brugge; **b** Pr. Doyon, Hospital Kremlin Bicêtre, Paris)

Ophthalmic nerve (V¹) 87

Superior orbital fissure, course of the ophthalmic nerve (V¹)

Axial computed tomography (CT)

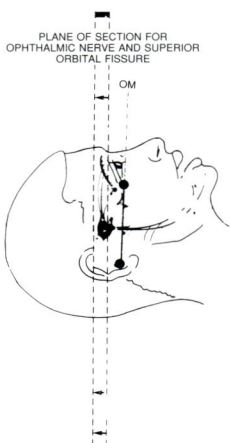

Fig. 5.28. Centering for scanning (CT) and magnetic resonance imaging (MRI)

Note: For a lesion situated in the region of the trigeminal ganglion, cavernous sinus or ophthalmic nerve, whether due to a petrous apex syndrome, an aneurysm of internal carotid artery or a meningioma of the lesser wing of the sphenoid, it is necessary to perform a computed tomographic study (CT), or axial magnetic resonance imaging (MRI), in the axis of the ophthalmic nerve, i.e., clearly parallel to the orbitomeatal plane (OM) (Fig. 5.28).

Displayed: the entire course of V, from its origin as far as the ophthalmic nerve in its superior orbital fissure (Fig. 5.29 a, b).

Fig. 5.29 a, b. Axial computed tomographic (CT) (**a**) and anatomic (**b**) sections of ophthalmic nerves and superior orbital fissures (see sagittal MRI: Fig. 5.6 a)

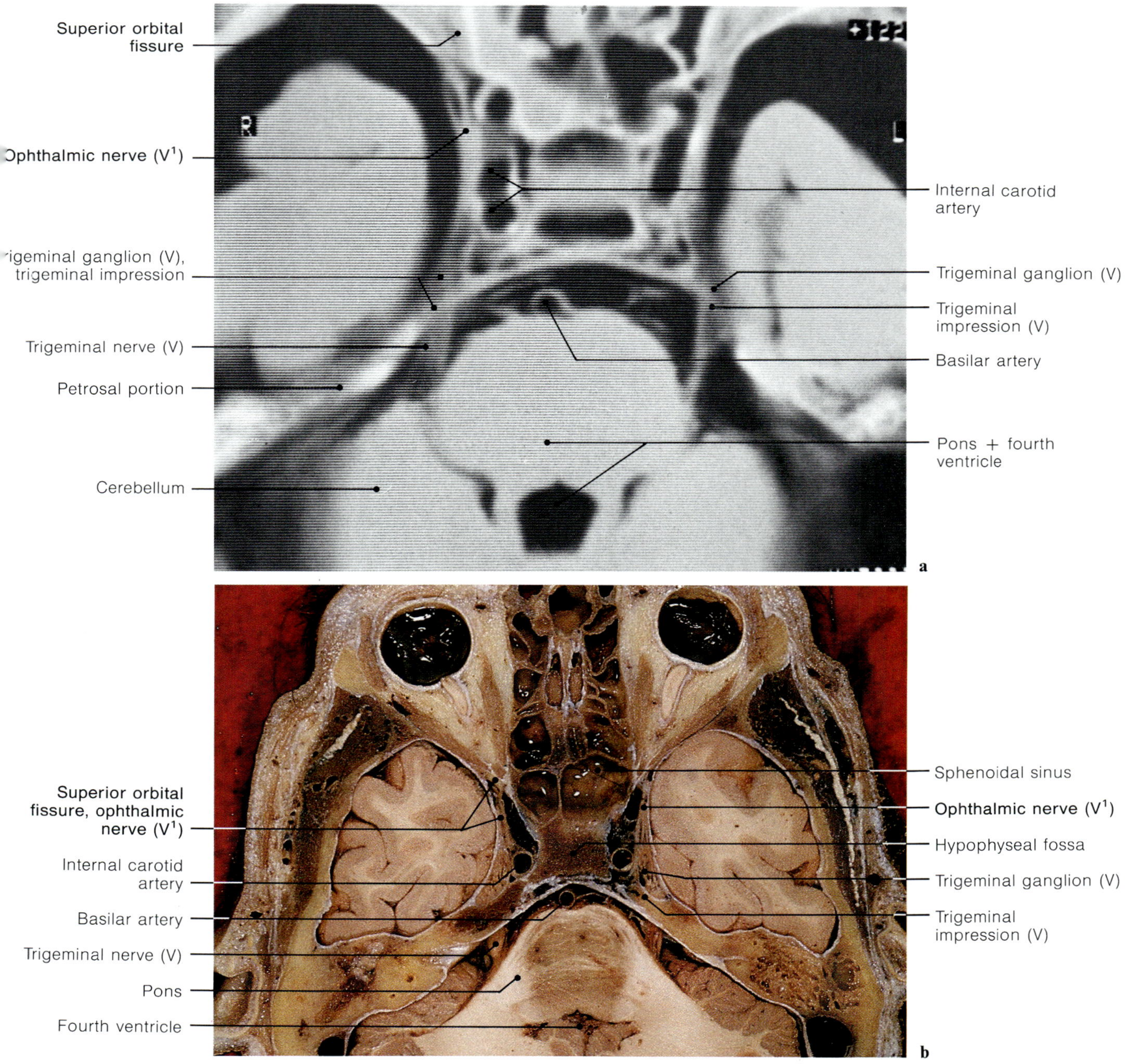

Topography

Posterior ethmoidal nerve (V¹)
- Posterior ethmoidal foramen

Anterior ethmoidal nerve (V¹)
- Anterior ethmoidal foramen

Pathology

- Syndrome of ciliary ganglion (Charlin) or syndrome of nasal nerve,
- tumor of ethmoid,
- tumor of orbit,
- fracture of anterior fossa extending towards the ethmoidal cells and the cribriform plate of ethmoid,
- frontal fractures of the superior orbital margin and of the nasal cavity,
- fracture of anterior cranial fossa.

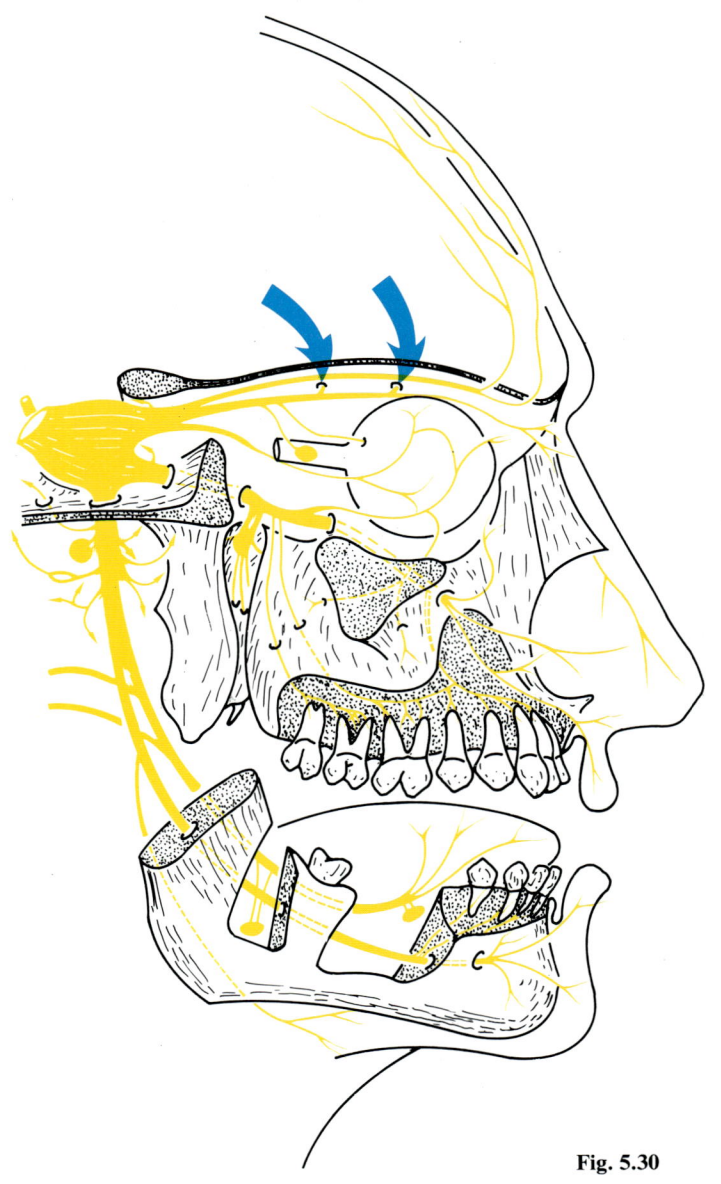

Fig. 5.30

Posterior and anterior ethmoidal nerves: Posterior and anterior ethmoidal foramina

Anatomy

After having traversed the superior orbital fissure, the nasociliary nerve crosses the optic nerve from within outwards, passing above it; then it accompanies the ophthalmic artery along the inferior border of the superior oblique muscle. It divides into two terminal branches: the infratrochlear nerve and the anterior ethmoidal nerve (Fig. 5.3; 5.31 f).

Collateral branches

During its course the nasociliary nerve gives off:

- a branch to the ciliary ganglion, the long or sensory root of the ganglion,
- the long ciliary nerves, often two in number, enter the eyeball,
- the *posterior ethmoidal* strand or *nerve* (V^1), which traverses the posterior ethmoidal foramen to be distributed to the posterior ethmoidal cells and the sphenoidal sinus (Fig. 5.31 f; 5.33; 5.34 b).

Terminal branches

The anterior ethmoidal nerve enters the anterior ethmoidal foramen and then traverses the ethmoidal sulcus.
It then traverses the ethmoidal foramen (Fig. 5.31 f; 5.33; 5.35 a, b) to be distributed in the nasal cavity as two strands, one medial and the other lateral (Fig. 5.31 f).
The lateral branch (nerve to the levator labii superioris muscle) glides in the posterior groove of the nasal bone and ends in the skin of the nasal ala.
The *infratrochlear nerve* continues the course of the nasociliary nerve, accompanied by the ophthalmic artery. Having arrived beneath the trochlea of the superior oblique muscle, it divides into descending strands supplying the skin of the root of the nose and the lacrimal pathways (Fig. 5.33; 5.34 c).

Imaging

The anterior and posterior ethmoidal foramina are hollowed out in the upper part of the ethmoid (Fig. 5.31 b, c, e, f; 5.35 a, c) and open laterally at the ethmoidofrontal suture in the orbit and medially at the lateral margin of the cribriform plate of ethmoid (Fig. 5.31 e, f).

EXAMINATION

- Radiographic (survey) study of the ethmoid in the Hirtz and sagittal views,
- horizontal tomographic or computed tomographic (CT) sections of the anterior and posterior ethmoidal foramina.

TECHNIQUE

Tomographic and computed tomographic (CT) study of the anterior and posterior ethmoidal foramina:

- The subject is in dorsal decubitus, with the back elevated on pillows and the head turned to give the Hirtz view, the orbitomeatal plane (OM) making an angle of 5° to 8° in relation to the horizontal (Fig. 5.31 a);
- the centering point is situated at the median line 3 cm from the mandibular symphysis;
- the planes of section are made every 2 or 3 mm, starting from 1 cm below the supraorbital margin and extending towards the inferior orbital margin.

A series of 4 films should be obtained.

Anterior and posterior ethmoidal nerves: Anterior and posterior ethmoidal foramina

Imaging

TECHNIQUE (AXIAL VIEW)

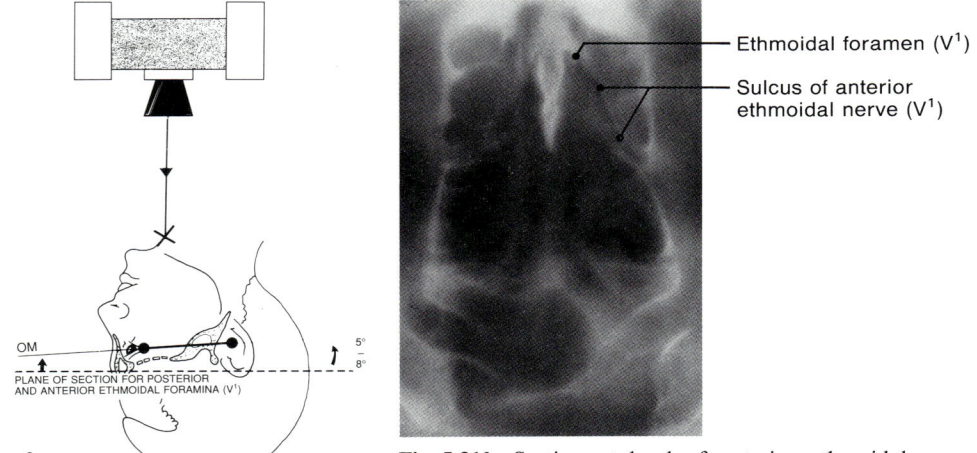

Fig. 5.31 a. Centering diagram for axial imaging of ethmoidal canals

Fig. 5.31 b. Section at level of anterior ethmoidal nerve up to ethmoidal foramen

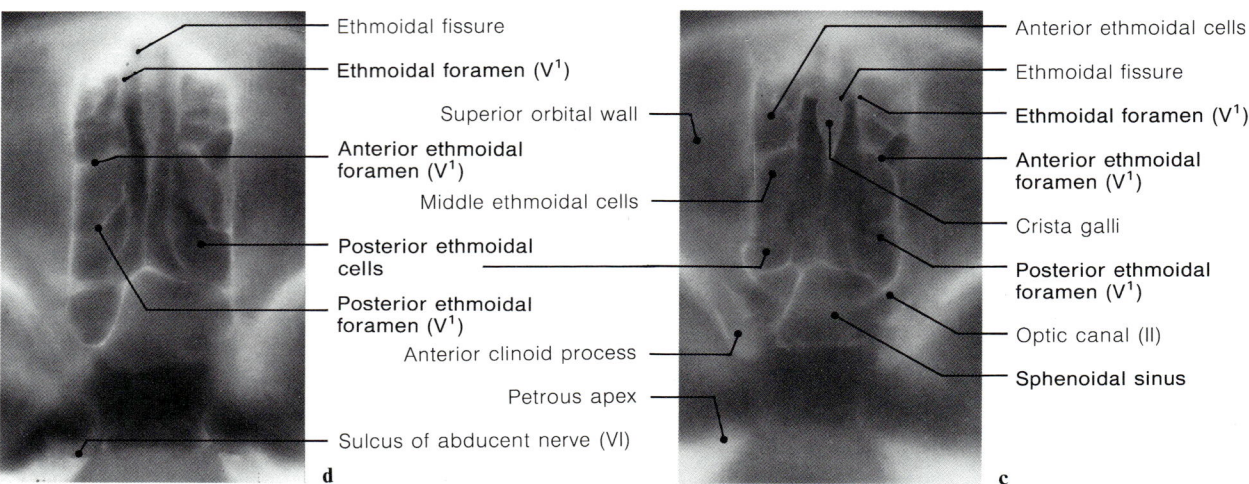

Fig. 5.31 c, d. Axial tomograms of anterior and posterior ethmoidal foramina

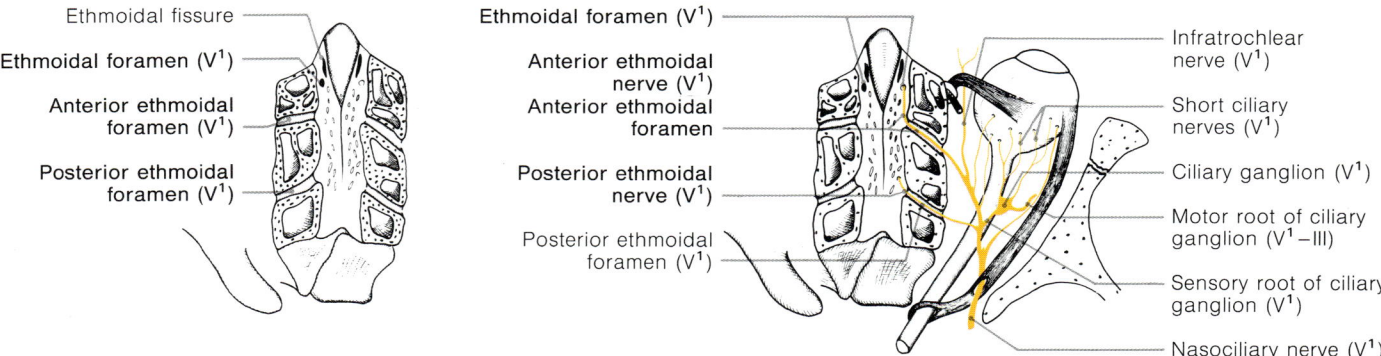

Fig. 5.31 e. Diagram of tomogram

Fig. 5.31 f. Diagram of tomogram of ethmoidal foramina with diagram of nasociliary nerve

Ophthalmic nerve (V¹) 91

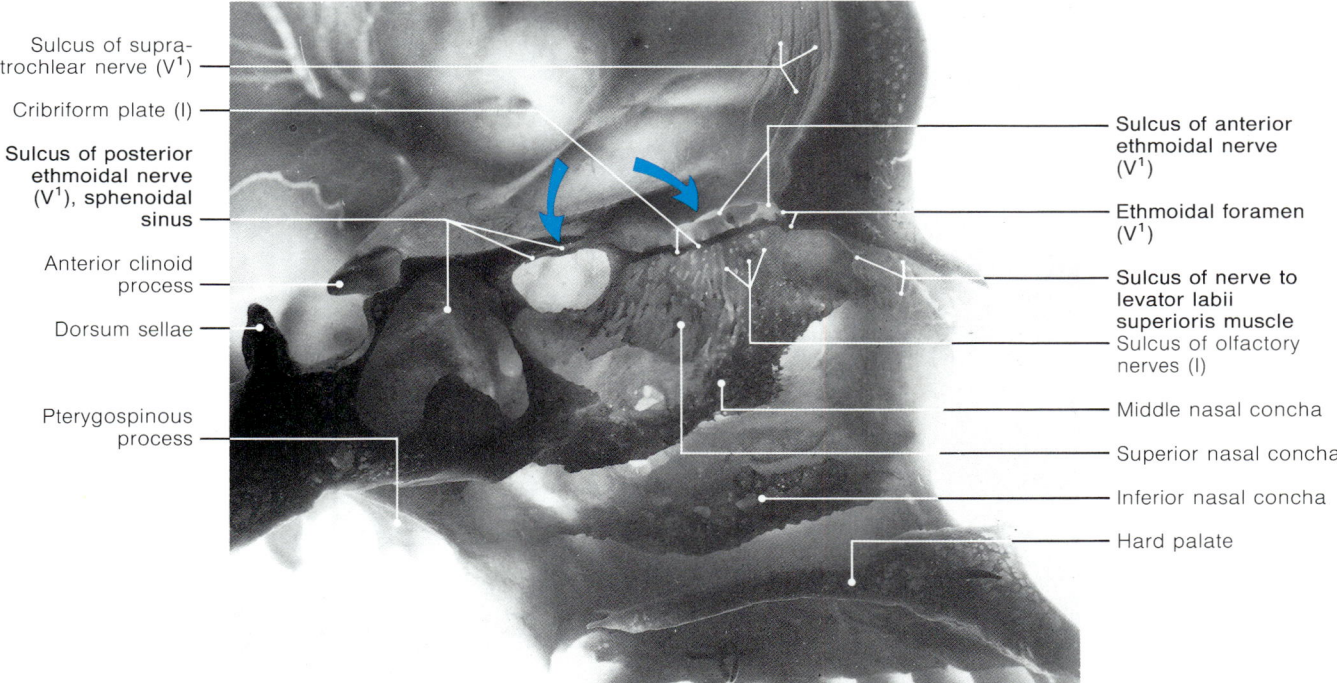

Fig. 5.32. Sagittal section of nasal cavity at level of sulci of anterior and posterior ethmoidal nerves

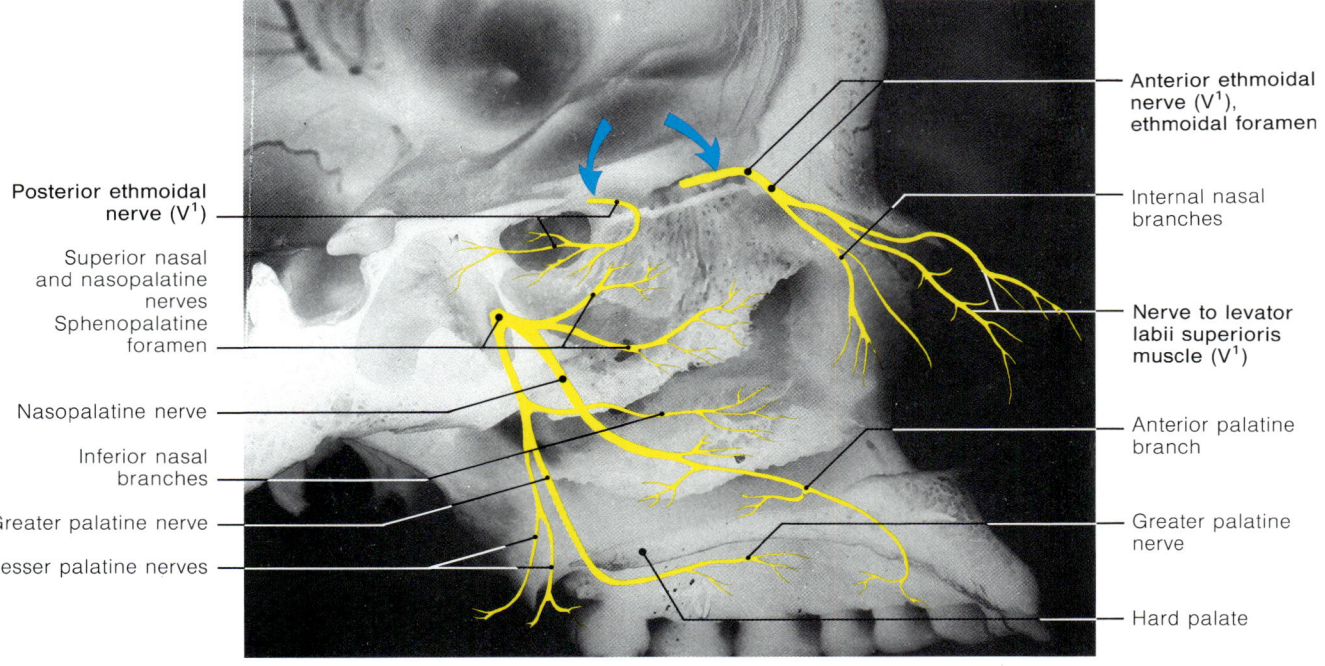

Fig. 5.33. Diagram of anterior and posterior ethmoidal nerves

Anterior and posterior ethmoidal foramina (V¹)

Fig. 5.34 a–c. Diagram of ophthalmic nerve showing origins of anterior and posterior ethmoidal nerves (**a**), their courses to the nasal cavity (**b**), with anatomic dissection (**c**) of nerve to levator labii superioris muscle

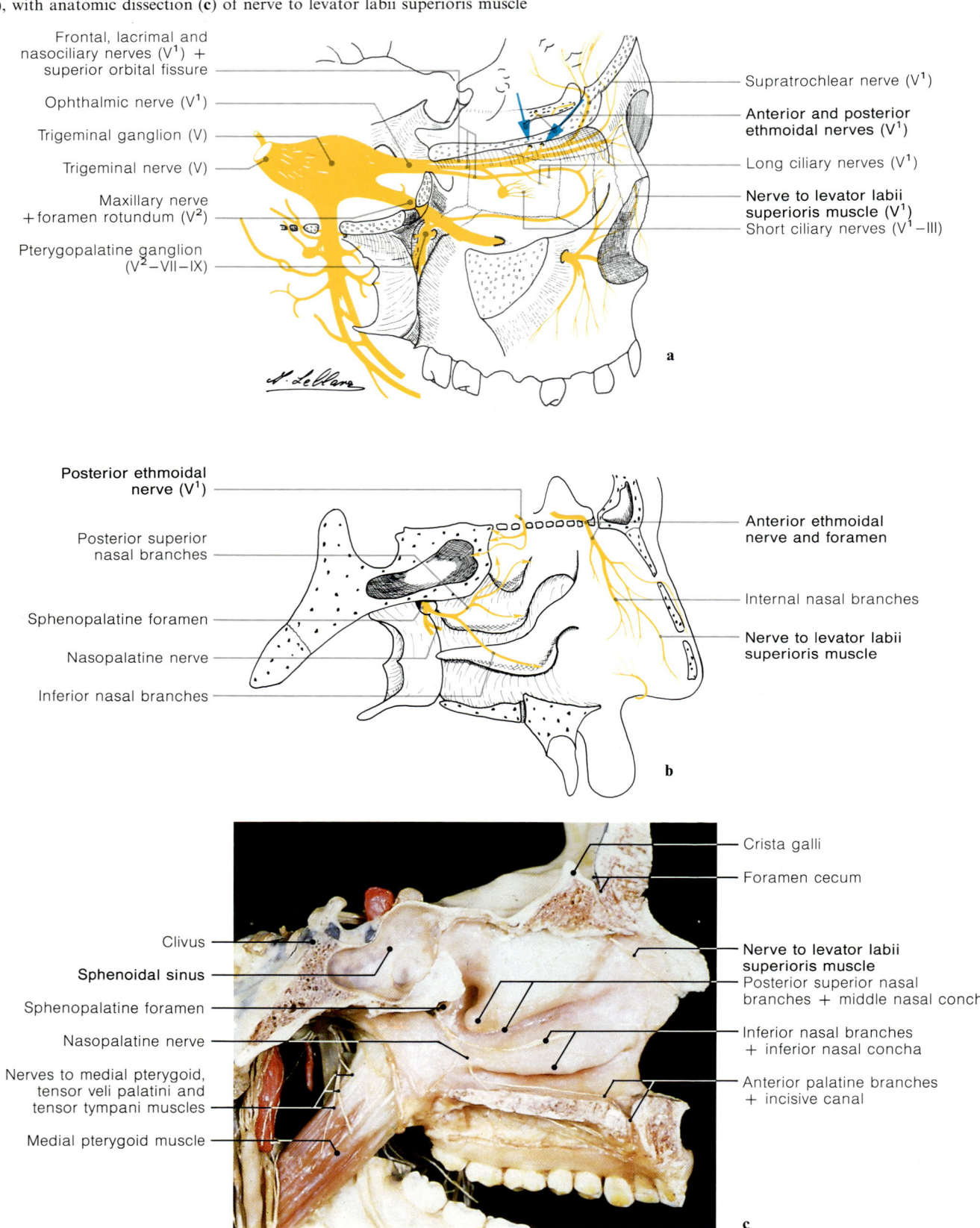

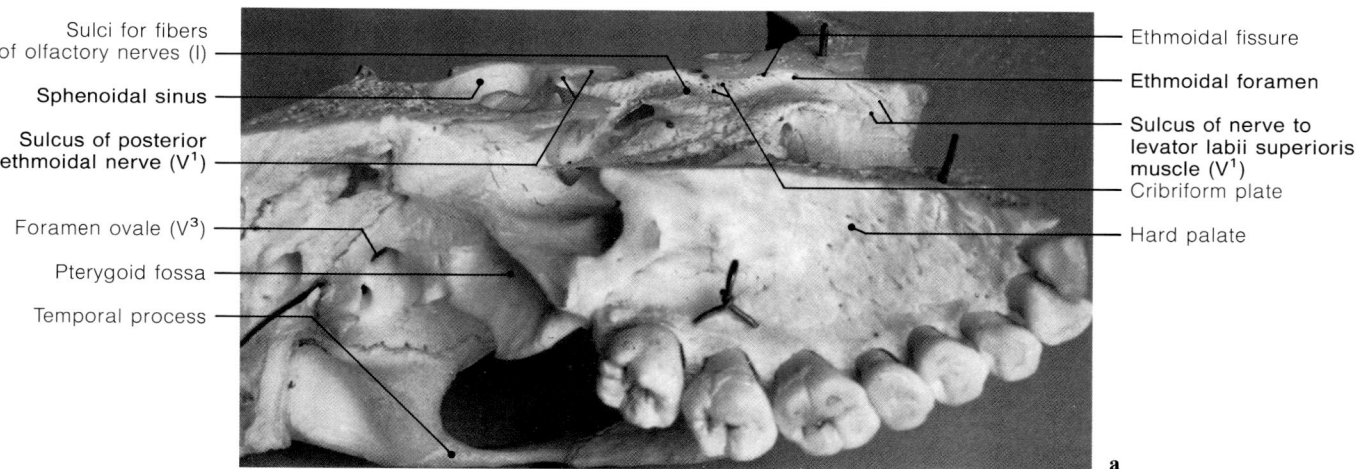

Fig. 5.35 a–c. Inferior (**a**) and superior (**b**) anatomic views of the nasal cavity and intraorbital view (**c**), showing foramina and sulci of the anterior and posterior ethmoidal nerves (V^1)

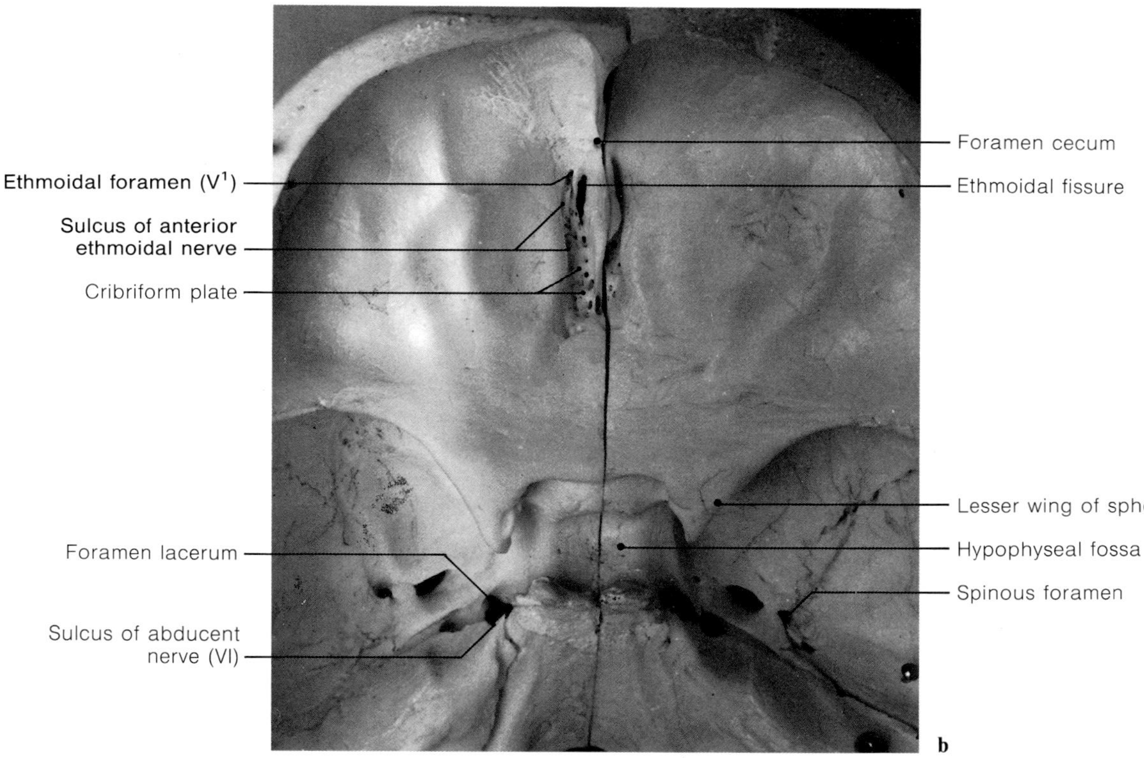

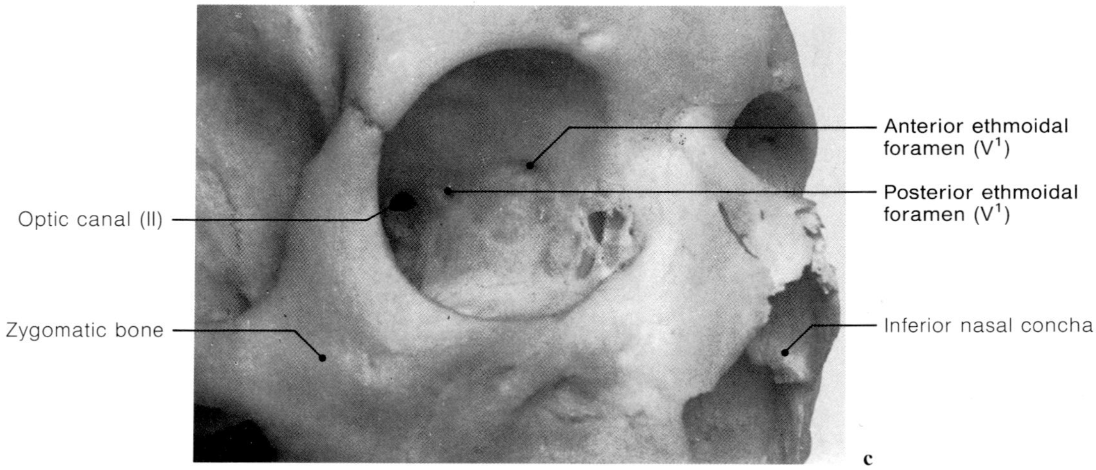

Anterior and posterior ethmoidal arteries and nerves (V¹)

(See vascular relations, p. 278)

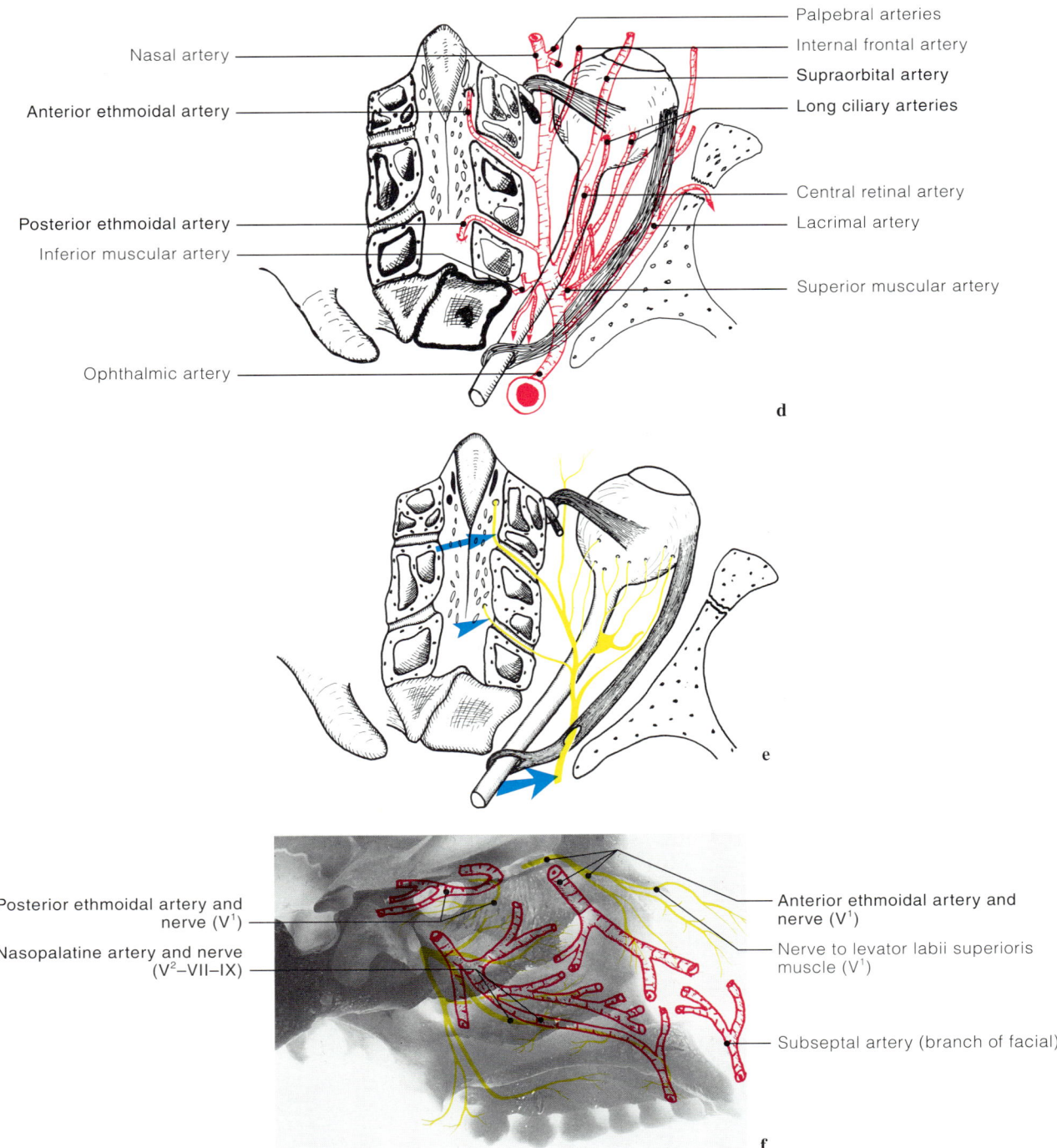

Fig. 5.35d–f. Axial and sagittal diagrams showing course and vascular relations of anterior and posterior ethmoidal nerves (**d**) (V¹).
e Nasociliary nerve (*large arrow*), posterior ethmoidal nerve (*arrowhead*), anterior ethmoidal nerve (*straight arrow*). (See annotations, p. 90)

Trigeminal nerve (V)

Maxillary nerve (V^2)
Foramen rotundum (V^2)
Pathology 96
Anatomy and imaging (examination) 98
    Frontal view (radiography, CT) 99
    Anatomy (extracranial and intracranial views) 100
    Oblique view (radiology) 102
    Discontinuous scanning (radiology) 103
    Frontal views (MRI) 103
    Diagram (anatomy, intraorbital view) 104
    Sagittal view (radiology) 105
    Axial view (radiology) 106
    Computed tomography (CT) 107
    Axial views (CT, radiology) 108
    Axial view (MRI) 109

Infraorbital nerve (infraorbital sulcus)
Pathology 110
Anatomy and imaging (examination) 112
    Axial views (MRI) 112
    Axial view (CT) 113
    Worms-Bretton view (radiology) 114
    Anatomy (infraorbital view) 115
    Termination and collaterals (diagram) 116

Infraorbital nerve (labial, palpebral and nasal branches, infraorbital canal and foramen)
Pathology 117
Anatomy and imaging (examination) 118
    Frontal view (CT) 119
    Discontinuous scanning (radiology) 120
    Sagittal view (radiology, CT, MRI) 121
    Diagram of orbital cavity 123

Pterygopalatine ganglion (pterygopalatine fossa) and palatine nerves
Pathology 124
Anatomy and imaging (examination) 126
    Sagittal views (MRI) 126
    Sagittal view (radiology) 127
    Sections of the nasal cavity (diagram) 128
    Axial and sagittal views (MRI, CT, radiography) . 130
    Frontal and sagittal views (MRI, CT) 134

Vascular relations:
Cavernous sinus 167, 290
Vein of the foramen rotundum 276, 277
Artery of the foramen rotundum 279
Arterial pedicles to the soft palate 280
Superior alveolar and infraorbital arteries 280
Labial, palpebral, and nasal branches 281
Greater, lesser, and accessory palatine arteries 287

Topography

Maxillary nerve (V^2)
- Foramen rotundum

Pathology

- Syndrome of lateral wall of cavernous sinus (Foix's syndrome),
- trigeminal neuralgia (type V^2),
- syndrome of foramen rotundum,
- aneurysm of internal carotid artery, carotid siphon (cavernous sinus),
- tumor of skull base,
- neurinoma of foramen rotundum,
- fracture of body of sphenoid,
- fracture of greater wing of sphenoid (vertical),
- fracture of inferior orbital wall and greater wing of sphenoid.

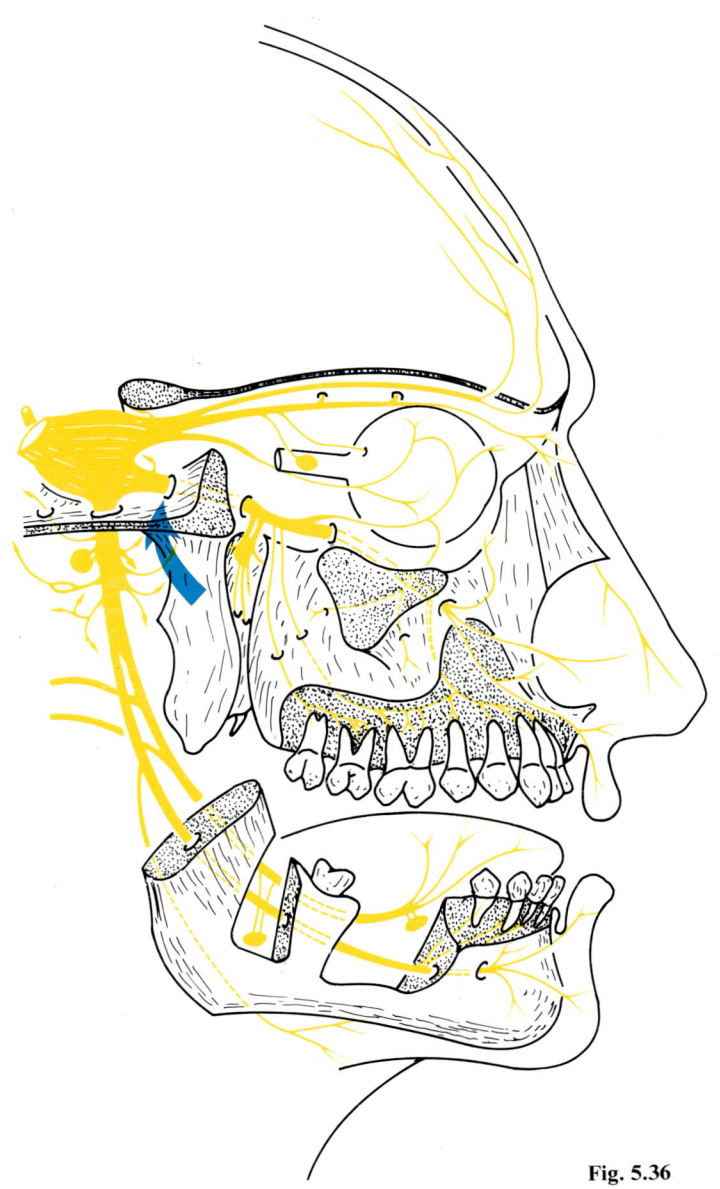

Fig. 5.36

Maxillary nerve (V²): Foramen rotundum

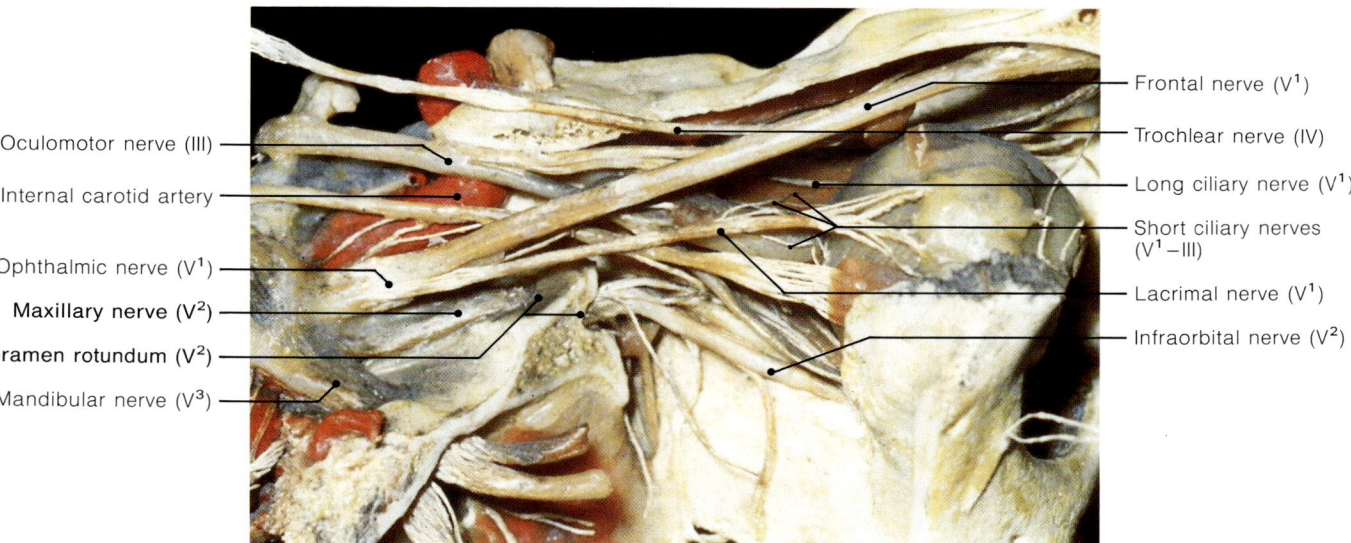

Fig. 5.37. Anatomic dissection showing the course of the maxillary nerve (V²)

Maxillary nerve (V^2): Foramen rotundum

(MRI sagittal view of maxillary nerve V^2: p. 144)

Anatomy

The maxillary nerve (V^2) takes a straight course to traverse the foramen rotundum and skirt the medial border of the inferior orbital fissure (Fig. 5.36; 5.37; 5.45a, b; 5.50). It then swerves to enter the infraorbital sulcus.

At its exit from the foramen rotundum it gives off six collateral branches:

- the meningeal branch, distributed to the adjacent dura mater,
- the orbital branch, which anastomoses with a branch of the lacrimal nerve (Fig. 5.45a), to give off the lacrimal fibers to the lacrimal gland, and the zygomatic nerve which gives off:
* a malar strand for the skin of the cheek (Fig. 5.45a),
* a temporal strand supplying the skin of the temporal region (Fig. 5.45a),
* the pterygopalatine nerve, which anastomoses with the pterygopalatine ganglion (Fig. 5.66; 5.67),
* the posterior superior, middle superior and anterior superior alveolar branches (Fig. 5.3; 5.57).

On leaving the infraorbital foramen, it gives off three terminal branches: the labial, palpebral and nasal branches (Fig. 5.3; 5.59).

The foramen rotundum is situated in the vertical portion of the greater wing of the sphenoid beneath the superior orbital fissure and lateral to the sphenoidal sinuses (Fig. 5.36; 5.37; 5.38f; 5.41b).

Imaging

EXAMINATION

- Examination and computed tomography (CT) in symmetric frontal view,
- radiologic study in unilateral oblique view,
- study in "discontinuous scanning",
- sagittal computed tomography (CT) of foramen rotundum,
- computed tomography (CT) of foramina rotunda in axial asymmetric view.

TECHNIQUE

Frontal tomographic study, symmetric view:

- The subject is in dorsal decubitus, the head strictly facing forward, with sufficient extension that the orbitomeatal plane (OM) makes an angle of 35° open downwards in relation to the incident beam (Fig. 5.38a);
- the centering point is at the midline;
- the beam must cut the line at the level of a point situated 3 cm outside the zygomatic process of the frontal bone (Fig. 5.38a, b). This point is still contained in the plane of the foramina rotunda. Tomographic sections should be made every 2 mm from this point, proceeding downwards.

Imaging

TECHNIQUE (FRONTAL VIEW)

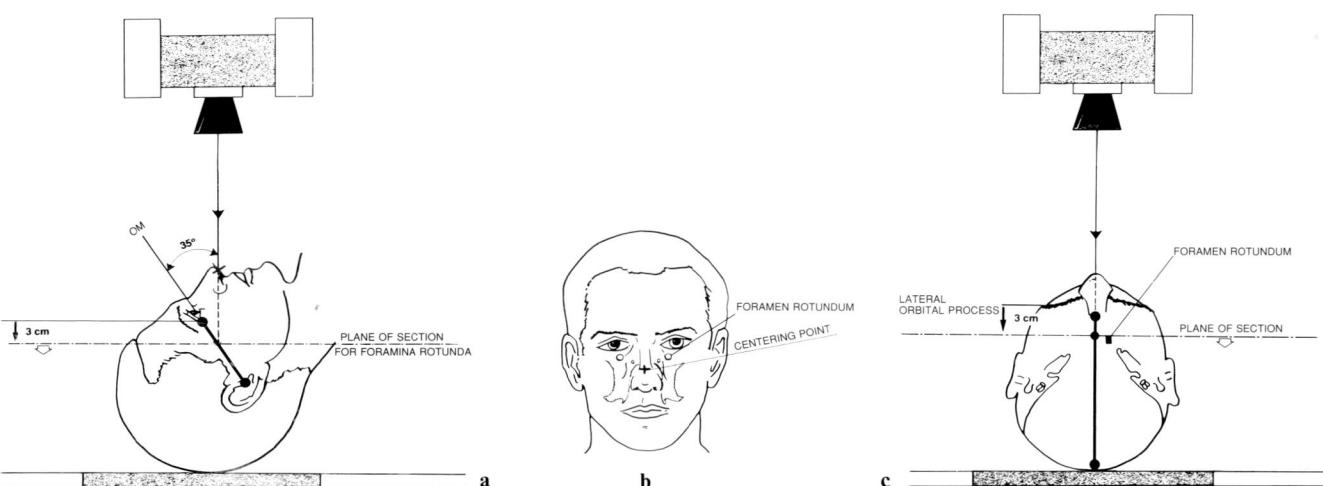

Fig. 5.38 a–c. Centering diagrams for tomographic and CT study of foramina rotunda in frontal view

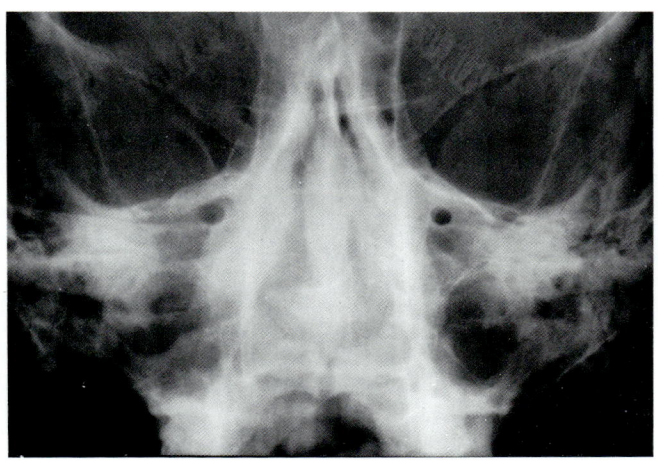
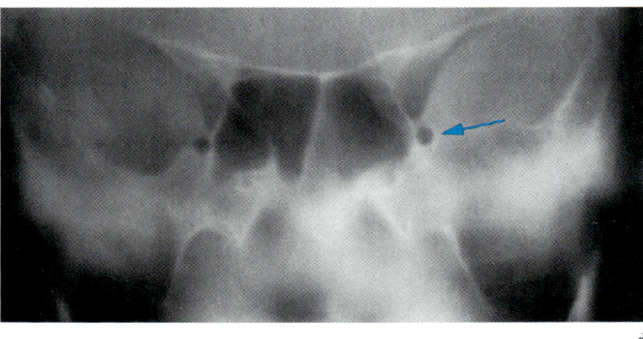

- Lesser wing of sphenoid
- Foramen rotundum (V²)
- Coronoid process of mandible
- Medial and lateral laminae of pterygoid process
- Anterior clinoid process
- Superior orbital fissure (V¹–III–IV–VI)
- Greater wing of sphenoid
- Pterygoid canal (VII–IX)
- Vomerovaginal canal

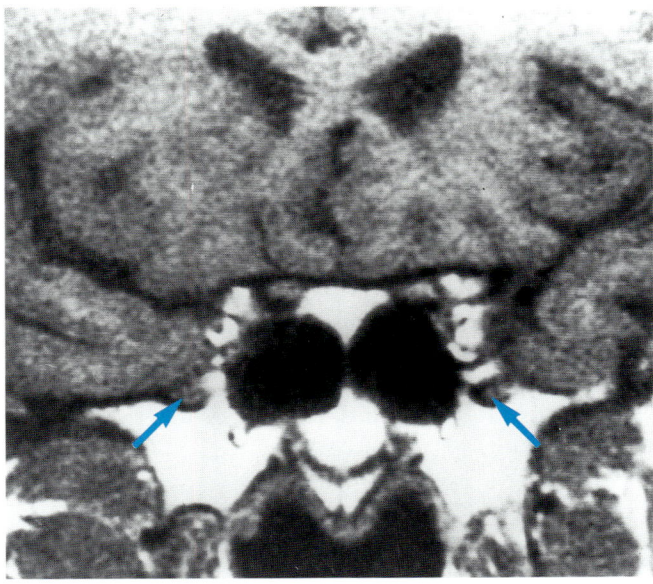

Fig. 5.38 d–g. Radiograph (**d**), tomogram (**e**) and diagram (**f**) of foramina rotunda; magnetic resonance imaging (**g**) frontal view of maxillary nerves in their foramina rotunda (V²) (arrows). (MRI: Pr. Doyon, Hospital Kremlin Bicêtre, Paris)

Maxillary nerve (V²): Foramen rotundum

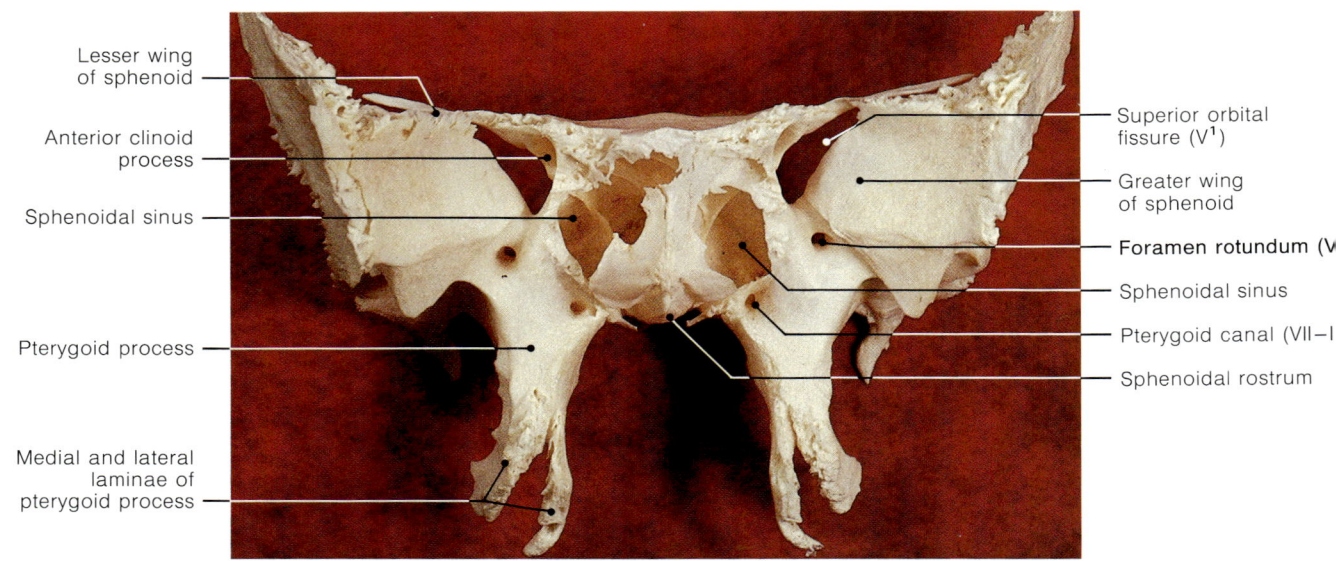

Fig. 5.39. Extracranial view of foramina rotunda

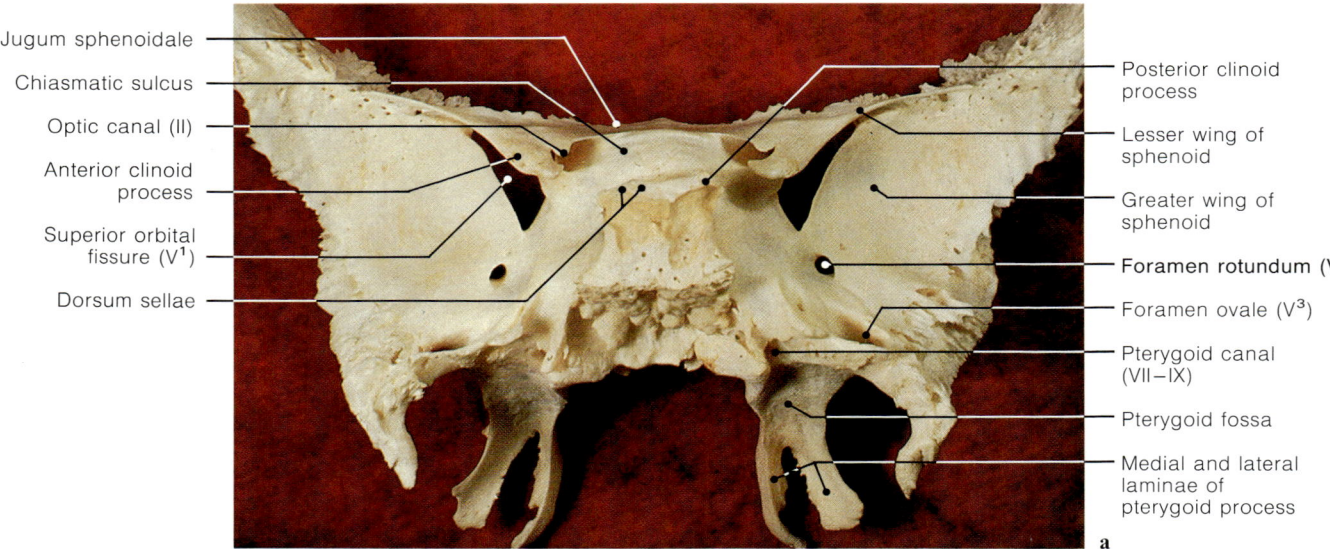

Fig. 5.40 a. Intracranial view of foramina rotunda

Fig. 5.40 b, c. MRI view (b) and sagittal anatomic section (c) of maxillary nerve (V²)

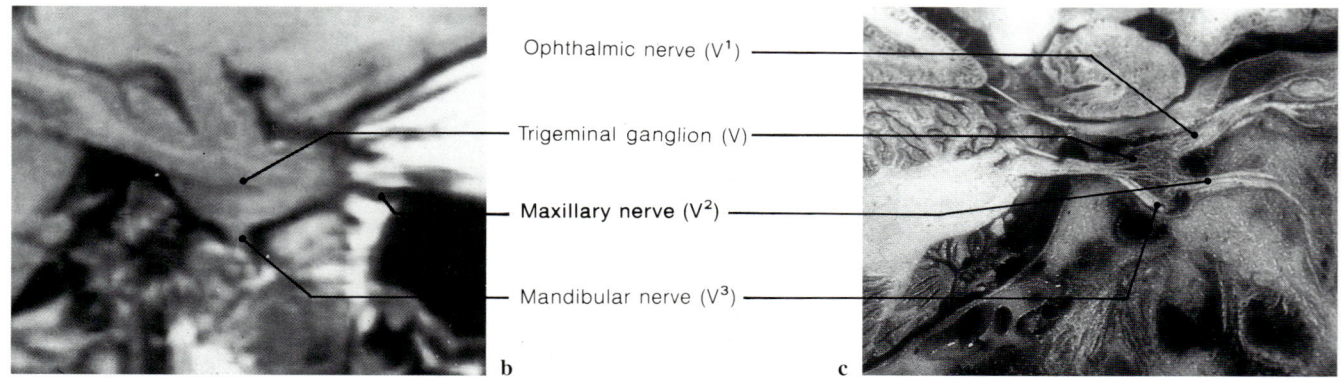

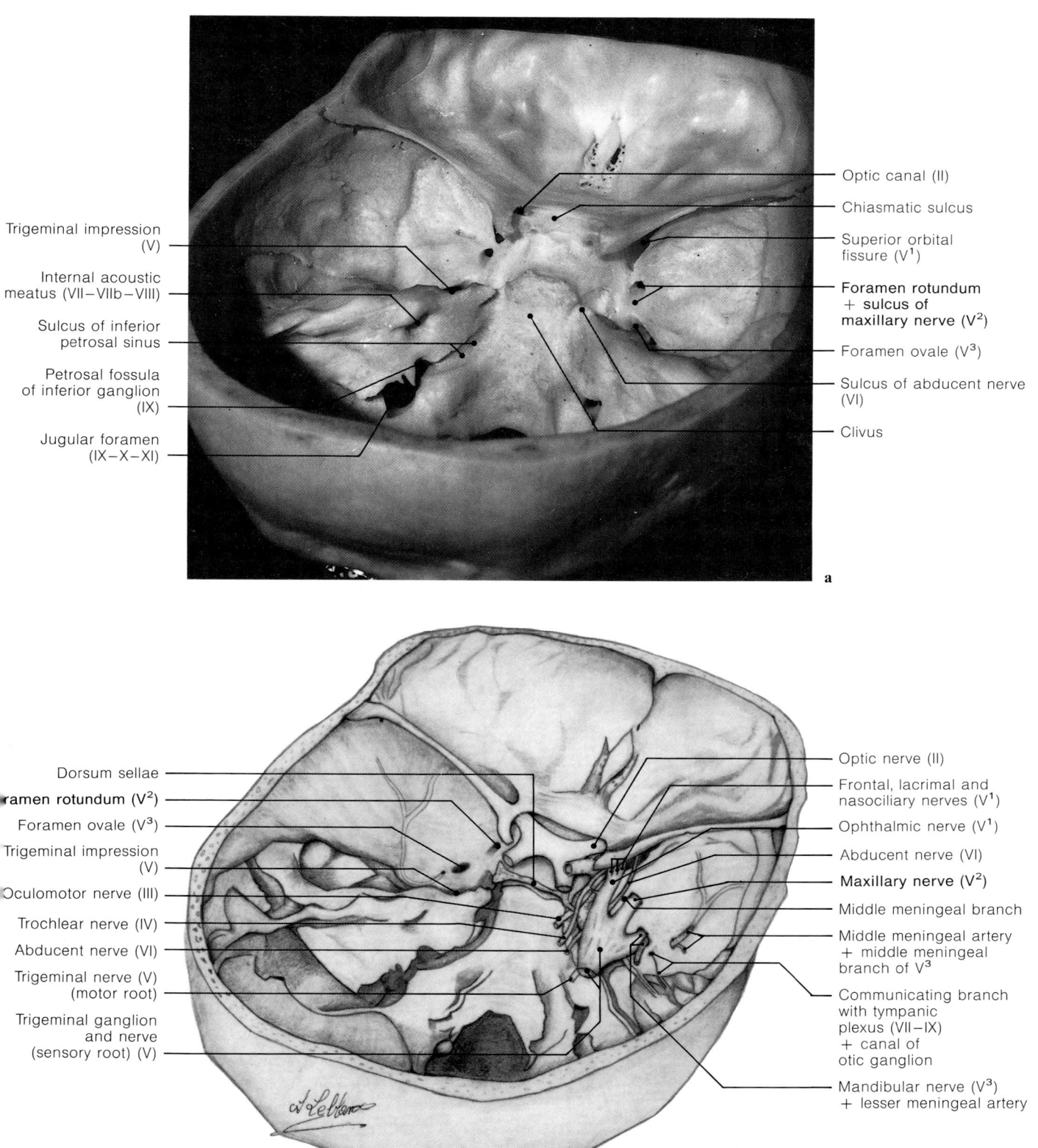

Fig. 5.41. a Superolateral intracranial view for foramina of trigeminal nerve; b diagram of trigeminal nerve and collaterals

Maxillary nerve (V^2): Foramen rotundum

Imaging

TECHNIQUE (OBLIQUE VIEW)

Study of foramen rotundum in unilateral oblique view:

- The subject is in dorsal decubitus, the head extended so that the vertical beam makes an angle of 35° with the orbitomeatal plane (OM);
- the head is turned away from the side to be examined by 5° in relation to the sagittal plane, so as to free the foramen rotundum from any overlying structures (Fig. 5.42c);
- the centering point is situated beneath the infraorbital rim, 2.5 cm lateral to the median plane (Fig. 5.42b).

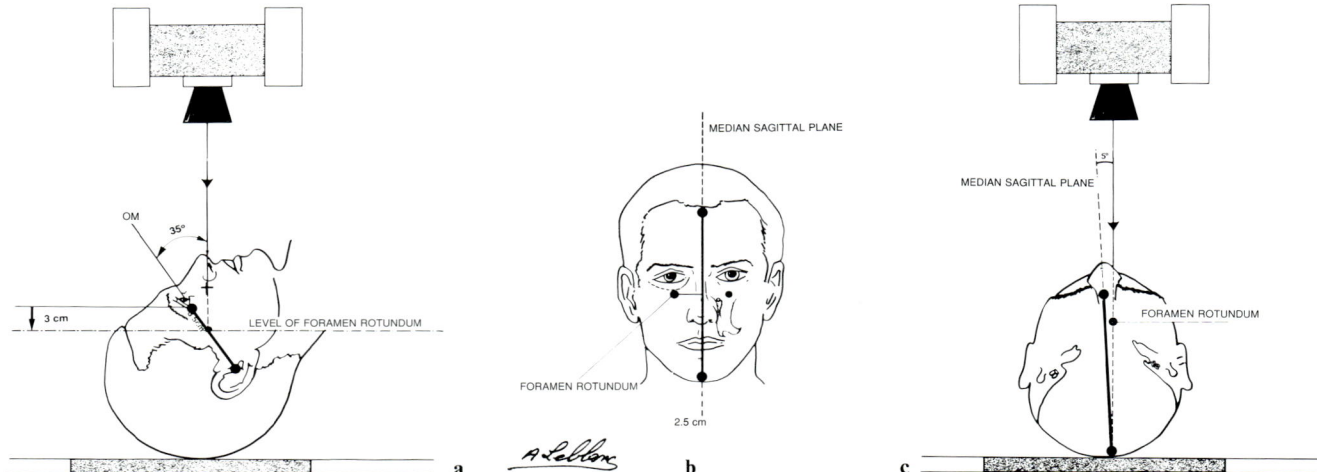

Fig. 5.42a–c. Centering diagrams for study of foramen rotundum in unilateral oblique view

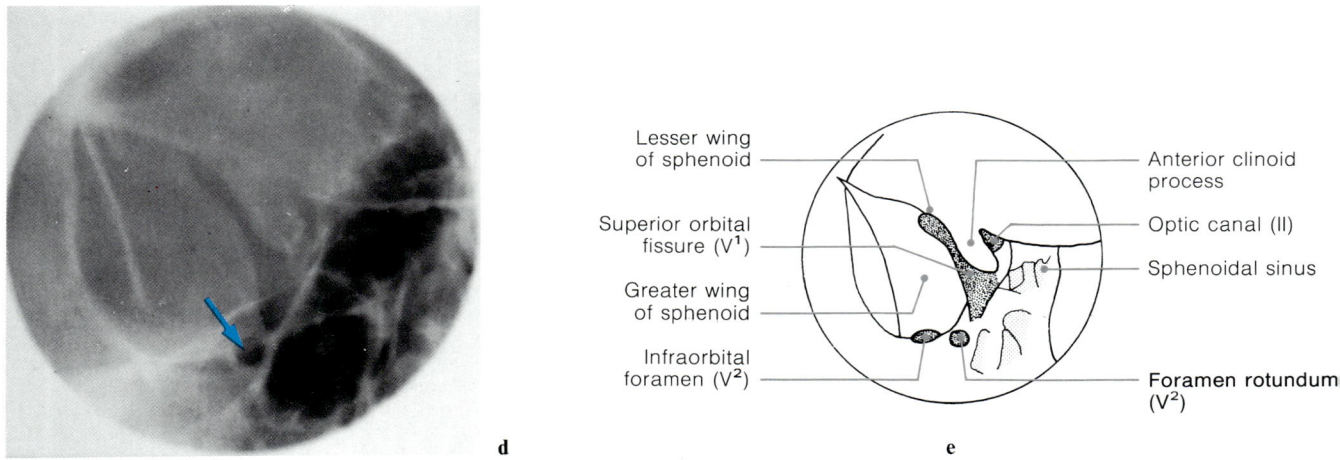

Fig. 5.42d, e. Radiograph (d) and diagram (e) of foramen rotundum in oblique view

Maxillary nerve (V²): Foramen rotundum

Imaging

TECHNIQUE (DISCONTINUOUS SCANNING)

Study of foramen rotundum in unilateral view:

- The patient's head remains in the same position as for the previous view (Fig. 5.42a–c);
- but the tube is now inclined by about 5° in relation to the centering point (Fig. 5.43);
- several films are taken in succession after each rotation of the tube (Fig. 5.54).

Note: This examination is easy to perform and provides good films of the walls of the foramen rotundum.

Fig. 5.43. Centering diagram for study of foramen rotundum by "discontinuous scanning"

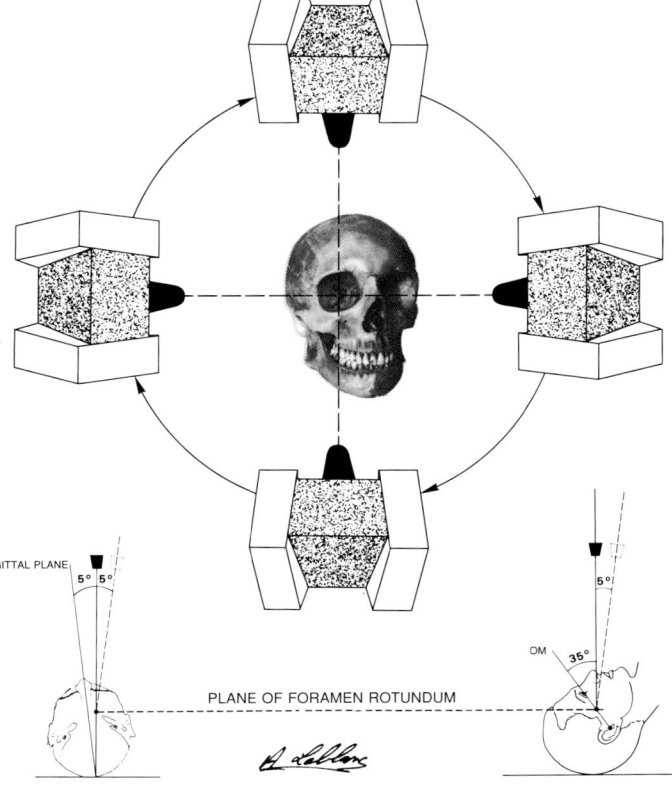

Fig. 5.44. Frontal magnetic resonance imaging (MRI) of maxillary nerve at foramen rotundum (V²). (MRI: Dr. J.W. Casselman, A.Z. St-Jan, Brugge)

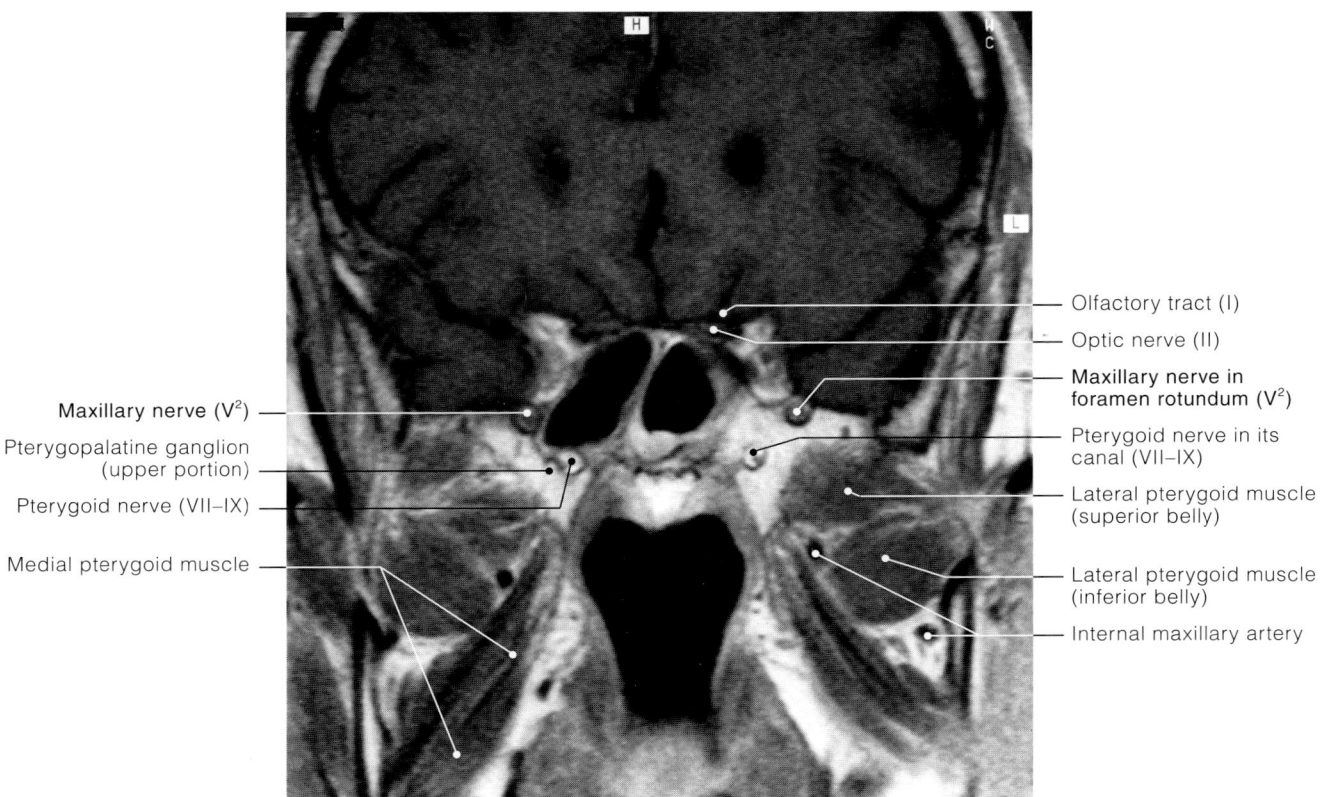

Maxillary nerve (V²): Foramen rotundum (See vascular relations, p. 279)

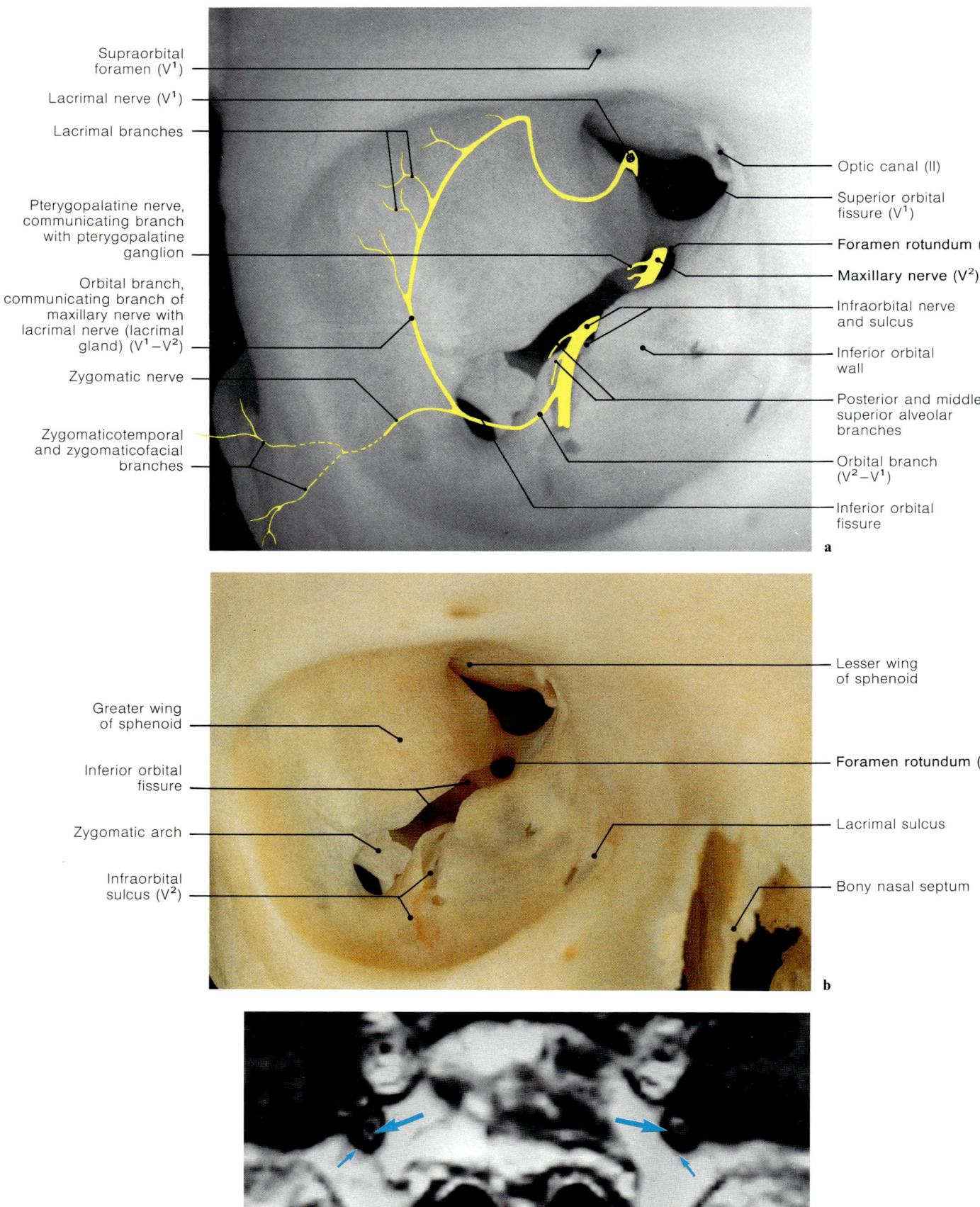

Fig. 5.45 a, b. Infraorbital views and diagram of anastomotic branch, orbital branch (V¹–V²); c frontal magnetic resonance imaging (MRI) of maxillary nerve (V²) (arrows) in its foramen rotundum (small arrows)

Maxillary nerve (V²): Foramen rotundum

Imaging

TECHNIQUE (SAGITTAL VIEW)

Sagittal tomographic study of foramen rotundum:
The technique and centering point are very much the same as for the sagittal view of the pterygopalatine fossa.

- The subject is in lateral decubitus in the "gun-dog" position. The head is in strict lateral position, resting on non-opaque blocks and well immobilized by flour bags;

- after having identified the orbitomeatal plane (OM), a centering point "A" is traced 3.5 cm in front of the external acoustic meatus;
- a point "B" is marked 1.5 cm away from the median sagittal plane on the side to be examined (Fig. 5.46 a);
- after centering on "A", a series of sections is made every 3 mm starting from "B" and travelling towards the outer side.

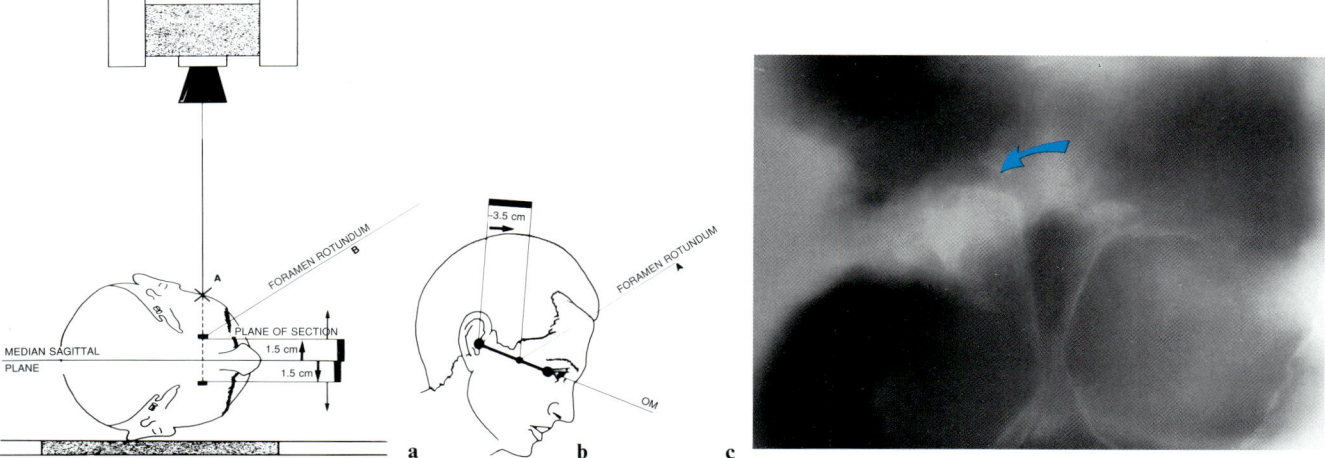

Fig. 5.46a, b. Centering diagrams for tomographic study of the foramen rotundum in sagittal view

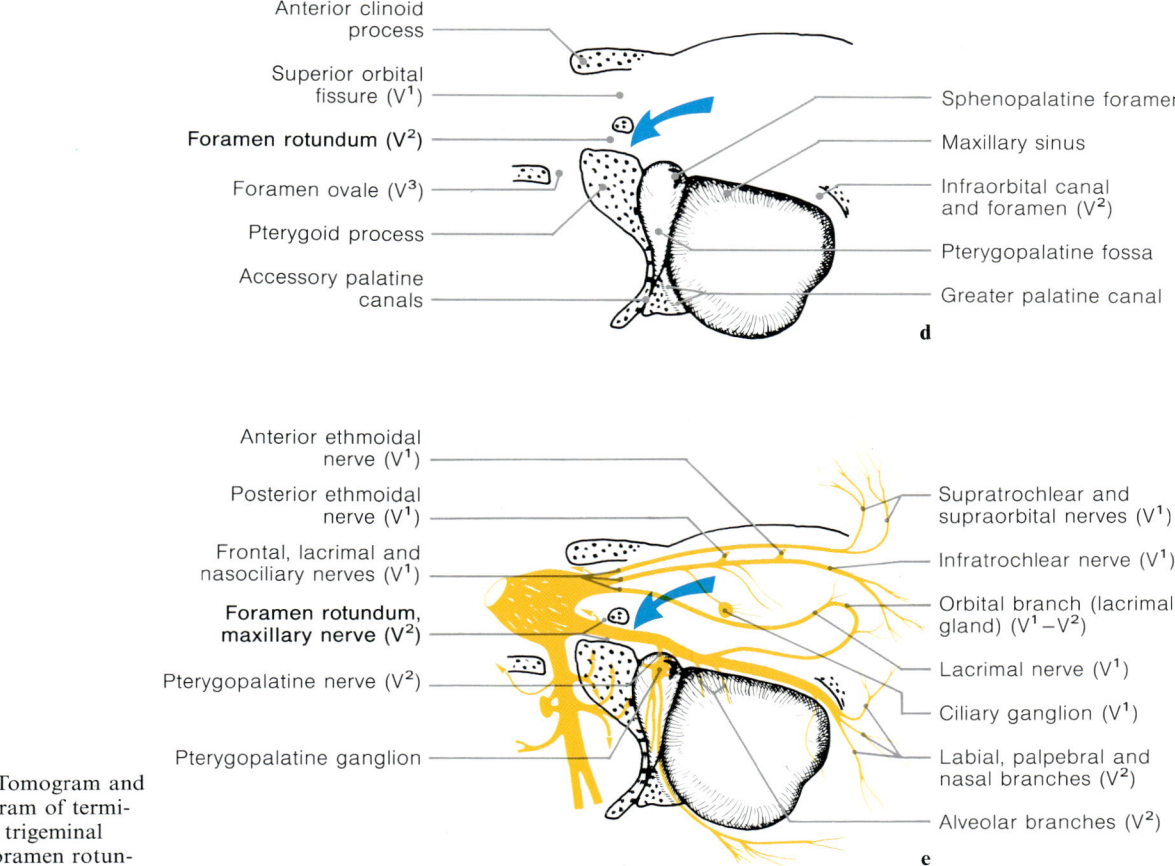

Fig. 5.46. c, d Tomogram and diagram; **e** diagram of terminal branches of trigeminal nerve; arrow: foramen rotundum

Maxillary nerve (V²): Foramen rotundum

Imaging

TECHNIQUE (AXIAL VIEW)

Axial imaging of foramina rotunda in symmetric view:

- The subject is in dorsal decubitus, the back raised on pillows and the head extended in extreme Hirtz view;
- the orbitomeatal plane (OM) makes an angle of about 15° to the horizontal;
- the plane of section passes through a point "A" situated at 3.5 cm on the orbitomeatal plane (OM) starting from the external acoustic meatus; "A" is also the centering point;
- the sections start from "A" and are made every 3 mm rising towards the chin over a depth of 1 cm.

Note: This examination of the foramina rotunda in axial view is practicable only by computed tomography (CT) or spiral scanning tomography (Fig. 5.48–5.50).

Figures 5.47 and 5.49 represent tomographic and computed tomographic (CT) sections of the foramina rotunda with superimposition of the diagram of the maxillary nerve (V²) in bayonet shape, traversing the foramen rotundum, skirting the inferior orbital fissure, entering the infraorbital sulcus and infraorbital foramen, and giving rise at its exit to the labial, palpebral and nasal branches.

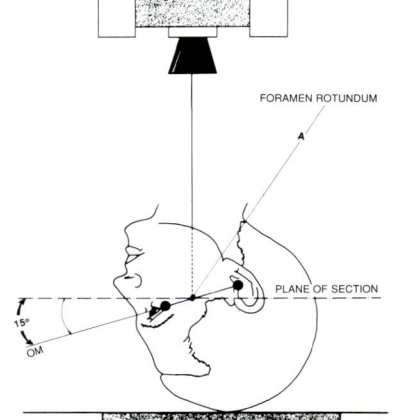

Fig. 5.47a, b. Centering diagram for tomographic study (**a**); axial tomogram of foramina rotunda with diagram of course of maxillary nerve (V²) (**b**)

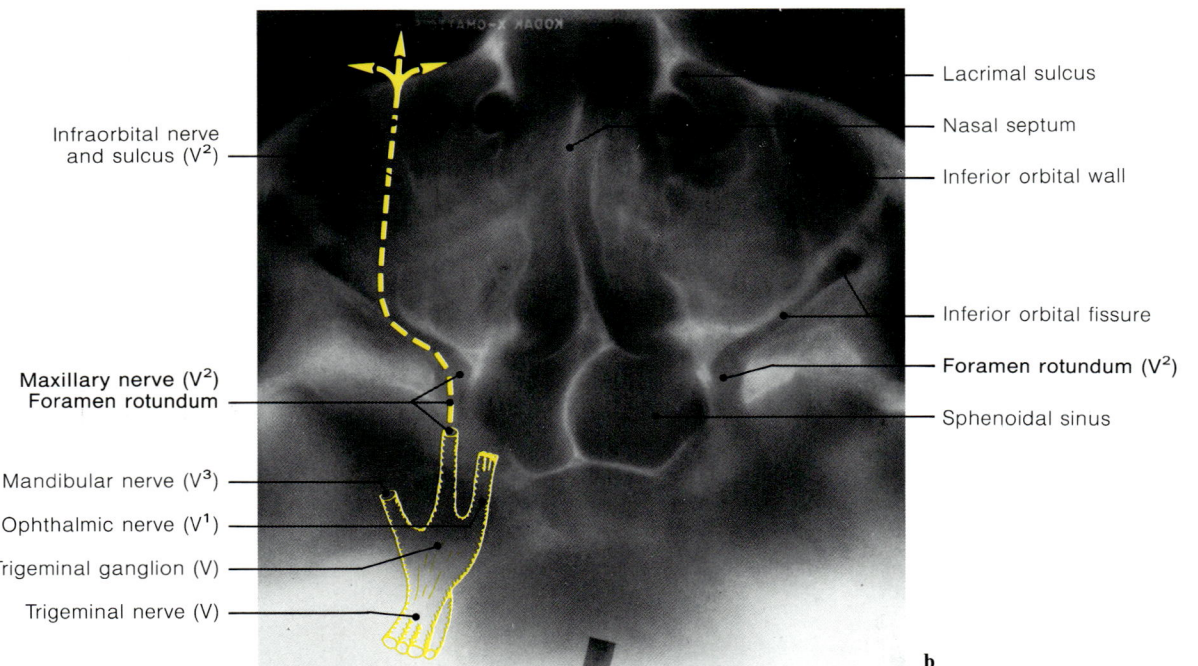

Maxillary nerve (V²): Foramen rotundum

Computed tomography (CT)

For computed tomography (CT) or magnetic resonance imaging (MRI) of the maxillary nerve (Fig. 5.48), the head is extended more than for the study of the foramen rotundum of Fig. 5.47a. This permits display of the entire course of the maxillary nerve (V²), from its origin as far as the infraorbital nerve.
For this study, the head is extended in extreme Hirtz view, so that the orbitomeatal plane makes an angle of about 20° to 30° to the centering plane.
(For the plane of section, see previous p. 106.)

Displayed: the course of the maxillary nerve from the trigeminal ganglion to the foramen rotundum, infraorbital sulcus and sometimes as far as the infraorbital foramen, the cavernous sinus, internal carotid artery, hypophysis, infundibulum and optic tracts.

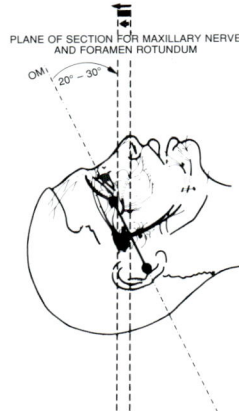

Fig. 5.48. Centering diagram for computed tomography (CT) and magnetic resonance imaging (MRI)

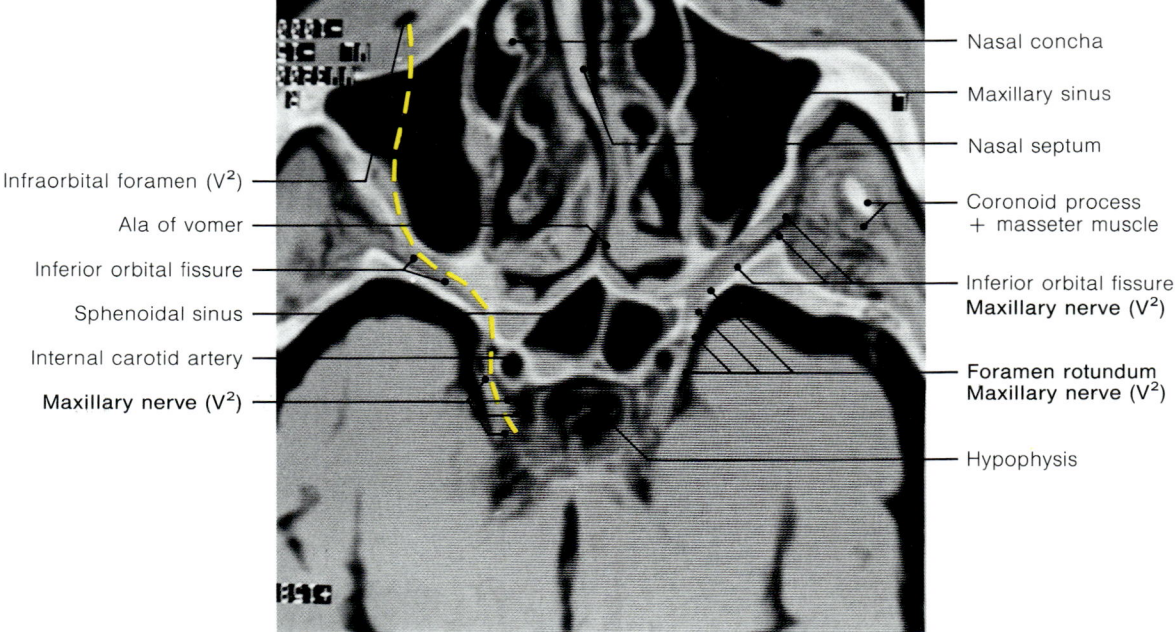

Fig. 5.49. Axial computed tomographic (CT) section of foramina rotunda and maxillary nerves (V²)

Maxillary nerve (V^2): Foramen rotundum

Magnetic resonance imaging (MRI) and computed tomography (CT)

Axial views

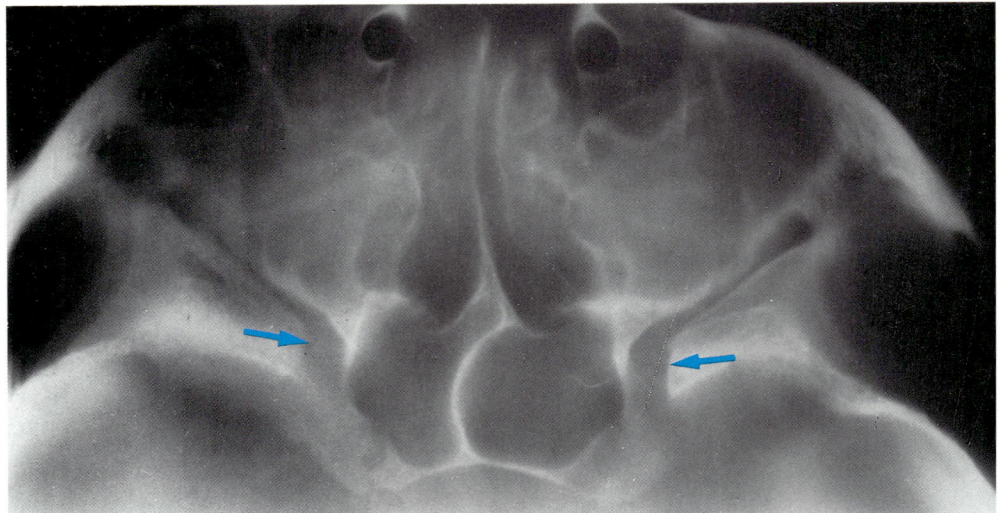

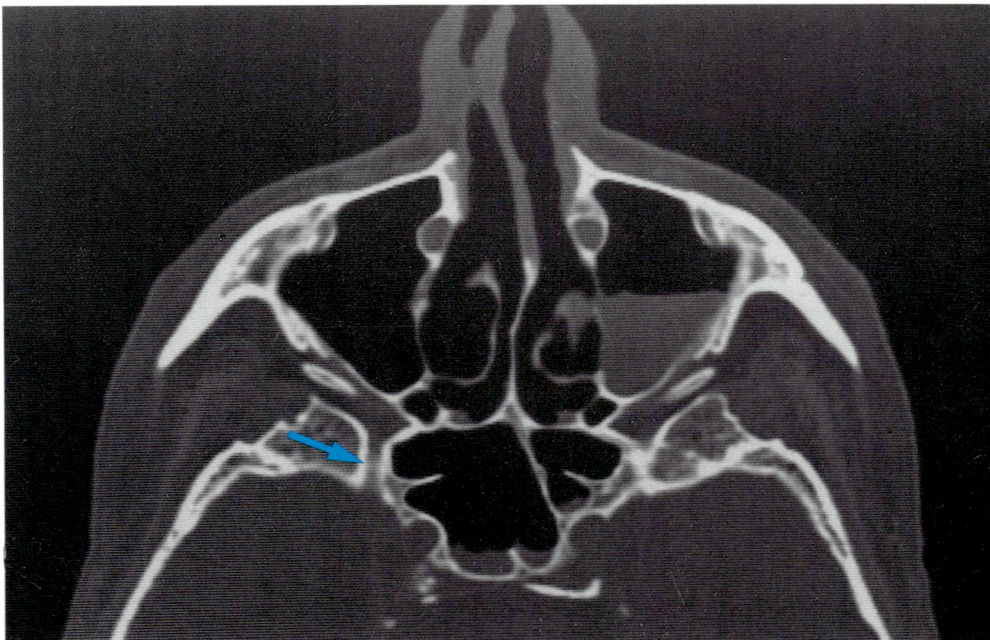

Fig. 5.50. a–c Conventional axial tomograms of foramina rotunda; **d** axial computed tomography (CT) of foramina rotunda and maxillary nerves (V^2); *dots*, course of maxillary nerve (V^2); *arrows*, foramen rotundum (V^2); **e** axial magnetic resonance imaging (MRI) of trigeminal recess ensheathing the trigeminal ganglion and of the mandibular nerve, visualizing throughout its passage in the foramen rotundum (V^2). (MRI and CT: Pr. Doyon, Hospital Kremlin Bicêtre, Paris)

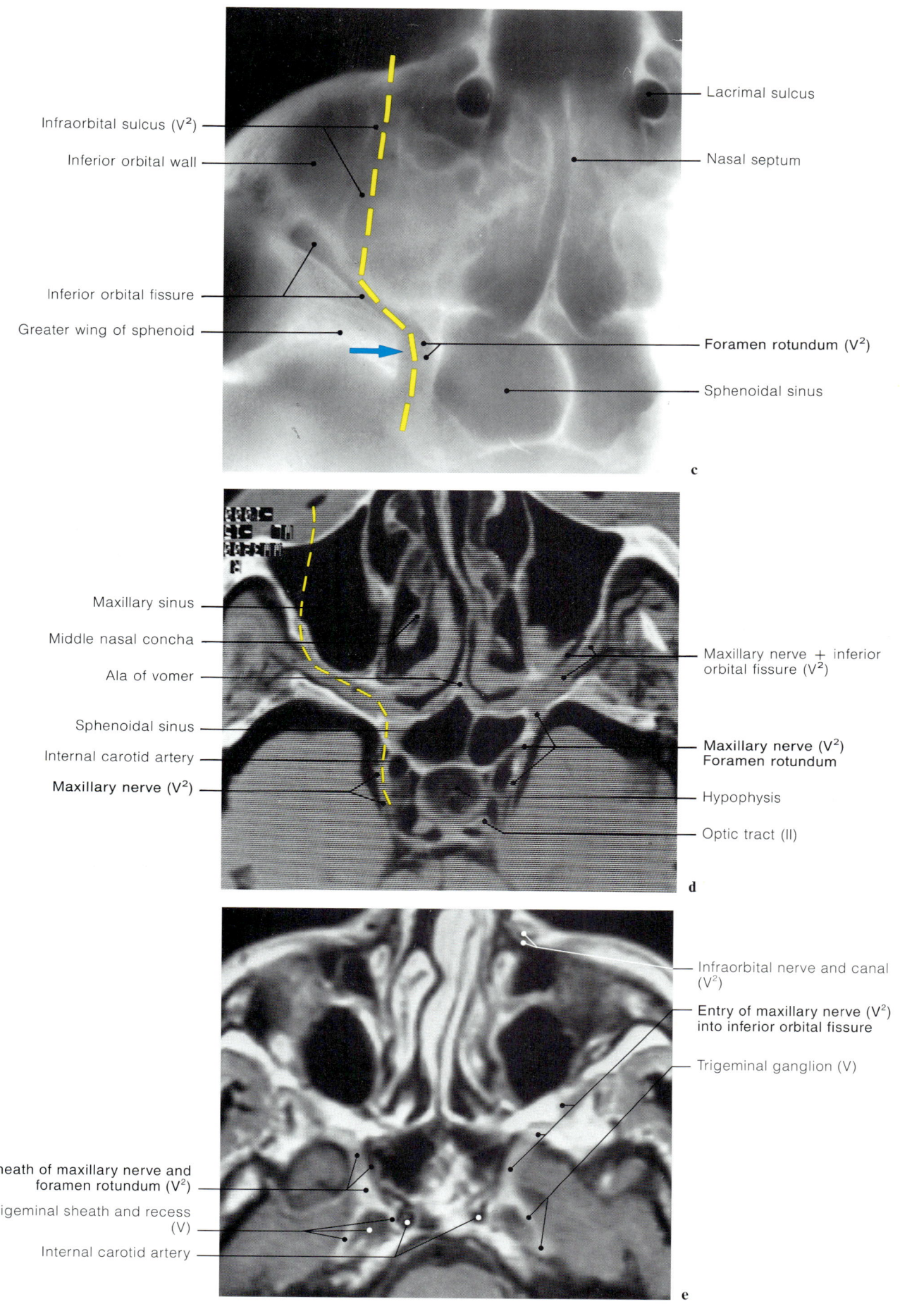

Topography

Infraorbital nerve (V²)
– Infraorbital sulcus

Pathology

– Orbital tumor,
– tumor of maxillary sinus,
– fracture of infraorbital wall,
– fracture of the superior wall of the maxillary sinus,
– neurinoma of infraorbital sulcus,
– trigeminal neuralgia (type V²).

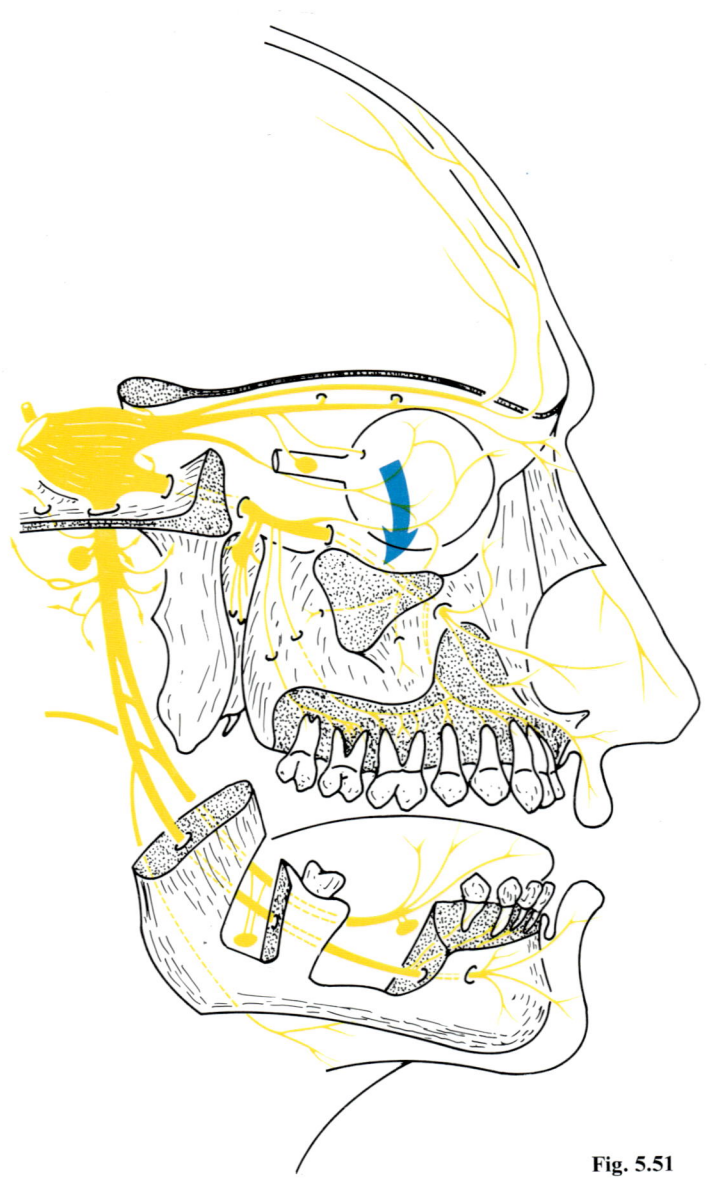

Fig. 5.51

Infraorbital nerve (V²): Infraorbital sulcus

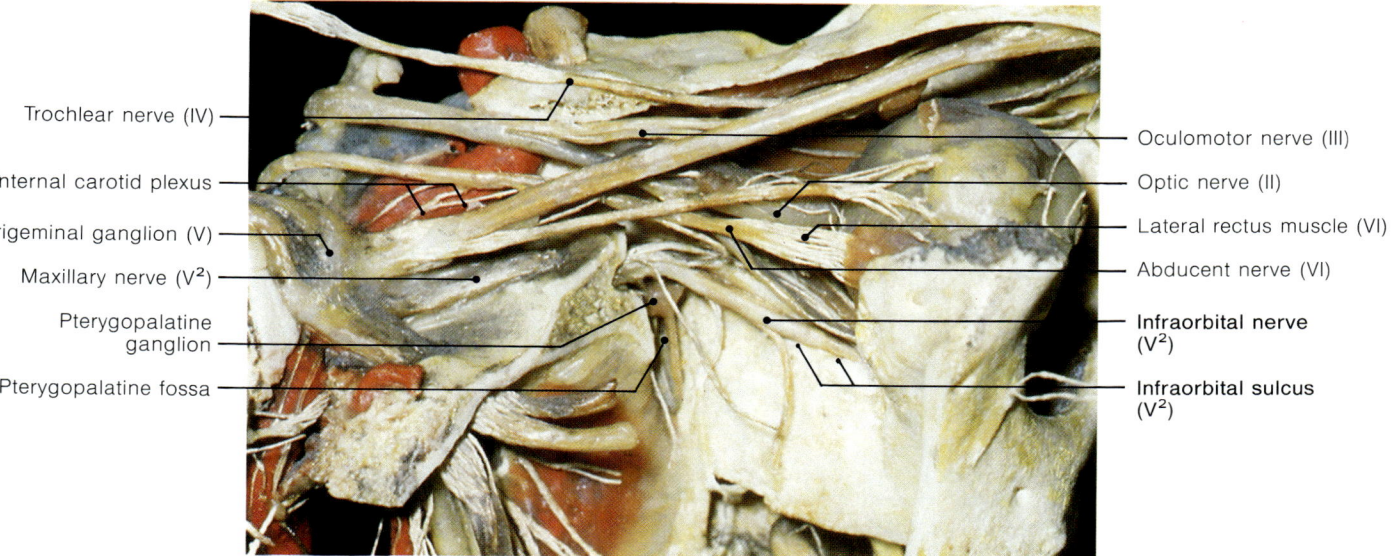

Fig. 5.52a. Anatomic dissection displaying infraorbital nerve (V²)

Infraorbital nerve (V²): Infraorbital sulcus (See vascular relations, p. 281)

Anatomy

The infraorbital or maxillary nerve (V²), after having traversed the foramen rotundum, enters the depths of the pterygopalatine fossa. Within this cavity it follows an oblique course downward, forward and outward, emerges from the depths into the pterygopalatine fossa proper, and then reaches the posterior end of the infraorbital sulcus.

The maxillary nerve then changes direction for the second time, entering first the infraorbital sulcus and then the infraorbital foramen to give rise at its exit to three terminal branches (Fig. 5.55b).

These two bends give the maxillary nerve the shape of a bayonet (Fig. 5.47b; 5.54).

The infraorbital sulcus traverses the inferior orbital wall diagonally and penetrates the superior wall of the maxillary sinus (Fig. 5.51; 5.55b).

Note: The orbit is separated from the maxillary sinus by a thin bony wall housing the infraorbital sulcus.

Morphologic variations sometimes exist, notably when the infraorbital nerve penetrates the maxillary sinus directly and the sulcus is absent.

The inferior orbital fissure separates the posterior wall of the orbit from the orbital floor (Fig. 5.55a).

Imaging

EXAMINATION

– Horizontal tomographic study in symmetric view of the infraorbital sulci and inferior orbital fissures.

TECHNIQUE

Axial tomographic or computed tomographic (CT) studies of the infraorbital sulci:

- The subject is in dorsal decubitus, the back raised on pillows, the head extended in extreme Hirtz view, the orbitomeatal plane (OM) making an angle of 40° to the horizontal in such a way that the infraorbital sulcus is parallel to the plane of the table;
- the centering point is situated on the median line 4 cm behind the mental symphysis;
- the tomographic sections are begun in the plane of the infraorbital rim, travelling towards the chin over a depth of 1 cm (Fig. 5.53a, b).

To obtain satisfactory films of the thin walls of the infraorbital sulcus when no scanner is available, it is essential for this examination to be conducted with a spiral scanning tomographic apparatus at 1 mm intervals.

Maxillary and infraorbital nerves (V²)

Magnetic resonance imaging (MRI)

AXIAL VIEWS

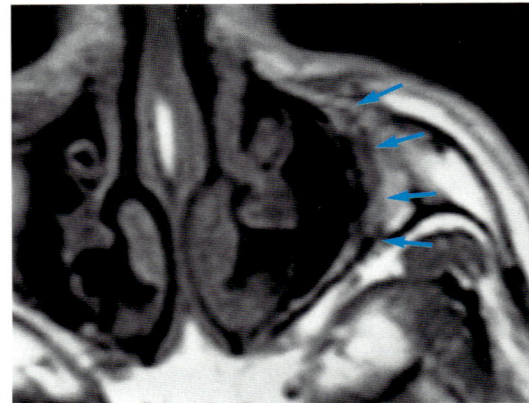

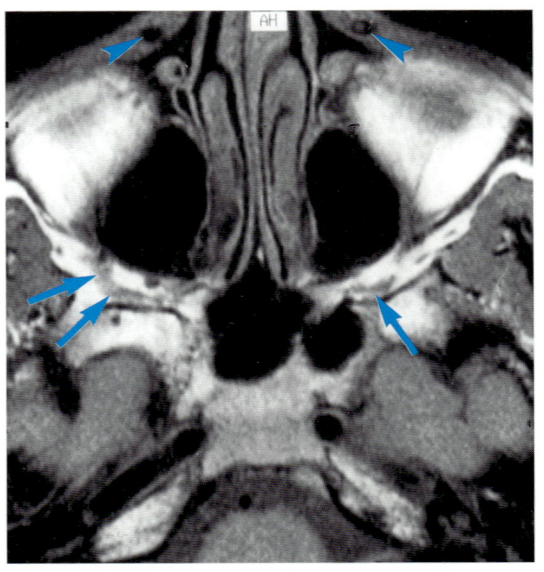

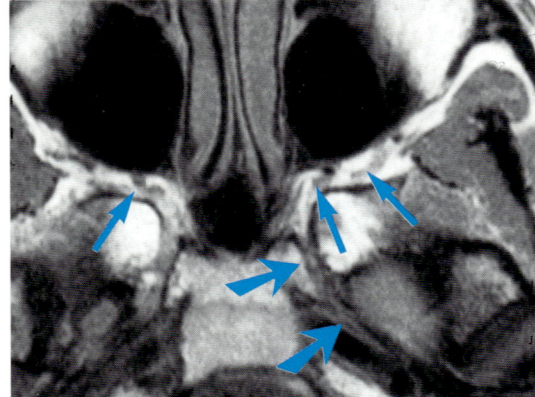

Fig. 5.52b–d. Axial magnetic resonance imaging (MRI) at level of inferior orbital fissures showing bayonet-shaped intersections of maxillary nerves (V²) (*straight arrows*), infraorbital nerves and grooves (*small arrows*), infraorbital nerves and canals (*arrowheads*), pterygoid nerve (*large arrows*). (MRI: Dr. J.W. Casselman, A.Z. St-Jan, Brugge)

Infraorbital nerve (V^2): Infraorbital sulcus

Tomography

AXIAL VIEW

4 cm
40°
1cm
PLANE OF SECTION
FOR INFRAORBITAL SULCI
OM

a

INFRAORBITAL
SULCUS
PLANE OF SECTION
1cm

b

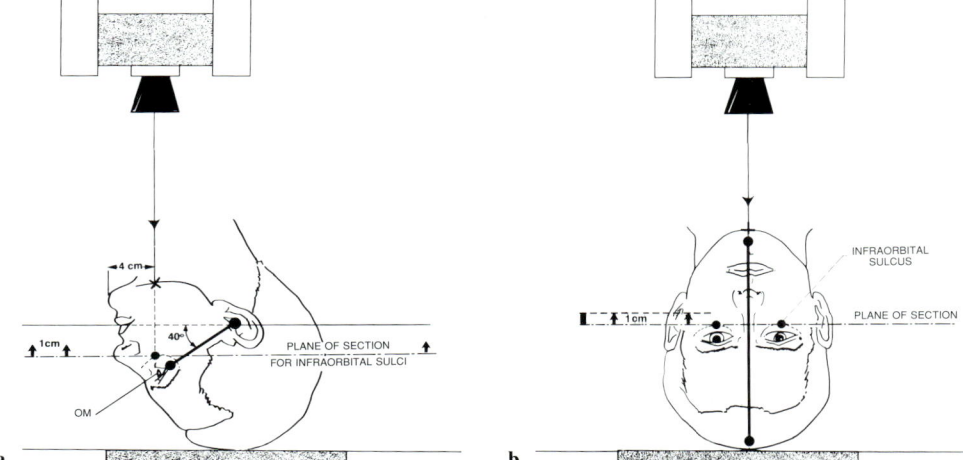

Fig. 5.53 a, b. Centering diagrams for computed tomographic (CT) or tomographic study of the infraorbital sulci in axial and symmetric views

Fig. 5.53 c–e. Tomography and diagram of infraorbital sulcus (V^2) in axial view; dotted: course of maxillary nerve

c

d

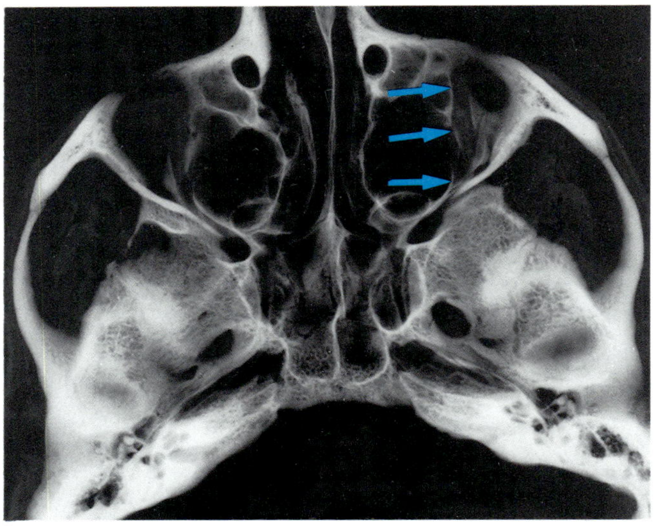

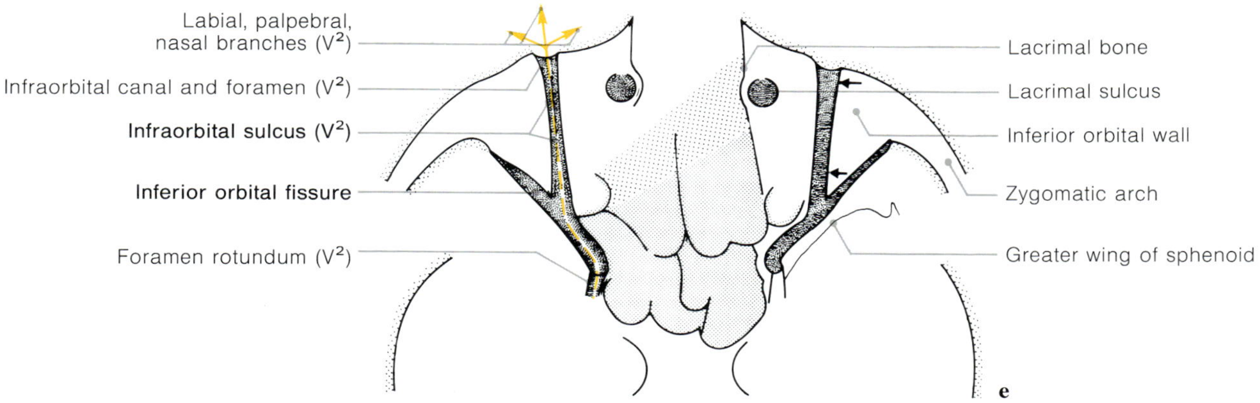

Labial, palpebral,
nasal branches (V²)
Infraorbital canal and foramen (V²)
Infraorbital sulcus (V²)
Inferior orbital fissure
Foramen rotundum (V²)
Lacrimal bone
Lacrimal sulcus
Inferior orbital wall
Zygomatic arch
Greater wing of sphenoid

e

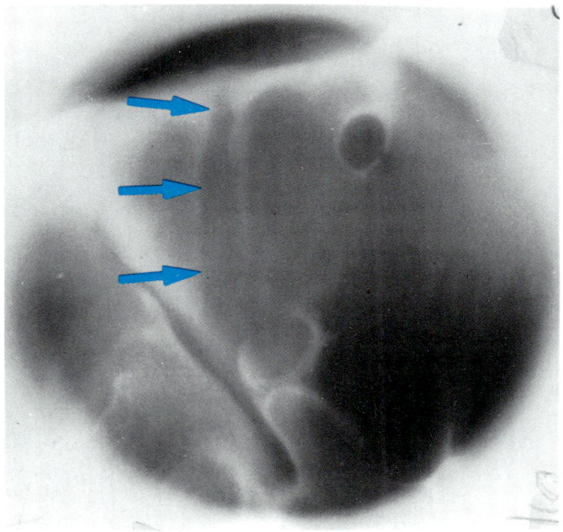

114 Trigeminal nerve (V)

Infraorbital nerve (V²): Infraorbital sulcus

Radiography

WORMS-BRETTON VIEW

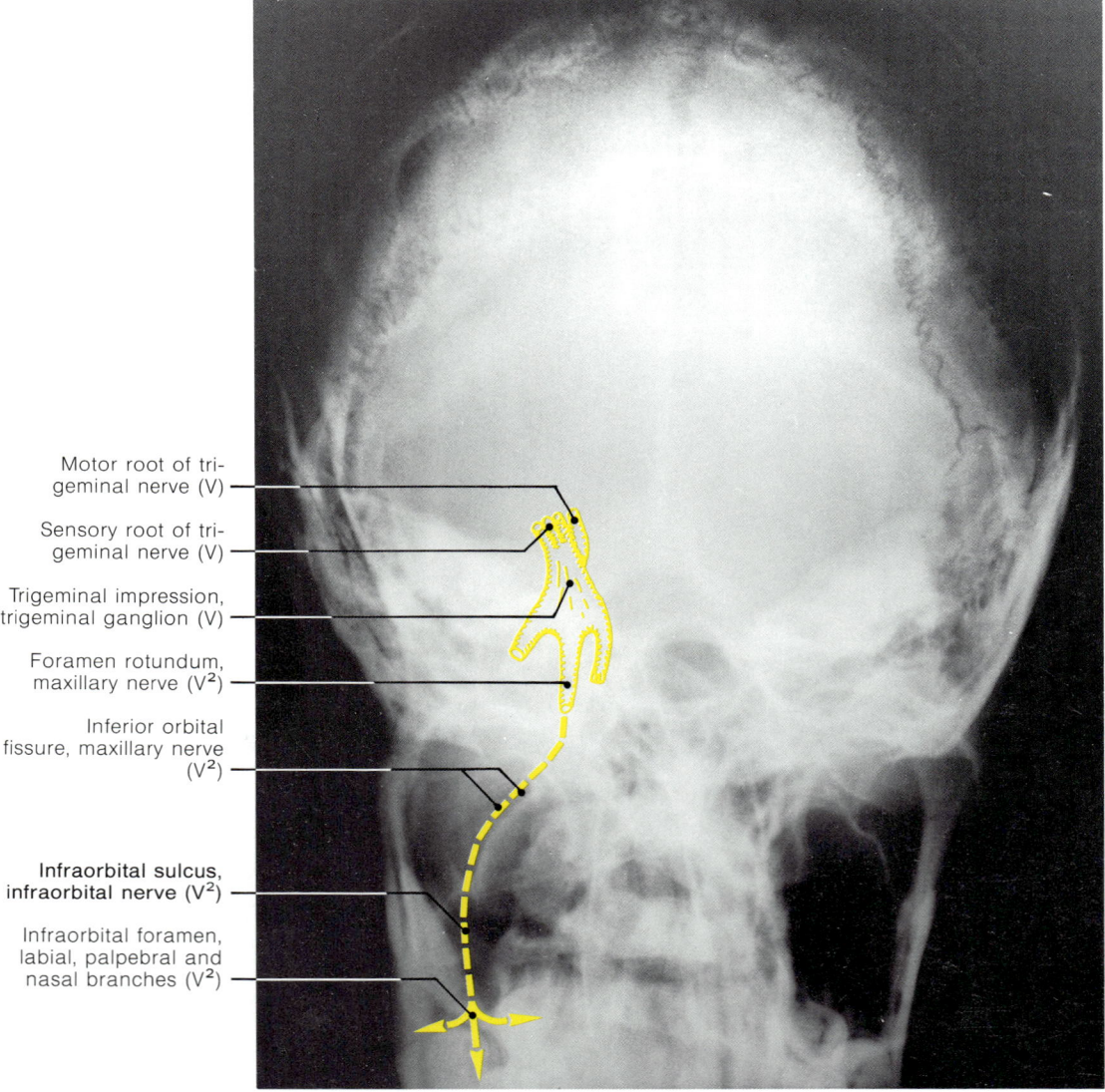

Fig. 5.54. Radiograph in Worms-Bretton view with diagram of the trigeminal nerve and course of the infraorbital nerve (V²) up to its terminal branches

Fig. 5.55 a, b. Intraorbital views with diagram of infraorbital nerve (V²)

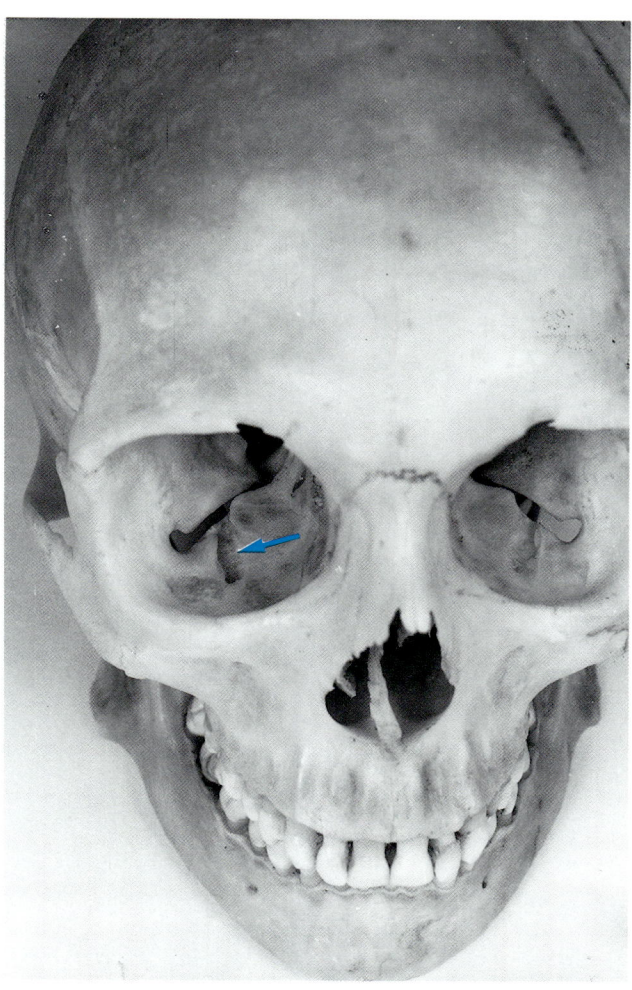

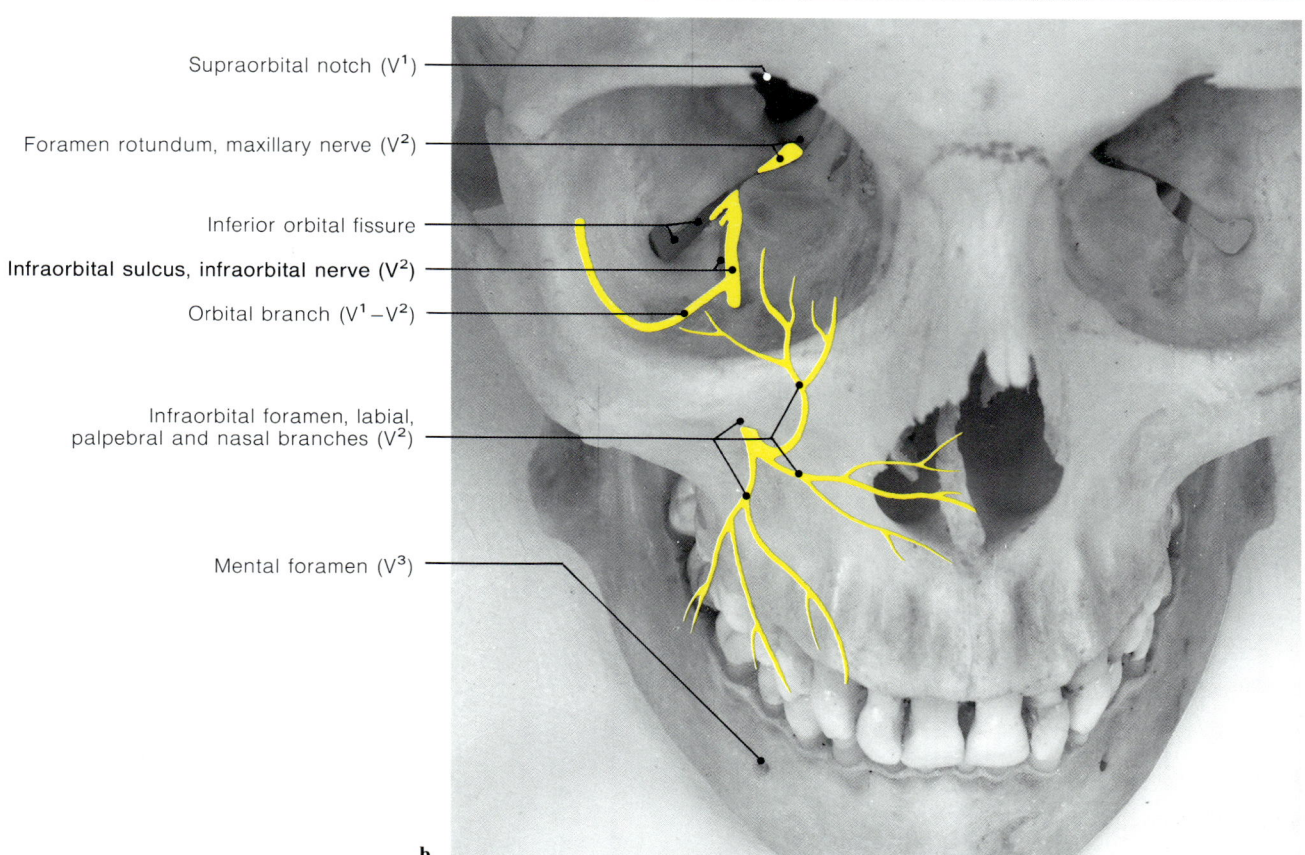

Infraorbital nerve (V²): Infraorbital sulcus

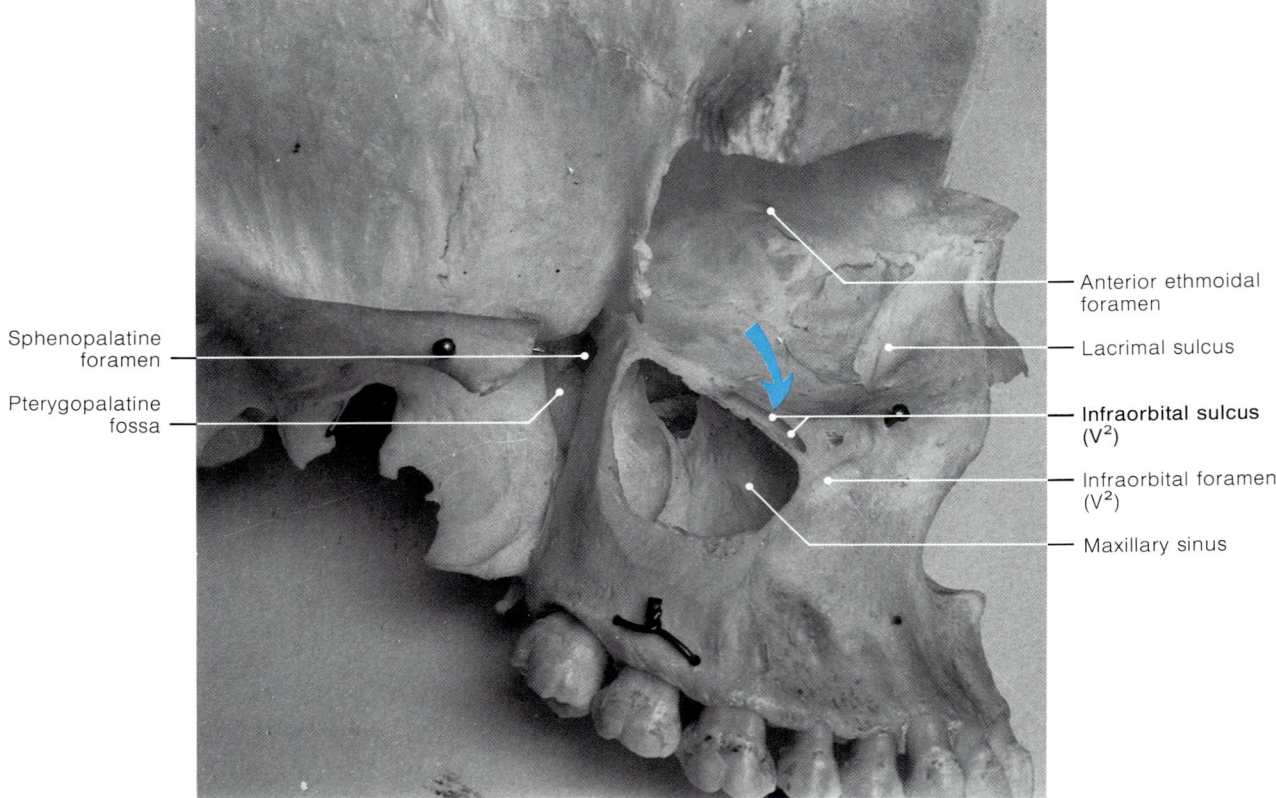

Fig. 5.56. Sagittal section of facial massif at level of infraorbital sulcus (V²)

Fig. 5.57. Diagram of infraorbital nerve, termination and collaterals

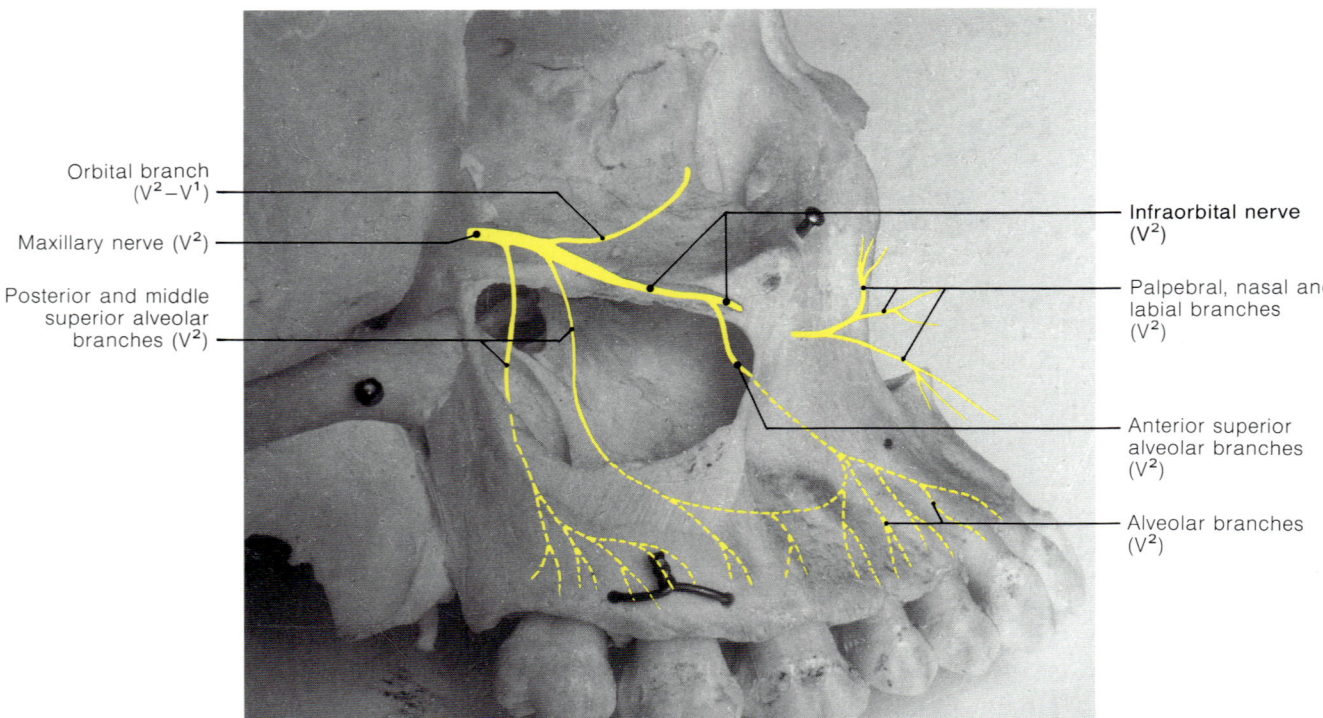

Maxillary nerve (V²)   117

Topography

Infraorbital nerve (V²)
- Infraorbital canal and foramen
- Labial, palpebral and nasal branches

Pathology

- Trigeminal neuralgia (type V²),
- depressed fracture of zygomatic bone,
- fractures of infraorbital margin,
- tumors of maxillary sinus.

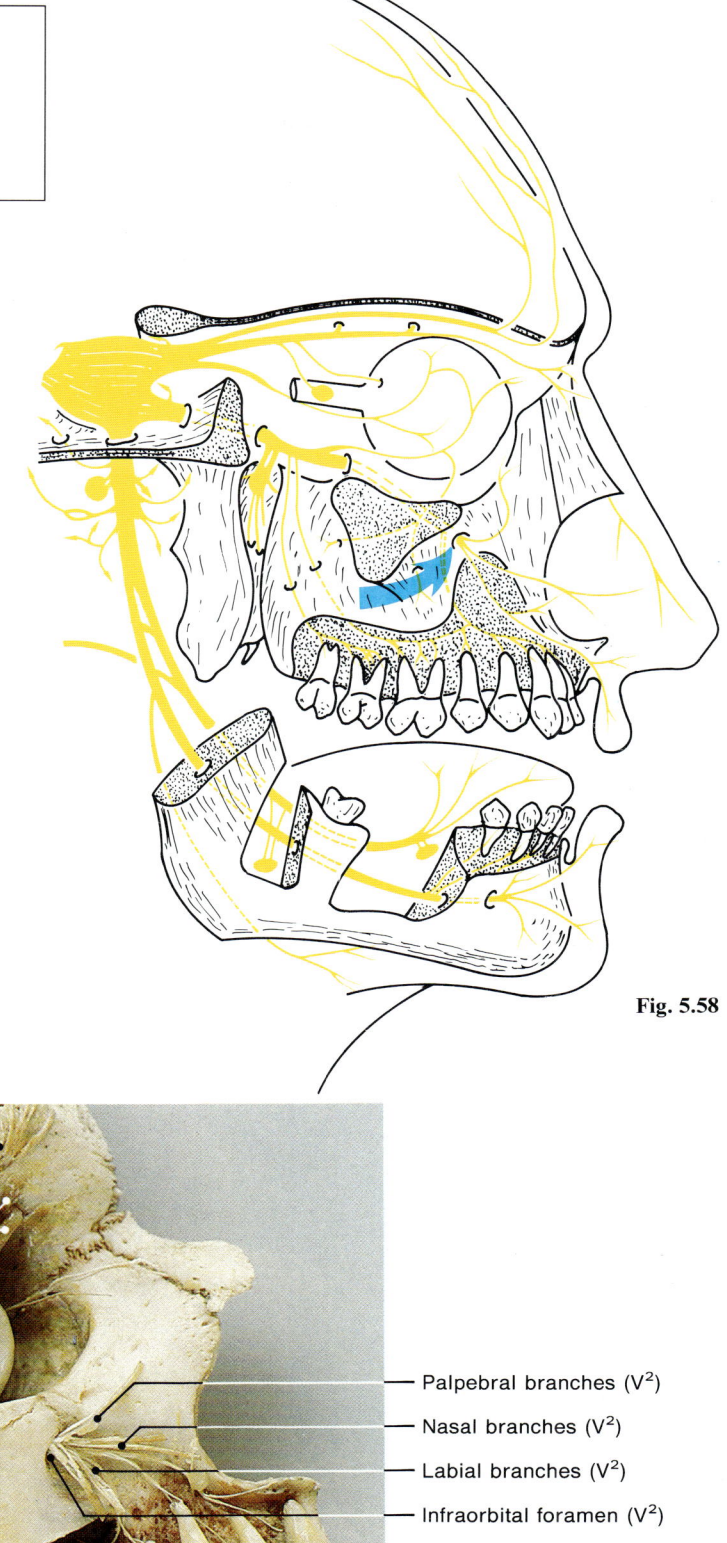

Fig. 5.58

Fig. 5.59. Anatomic dissection of infraorbital branches

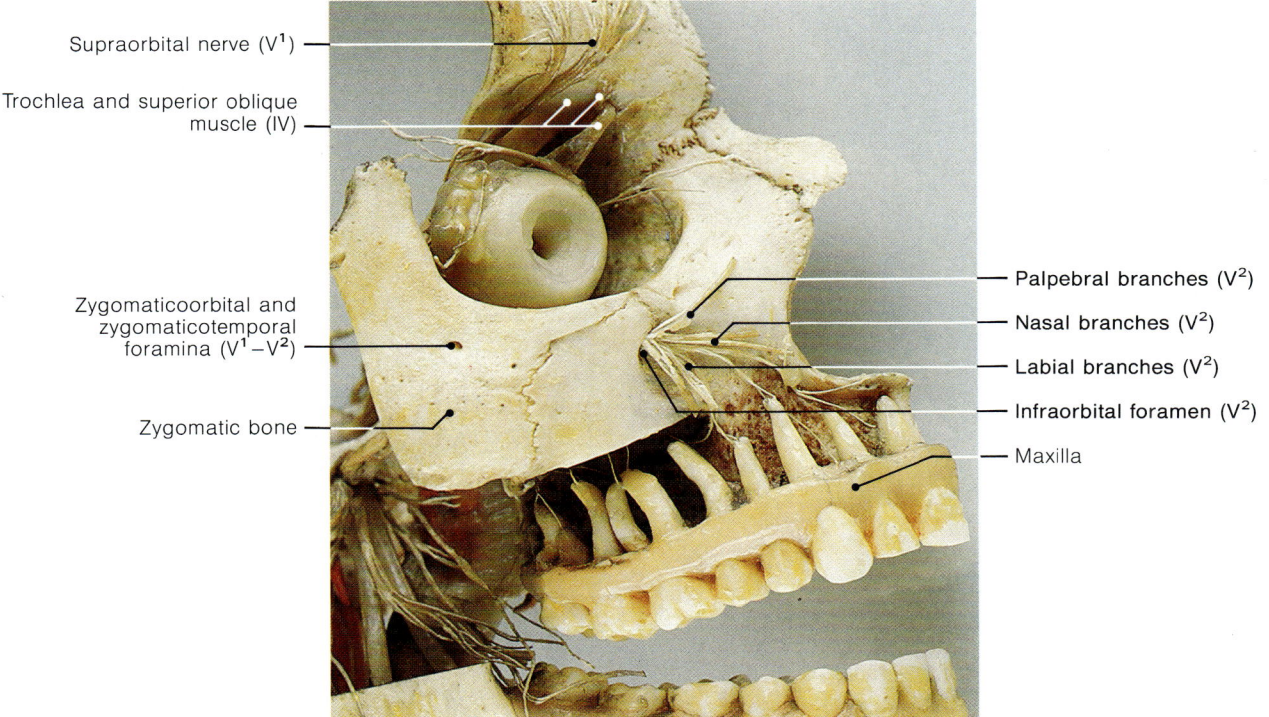

Infraorbital canal and foramen: Labial, palpebral and nasal branches (V^2)

Anatomy

After emerging from the infraorbital canal and foramen, the maxillary nerve (V^2) divides into several terminal branches:

- the descending or labial branches,
- the ascending or palpebral branches,
- the medial or nasal branches (Fig. 5.59).

The *labial branches* travel to the skin and mucosa of the cheek and upper lip, the *palpebral branches* travel to the lower eyelid, and the *nasal branches* ramify over the nasal coverings.

The infraorbital foramen marks the end of the infraorbital sulcus beneath the infraorbital rim, taking a vertical direction (Fig. 5.63 b, c).

It is situated about 2.5 cm lateral to the sagittal plane, 1 cm below the infraorbital margin (Fig. 5.60 b, c).

Imaging

Examination

- Survey study in Blondeau view (Fig. 5.60 d, e),
- frontal and symmetric radiographs and computed tomographic (CT) sections,
- unilateral radiographic study of infraorbital foramen in "discontinuous scanning",
- CT scan or tomographic study in sagittal view.

Technique

Radiologic and computed tomographic study of infraorbital foramina in frontal and symmetric view:

- The subject is in dorsal decubitus, the back elevated on pillows, the head facing directly forward and extended so that the incident beam makes an angle of 70° with the orbitomeatal plane (OM) (Fig. 5.60);
- the centering point is situated at the median line, 1 cm below the infraorbital margin;
- the plane of section begins at the level of the infraorbital margin. The sections are made travelling towards the chin over an extent of about 1 cm (Fig. 5.60 a).

Maxillary nerve (V²)   119

Infraorbital canal and foramen: Labial, palpebral and nasal branches (V²)

Computed tomography (CT)

FRONTAL VIEW

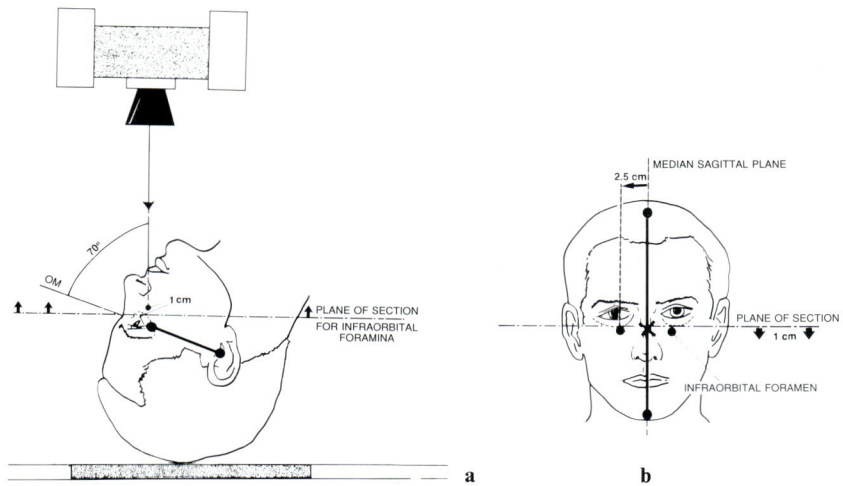

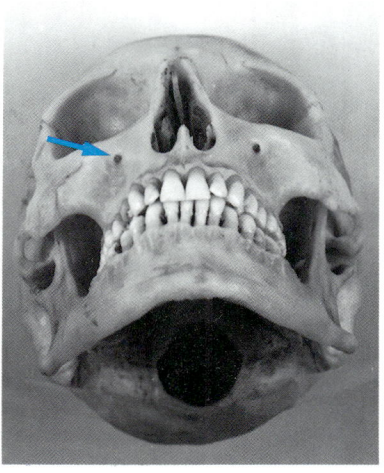

Fig. 5.60 a, b. Centering diagrams for computed tomographic (CT) and radiographic study of infraorbital canals and foramina

Fig. 5.60 c. Axis of infraorbital foramina (V²)

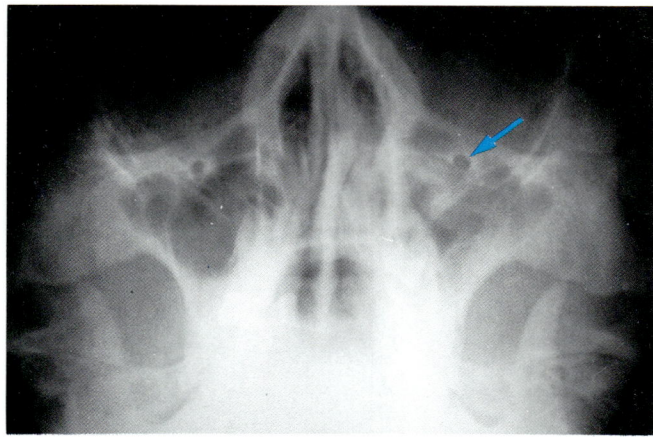

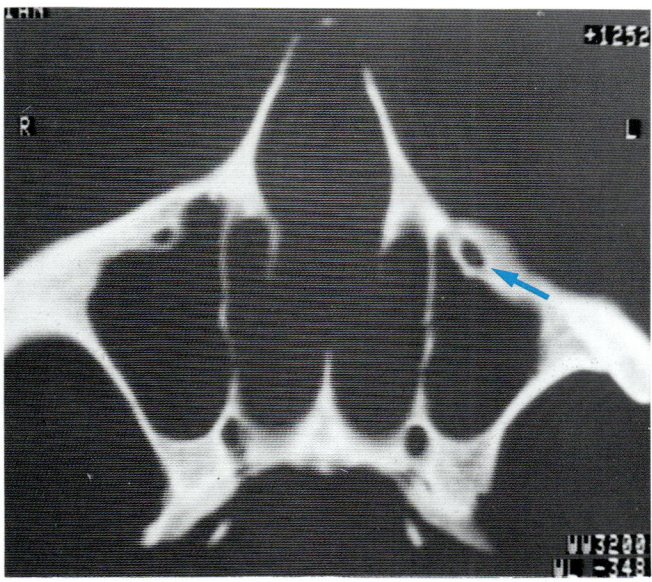

Fig. 5.60 d – g. Computed tomography (CT), tomography and conventional radiograph of infraorbital foramina (V²)

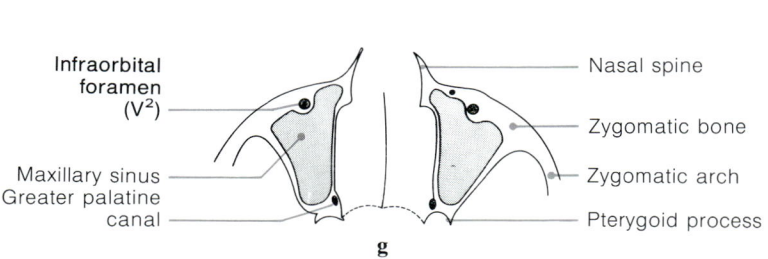

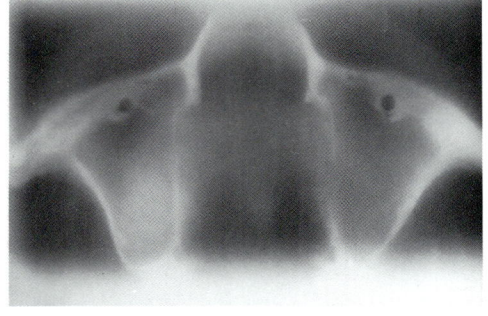

Infraorbital canal and foramen: Labial, palpebral and nasal branches (V²)

Imaging

TECHNIQUE (DISCONTINUOUS SCANNING)

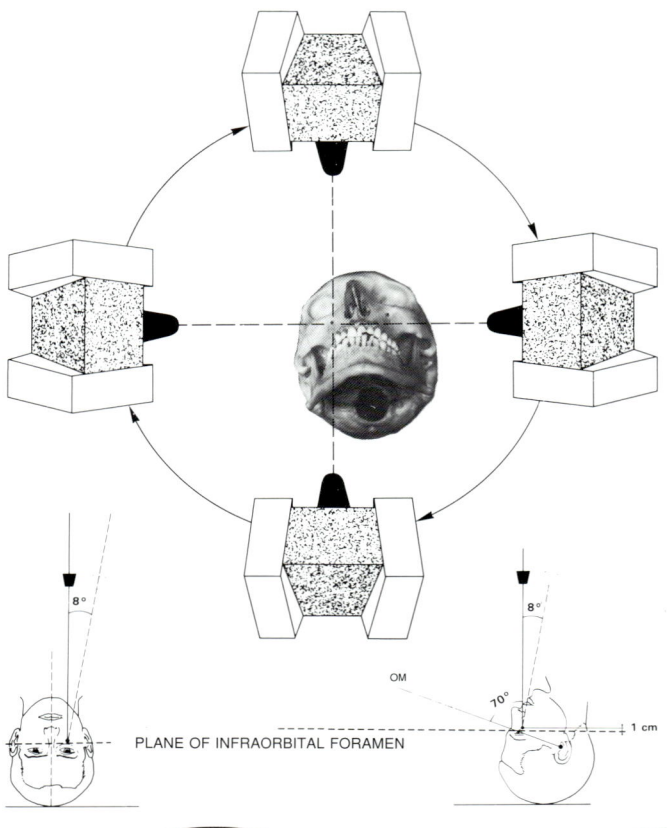

Unilateral study of infraorbital foramen:
The view is identical with that previously described (Fig. 5.60a). The tube is inclined by 7°. Four films are taken in succession during a complete rotation of the tube (Fig. 5.61).

Note: This technique gives good definition of all the margins of the infraorbital canal and foramen.
If the equipment does not allow circular movement of the tube, it is simple to incline the head very slightly (rotation before taking each film).

Fig. 5.61. Centering diagram for study of the infraorbital foramen by "discontinuous scanning"

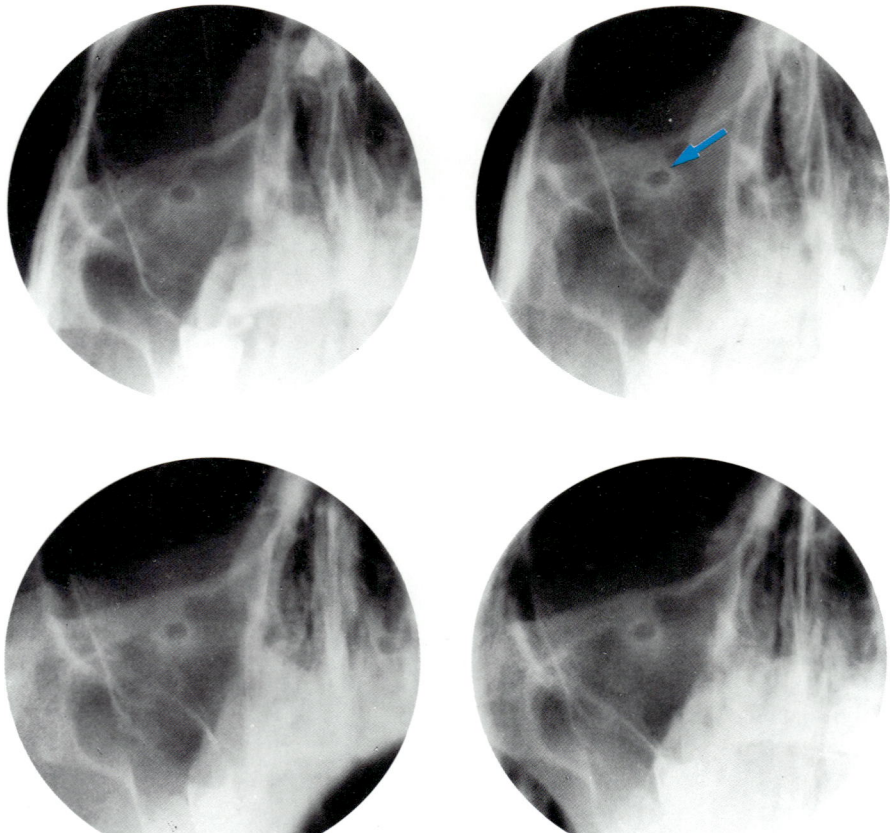

Fig. 5.62. Radiographs of infraorbital foramen by "discontinuous scanning"

Maxillary nerve (V²)   121

Infraorbital canal and foramen: Labial, palpebral and nasal branches (V²)

Imaging

(See vascular relations, p. 281)

TECHNIQUE (SAGITTAL VIEW)

- The subject is prone, the head strictly in side-view. Flour bags are placed in front of the facial massif to obtain good homogeneity of the region to be radiographed and to diminish diffused radiation;
- the centering point is situated at the inferolateral orbital angle (Fig. 5.63 a, b);
- the plane of section is situated 2.5 cm lateral to the median sagittal plane.

The sections are made starting from this plane and moving laterally for about 1 cm.

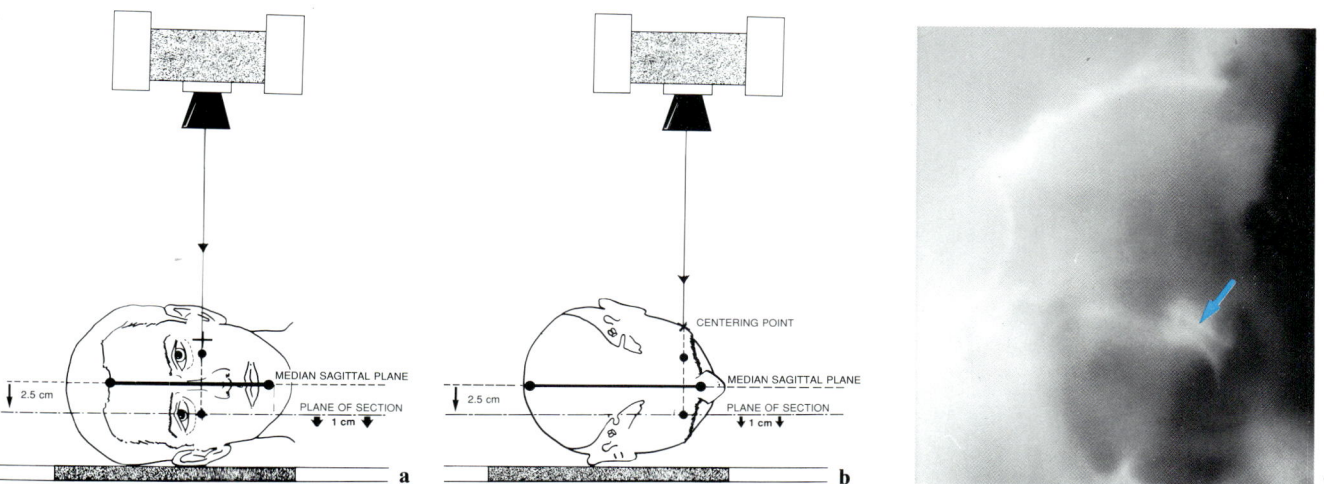

Fig. 5.63. a, b Centering diagrams for sagittal study of infraorbital canal and foramen; c sagittal tomographic section of infraorbital canal and foramen; d, e diagram of film and of infraorbital branches; f sagittal magnetic resonance imaging (MRI) of infraorbital nerve (V²) in its groove (*arrows*) and infraorbital canal (*curved arrows*).

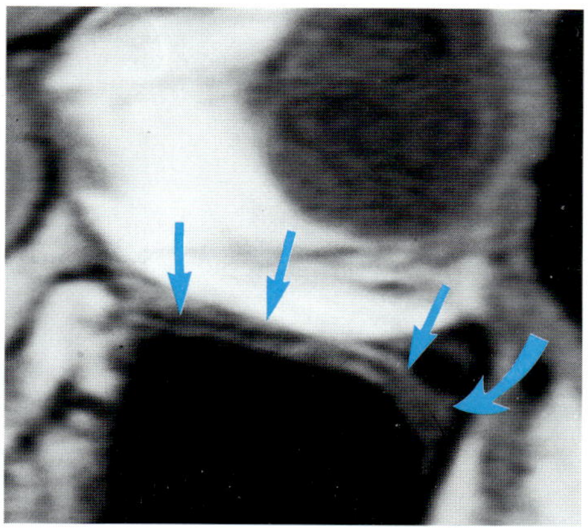

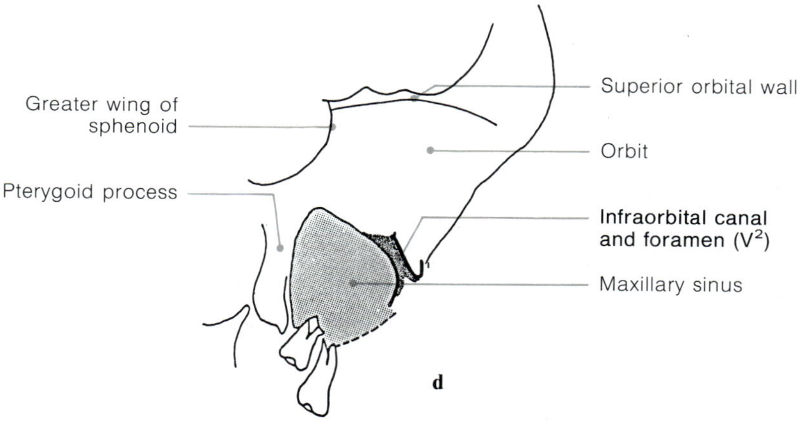

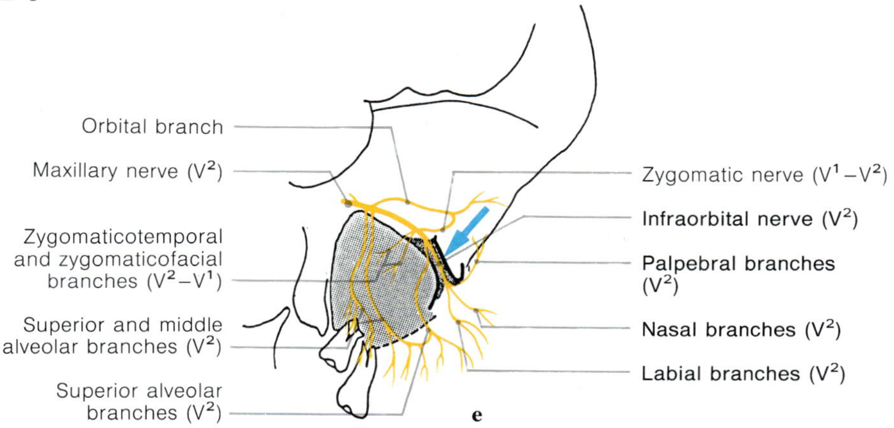

Infraorbital canal and foramen: Labial, palpebral and nasal branches (V²)

Computed tomography (CT)

SAGITTAL VIEW

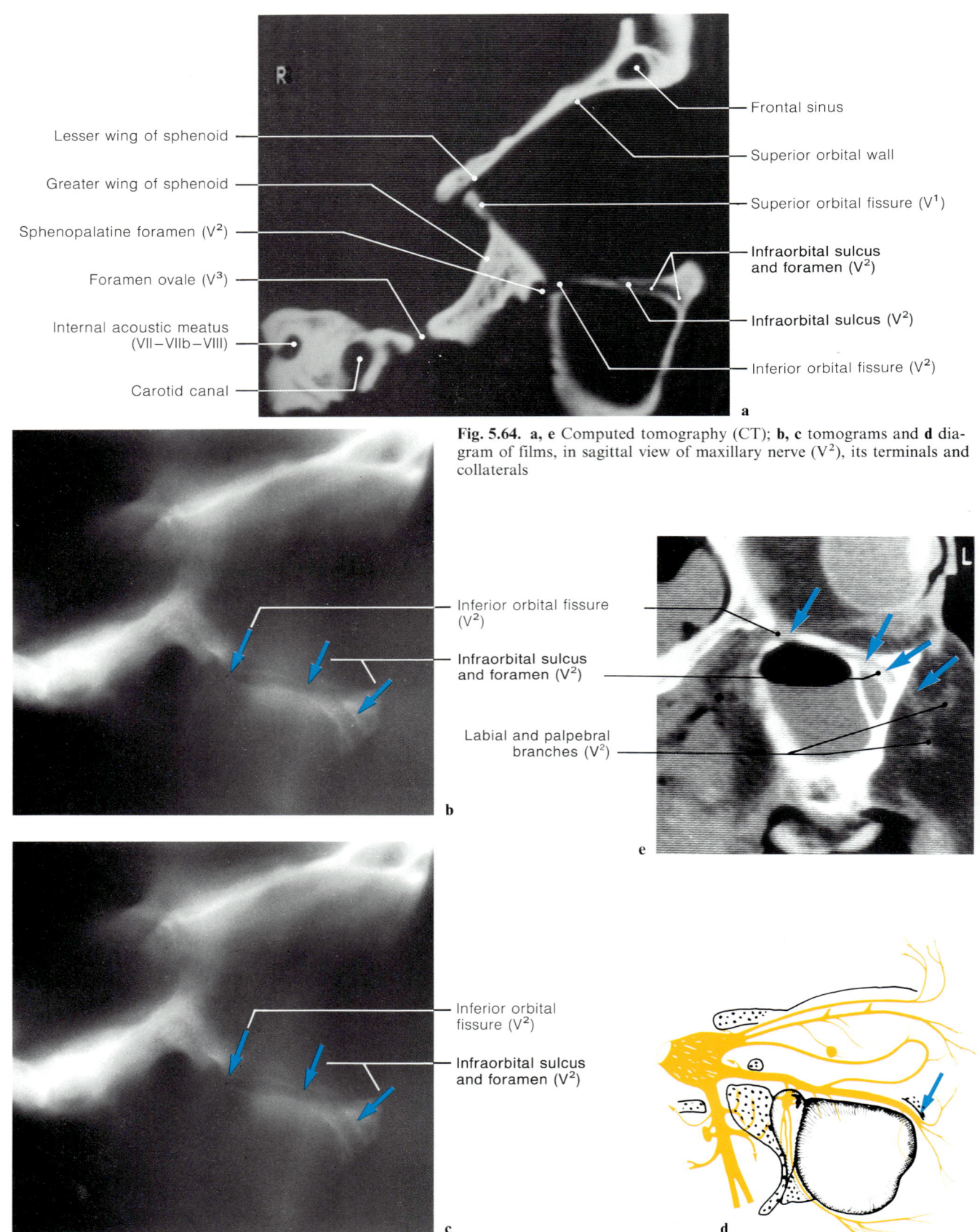

Fig. 5.64. **a, e** Computed tomography (CT); **b, c** tomograms and **d** diagram of films, in sagittal view of maxillary nerve (V²), its terminals and collaterals

Maxillary nerve (V²) 123

Fig. 5.65 a. Sagittal section of orbital cavity at level of infraorbital canal and foramen

Fig. 5.65 b. Diagram of nerves of orbital cavity

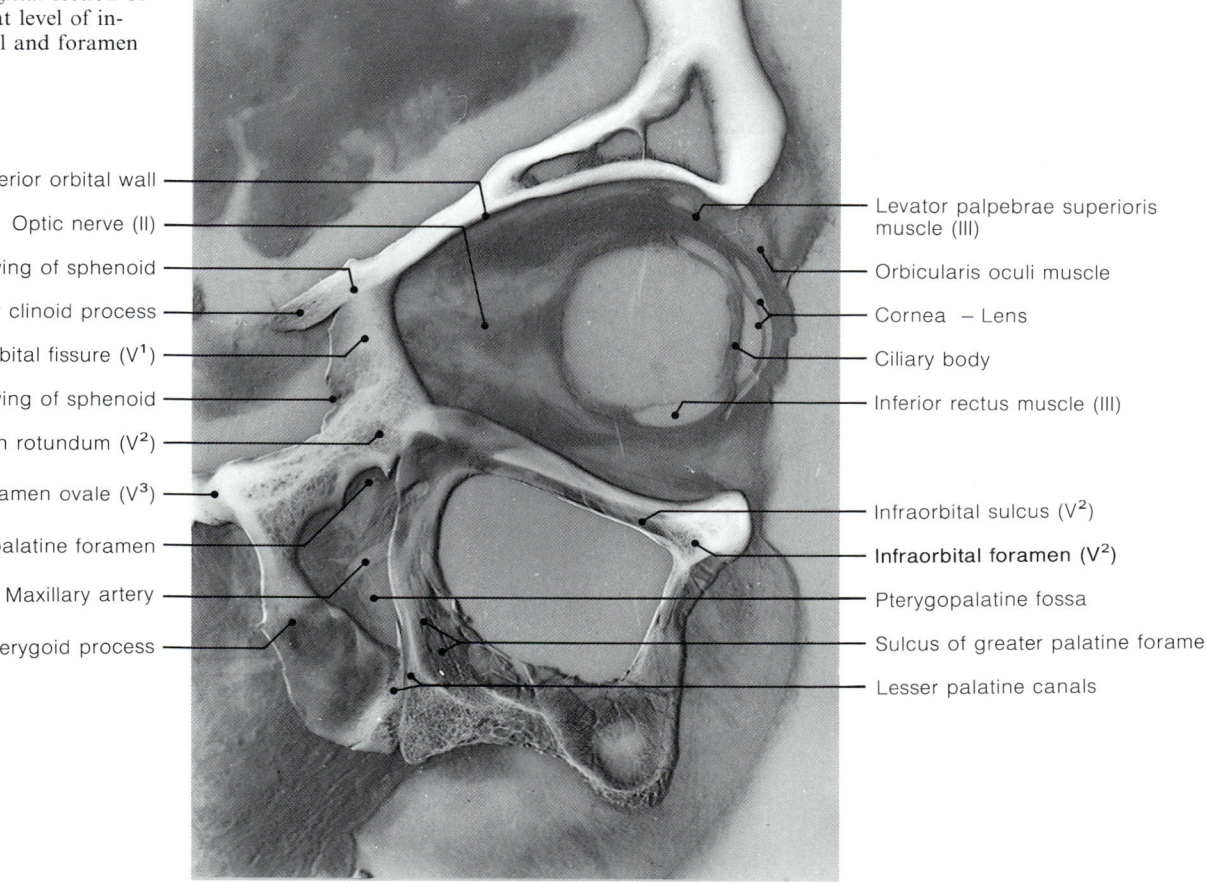

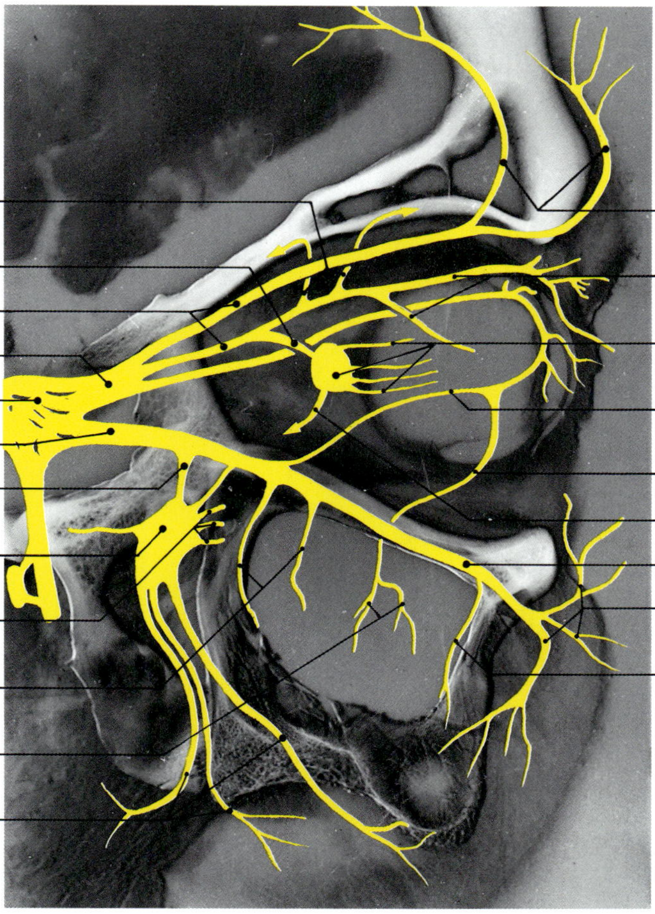

Topography

Pterygopalatine ganglion (V^2–VII–IX)
– Pterygopalatine fossa

Greater and lesser palatine nerves
– Greater and lesser palatine foramina

Pathology

– Syndrome of pterygopalatine ganglion (Sluder),
– tumors of cavum, auditory tube or pharyngeal recess,
– fracture of posterior wall of maxillary sinus,
– fracture of pterygoid process,
– tumor of maxillary sinus.

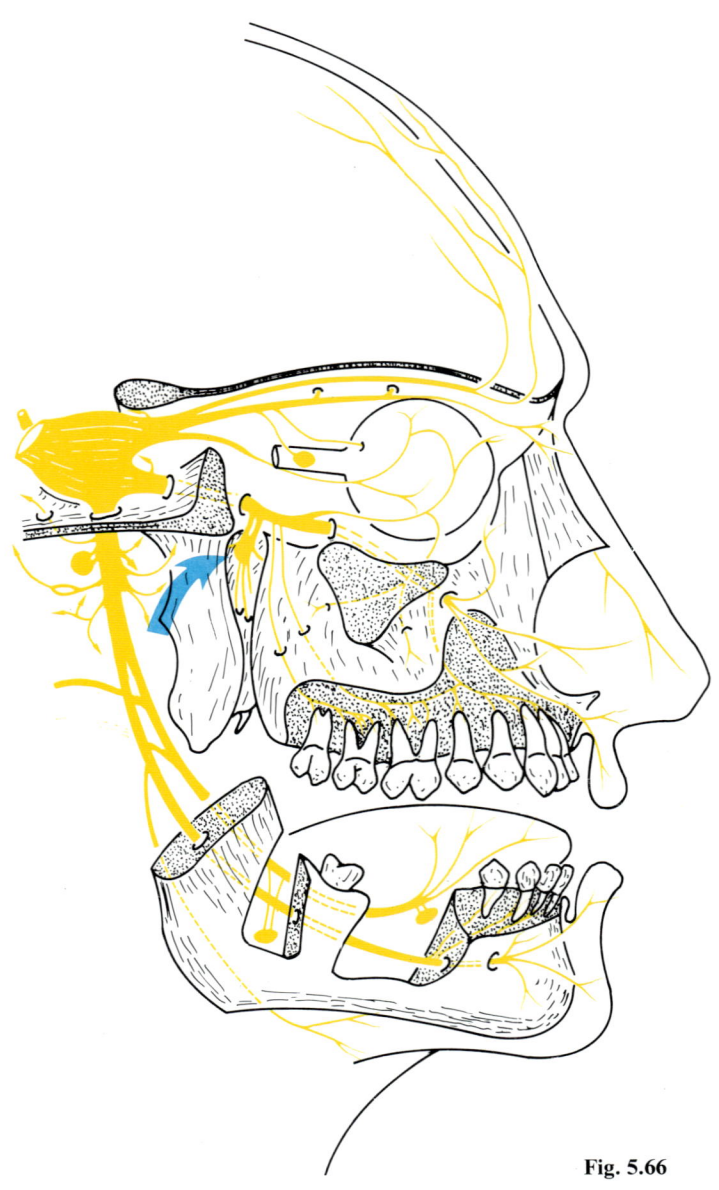

Fig. 5.66

Pterygopalatine ganglion (V^2–VII–IX): Pterygopalatine fossa
Anatomic, magnetic resonance imaging (MRI) and diagram
SAGITTAL AND FRONTAL VIEWS

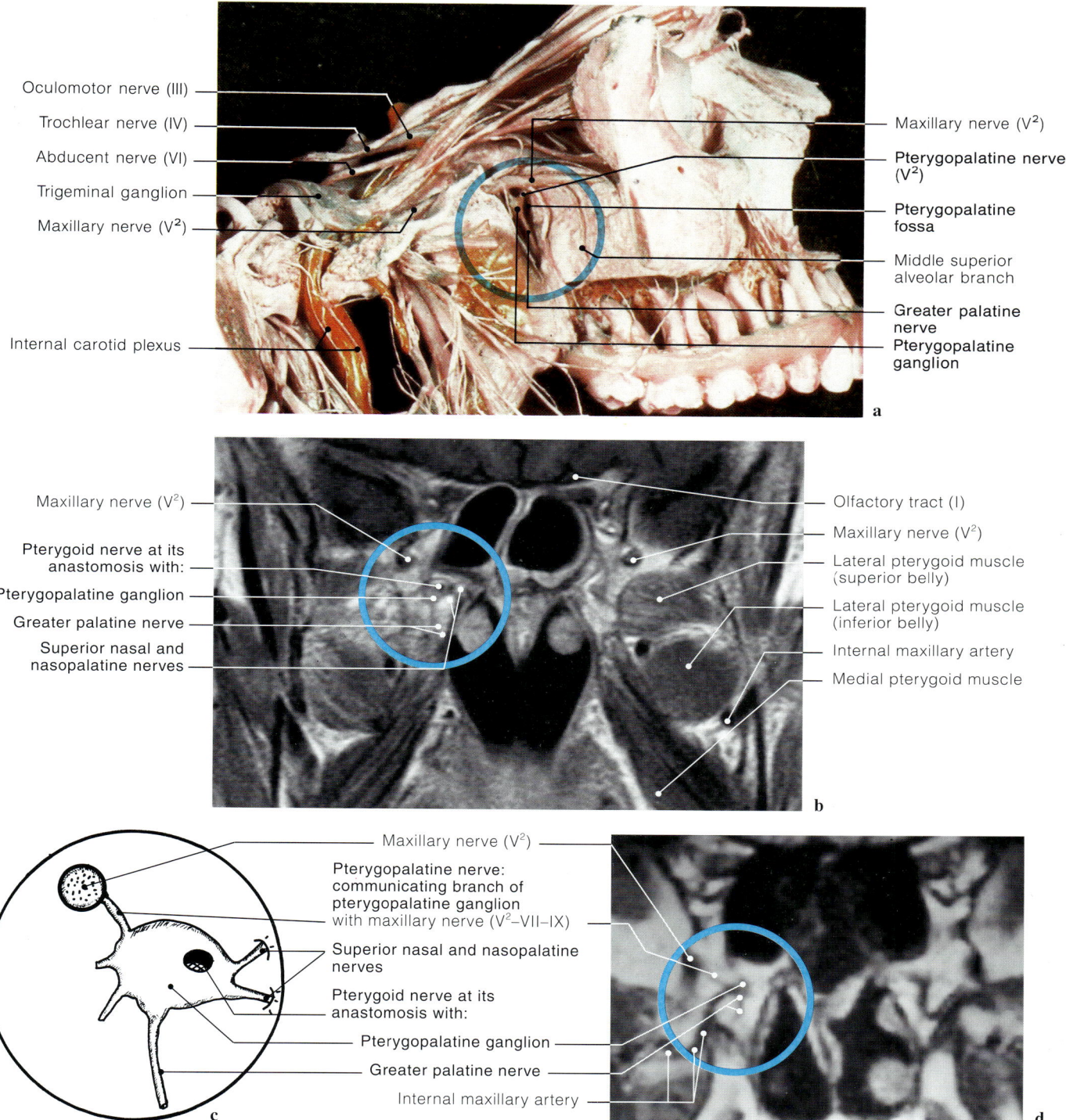

Fig. 5.67a–d. Sagittal anatomic dissection (**a**) to show pterygopalatine ganglion; frontal magnetic resonance imaging (MRI) (**b, d**) and diagram (**c**) clearly demonstrating the pterygopalatine ganglion and its collateral branches (V^2–VII–IX). (MRI: Dr. J.W. Casselman, A.Z. St-Jan, Brugge)

Pterygopalatine ganglion (V^2–VII–IX): Pterygopalatine fossa

Anatomy

The pterygopalatine nerve arises from the maxillary nerve (V^2) within the depths of the pterygopalatine fossa (Fig. 5.37; 5.69c). It enters into relationship with the pterygopalatine ganglion, to which it gives an anastomotic branch (sometimes two).
Beneath this ganglion it divides into numerous terminal branches:

- the superior nasal nerves,
- the nasopalatine nerve,
- the pterygopalatine nerve,
- the greater palatine nerve,
- the lesser palatine nerves.

The *superior nasal nerves*, composed of two branches, enter the sphenopalatine foramen (Fig. 5.71a) and then the nasal cavity.
They are distributed in the mucosa of the middle and superior nasal conchae (Fig. 5.70a). The nasopalatine nerve also enters the nasal cavity via the sphenopalatine foramen (Fig. 5.70b, c; 5.71a) and travels under the mucosa of the vault to reach the nasal septum.
Here it divides into numerous strands and traverses the incisive canal of the hard palate (Fig. 5.70b; 5.74c).
The *pterygopalatine nerve* terminates in the mucosa of the rhinopharynx.
The *greater palatine nerve* descends in the greater palatine sulcus, gives a branch to the inferior nasal concha, and then ramifies in the hard palate and the mucosa of the palatal arch.
The *lesser palatine nerves* descend in the lesser palatine foramina to reach the mucosa of the soft palate.

Imaging

The greater palatine nerve gives off branches distributed to the palatoglossus, tensor veli palatini and palatopharyngeal muscles. In addition to the nerves mentioned above, the pterygopalatine ganglion also receives the pterygoid nerve composed of the superficial greater petrosal (VII) and deep petrosal (IX) nerves.

Pterygopalatine fossa

This is a large hollow situated behind the maxillary antrum, lateral to the pterygoid process, below the vertical portion of the greater wing of the sphenoid, traversed by the foramen rotundum and just in front of the foramen ovale.

Regions to be studied:

- pterygopalatine fossa,
- sulcus of greater palatine canal,
- lesser palatine foramina,
- incisive canal.

EXAMINATION

- Computed tomographic (CT) or tomographic study in sagittal view of the pterygopalatine fossa and the greater and lesser palatine foramina (Fig. 5.69a–c),
- axial and symmetric tomographic and computed tomographic (CT) studies of the pterygopalatine fossae, greater and lesser palatine foramina and the incisive canals (Fig. 5.74a, b; 5.75a, d),
- frontal and symmetric computed tomographic (CT) study of the sulci of the greater palatine foramina (Fig. 5.76c, d).

Magnetic resonance imaging (MRI)

SAGITTAL VIEWS

Fig. 5.67e–g. Magnetic resonance imaging (MRI; sagittal views) to show pterygopalatine ganglion (*medium, straight arrow*), pterygoid nerve (*arrowhead*), greater palatine nerve (*large, straight arrows*), lesser and accessory palatine nerves (*small arrows*), hypoglossal nerve in its canal (XII) (*large arrow*)

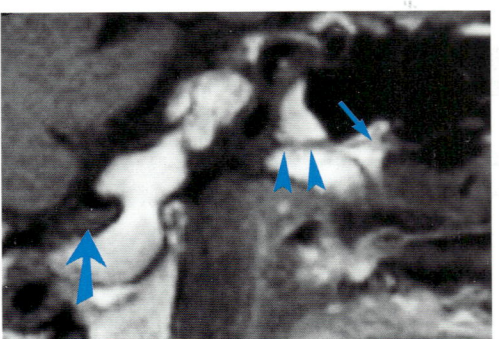

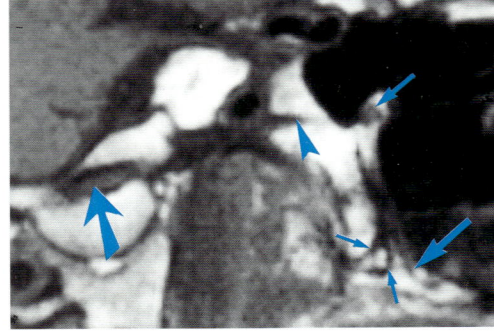

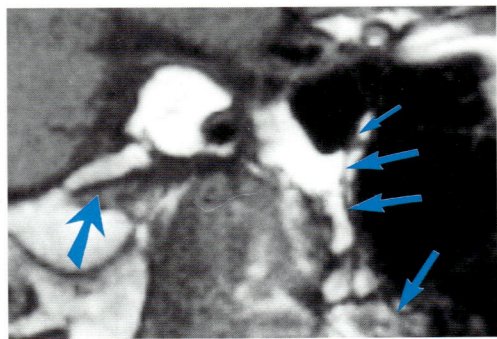

Pterygopalatine ganglion (V² – VII – IX): Pterygopalatine fossa

Imaging

TECHNIQUE (SAGITTAL VIEW)

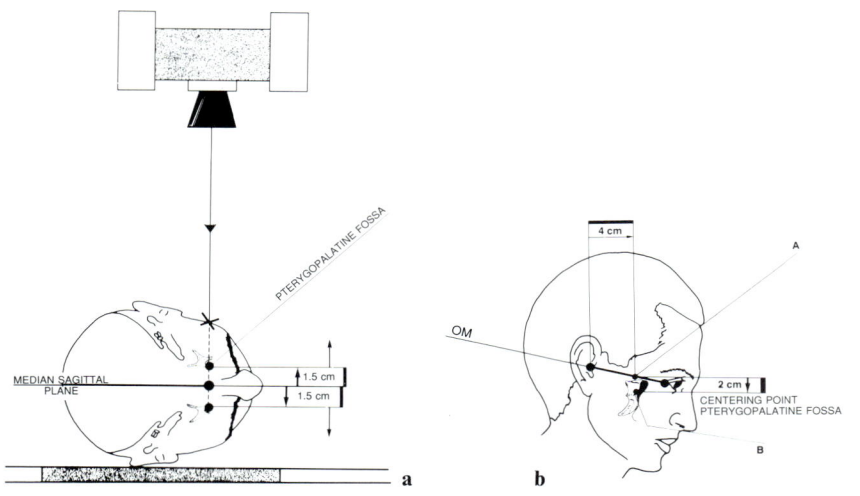

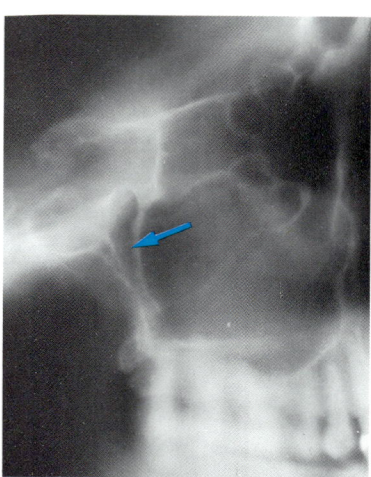

Fig. 5.68 a, b. Centering diagrams for sagittal CT scanning and tomography of the pterygopalatine fossa

Fig. 5.69 a

Fig. 5.69 a, b. Sagittal tomographic section of the pterygopalatine fossa

TECHNIQUE

Sagittal tomographic study:

- The subject is in lateral decubitus in the "gun-dog" position, the head in strict profile resting on plastic supports. Good stability is ensured by flour bags in contact with the back;
- after having located the orbitomeatal plane (OM), a point "A" is marked 4 cm from the external acoustic meatus in a direction towards the orbit, and then a point "B" 2 cm below this which will be the centering point (Fig. 5.68 b);
- starting from the median sagittal plane, a point "C" is marked 1.5 cm towards the outer side of the side to be examined (Fig. 5.68 a).

Centering on "B", sections are made every 3 mm from "C" to demonstrate successively:

- the pterygopalatine fossa,
- the sphenopalatine foramen,
- the sulcus of the greater palatine foramen,
- the lesser palatine foramina (Fig. 5.69 b).

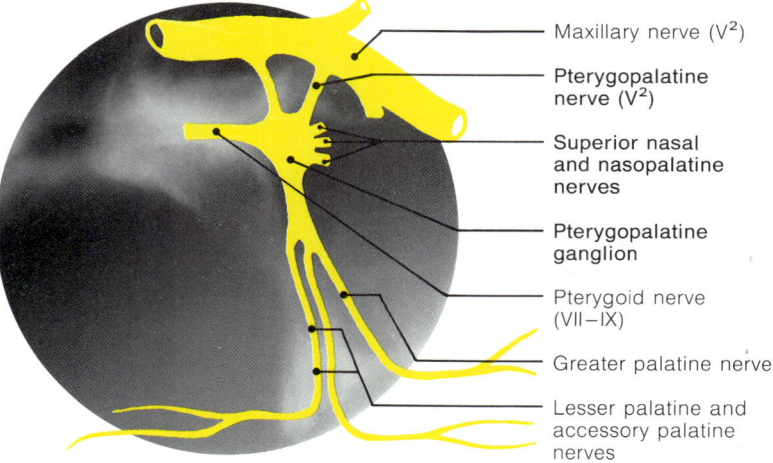

Fig. 5.69 c. Diagram of pterygoplatine ganglion and terminal branches (see anatomic view in Fig. 5.76 e)

Pterygopalatine ganglion (V^2–VII–IX): Pterygopalatine fossa

Fig. 5.70a–c. Sections of the nasal cavity at the level of the sphenopalatine foramen, with diagram and anatomic section of the nasal nerves distributed to the nasal conchae

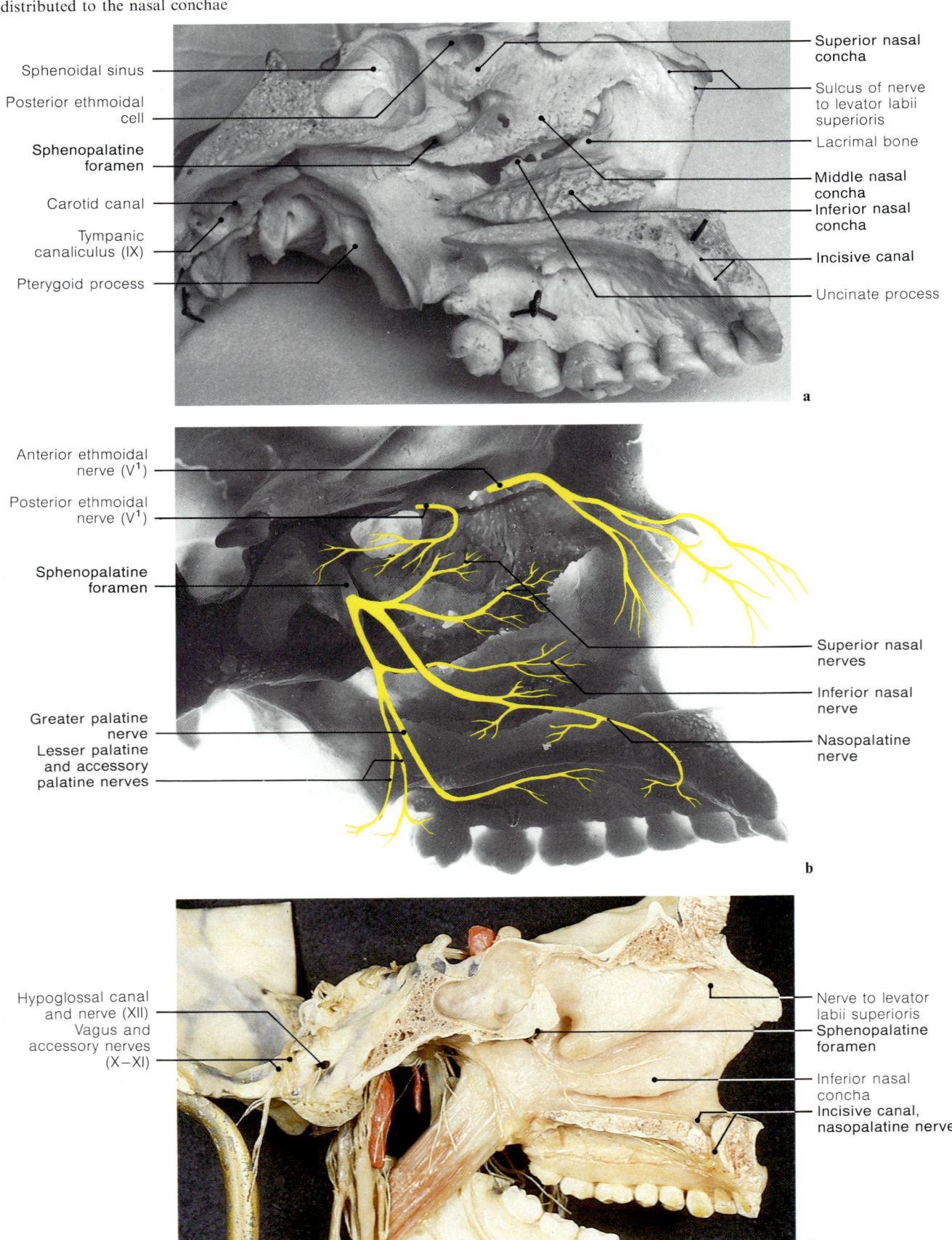

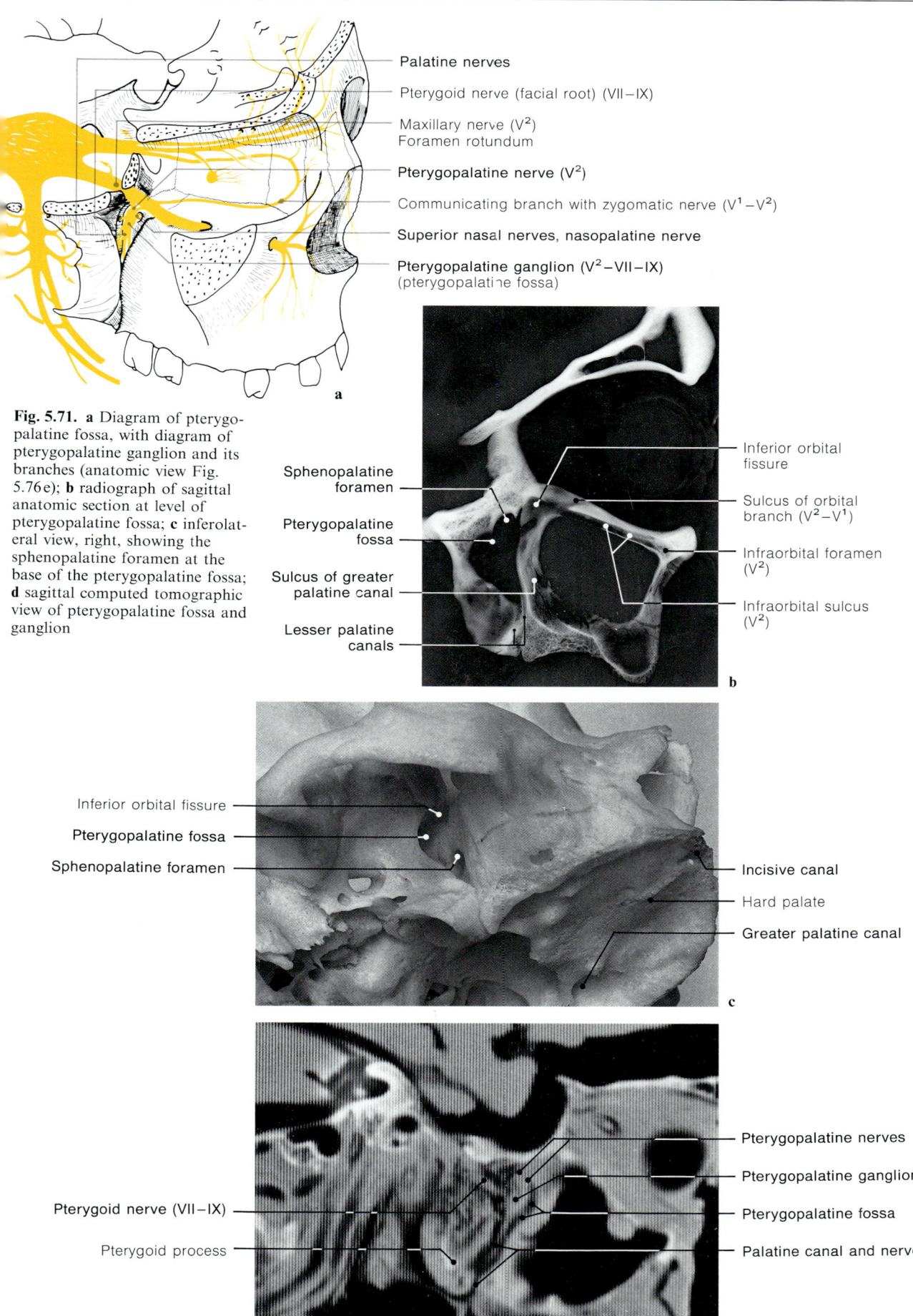

Fig. 5.71. a Diagram of pterygopalatine fossa, with diagram of pterygopalatine ganglion and its branches (anatomic view Fig. 5.76e); b radiograph of sagittal anatomic section at level of pterygopalatine fossa; c inferolateral view, right, showing the sphenopalatine foramen at the base of the pterygopalatine fossa; d sagittal computed tomographic view of pterygopalatine fossa and ganglion

Pterygopalatine ganglion (V^2–VII–IX): Pterygopalatine fossa

Imaging

TECHNIQUE (AXIAL VIEW)

Axial imaging of pterygopalatine fossa, greater and lesser palatine foramina:

- The subject is in dorsal decubitus, the back raised on pillows, the head turned as for the Hirtz view, the orbitomeatal plane (OM) parallel to the table (Fig. 5.72 a, b);
- the centering point is situated on a line 4 or 5 cm behind the mandibular symphysis;
- the planes of section are made starting from the orbitomeatal plane (OM) every 5 mm travelling towards the hard palate, so as to show successively:
  * the pterygopalatine fossa,
  * the sulcus of the greater palatine foramen,
  * the lesser palatine foramina and, finally,
  * the incisive canal (hard palate).

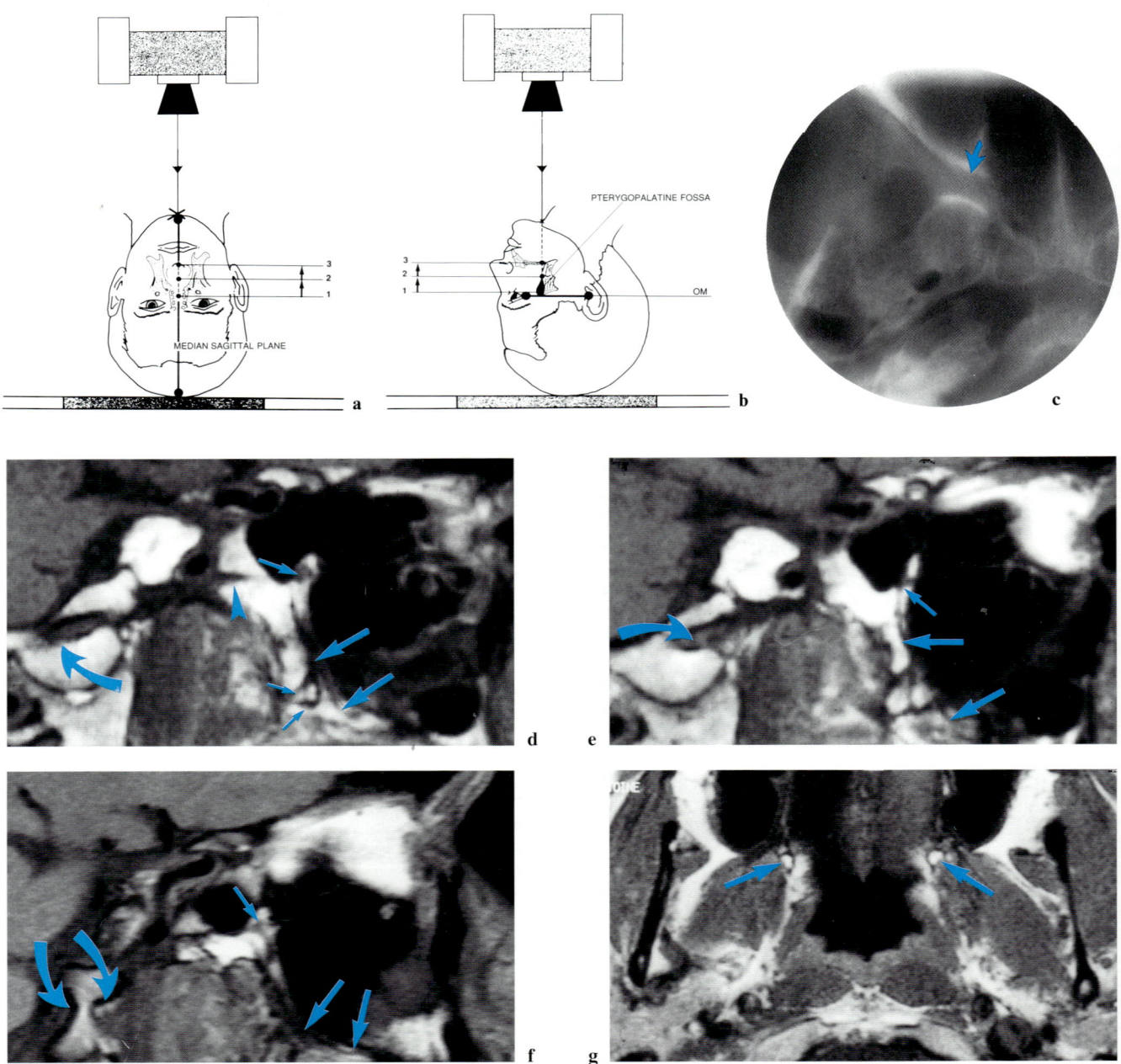

Fig. 5.72. **a, b** Centering diagrams for axial study of the pterygopalatine fossa (*1*), the sulcus of the greater palatine foramen (*2*) and the greater and lesser palatine foramina (*3*); **c** axial section of pterygopalatine fossa; **d–g** sagittal and axial magnetic resonance imaging (MRI) showing pterygopalatine ganglion (*medium, straight arrows*), pterygoid nerve (*arrowhead*), greater palatine nerve (*large, straight arrows*) and hypoglossal nerve in its canal (XII) (*curved arrows*)

Pterygopalatine fossa

Computed tomography (CT) and tomography

AXIAL VIEW

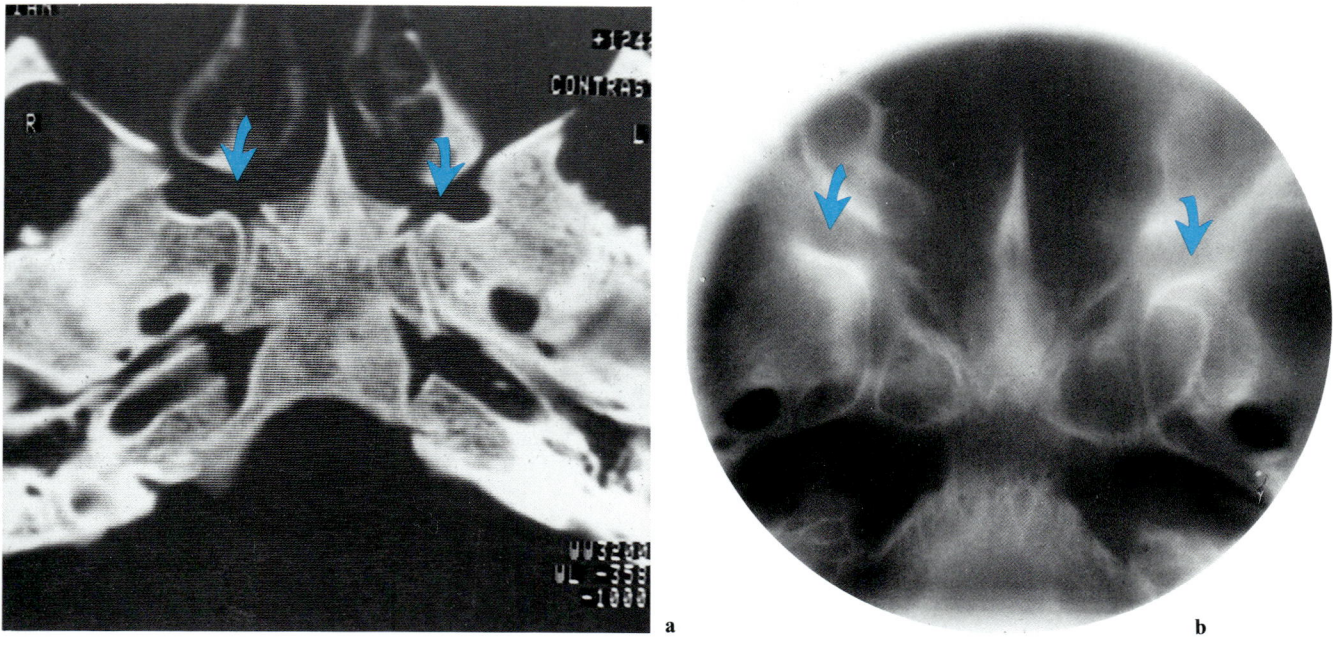

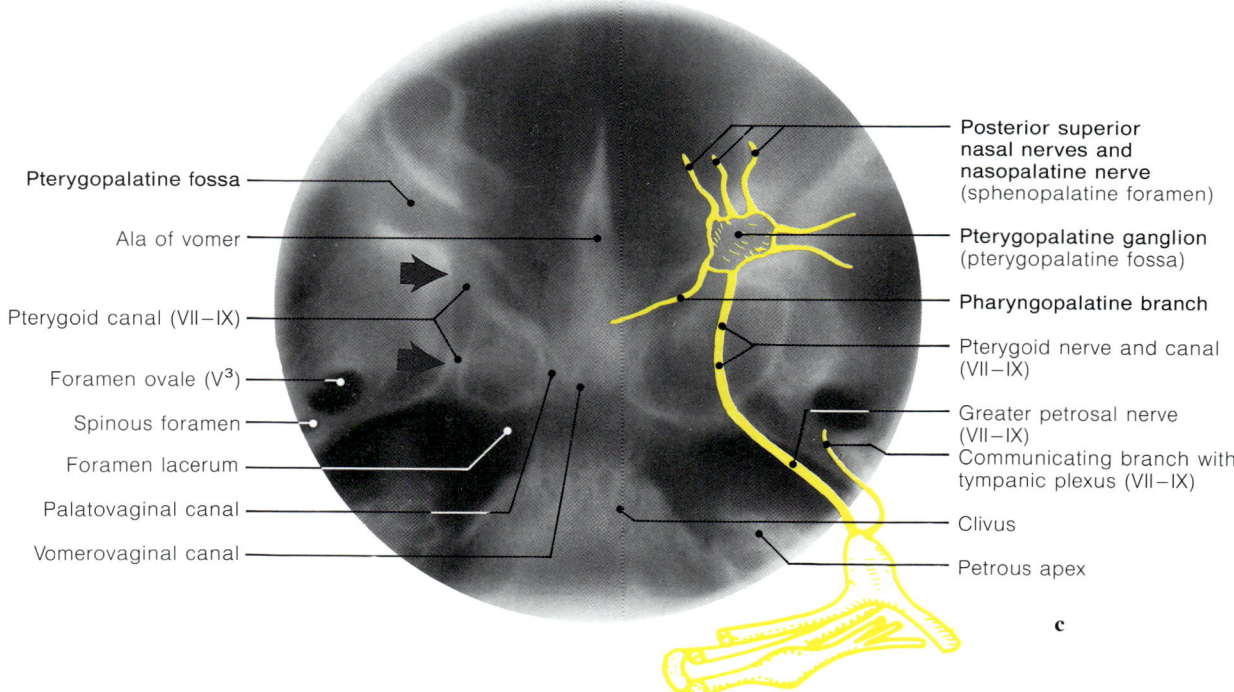

Fig. 5.73. a Axial computed tomography (CT) of pterygopalatine fossa; b, c axial tomographic section of pterygopalatine fossa with diagram of pterygopalatine ganglion and its collateral and anastomotic branches. Arrows: pterygopalatine fossa

Pterygopalatine ganglion (V^2–VII–IX): Pterygopalatine fossa, palatine foramina
Computed tomography (CT) and tomography
AXIAL VIEW

Fig. 5.74 a–c. Axial tomography (**a**) and computed tomography (CT) (**b**) of palatine foramina; view of hard palate, with diagram (**c**) of terminal branches of pterygopalatine ganglion

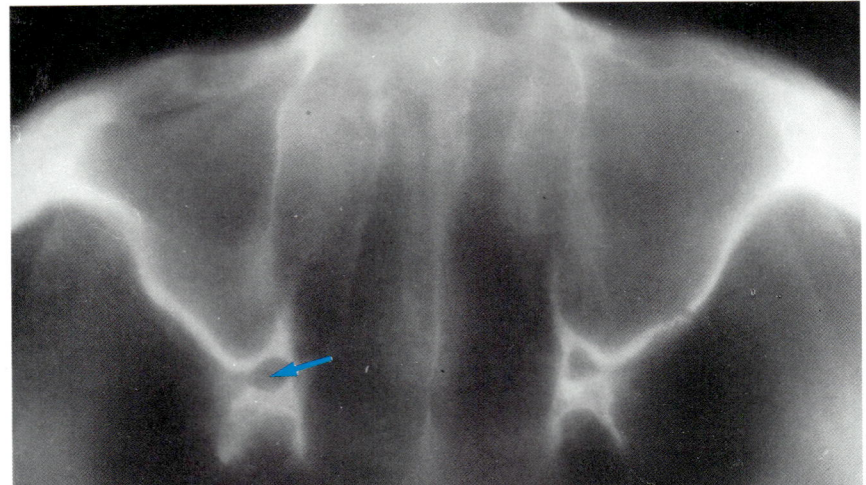

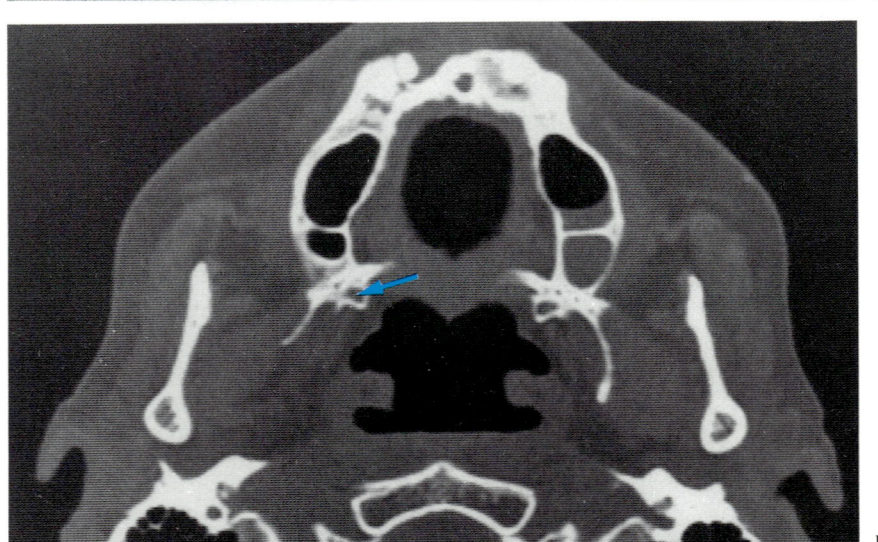

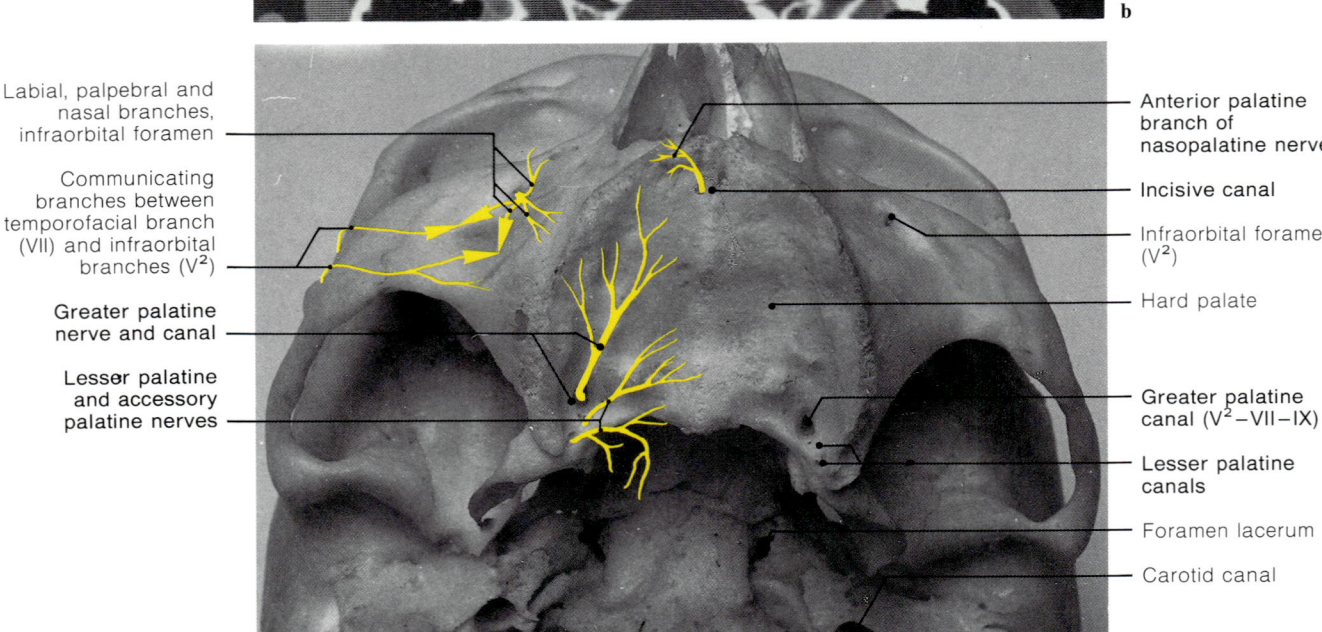

Palatine and incisive foramina

Computed tomography (CT)

AXIAL VIEW

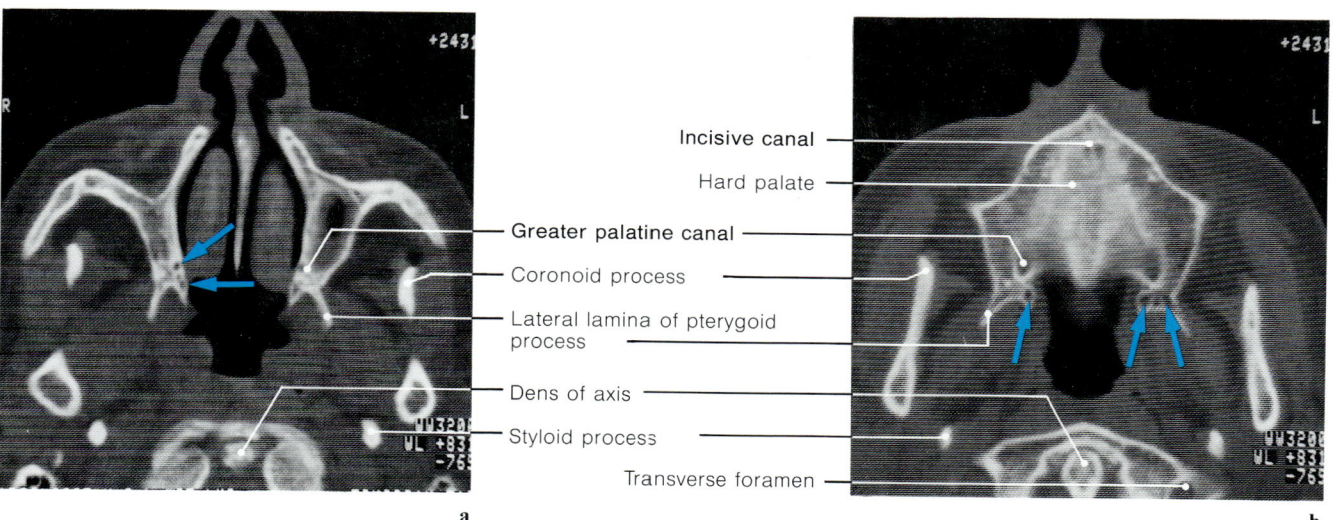

Fig. 5.75 a–d. Axial computed tomographic (CT) (**a–c**) and conventional (**d**) sections of hard palate to show palatine foramina, with diagram of terminal branches of the pterygopalatine ganglion

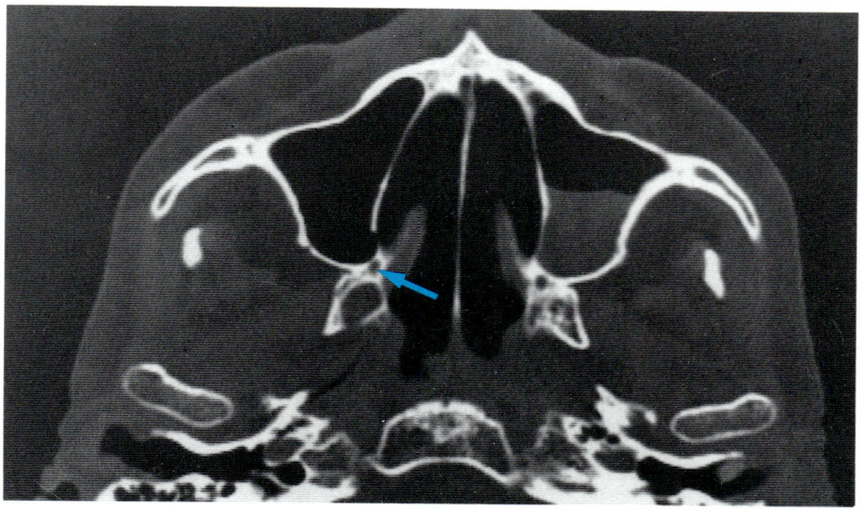

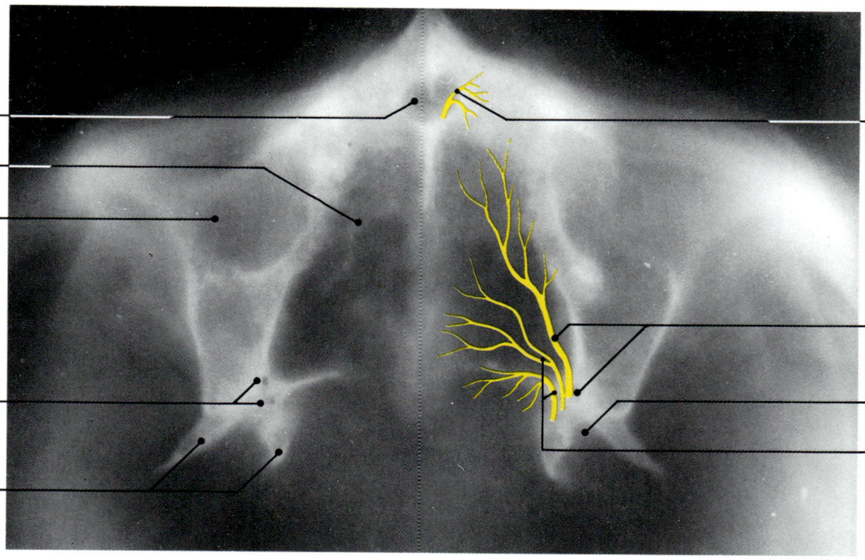

Nerve and sulcus of greater palatine foramen

Magnetic resonance imaging (MRI) and computed tomography (CT)

FRONTAL AND SAGITTAL VIEWS

Frontal CT and tomographic studies of sulcus of greater palatine foramen:

- The subject is in dorsal decubitus, the head strictly face forward, supported by flour bags; the orbitomeatal plane (OM) is to be seen as perpendicular to the plane of the table;
- the centering point is situated at the middle of the nose, at the level of the outer angle of the orbit (Fig. 5.76 b);
- after having located the inferolateral border of the orbit, a point is marked 3 cm below this, the plane of section passing through this point;
- the CT or ordinary tomographic sections are made starting from this point, at every 3 mm moving towards the nasal cavity (Fig. 5.76a) so as to visualize the pterygoid process and the sulcus of the greater palatine canal.

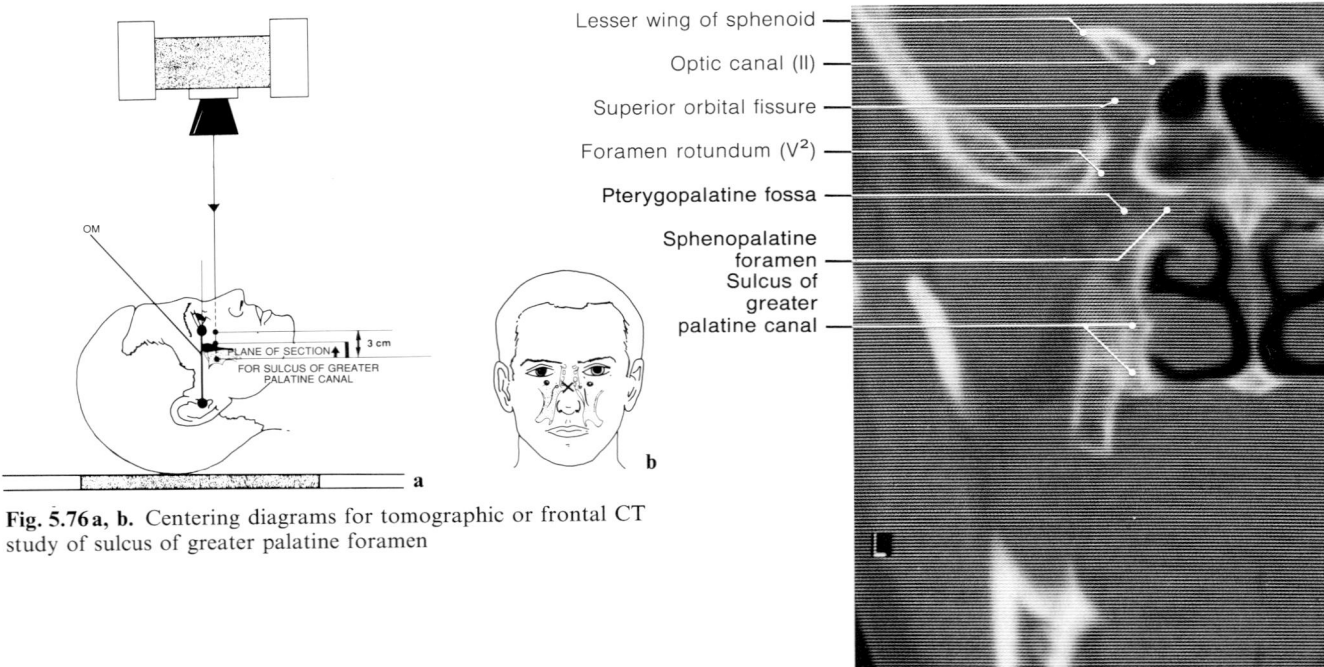

Fig. 5.76 a, b. Centering diagrams for tomographic or frontal CT study of sulcus of greater palatine foramen

Fig. 5.76 c–e. Frontal CT (c) of sulcus of greater palatine foramen; sagittal MRI (d) and anatomic view (e) of the pterygopalatine fossa, displaying the ganglion and the palatine nerves

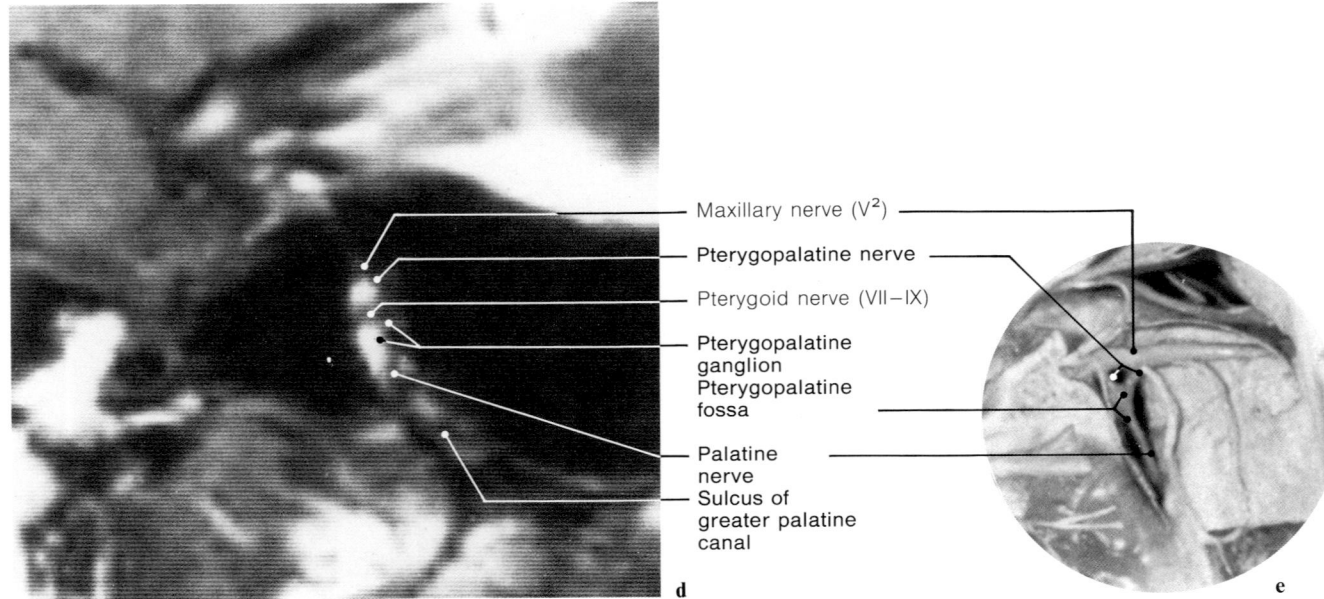

Trigeminal nerve (V)

Mandibular nerve (V^3)
Foramen ovale (V^3)
Pathology 136
Anatomy and imaging (examination) 138
   Axial views (MRI) 138
   Axial view (CT) 139
   Oblique view (radiography) 140
   Oblique view, discontinuous scanning (radiology) . 141
   Frontal view (MRI) 141
   Sagittal and frontal views (CT) 142
   Frontal views (CT, MRI) 143
   Skull base (radiography, sagittal MRI) 144
   Superolateral view and diagram 145

Inferior alveolar nerve (mandibular canal)
and mental nerve (mental foramen)
Pathology 146
Anatomy and imaging (examination) 148
   Diagram and anatomic view 149
   Anatomic medial view of mandible 150
   Frontal and sagittal views (radiology) 151
   Dental surveys (radiology) 152
Terminal branches, sensory territories 153

Vascular relations:
Cavernous sinus 167, 290
Accessory meningeal artery 276, 277
Lingual nerve arterial branch 276, 277
Vein of the foramen ovale 276, 277
Lingual branch 283
Medial mandibular artery and submental artery 283
Inferior alveolar artery 285

Topography

Mandibular nerve (V³)
– Foramen ovale

Pathology

– Trigeminal neuralgia (type V³),
– neurinoma of foramen ovale or foramen lacerum,
– aneurysm of carotid siphon (cavernous sinus),
– fracture of greater wing of sphenoid,
– tumors of cavum, rhinopharynx, auditory tube.

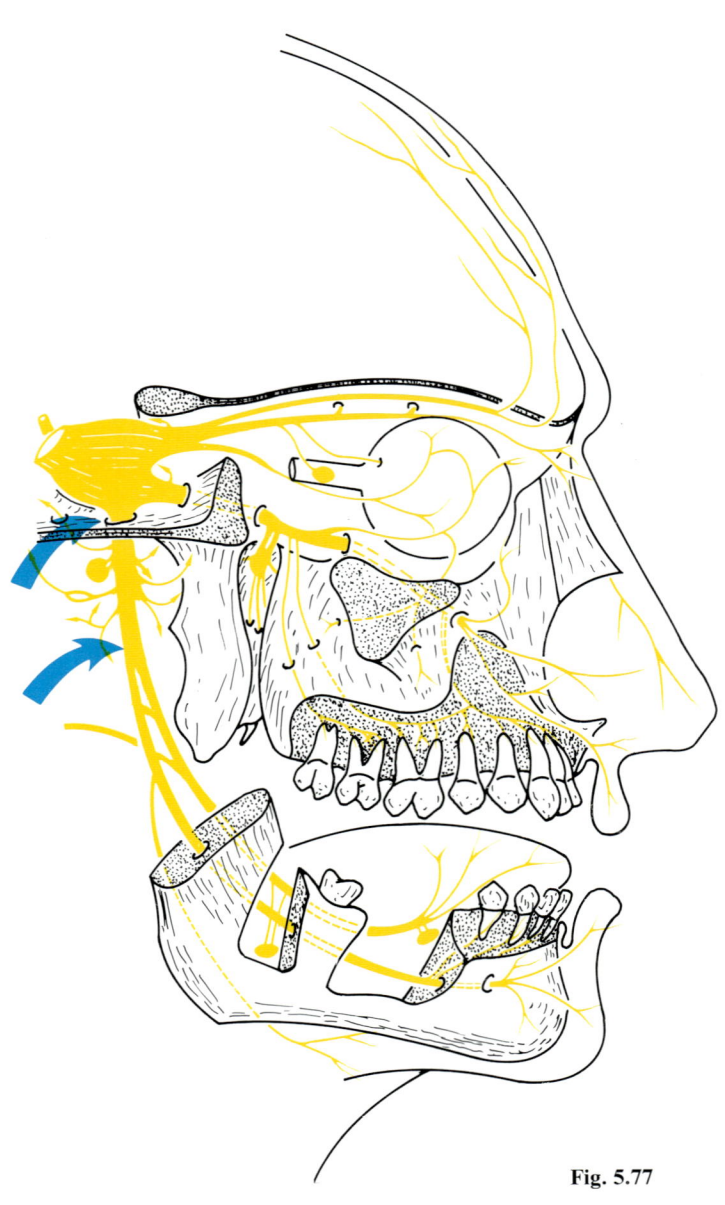

Fig. 5.77

Mandibular nerve (V³): Foramen ovale

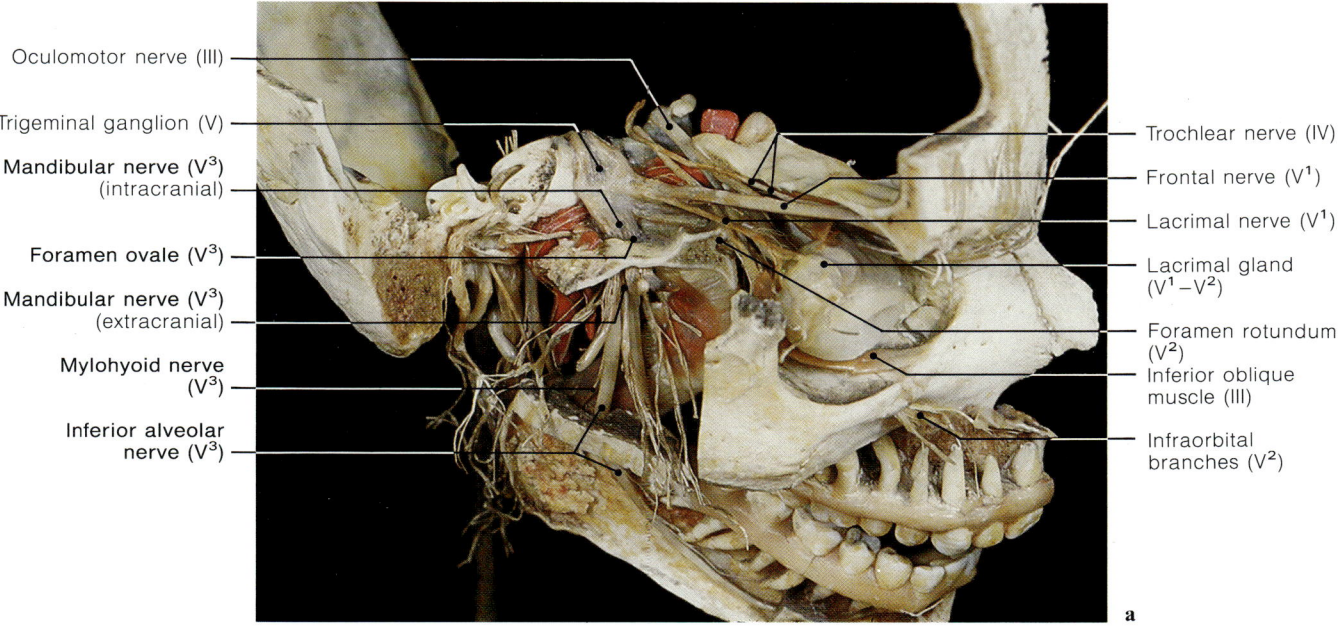

Fig. 5.78a. Anatomic dissection of mandibular nerve and foramen ovale (V³)

Mandibular nerve (V³): Foramen ovale

Anatomy

The mandibular nerve (V³) travels laterally to the foramen ovale, in company with the lesser meningeal artery.
At its exit it gives off:

- the meningeal branch,
- the auriculotemporal nerve which receives the lesser petrosal nerve,
- the inferior alveolar nerve which anastomoses with the lingual nerve and gives off the mental nerve,
- the lingual nerve, which is joined by the chorda tympani,
- the deep temporal nerve,
- the masseteric nerve,
- the buccal nerve,
- the media pterygoid nerve,
- the lateral ampullary nerve,
- the nerve to tensor tympani muscle (Fig. 5.3; 5.86 b).

Innervation

Its sensory supply is to:

- the skin of the temporoparietal region,
- the cheek,
- the chin,
- the lower lip,
- the anterior part of the external ear,
- the mucosa of the buccal floor, cheek, lower lip, lower gums, anterior two-thirds of the tongue and dental pulp of the lower teeth.

Its motor supply is to the masticatory muscles.

Imaging

The foramen ovale is situated in the greater wing of the sphenoid in its posterior horizontal portion, in front of the foramen lacerum and the petrous apex. The spinous foramen is behind and slightly lateral to the foramen ovale, while medially there is the canal of the otic ganglion (V³–VII–IX) (Fig. 5.79 b; 5.80 e; 5.86 a).

EXAMINATION

- Tomographic or computed tomographic (CT) study in symmetric Hirtz view,
- study of foramen ovale in its axis in unilateral oblique view,
- study of foramen ovale in unilateral view in "discontinuous scanning".

TECHNIQUE

Computed tomography (CT) or tomography of the foramen ovale in the Hirtz view:
- The subject is in dorsal decubitus, the shoulders elevated on pillows. The head is strictly face-forward and rests on the vertex in such a way that the orbitomeatal plane (OM) is parallel to the plane of the table (Fig. 5.79 a);
- the centering point is median, at two fingersbreadths behind the mental symphysis.

For tomography, the plane of section is identical with the orbitomeatal plane (OM).
Sections are made at the level of this plane, over 1 cm moving down to the vertex.

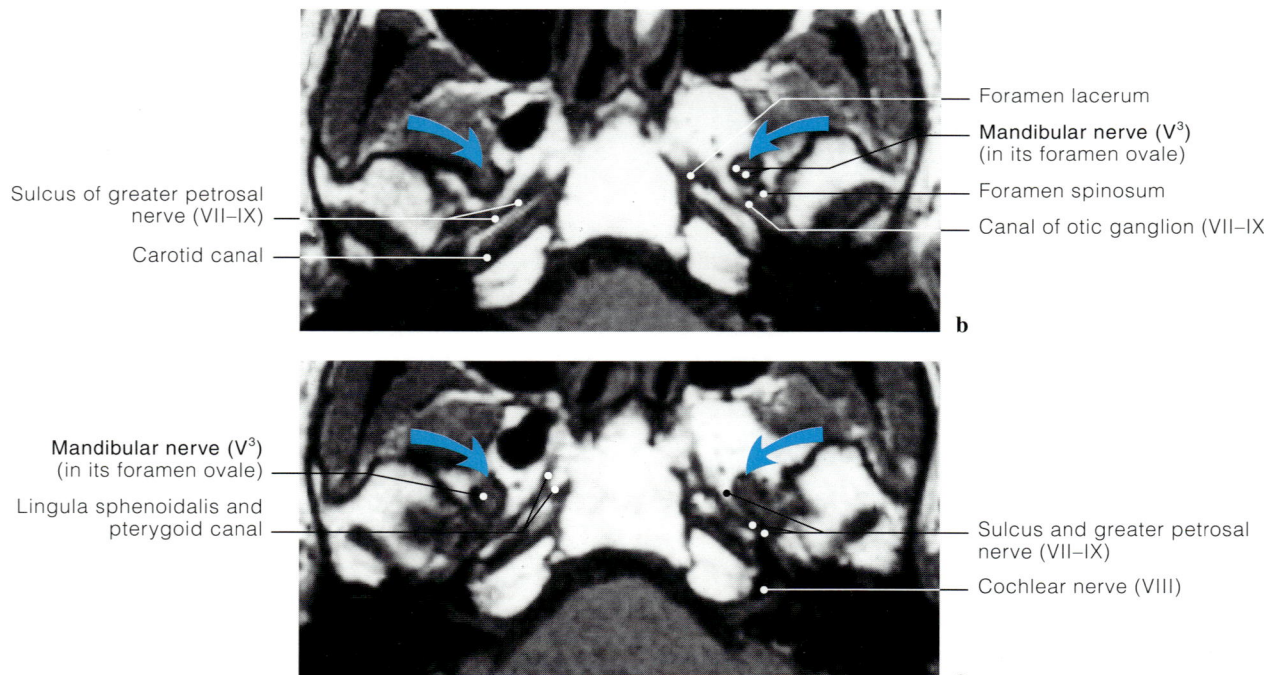

Fig. 5.78 b, c. Magnetic resonance imaging (MRI) with good visualization of mandibular nerve in foramen ovale (V³) (*curved arrow*). (MRI: Dr. J.W. Casselman, A.Z. St-Jan, Brugge)

Mandibular nerve (V³): Foramen ovale

Axial computed tomography (CT)

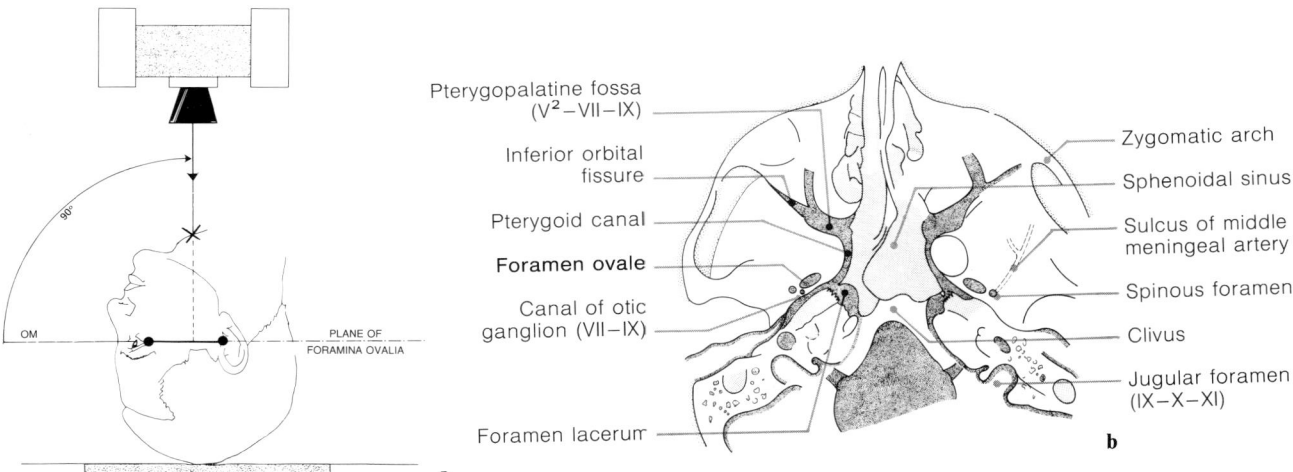

Fig. 5.79 a. Centering diagram for axial study of foramina ovalia

Fig. 5.79 b, c. Computed tomography (CT) and diagram of foramen ovale (in axial view)

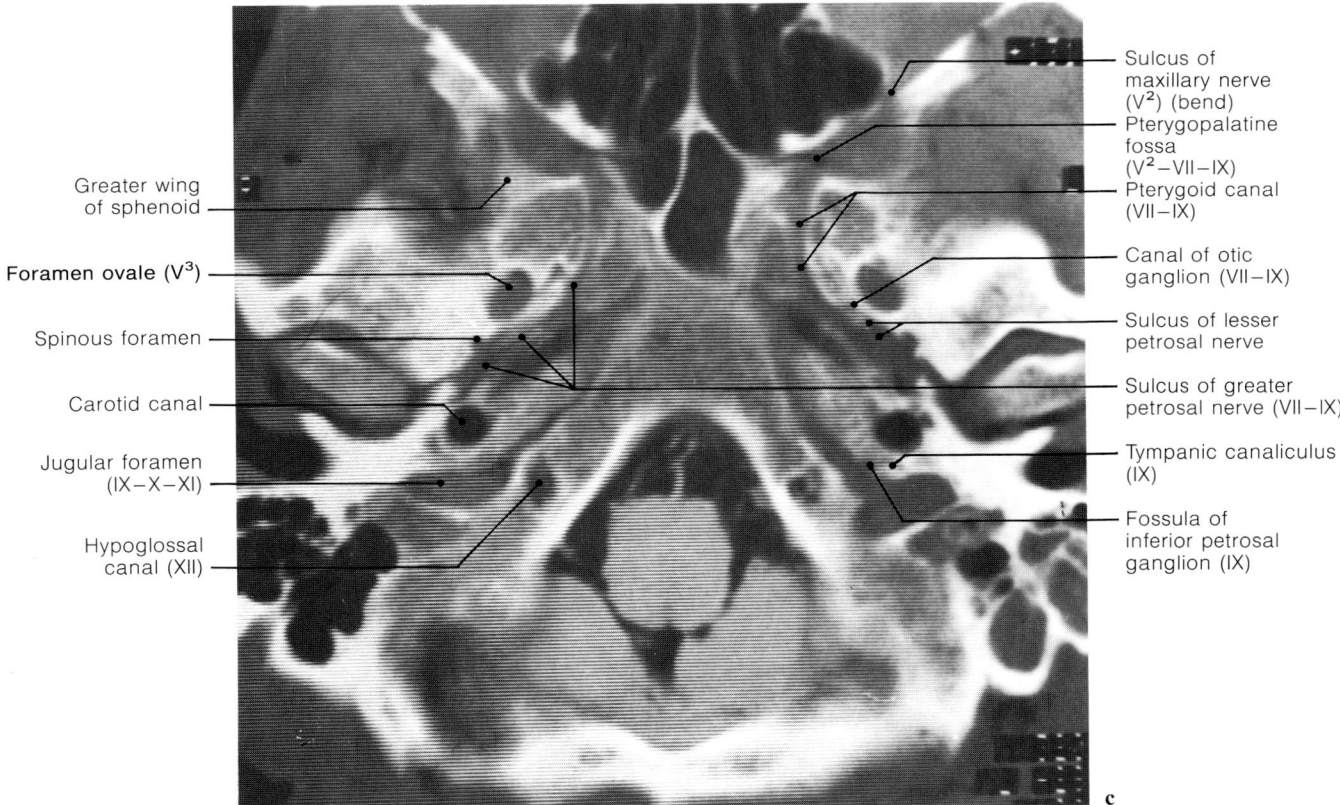

Note: It should be added that the foramen ovale is often masked by the lateral and medial laminae of the pterygoid process (Fig. 5.82a). It is therefore necessary to take comparable unilateral oblique views (Fig. 5.80a, b). This position has the advantage of being less uncomfortable for the patient. This technique also allows display of the trigeminal impression, projected under the foramen ovale (Fig. 5.80 d, e).

Mandibular nerve (V³): Foramen ovale

Imaging

TECHNIQUE (OBLIQUE VIEW)

Study of foramen ovale in unilateral oblique view:

- The subject is in dorsal decubitus, the back raised on pillows, the head extended so that the vertical incident beam makes an angle of 55° to the orbitomeatal plane (OM) (Fig. 5.80a);
- the head is subsequently turned by 45° towards the side opposite to that to be radiographed in relation to the median sagittal plane (Fig. 5.80b, c);
- the centering point is situated 1 cm under the zygomatic bone at the level of the mandibular angle.

Note: In the film, the foramen ovale should be projected in front of the mandibular ramus or antero-inferior edge of the coronoid process (Fig. 5.80d, e).

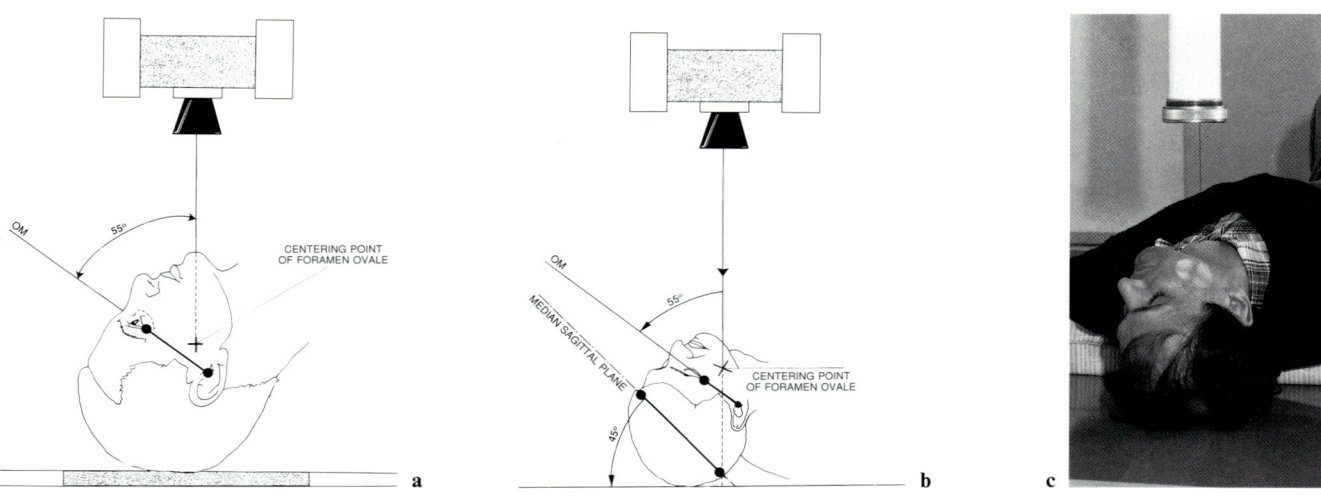

Fig. 5.80a–c. Centering diagrams for study of foramen ovale in unilateral oblique view

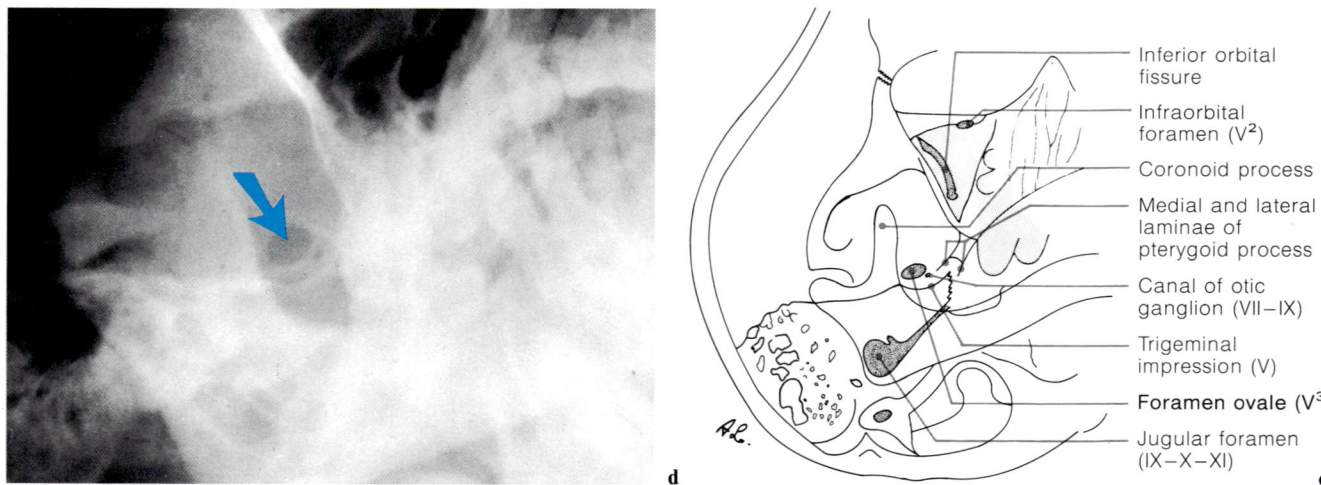

Fig. 5.80d, e. Radiograph and diagram of foramen ovale in its axis, in oblique view

Mandibular nerve V³: Foramen ovale

Imaging

TECHNIQUE (OBLIQUE VIEW IN "DISCONTINUOUS SCANNING")

Study of foramen ovale in "discontinuous scanning" in unilateral oblique view:

– The view is identical to that previously stated and only the angulation of the tube varies, the patient's head remaining in the same position; the tube is inclined by 5° to 8° in relation to the centering point and 4 films are taken in succession during the rotation of the tube (Fig. 5.81 a).

Note: This simple technique is particularly suitable for obtaining good definition of the margins of the foramen ovale around its axis and for displaying the trigeminal impression, its retrogasserian tubercle and the petrous apex (Fig. 5.81 b).

Fig. 5.81 a. Centering diagram for study of foramen ovale in "discontinuous scanning"

Mandibular nerve (V³)

Magnetic resonance imaging (MRI)

FRONTAL VIEW

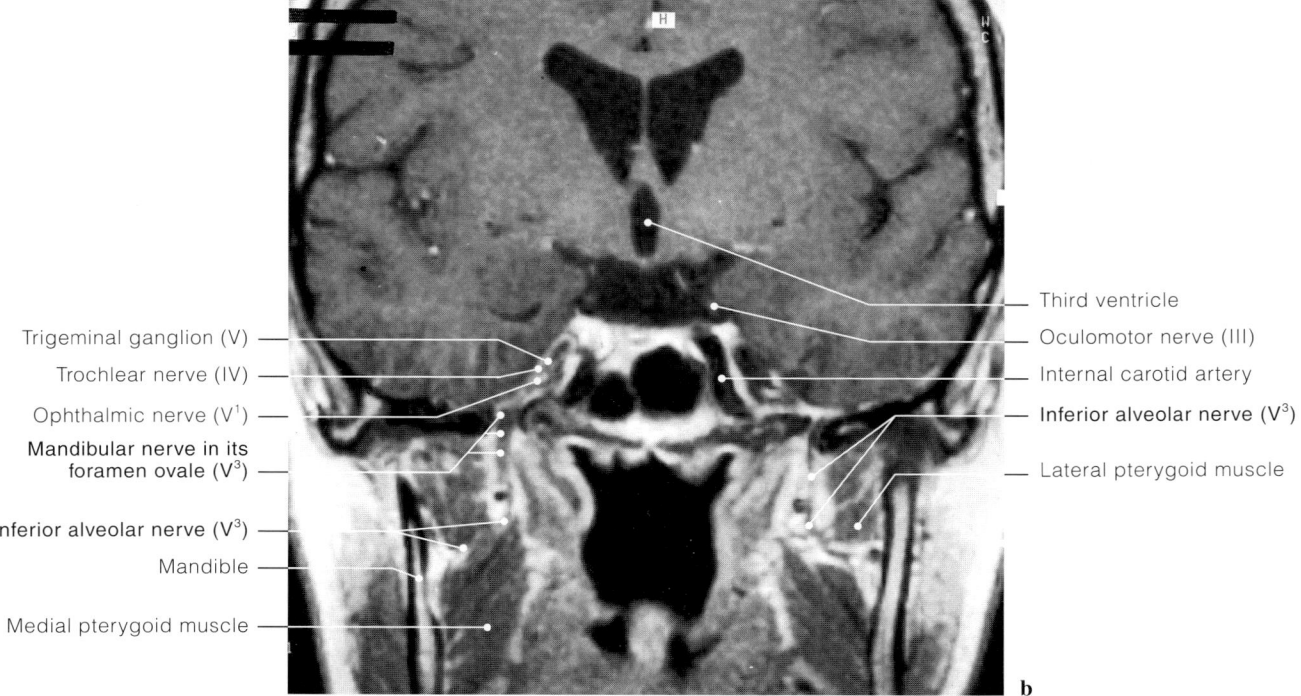

Fig. 5.81 b. Frontal magnetic resonance imaging (MRI) for study of mandibular nerve in its foramen ovale (V³). (MRI: Dr. J.W. Casselman, A.Z. St-Jan, Brugge)

Mandibular nerve (V³): Foramen ovale

Computed tomography (CT)

SAGITTAL AND FRONTAL VIEWS

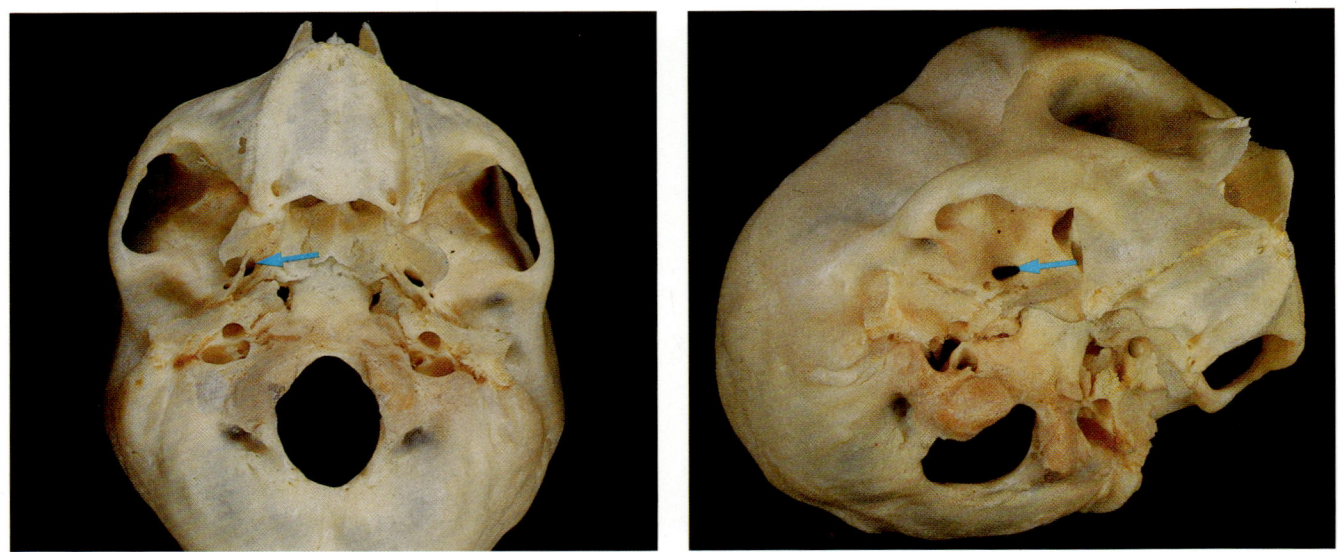

Fig. 5.82. a Poor orientation of skull: the foramina ovalia are not projected exactly in their axes and are often masked by the laminae of the pterygoid process; **b** good orientation of the foramen in its axis (Fig. 5.80)

Fig. 5.83 a, b. Computed tomography (CT) of foramen ovale (V³); **a** sagittal view; **b** frontal view

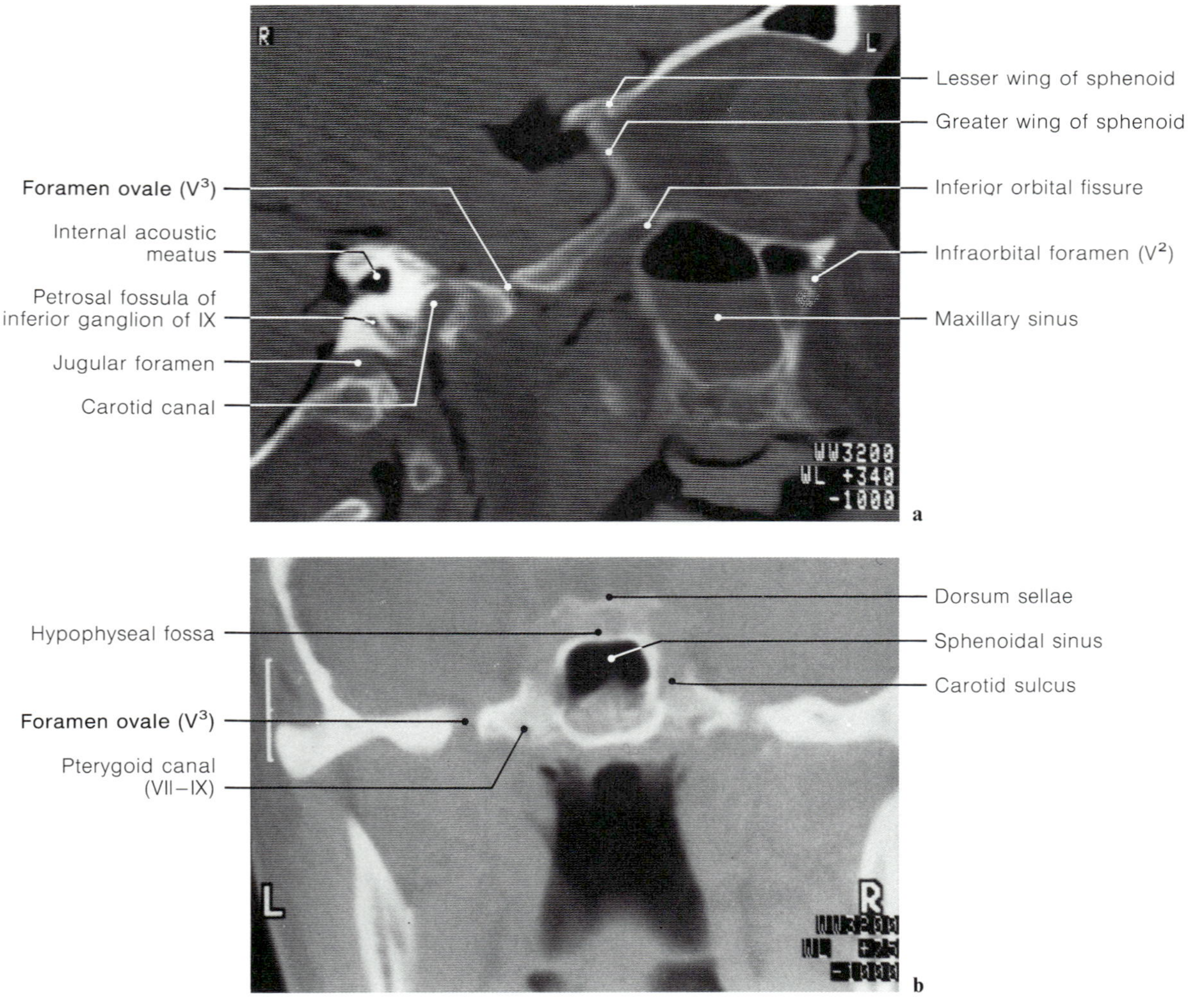

Mandibular nerve (V³): Foramen ovale
Computed tomography (CT) and magnetic resonance imaging (MRI)
FRONTAL VIEWS

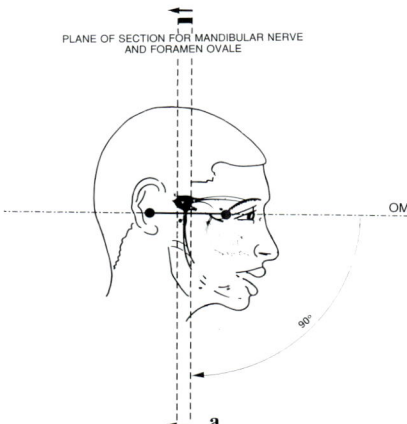

Fig. 5.84. a Centering diagram for study of MRI or CT scan of foramina ovalia and mandibular nerves; **b, c** computed tomography (CT) (**b**) and anatomic section (**c**) at the level of trigeminal ganglion showing course of mandibular nerve (in its foramen ovale) to alveolar nerve entering the mandibular canal (V³) in frontal views, MRI (**d**) of mandibular nerve (V³)

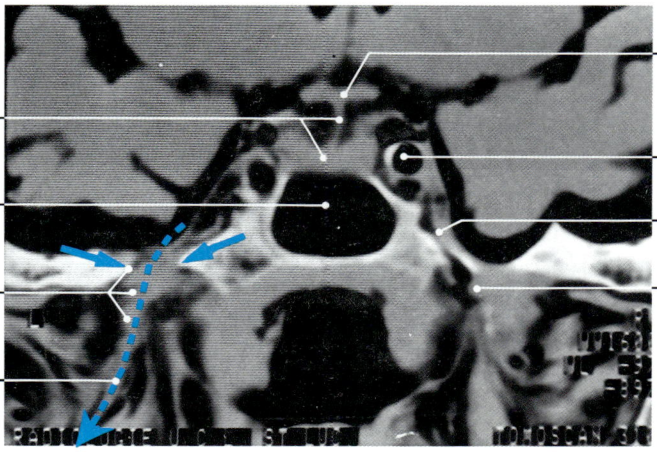

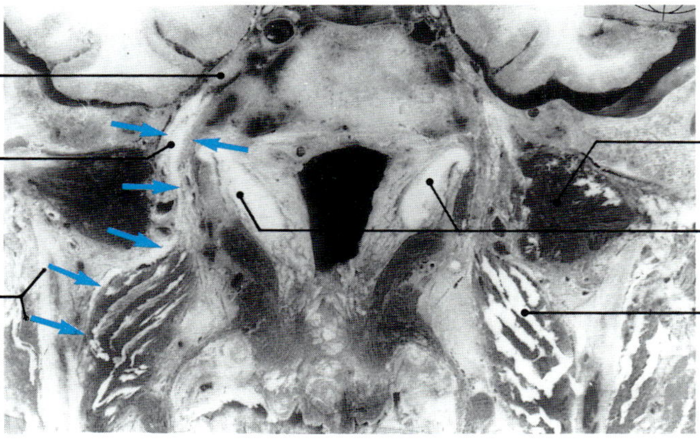

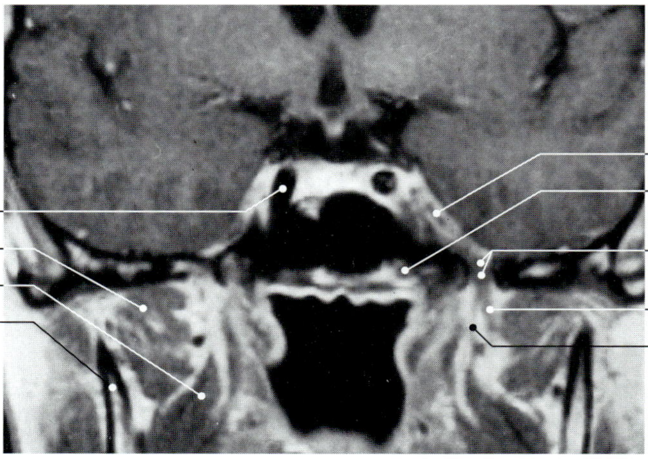

Mandibular nerve (V³): Foramen ovale

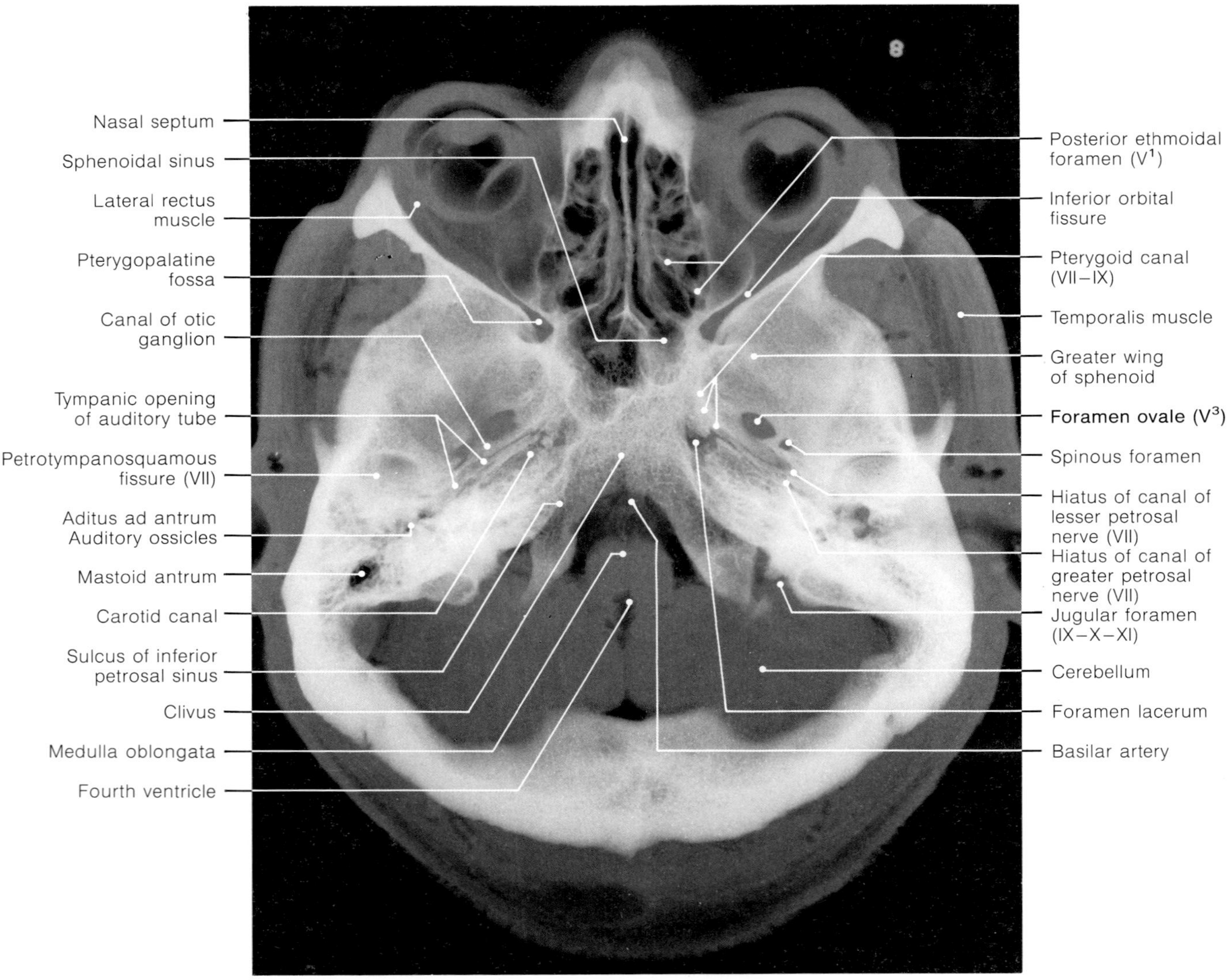

Fig. 5.85a. Radiograph of an anatomic section of skull base to show the foramina ovalia (V³)

Fig. 5.85b. Sagittal view of mandibular nerve (V³)

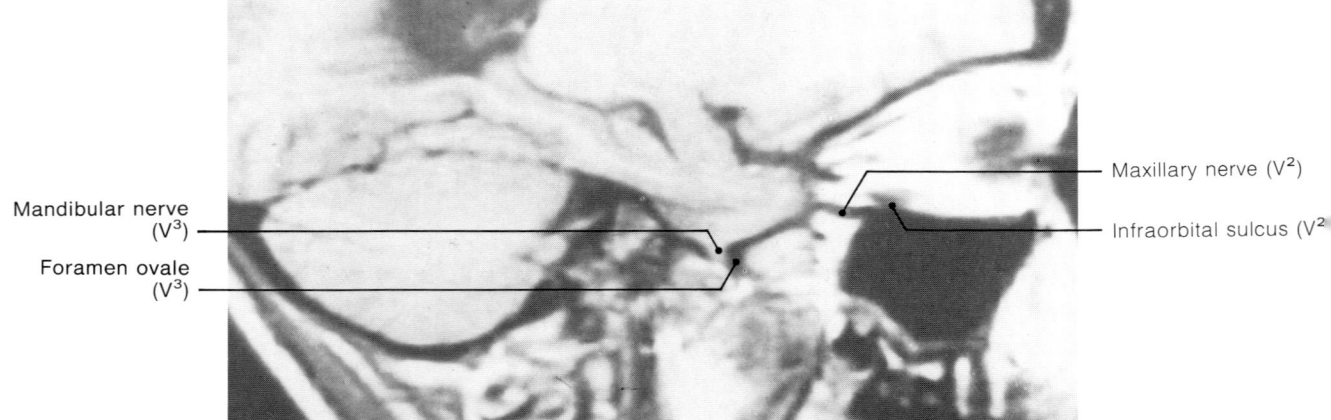

Mandibular nerve (V³): Foramen ovale

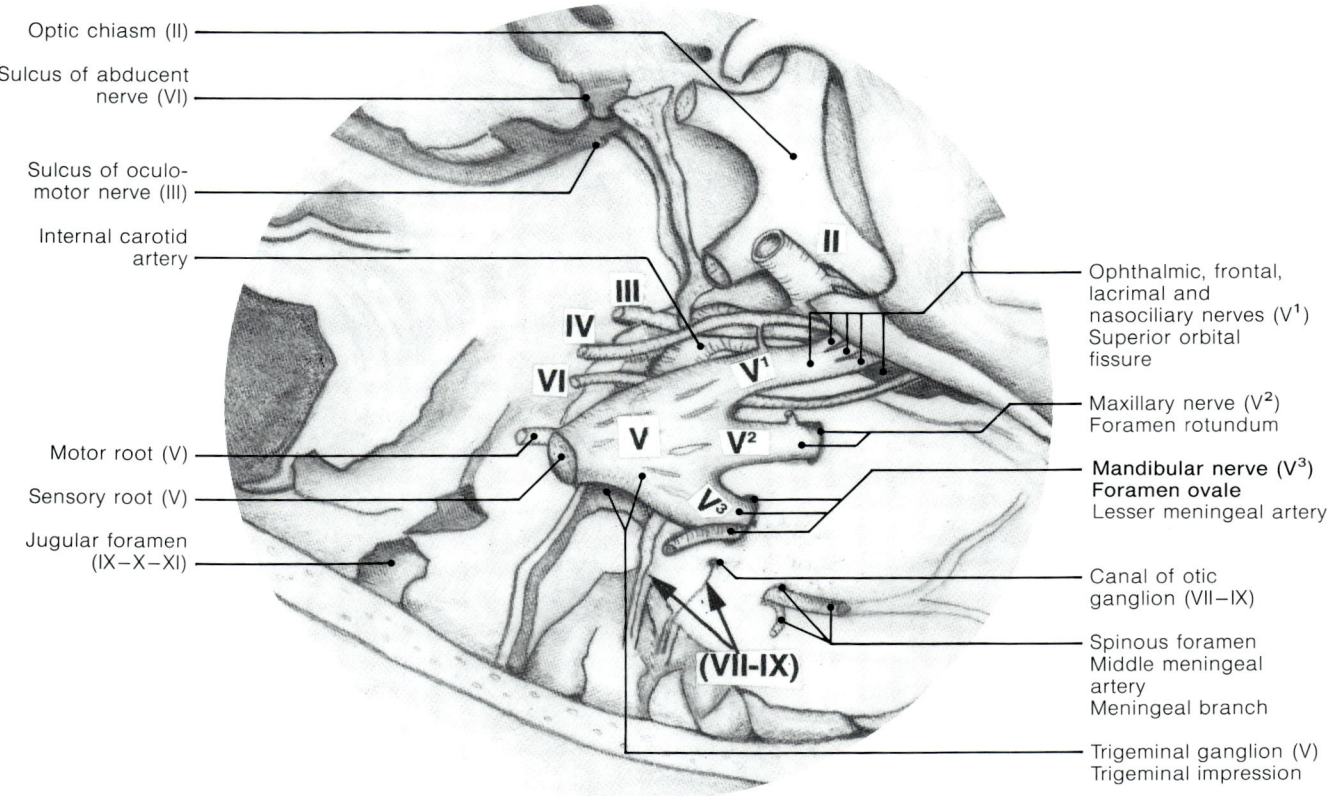

Fig. 5.86 a. VII–IX: Superficial and deep greater and lesser petrosal nerves

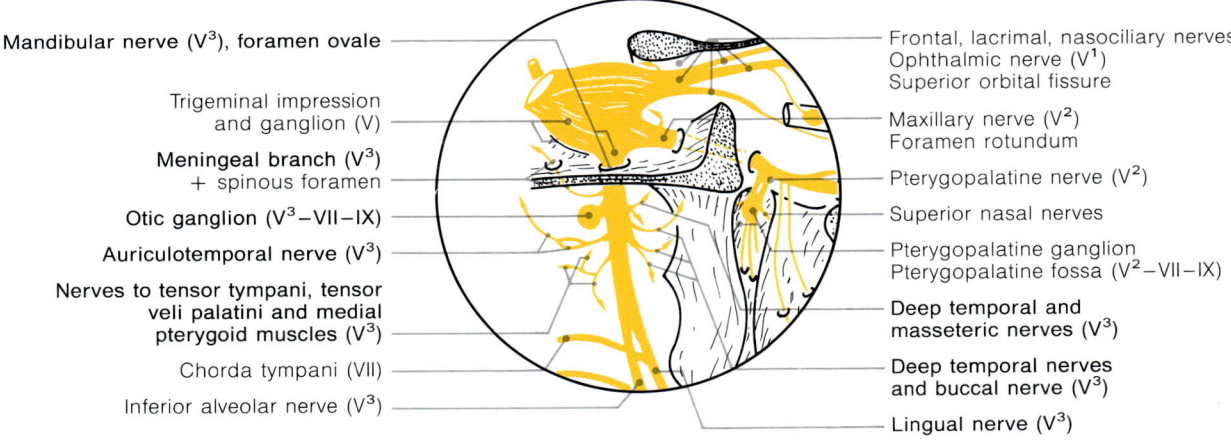

Fig. 5.86 a, b. Right superolateral and sagittal views with diagram of trigeminal nerve and its three branches entering their ostia

Topography

Inferior alveolar nerve (V³)
– Mandibular canal

Mental nerve (V³)
– Mental foramen

Pathology

– Alveolar cyst expanding towards the mandibular canal,
– mandibular tumor,
– fractures of mandible, mandibular ramus and mandibular symphysis,
– depressed fracture of mandibular symphysis.

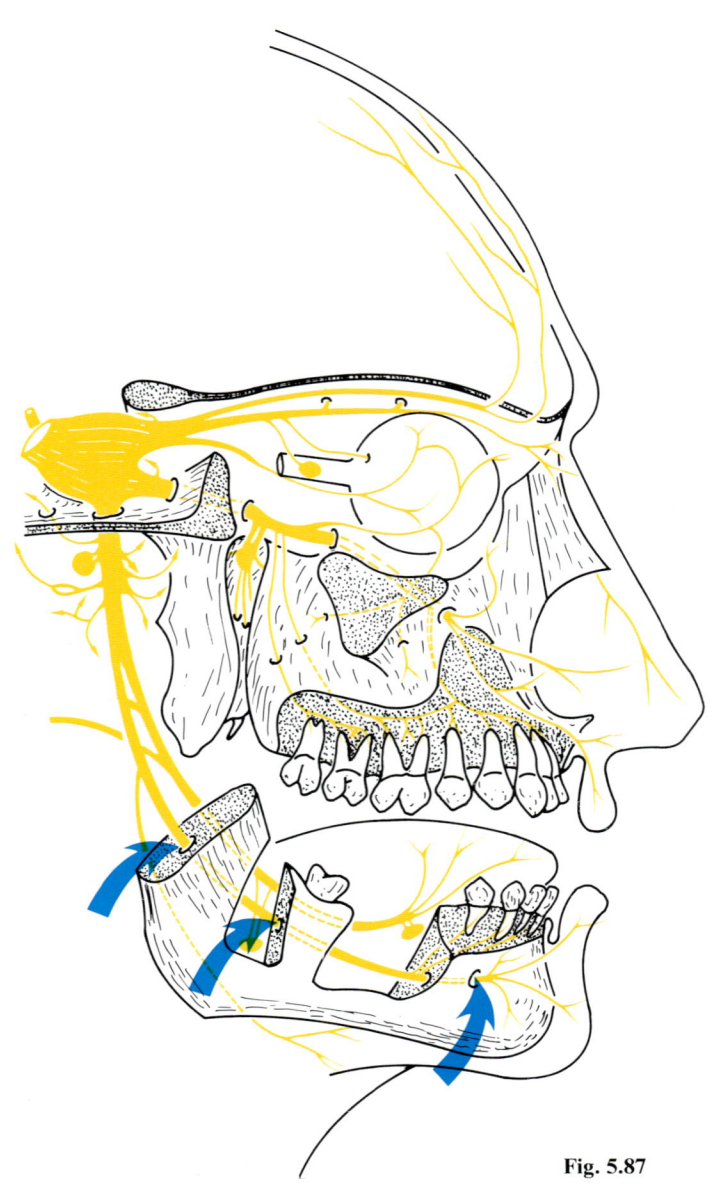

Fig. 5.87

Inferior alveolar nerve, mental nerve (V³): Mandibular canal, mental foramen

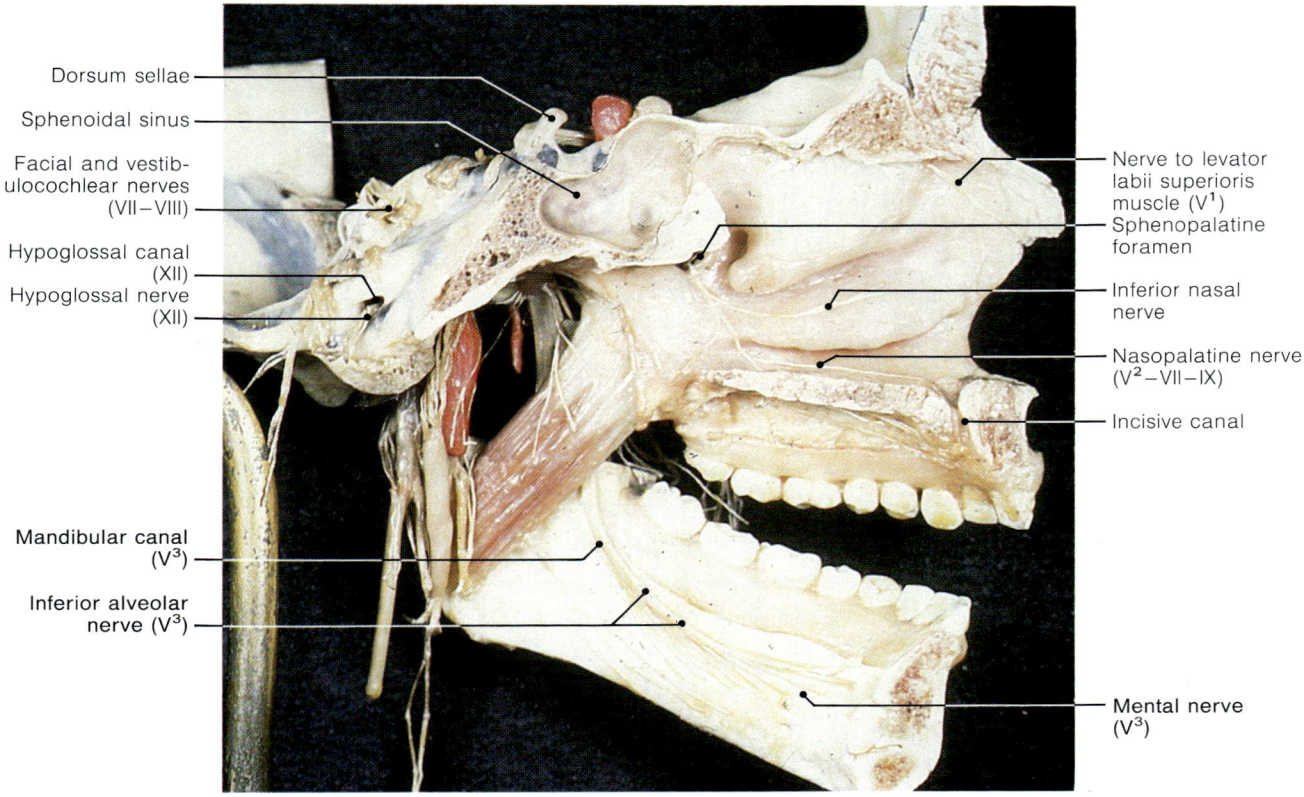

Fig. 5.88. Anatomic dissection showing course of inferior mandibular nerve (V³)

Inferior alveolar nerve, mental nerve (V³): Mandibular canal, mental foramen

Anatomy

The inferior alveolar nerve follows the mandibular canal and is the largest branch of the mandibular nerve.

It travels in its canal with the inferior alveolar vessels. After entering the canal, it sometimes divides into two terminal branches (Fig. 5.89c): the mental nerve, which reaches the mental foramen and divides into two terminal branches destined for the mucosa of the lower lip and for the chin (Fig. 5.89c), and the dental nerve, which gives off all the dental branches.

Before entering its canal, the mandibular nerve gives origin to several terminal branches:

- an anastomotic branch to the lingual nerve,
- the mylohyoid nerve, which leaves the inferior alveolar nerve to skirt the mylohyoid sulcus and the anterior belly of the digastric muscle (Fig. 5.77; 5.78; 5.89d),
- within the mandibular foramen it gives off collaterals to the molar and premolar teeth, also branches to the bone and gums (Fig. 5.89c). It divides into two terminal branches:
* the mental nerve, which emerges at the mental foramen (Fig. 5.87; 5.89d; 5.91d),
* the incisive nerve, which gives branches to the incisor teeth, gum and canine tooth (Fig. 5.89c).

The orifice of the mandibular canal is situated at the center of the inner aspect of the mandible (Fig. 5.90a–c); the canal travels obliquely forward and downward.

The entry orifice is extended as two prominences:

- an anterior prominence, the lingula of the mandible,
- a posterior, inconstant, prominence, the antilingula.

The mandibular canal transmits the alveolar and mental vessels and nerves (the mental structures traverse the mental foramen; Fig. 5.91b–d).

The pterygoid tuberosity is situated on the inner aspect of the mandible, behind the canal.

Imaging

EXAMINATION

- Survey in sagittal and lower frontal view,
- study of mandibular ramus for mandibular canal,
- study of mandibular angle, oblique view with chin supported, for mental foramen,
- dental survey view.

TECHNIQUE

Study of mandibular canal (mandibular ramus):

- The subject is prone, the thorax is raised on a pillow. The head is in profile with a support on the side to be examined and rests on a plane inclined by about 20°, with the forehead lower than the chin;
- the beam is angled 10°–15° towards the head and is centered at the mandibular angle of the side to be examined;
- the mandible must be in contact with the cassette (Fig. 5.89a).

Mandibular nerve (V³)   149

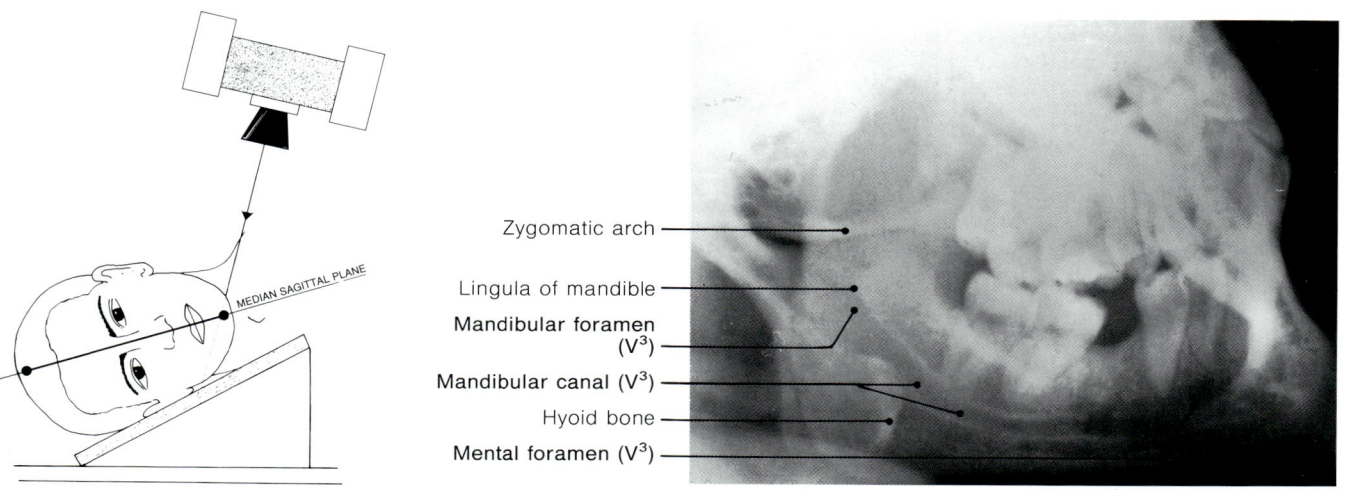

Fig. 5.89 a. Centering diagram for study of the mandibular canal

Fig. 5.89 b. Radiograph of the mandibular canal

Fig. 5.89 c, d. Diagram and anatomic view of mandibular canal and inferior alveolar nerve (V³)

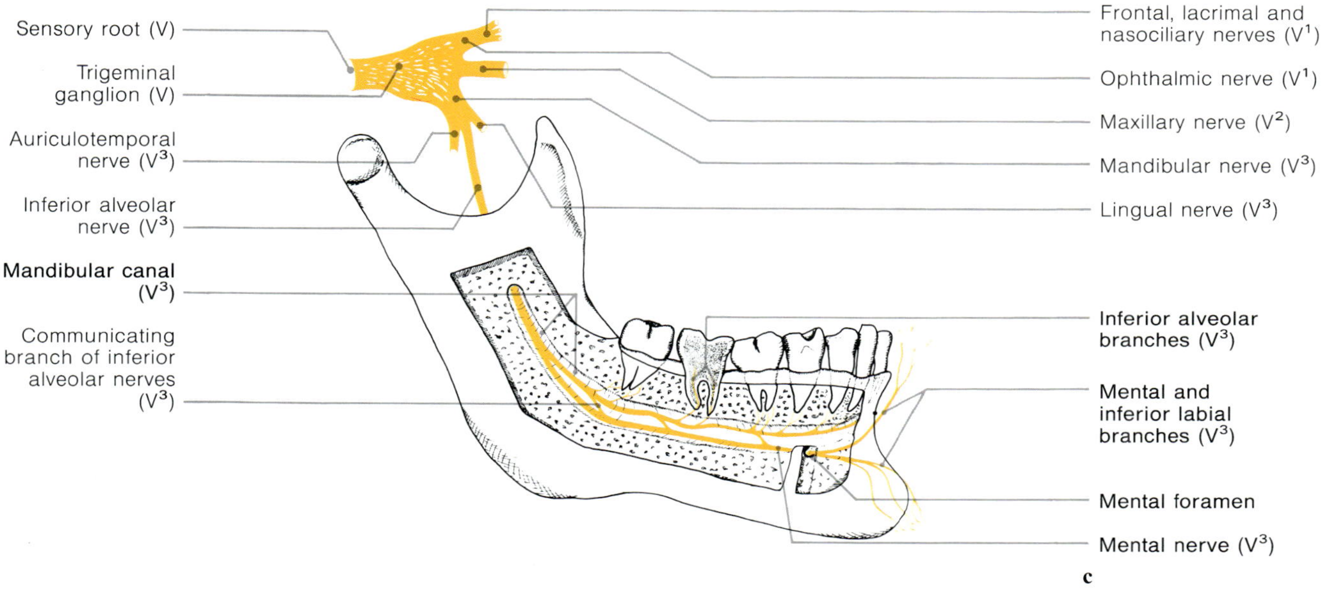

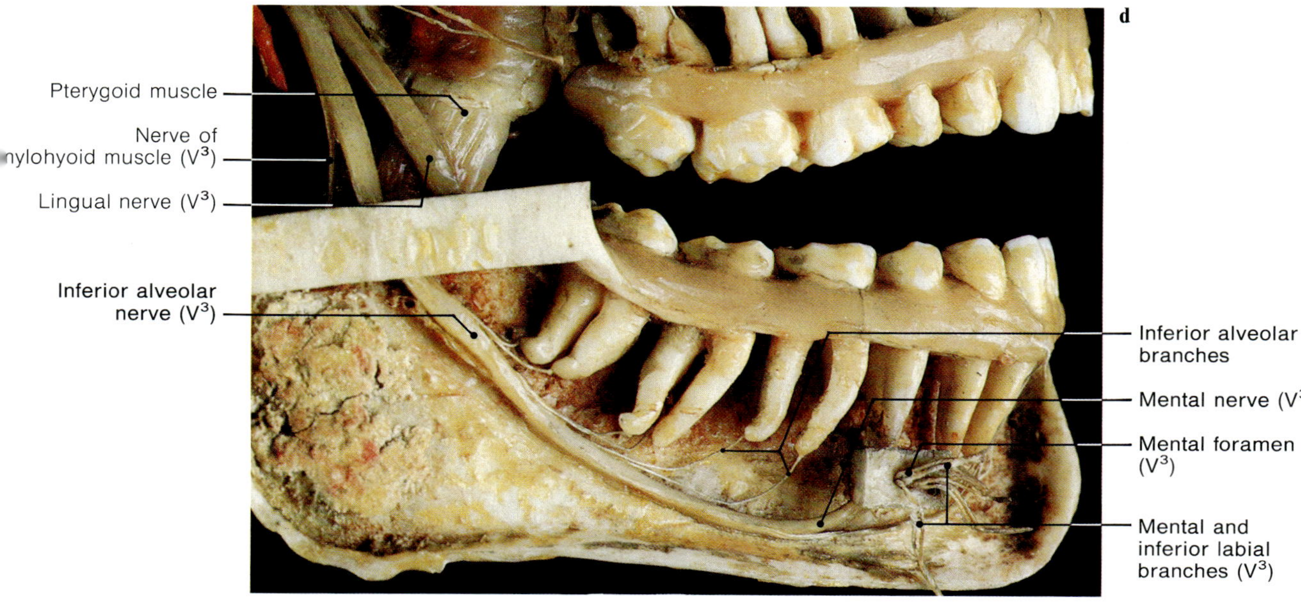

150 Trigeminal nerve (V)

Inferior alveolar nerve, mental nerve (V³): Mandibular canal, mental foramen

Fig. 5.90. a, b Medial views of the mandible showing orifice of mandibular canal; **c** medial and oblique view for orifice of mandibular canal, sulcus of mylohyoid nerve and fossae of attachment of muscles and ligaments; **d** lateral view for mental foramen and fossae of muscular attachments

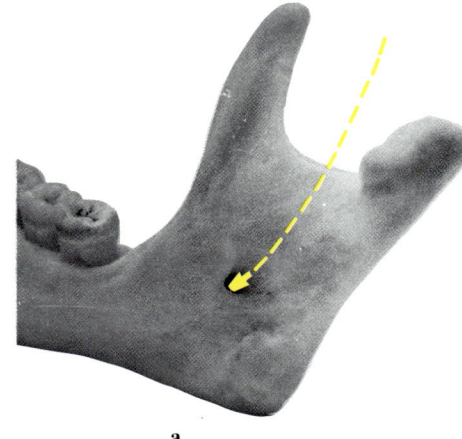

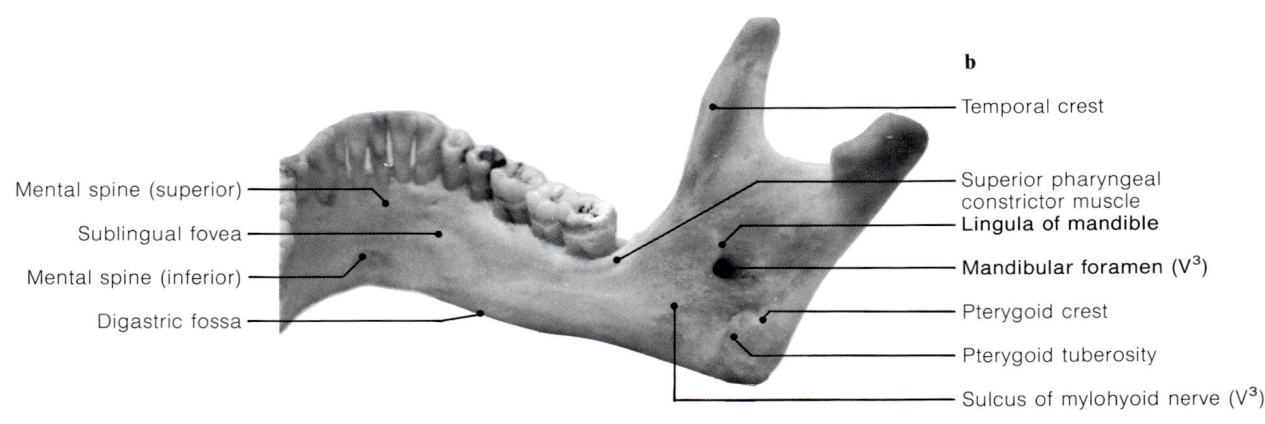

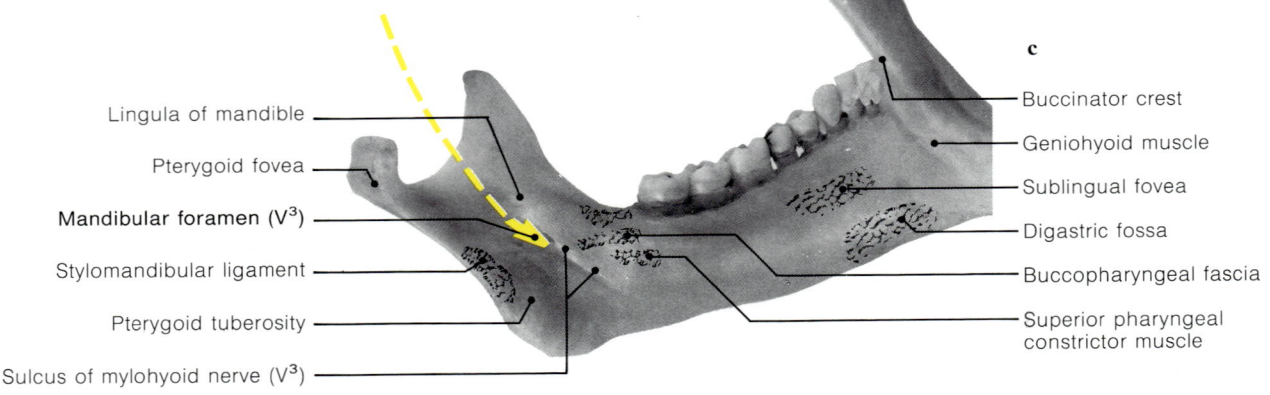

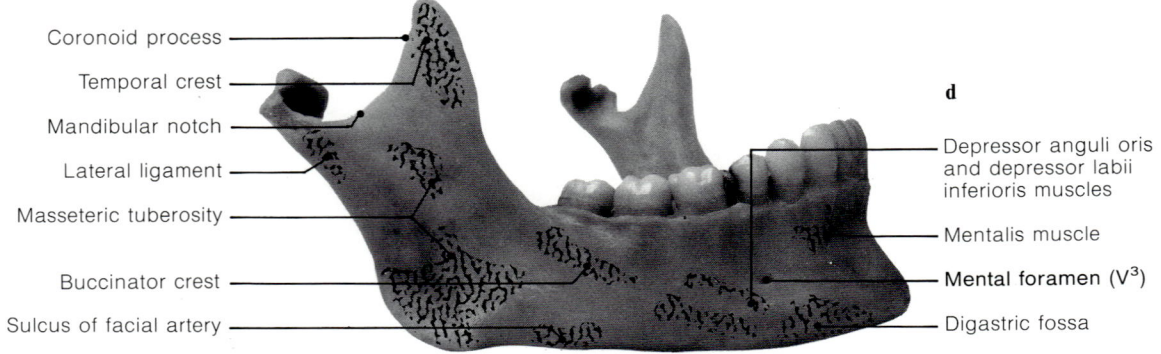

Mental foramen

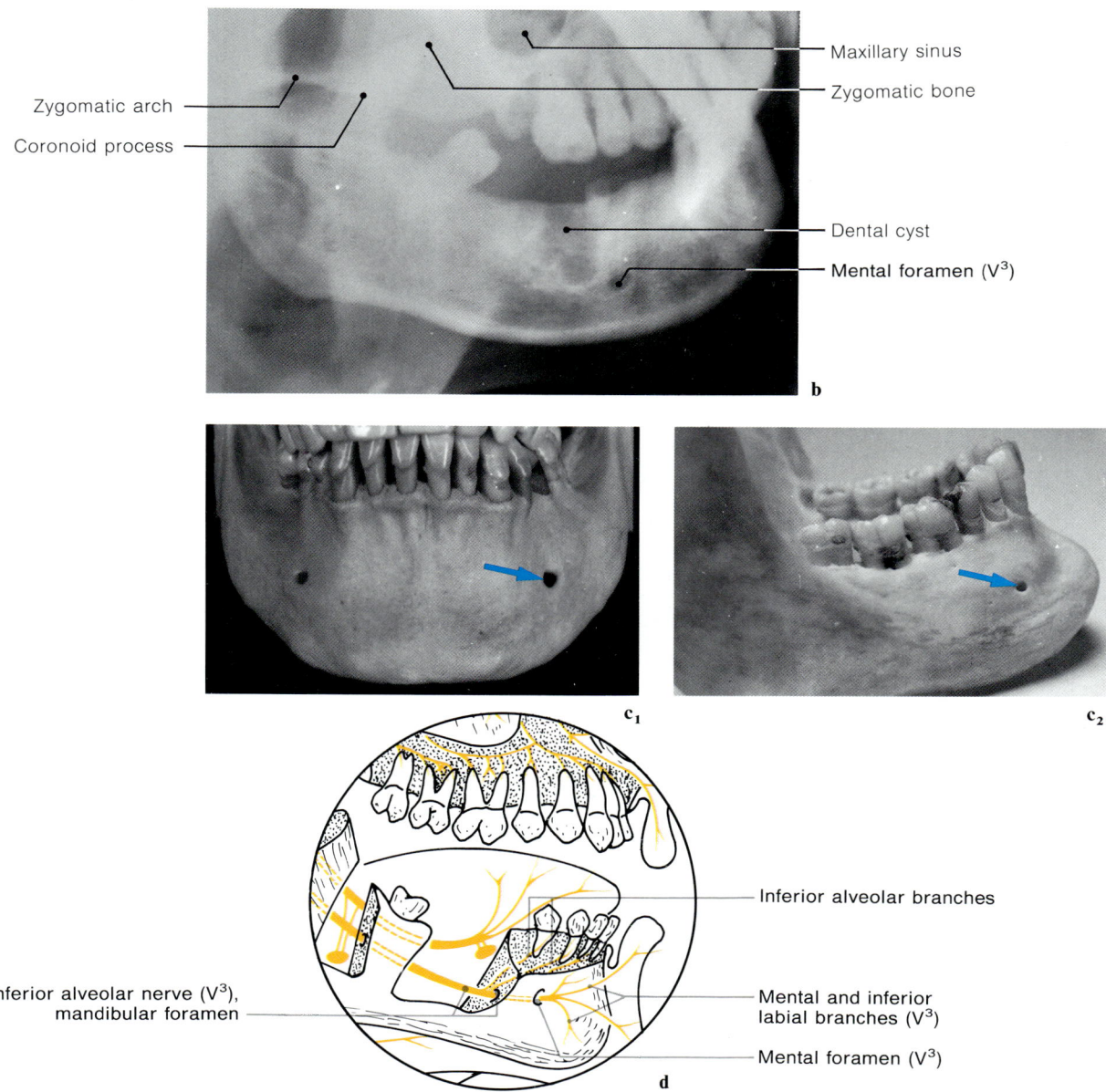

Fig. 5.91. Centering diagram for study of mental foramen

Fig. 5.91. a, b Radiographs of mental foramen; **c** frontal and sagittal views of mandible showing mental foramina; **d** diagram of terminal branches of inferior alveolar nerve at its exit from mental foramen

152   Trigeminal nerve (V)

Inferior alveolar nerve, mental nerve (V³): Mandibular canal, mental foramen

Imaging

TECHNIQUE (DENTAL SURVEY)

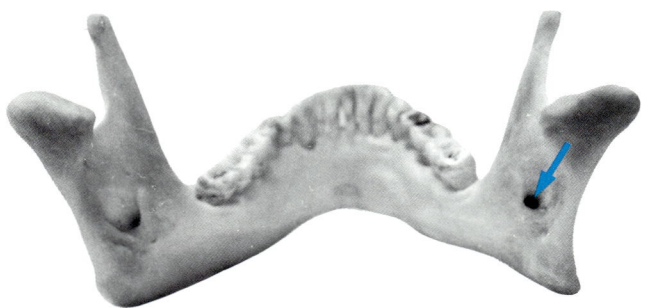

Fig. 5.92 a. Anatomic view of mental foramen

Fig. 5.92 b, c. Dental surveys of mental foramina and mandibular canals

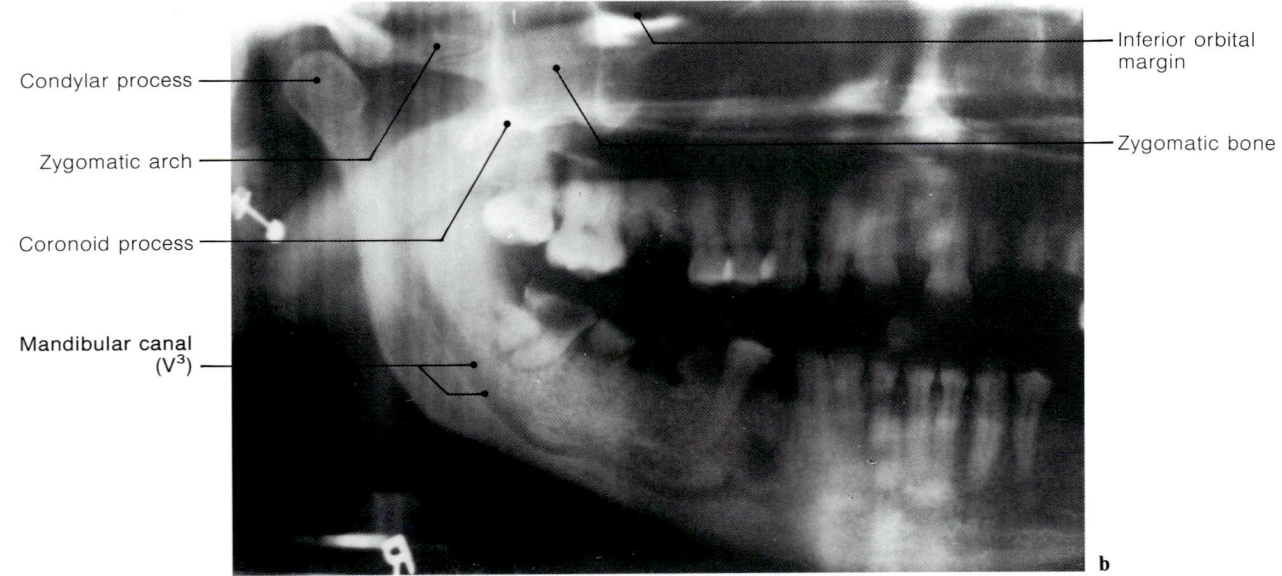

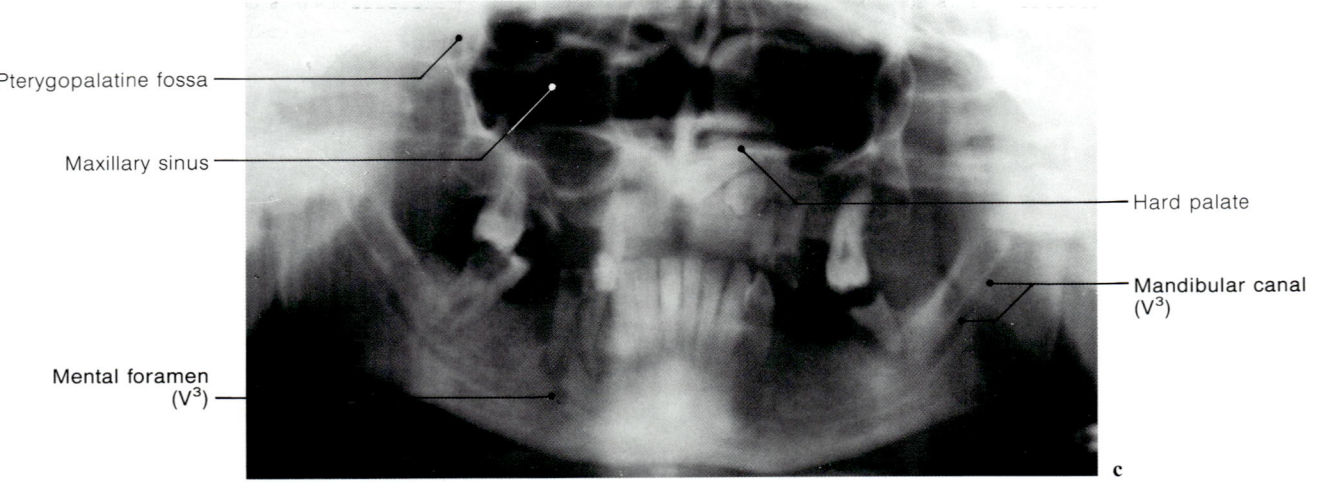

Trigeminal nerve (V): Trigeminal branches, sensory territories

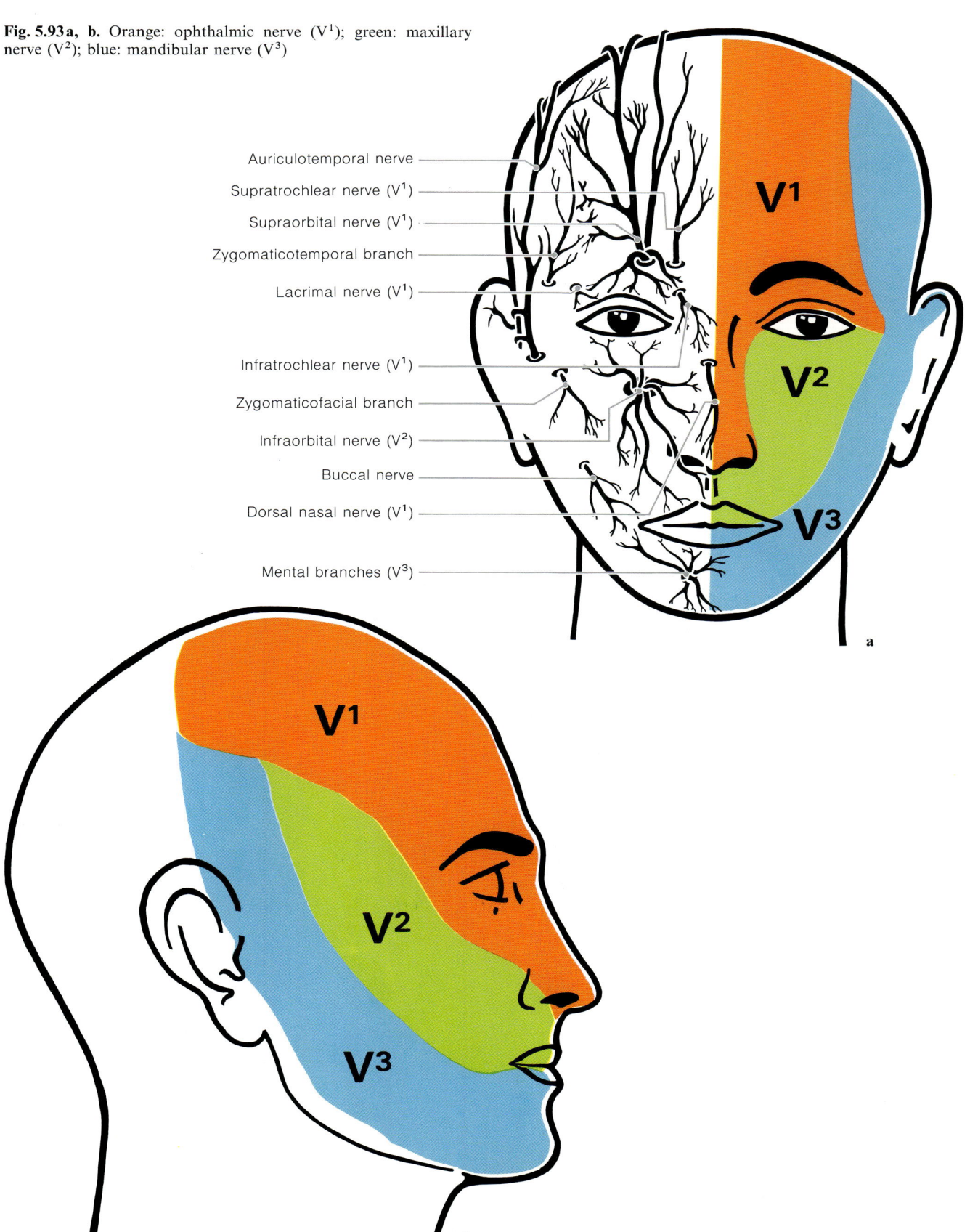

Fig. 5.93 a, b. Orange: ophthalmic nerve (V¹); green: maxillary nerve (V²); blue: mandibular nerve (V³)

Abducent nerve (VI)
(or lateral oculomotor nerve)

Anatomy (course – terminals – collaterals) 157
Imaging (regions examined) 157
Pathology 157
Apparent origin of abducent nerve (medullopontine sulcus, cistern of cerebellopontine angle)
    Anatomy and imaging (examination) 159
    Sagittal view (MRI) 160
Course and sulcus of abducent nerve
    Anatomy and imaging (examination) 162
    Axial views (MRI, CT) 162
    Axial view (MRI) 163
    Frontal and axial views (MRI, CT) 163
    Axial and oblique views (radiology, CT) 165
Intracavernous course
    Frontal (CT) and axial (MRI) views
    Reference diagram 166
Superior orbital fissure
    Diagram and sagittal view (MRI) 167
Termination of abducent nerve (lateral rectus muscle)
    Frontal, oblique and axial views (CT) 168
    Sagittal and intracranial anatomic dissections 169
Course of abducent nerve (diagram) 170

Vascular relations:
Cavernous sinus
    Venous drainage at the skull base 167, 290
    Ascending pharyngeal artery 276, 277
    Inferolateral trunk 276, 277
Communicating branch of the abducent nerve
with carotid sympathetic plexus 169, 210

The abducent nerve (or lateral oculomotor nerve), the VIth cranial nerve, is a motor nerve which supplies the lateral rectus muscle exclusively.
It arises in the pons and ends in the orbital cavity.
Its nucleus of origin is situated in the inferior region of the pons, beneath the fourth ventricle and close to the fibers of the facial nerve. Its paralysis produces loss of abduction movement of the eye.

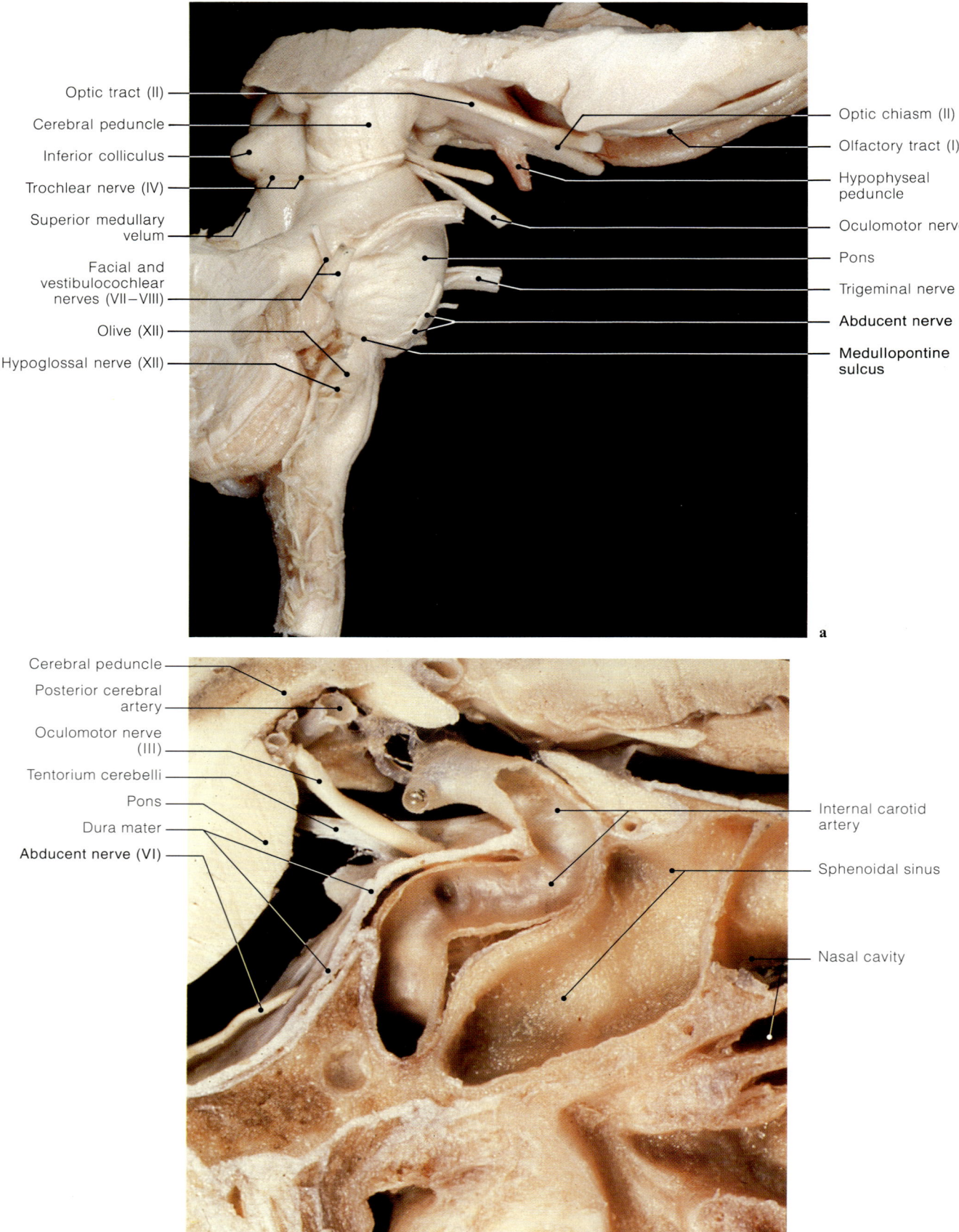

Fig. 6.1. a Right lateral view of brain-stem showing apparent origin of abducent nerve (VI); **b** sagittal anatomic section at level of left abducent nerve (VI). (Anatomic section: Pr. J.P. Francke, Faculty of Medicine, Lille)

Anatomy

COURSE – TERMINALS – COLLATERALS

Apparent origin and intracranial course

Sulcus of abducent nerve

Intracavernous course

Passage of abducent nerve through superior orbital fissure

Intraorbital course and lateral rectus muscle (VI)

Imaging

REGIONS EXAMINED

Medullopontine sulcus

Imaging of cerebellopontine angle and pontine cistern

Examination of petrous apex for sulcus of abducent nerve

Imaging of cavernous sinuses and lateral walls of sphenoidal sinuses

Study of superior orbital fissure

Study of ocular muscles (lateral rectus muscle VI)

Pathology

Lower pons:
– Syndrome of lower pons,
– tumor of cerebellopontine angle.

Sulcus (petrous apex):
– Osteitis of petrous apex (neuralgia of V and paralysis of VI; Gradenigo's syndrome),
– fracture of petrous apex.

Cavernous sinus:
– Syndrome of lateral wall of cavernous sinus (Foix's syndrome),
– fractures of sphenoidal sinuses.

Superior orbital fissure:
– Syndrome of superior orbital fissure (Rochon-Duvigneaud's syndrome),
– syndrome of petrosphenoidal junction (Garcin's syndrome),
– meningioma of lesser wing of sphenoid,
– fractures and sarcoma of anterior cranial fossa.

Intraorbital – lateral rectus muscle:
– Orbital fracture,
– intraorbital tumors.

Topography

Apparent origin of abducent nerve (VI)
- Medullopontine sulcus
- Cistern of cerebellopontine angle

Course of abducent nerve
- Petrous apex
- Sulcus of abducent nerve
- Cavernous sinus
- Superior orbital fissure
- Intraorbital and lateral rectus muscle (VI)

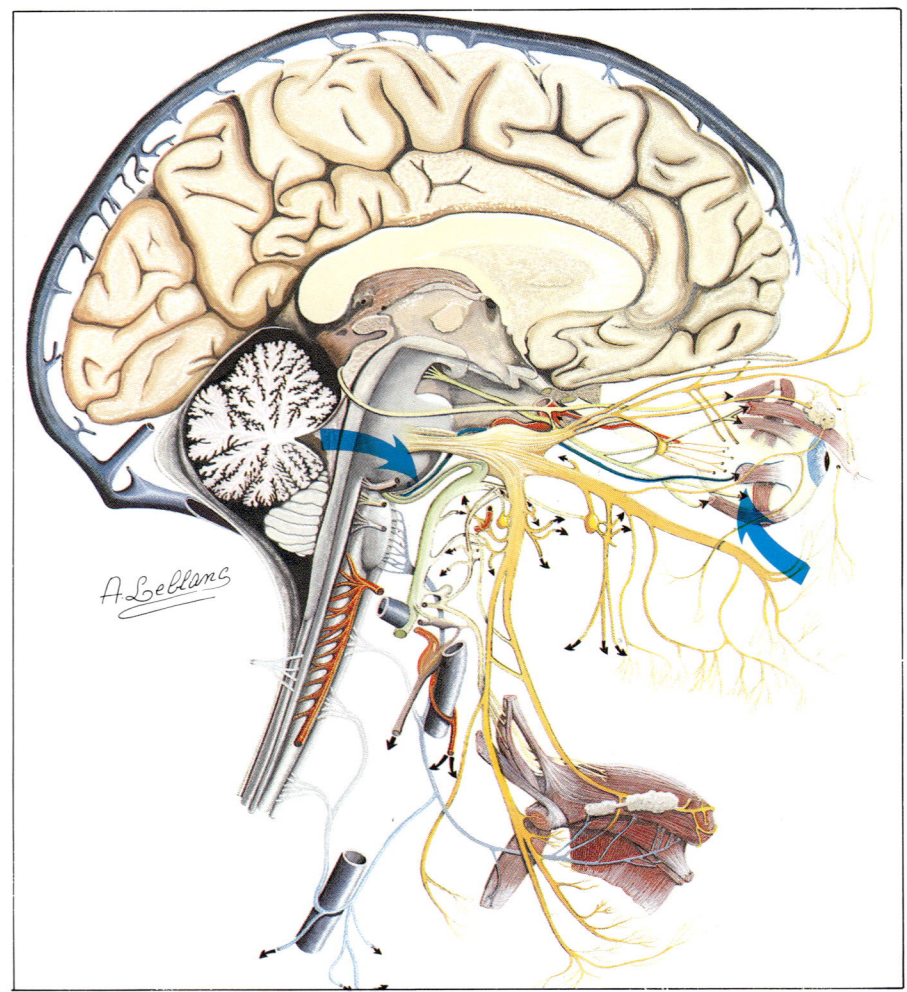

Fig. 6.2

Apparent origin of abducent nerve, medullopontine sulcus, cistern of cerebellopontine angle

Anatomy

The abducent nerve (VI) emerges at the anterior aspect of the brain-stem, from the medullopontine sulcus, immediately above the pyramids (Fig. 6.1; 6.2; 6.4).
Its radicular fibers derive from a nucleus situated in the floor of the fourth ventricle opposite the median eminence.

Imaging

CLINICAL FEATURES

– Homolateral paralysis of lateral ocular movements, peripheral facial paralysis, paralysis of abducent nerve (VI) with a hemiplegia on the side opposite the lesion not involving the face.

POSSIBLE CAUSES

– Syndrome of inferior protuberance (Foville's syndrome),
– fracture of clivus (hematoma compressing VI after its emergence).

EXAMINATION

– Magnetic resonance imaging (MRI) and computed tomography (CT) of cerebellopontine angle and prepontine cistern visualizing the medullopontine sulcus for the apparent origin of the abducent nerve (VI), in sagittal (Fig. 6.3a, b; 6.4b) and axial views (Fig. 6.5a; 6.6; 6.7).

Cerebellopontine angle

Magnetic resonance imaging (MRI)

SAGITTAL VIEW

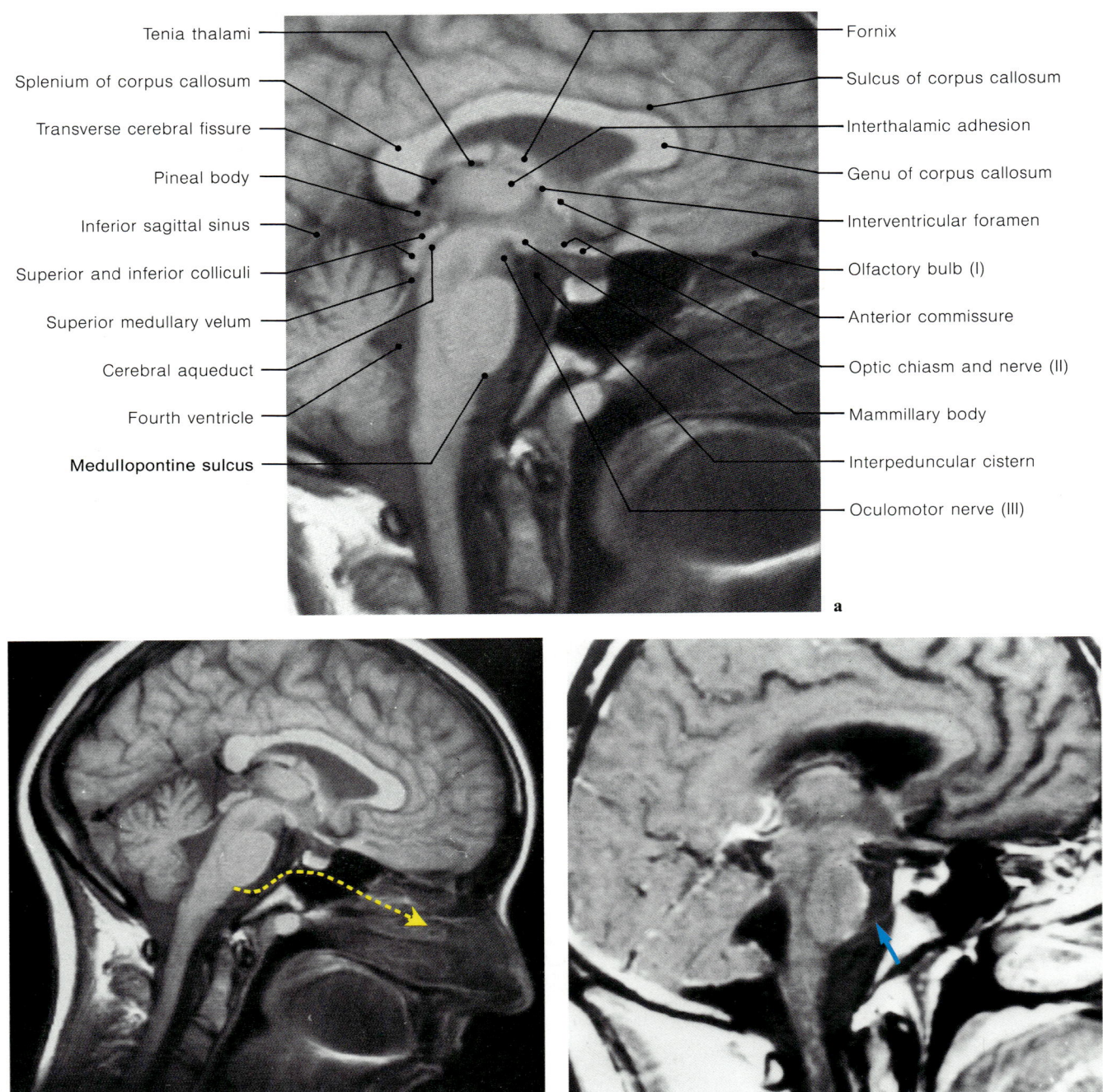

Fig. 6.3 a–c. Sagittal magnetic resonance imaging of prepontine cistern and medullopontine sulcus for apparent origin of the abducent nerve (VI); arrow: apparent origin of VI; dotted: course of VI

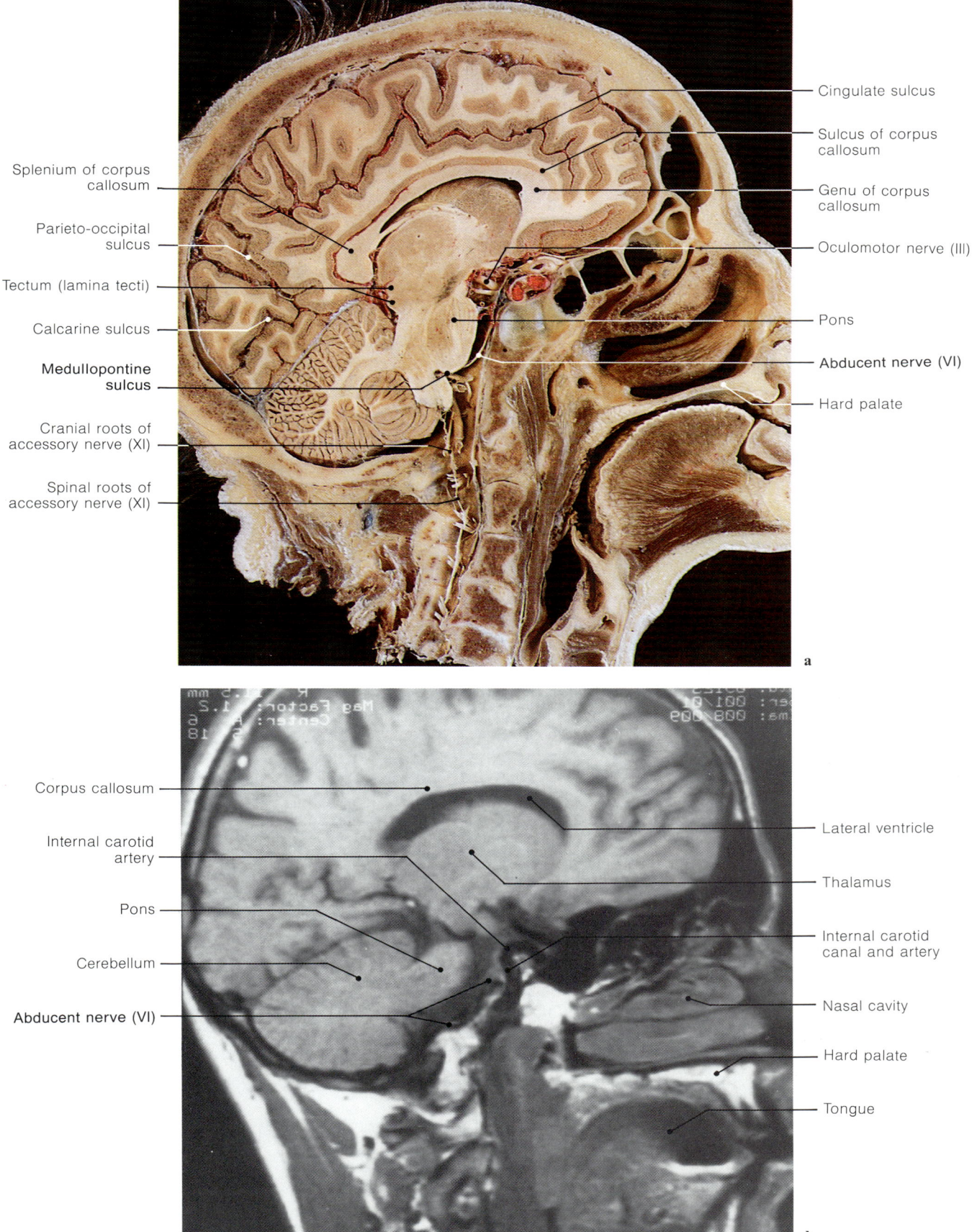

Fig. 6.4a, b. Anatomic section (a) and magnetic resonance imaging (b), both sagittal, at the apparent origin of the abducent nerve (VI)

Course of abducent nerve

Note: Apart from their true and apparent origins, the study of the three nerves controlling ocular movements calls for virtually the same radiologic techniques, while lesions of these nerves give rise to much the same clinical picture, their vulnerable points being similar (cavernous sinus, superior orbital fissure, orbit).

Anatomy

The trunk of the abducent nerve (VI) is ensheathed by a prolongation of the pia mater. It runs upwards, forwards and laterally. After having traversed the dura mater, it travels successively over the clival sulcus and the petrobasilar suture and creates a sulcus situated between the petrous apex and the trigeminal impression (V).
It enters the lateral wall of the cavernous sinus and travels within this, gliding along the lateral aspect of the internal carotid artery (Fig. 6.5b; 6.14a, b).
The abducent nerve (VI) traverses the superior orbital fissure and the common tendinous ring. In the orbital cavity, it reaches the lateral rectus muscle, which it innervates. It allows abduction of the eyeball.

Imaging

Course of abducent nerve (VI):
– Study by magnetic resonance imaging (MRI) or computed tomography (CT) in axial view, showing the course of the abducent nerve (VI) from its cerebral origin up to the lateral rectus muscle (Fig. 6.5a; 6.6).

Sulcus of abducent nerve (VI):
– Computed tomographic (CT) or tomographic study of petrous apex (Fig. 6.6; 6.8a–e).

Cavernous sinuses:
– Magnetic resonance imaging (MRI) and computed tomography (CT) of cavernous sinuses in frontal and axial views (Fig. 6.5a; 6.6; 6.10).

Superior orbital fissure (or sphenoidal cleft):
– Computed tomography (CT) or tomographic study of the superior orbital fissures.

Lateral rectus muscle:
– Magnetic resonance imaging (MRI) or computed tomography (CT) of the orbital cavity for the lateral rectus muscle (VI) in frontal, axial and oblique sagittal views in its axis (Fig. 6.13a–c).

Magnetic resonance imaging (MRI) and computed tomography (CT)

AXIAL VIEWS

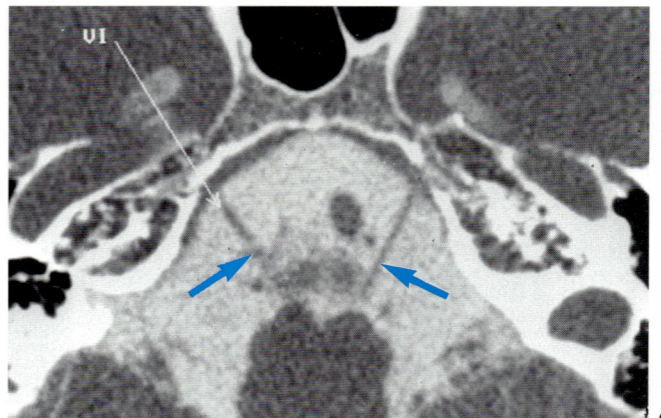
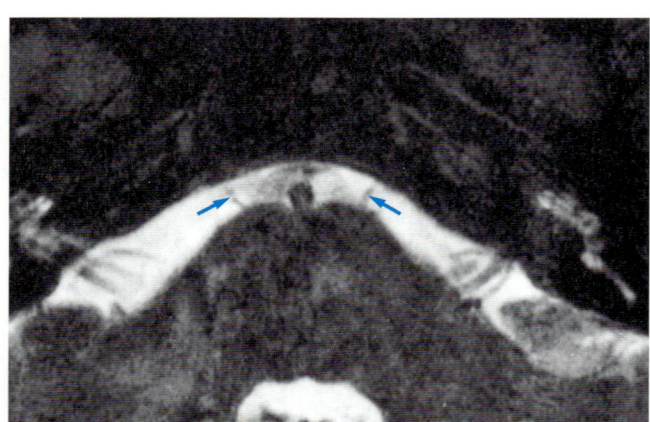
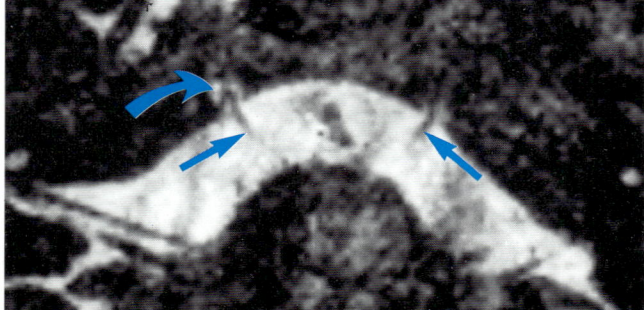

Fig. 6.4c–e. Computed tomography (CT; **c**) and magnetic resonance imaging (MRI) (**d, e**): axial views of abducent nerve (VI) (*arrows*) in Dorelli's canal (*curved arrow*). (CT: Pr. Doyon, Hospital Kremlin Bicêtre, Paris; MRI: Dr. J.W. Casselman, A.Z. St-Jan, Brugge)

Cerebellopontine angle, course of abducent nerve
Magnetic resonance imaging (MRI)
AXIAL VIEW

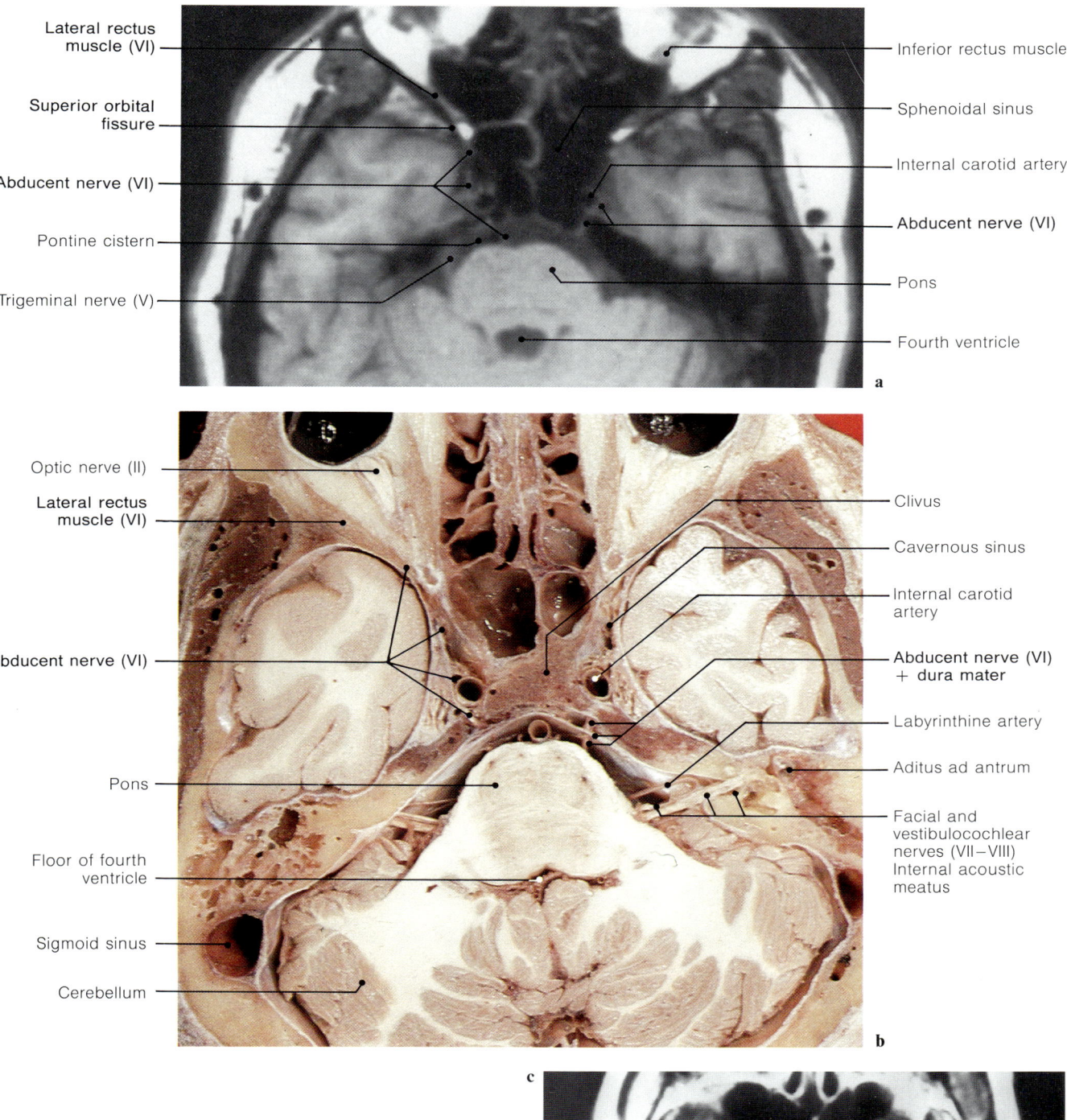

Fig. 6.5. a Magnetic resonance imaging and **b** anatomic section, both axial, at the level of the cavernous sinuses, showing course of abducent nerve (VI); **c** MRI axial view of apparent origins of VI (*arrows*). (MRI: Pr. Doyon, Hospital Kremlin Bicêtre, Paris)

Cerebellopontine angle, cavernous sinus, course of abducent nerve
Magnetic resonance imaging (MRI) and computed tomography (CT)
AXIAL VIEW

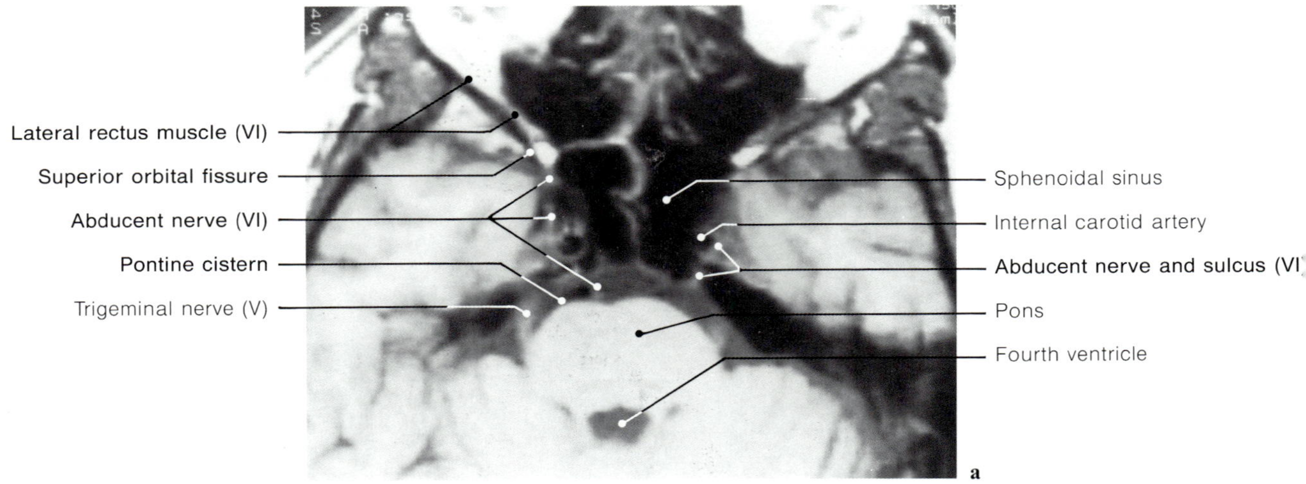

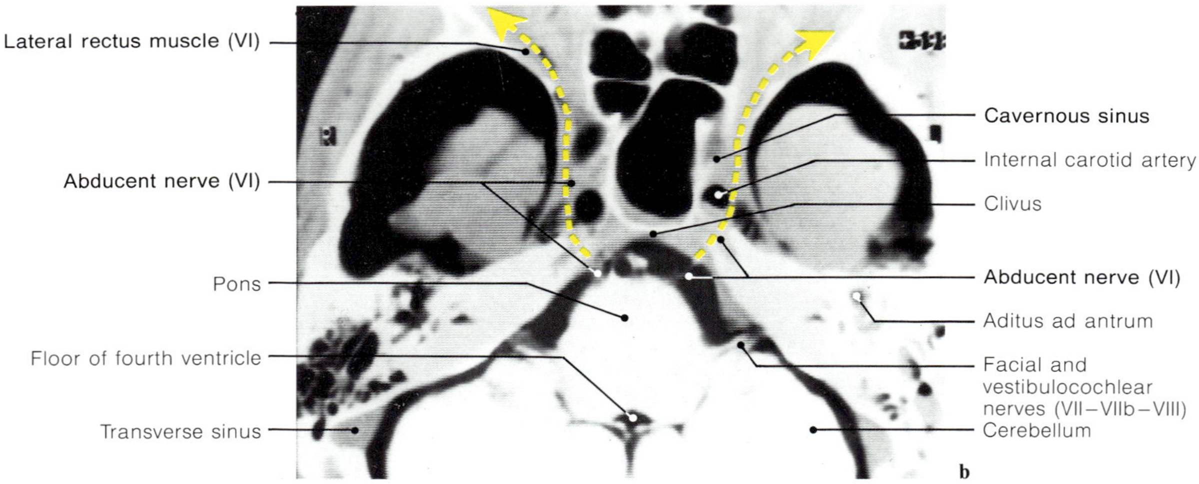

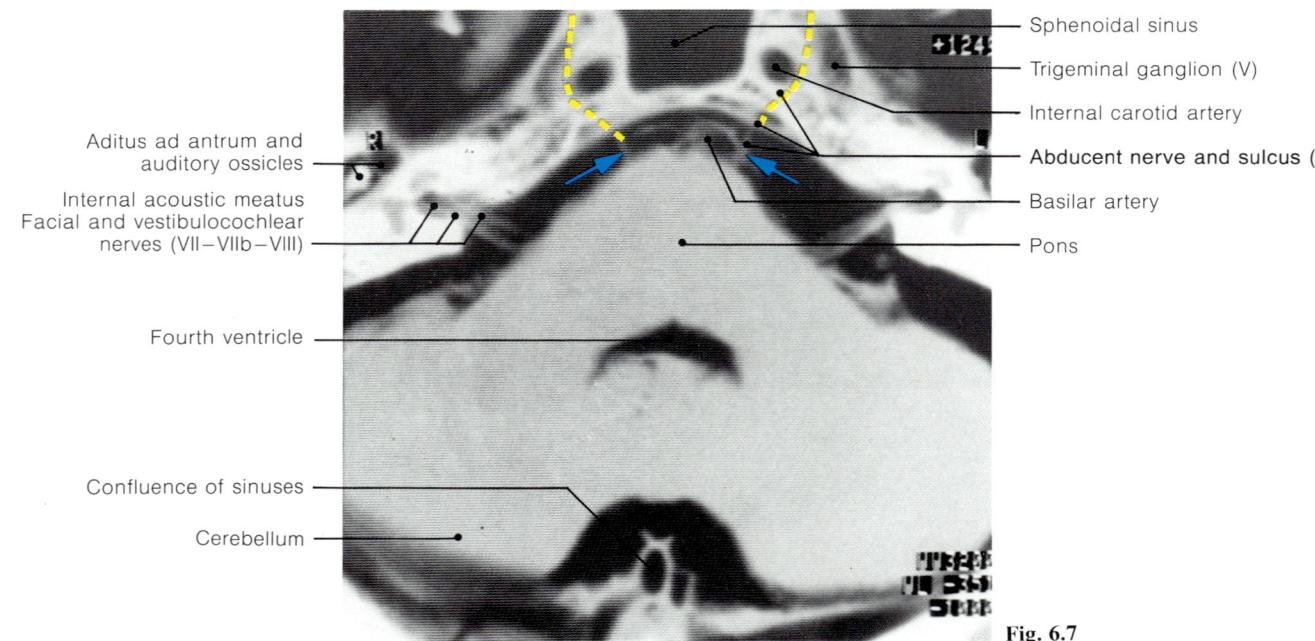

Fig. 6.6 a, b; 6.7. Magnetic resonance imaging (MRI) and computed tomography (CT) of course of abducent nerve (VI) in axial view

Sulcus of abducent nerve

Imaging

CLINICAL FEATURES

– Paralysis of abducent nerve (VI) associated with a lesion of the trigeminal nerve (V) causing atypical facial neuralgia.

POSSIBLE CAUSES

– Gradenigo's syndrome, due to osteitis or fracture of the petrous apex,
– aneurysm of internal carotid artery.

EXAMINATION

– Tomographic or computed tomographic (CT) examination of the petrous apex to display the sulcus of the abducent nerve (VI) (Fig. 6.8a–e).
The technique is identical with that for the trigeminal impression (Fig. 5.13; 5.15; 5.17).

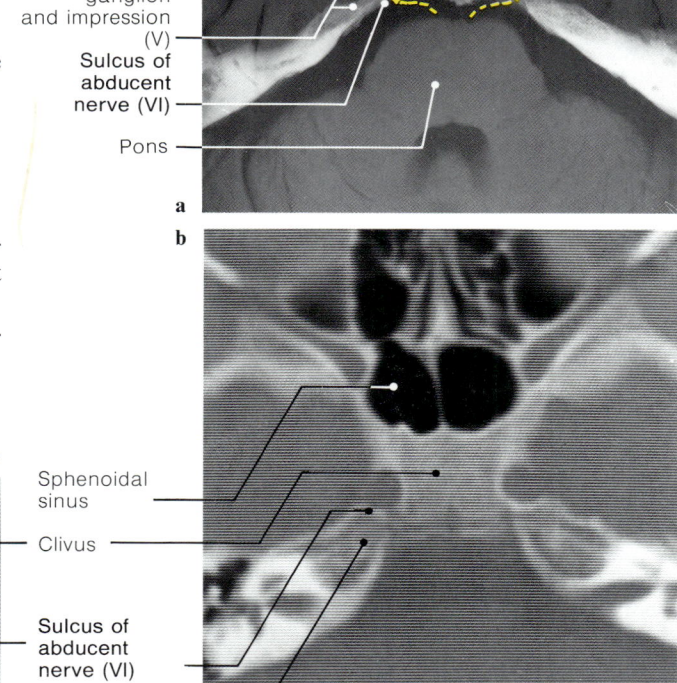

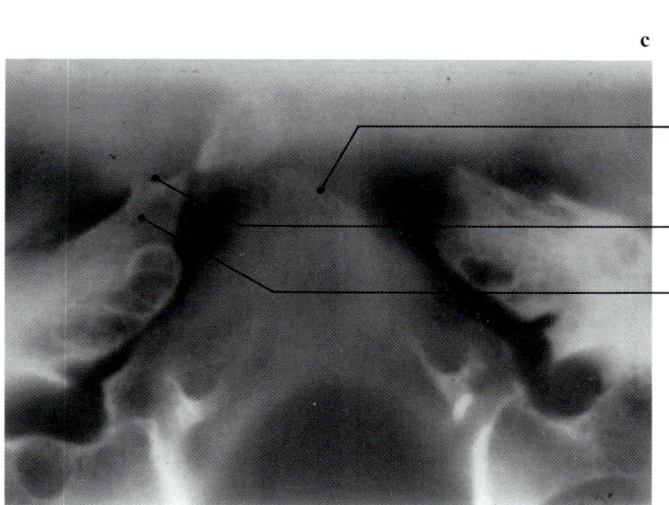

Fig. 6.8. a Axial section showing course of abducent nerve (VI) and its sulcus; b, c tomographic and computed tomographic (CT) studies of the sulci of the abducent nerves (VI) (petrous apex)

Tomography and computed tomography (CT)

OBLIQUE AND AXIAL VIEWS

Fig. 6.8d, e. Dry bone specimen and diagram of region of petrous apex for abducent nerve and sulcus (VI)

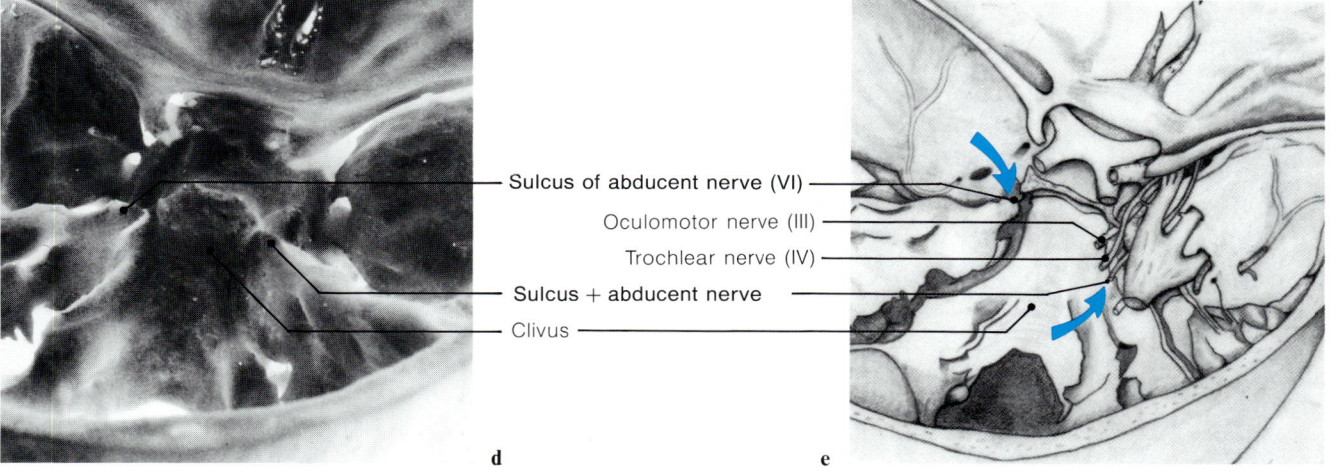

Intracavernous course (See diagram of the venous drainage, p. 290)

Imaging

CLINICAL FEATURES

– Paralysis of cranial nerves III, IV and VI with involvement of the ophthalmic (V^1) and maxillary (V^2) branches of the trigeminal nerve (V).

POSSIBLE CAUSES

– Syndrome of the lateral wall of the cavernous sinus (Foix's syndrome), which may be associated with a hypophyseal tumor, a phlebitis of the cavernous sinus or an aneurysm of the internal carotid artery (siphon).

EXAMINATION

– Magnetic resonance imaging (MRI) and computed tomography (CT) in frontal and axial views of the cavernous sinuses (Fig. 6.5a; 6.6; 6.10).

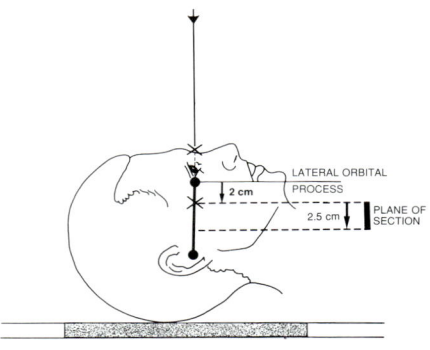

Fig. 6.9. Reference diagram for frontal imaging of cavernous sinuses

Computed tomography (CT) and magnetic resonance imaging (MRI)

FRONTAL AND AXIAL VIEWS

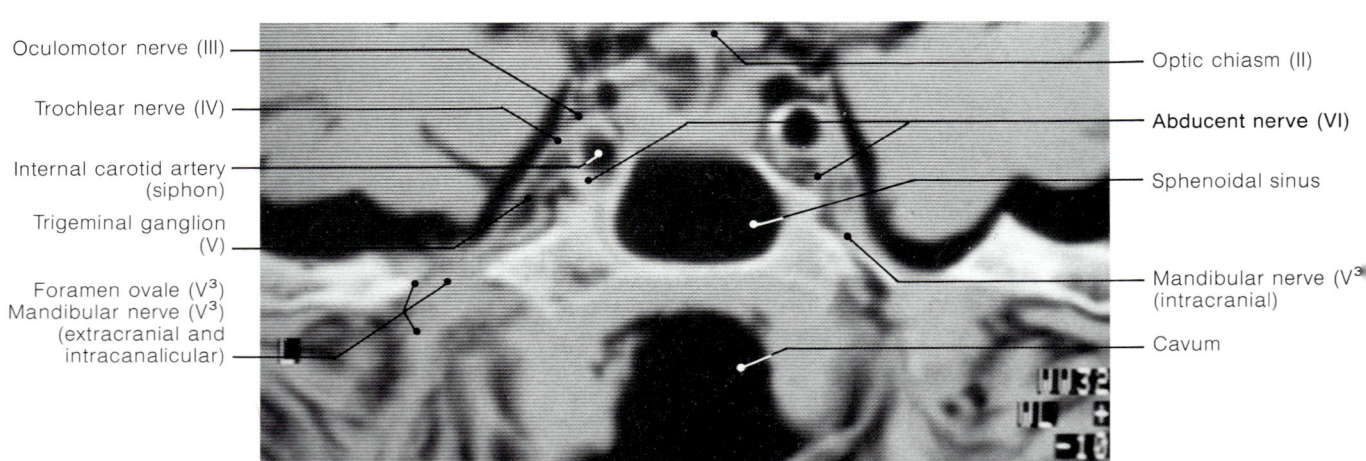

Fig. 6.10. Frontal computed tomographic (CT) section of cavernous sinuses showing arrangement of abducent nerves (VI)

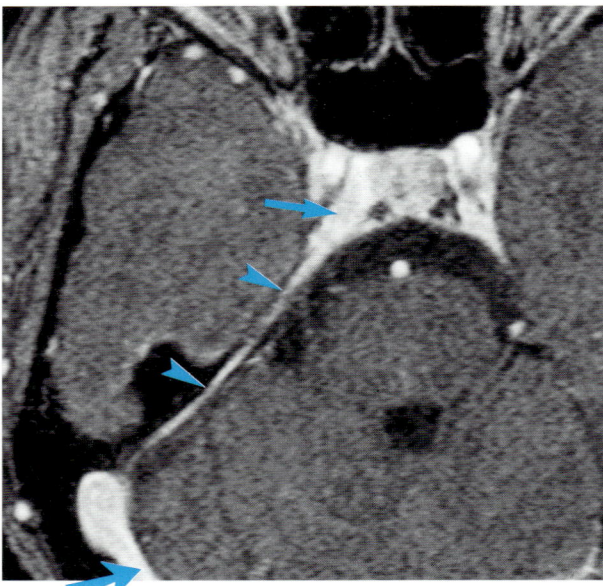

Fig. 6.11. Axial magnetic resonance imaging (MRI) of cavernous sinus (*straight arrow*), superior petrosal sinus (*arrowheads*) and lateral sinus (*large arrow*)

Abducent nerve (VI) 167

Superior orbital fissure

Imaging

CLINICAL FEATURES

– Paralysis of cranial nerves III, IV and VI, involvement of the ophthalmic (V^1) branch of the trigeminal nerve (V) with simultaneous complete intrinsic and extrinsic ophthalmoplegia, plus anesthesia of the root of the nose, upper eyelid, forehead and cornea with loss of corneal reflex.

POSSIBLE CAUSES

– Rochon-Duvigneaud's syndrome or syndrome of the superior orbital fissure, the possible result of a fracture of the lesser wing of the sphenoid, an aneurysm of the internal carotid artery or an adjacent tumor.

EXAMINATION

– Frontal and symmetric imaging of superior orbital fissures (see centering diagrams: Fig. 5.25a, b, p. 85).

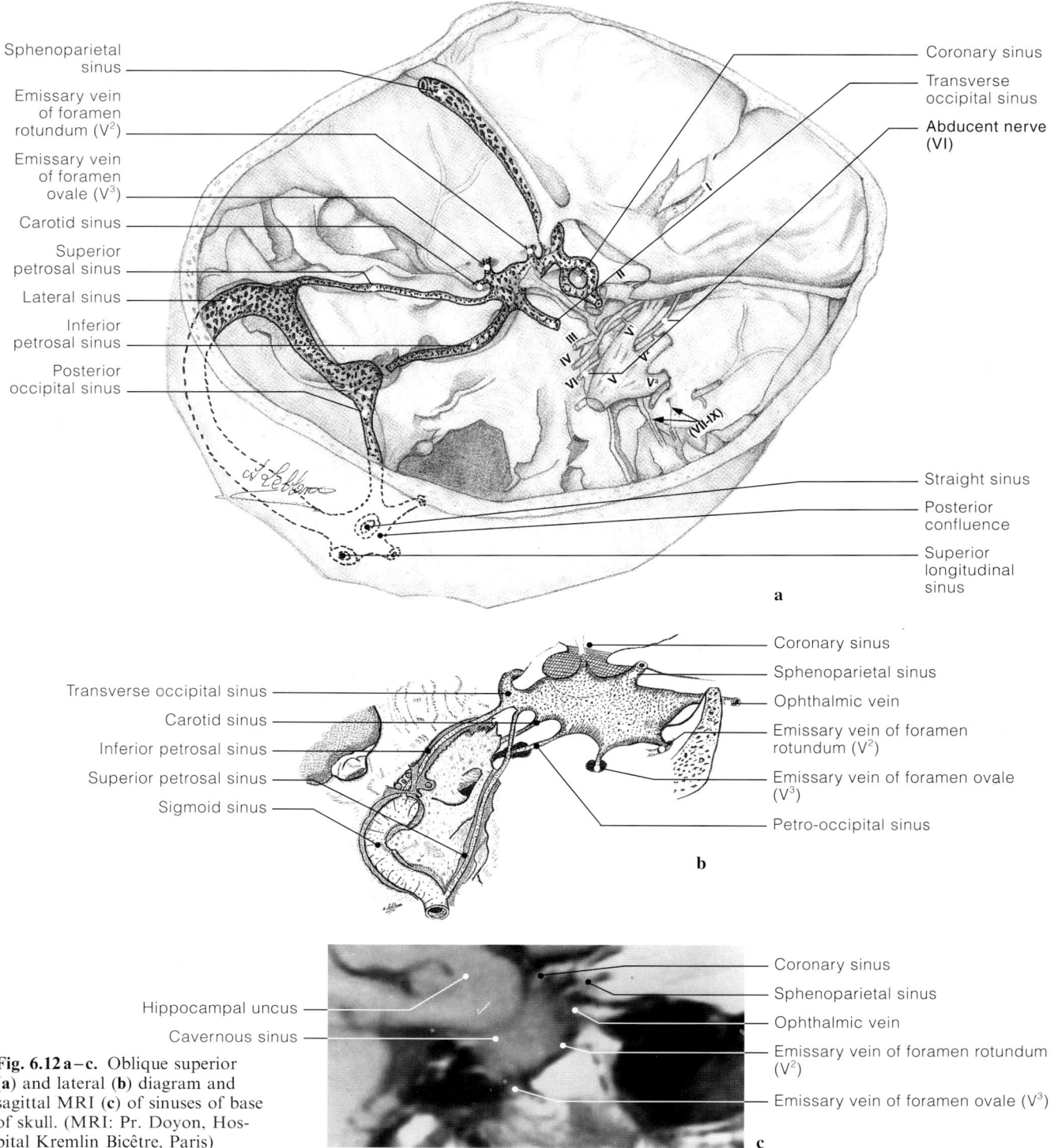

Fig. 6.12a–c. Oblique superior (**a**) and lateral (**b**) diagram and sagittal MRI (**c**) of sinuses of base of skull. (MRI: Pr. Doyon, Hospital Kremlin Bicêtre, Paris)

Termination of abducent nerve, lateral rectus muscle

Imaging

If the patient is affected by a paralysis of the lateral rectus muscle without involvement of the abducent nerve (VI) it is a matter of orbital pathology (intraorbital tumor with exophthalmos, head injury with fracture of the lateral orbital wall), and frontal, axial and sagittal computed tomographic (CT) studies of the orbits must be performed to visualize the orbital muscles (Fig. 6.13 a–c).

Computed tomography (CT)

AXIAL, OBLIQUE AND FRONTAL VIEWS

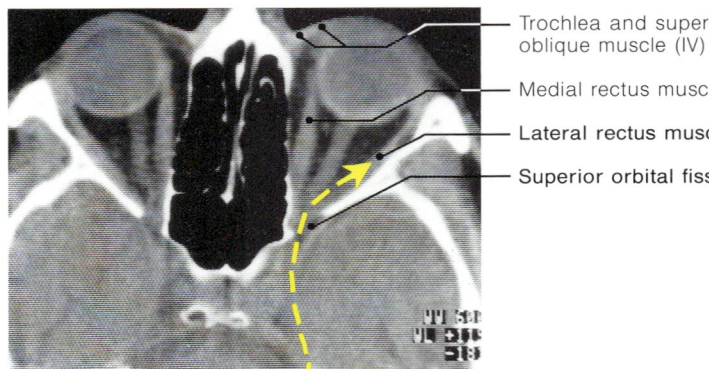

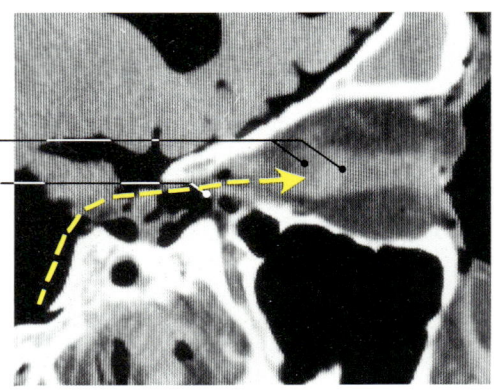

Fig. 6.13a. Axial computed tomography (CT) of lateral rectus muscles

Fig. 6.13b. Oblique computed tomography (CT) in the axis of the lateral rectus muscle

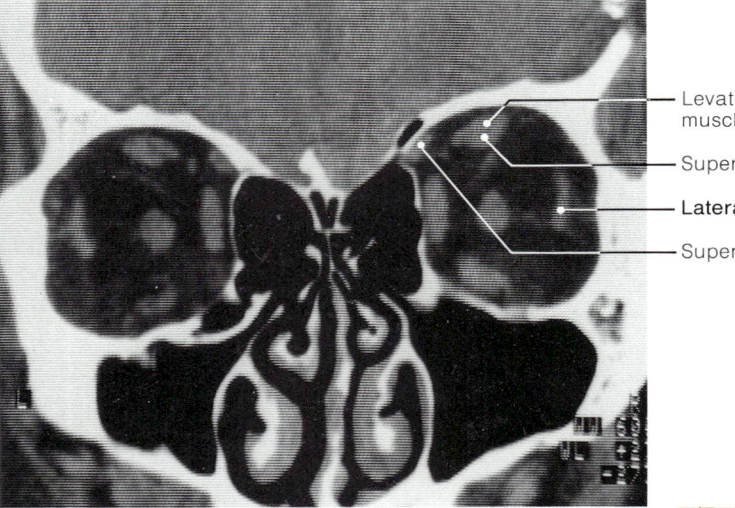

Fig. 6.13c. Frontal computed tomography (CT) of lateral rectus muscles

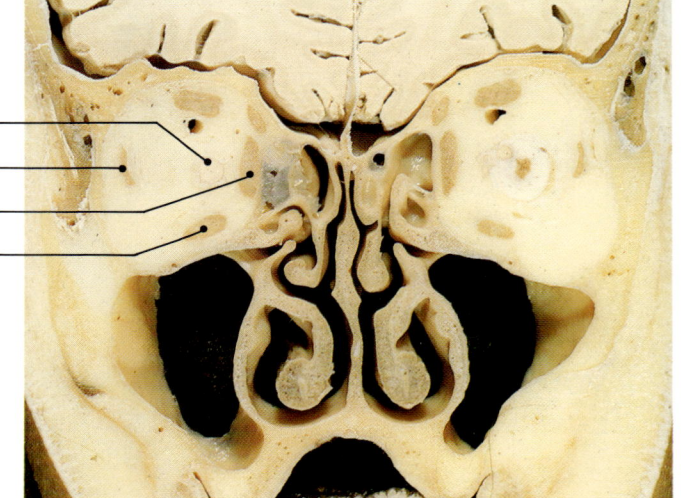

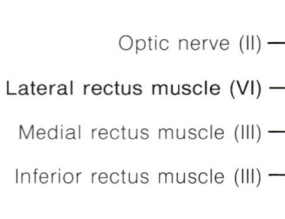

Fig. 6.13d. Frontal section at posterior pole of eye showing ocular muscles

Course of abducent nerve from its origin to lateral rectus muscle
Anatomic dissections

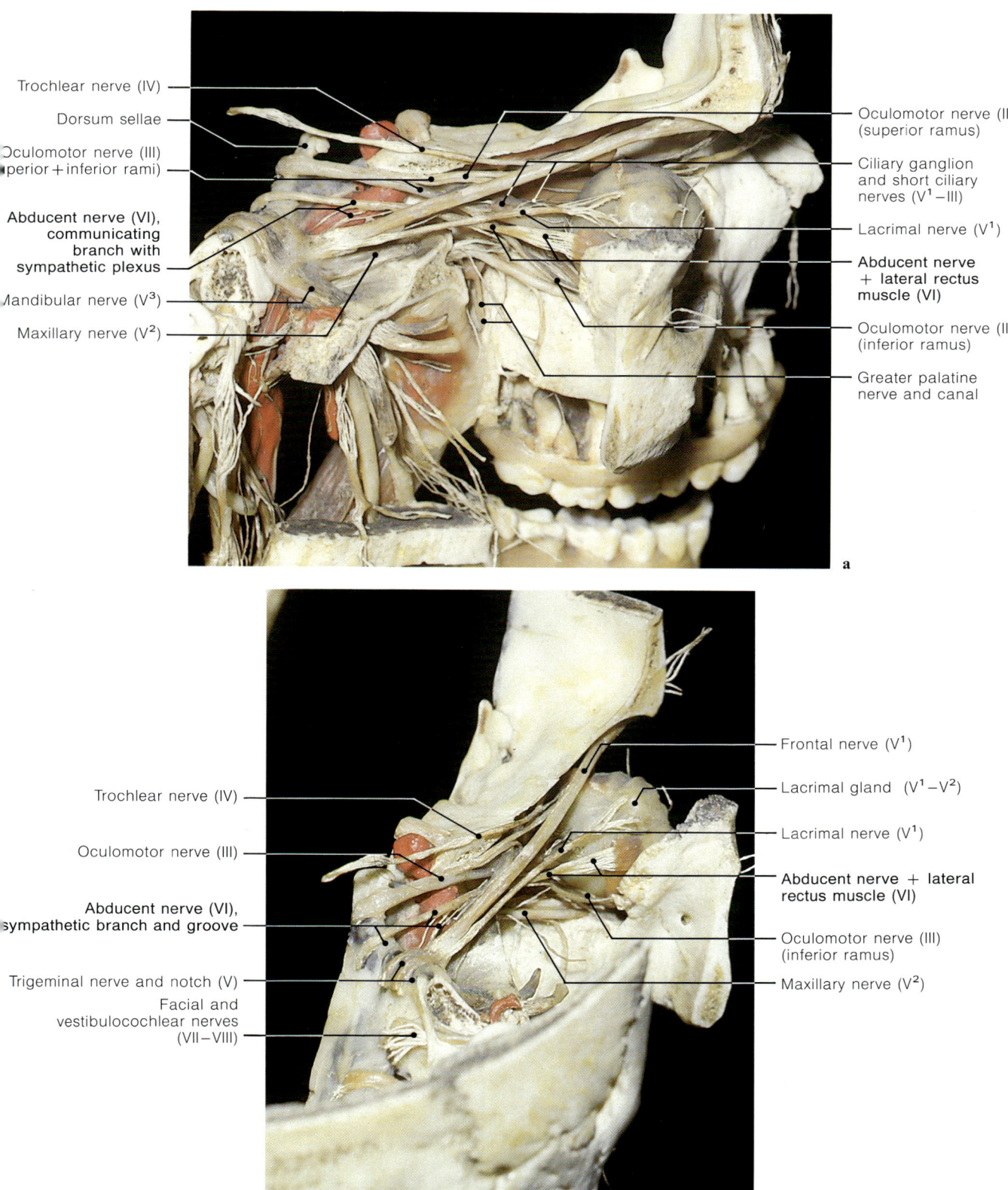

Fig. 6.14a, b. Anatomic dissections in sagittal and intracranial views showing course of abducent nerve (VI) to its termination

Course of abducent nerve

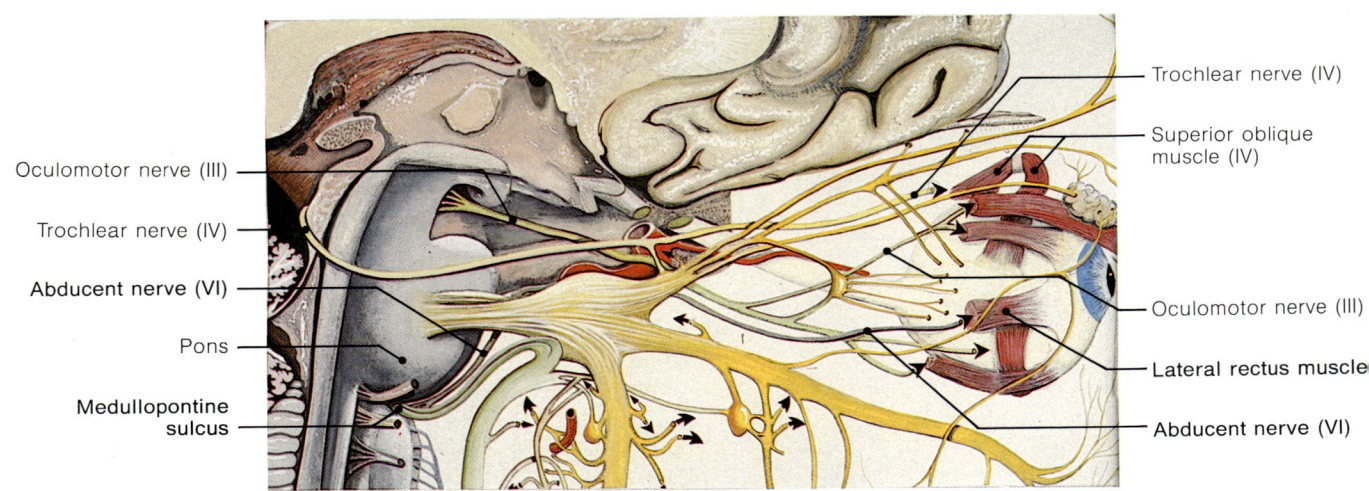

Fig. 6.15. Diagram of the course of abducent nerve (VI) up to lateral rectus muscle (VI)

Facial nerve (VII)

Anatomy (course – terminals – collaterals)	173
Imaging (regions examined)	173
Pathology	173
Collateral branches and orifices	
Intrapetrous branches	175
Extrapetrous branches	175
Terminal branches	175
Apparent origin of facial nerve (VII – VIIb), medullopontine sulcus	
Anatomy and imaging (examination)	176
Axial and frontal views (MRI)	177
Axial views (MRI)	178
Anatomic section, axial view (MRI)	179
Intrapetrous course and collaterals	
Course	180
Collaterals	180
Terminals	181
Anastomoses	182
Course (anatomic diagram)	183
Extrapetrous course	
Diagram of facial nerve with infraorbital branches	184
Facial nerves and collaterals	
Clinique and imaging	185
Imaging views	187
Intrapetrous course of facial nerve, internal acoustic meatus, intermedius nerve (VII – VIIb)	
Oblique view (CT)	188
Worms-Bretton view	189
Axial and sagittal views (radiology, CT, MRI)	189
First part of facial canal, compartment of geniculate ganglion	
Sagittal view (CT)	190
Hiatuses of canals and greater and lesser petrosal nerves (VII)	
CT and MRI	190
Facial canal	
Prestudied inclined sagittal view of Cornélis and Vignaud (MRI, CT)	191
Sulci and course of superficial and deep greater and lesser petrosal nerves (VII – IX)	
Oblique view (radiology)	192
Pterygoid canal, pterygoid nerve (VII – IX)	
Frontal and sagittal views (MRI, CT)	194
Pterygoid canal and canal of otic ganglion, superficial and deep greater and lesser petrosal nerves (VII – IX)	
Axial views (MRI)	196
Oblique view (radiology)	198
Unilateral oblique view (radiology)	199
Dissection of facial, trigeminal, oculomotor nerves and section of petrous bone	200
Second part of facial canal	
Varied sagittal views (radiology, CT)	201
Orifice of nerve to stapedius muscle	
Prestudied sagittal view (radiology, CT)	201
Petrotympanosquamous fissure, chorda tympani	
Varied sagittal views (radiology)	202
Axial view (radiology)	202
Anatomic view	203
Ostium introitus, auricular branch of vagus nerve (VII – X)	
Prestudied varied sagittal view	204
Sulcus of auricular branch of vagus nerve (VII – X) and communicating branch with glossopharyngeal nerve (VII – IX)	
Anatomic views	205
Stylomastoid foramen	
Sagittal and axial views (radiology)	206
Axial views (CT)	207
Anatomic and physiologic review, motor and sensory components	208
Salivary (V^3 – VII – IX) and lacrimomuconasal (V^2 – VII – IX) secretory pathways (diagrams)	209
Carotid sympathetic plexus (anastomotic branches)	
Anatomic views	210

Vascular relations:

Inferior anterior cerebellar artery	212, 215, 226
Petrous branch of the middle meningeal artery	276, 277
Vidian artery	279
Linguofacial collateral pattern	282
Stylomastoid foramen, chorda tympani, posterior auricular artery, inferior tympanic artery	286

This is formed of two roots: one motor, the facial nerve properly so-called, the other sensory, the intermedius nerve (VIIb). They contain autonomic fibers which stimulate muconasal and lacrimal secretion and submandibular and sublingual salivary secretion.

The facial nerve arises in the pons and emerges from the medullopontine sulcus. It follows an intracranial intrapetrous course and then becomes extracranial in the parotid conpartment, where it terminates in two branches destined for the facial muscles.

172 Facial nerve (VII)

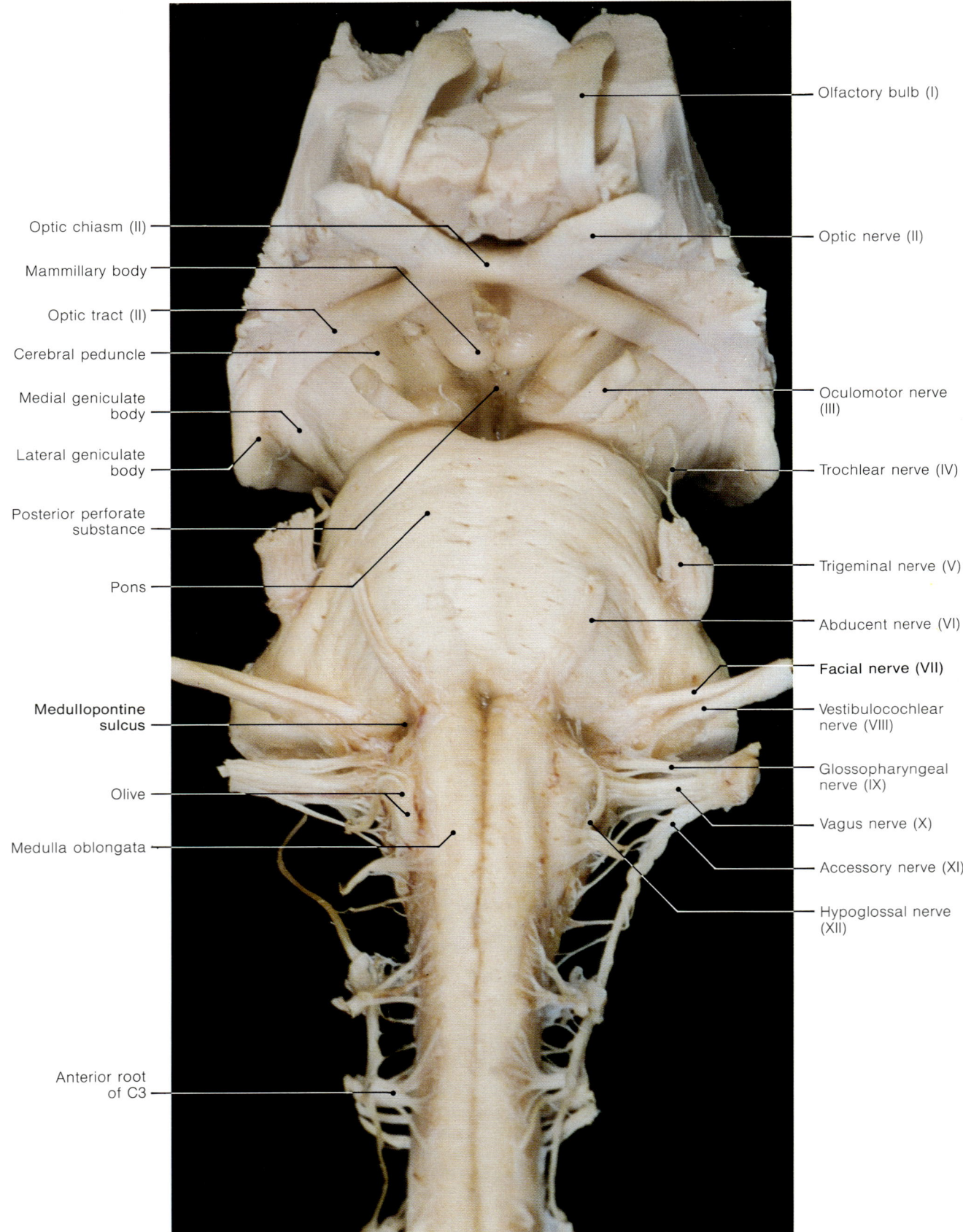

Fig. 7.1. Apparent origin of facial nerve in anterior frontal view of brain-stem

Facial nerve (VII)

Anatomy

COURSE – TERMINALS – COLLATERALS

Apparent origin in medullopontine sulcus and intracranial course

Course in internal acoustic meatus

Intrapetrous course and collaterals

Imaging

REGIONS EXAMINED

Study of cerebellopontine angle (pontine cistern)

Imaging of internal acoustic meatuses

Examination of facial canal and collateral ostia:

- hiatuses of canals of greater and lesser petrosal nerves,
- compartment of geniculate ganglion,
- ostium of nerve to stapedius muscle,
- petrotympanosquamous fissure,
- ostium introitus,
- stylomastoid foramen

Pathology

Lower pons:
- Syndrome of lower pons,
- syndrome of inferior protuberance (Foville's syndrome).

Posterior fossa:
- Tumor of cerebellopontine angle,
- extra- and intracanalicular neurinomas of cranial nerves VII, VIIb and VIII.

Petrous bone:
- Antral cholesteatoma extending towards the facial canal or compartment of geniculate ganglion,
- antro-adito-attical cholesteatoma involving the chorda tympani,
- peripheral facial paralysis (Bell's palsy),
- otosclerosis of the base of the stapes (stage 4 or 5) extending towards the second part of VII and sometimes involving the lateral semicircular canal,
- fracture of petrous bone.

Facial nerve (VII)

Topography

Apparent origin of facial nerve (VII–VIIb)
– Medullopontine sulcus

Intracanalicular course
– Internal acoustic meatus
– Facial nerve and intermedius nerve

Geniculate ganglion
– First part of facial canal

Intrapetrous part of facial nerve
– Facial canal

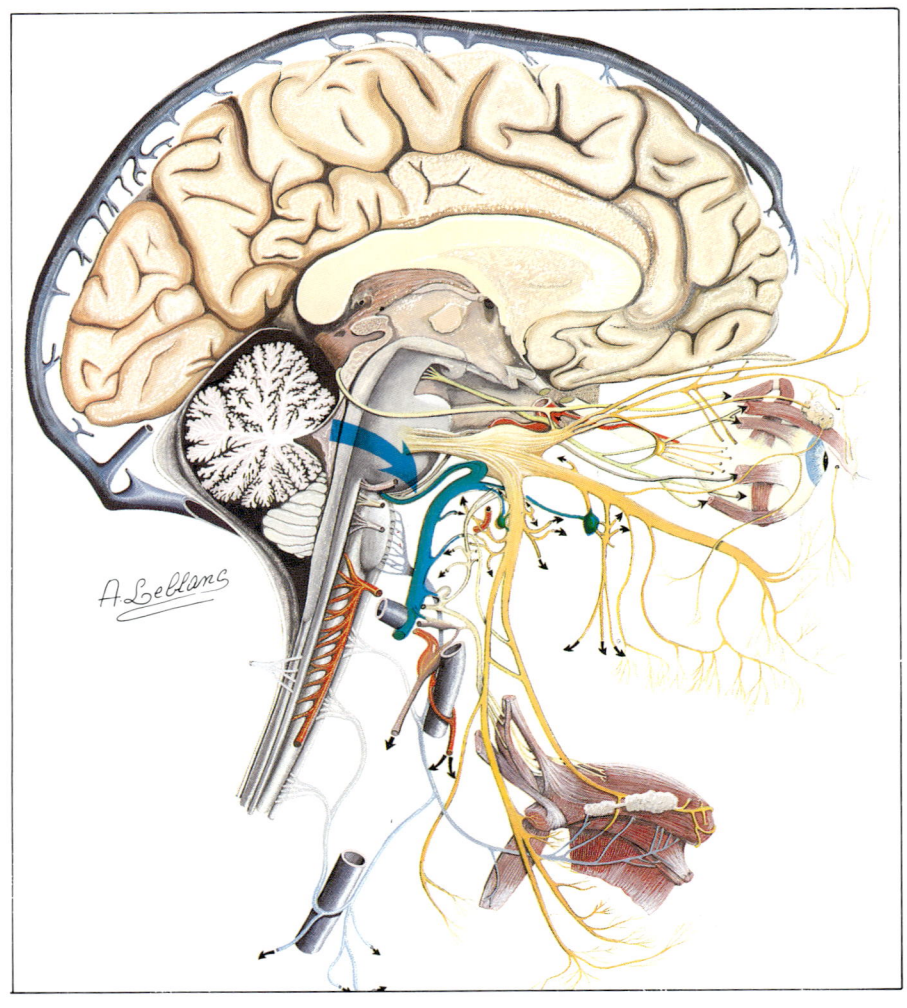

Fig. 7.2 a

Collateral branches and orifices

Intrapetrous collateral branches

NERVES	ORIFICES
Facial nerve and intermedius nerve	Internal acoustic meatus
Geniculate ganglion	First part of facial canal
Superficial greater petrosal nerve	Hiatus of canal of greater petrosal nerve
Superficial lesser petrosal nerve	Hiatus of canal of lesser petrosal nerve
Superficial and deep greater petrosal nerves and nerve of pterygoid canal	Sulcus of superficial and deep greater petrosal nerves, pterygoid canal
Superficial and deep lesser petrosal nerves, communicating branch with tympanic plexus	Sulcus of superficial and deep lesser petrosal nerves, canal of otic ganglion
Facial nerve	Facial canal
Nerve to stapedius muscle	Orifice of nerve to stapedius muscle
Chorda tympani	Posterior orifice of chorda tympani and petrotympanosquamous fissure
Auricular branch of vagus nerve, communicating branch with vagus nerve	Ostium introitus
Sensory branch of external acoustic meatus	Sulcus of auricular branch of vagus nerve and jugular foramen Stylomastoid foramen (exit)

Extrapetrous collateral branches

NERVES	ORIFICES
Communicating branch with glossopharyngeal nerve and its inferior ganglion	Roof of jugular foramen with petrosal fossula and sulcus of glossopharyngeal nerve
Posterior auricular branch, branch to stylohyoid and to posterior belly of digastric muscles Lingual branch	Stylomastoid foramen

Terminal branches

NERVES	ORIFICE
Temporofacial and cervicofacial branches	Stylomastoid foramen, exit of facial nerve

Apparent origin of facial nerve (VII–VIIb), medullopontine sulcus

Anatomy

The motor root arises from the motor nucleus of the facial nerve situated in the medial eminence of the floor of the fourth ventricle. After having passed around the motor nucleus of the abducent nerve (VI), it emerges from the neuraxis at the lateral part of the medullopontine sulcus (Fig. 7.1–7.5).

The autonomic fibers arise from two nuclei situated behind and lateral to the motor nucleus: the lacrimomuconasal nucleus and the superior salivary nucleus (Fig. 7.48; 7.49). The sensory root has its origin in the geniculate ganglion, which is situated on the course of the facial nerve at the level of its first intrapetrous bend (Fig. 7.2; 7.7; 7.17).

The prolongations of the cells of the geniculate ganglion form the sensory fibers of the intermedius nerve (VIIb), which enter the neuraxis at the medullopontine sulcus, medial to the vestibulocochlear nerve (VIII) and lateral to the facial nerve (Fig. 7.5). They terminate in the upper part of the salivary nucleus.

Imaging

When the patient presents a posterior fossa syndrome with involvement of the facial nerve associated with involvement of the vestibulocochlear (VIII) and glossopharyngeal (IX) nerves, typical of a syndrome of the cerebellopontine angle or other protuberantial syndromes, it is necessary to practise a study of the cerebellopontine angle. This displays the apparent origin of facial nerve in the medullopontine sulcus.

EXAMINATION

– Magnetic resonance imaging (MRI) or computed tomography (CT) of the cerebellopontine angle (medullopontine sulcus) for the apparent origin of the facial nerve and intermedius nerve, in sagittal, frontal and axial views (Fig. 7.3a–c; 7.4a, b).

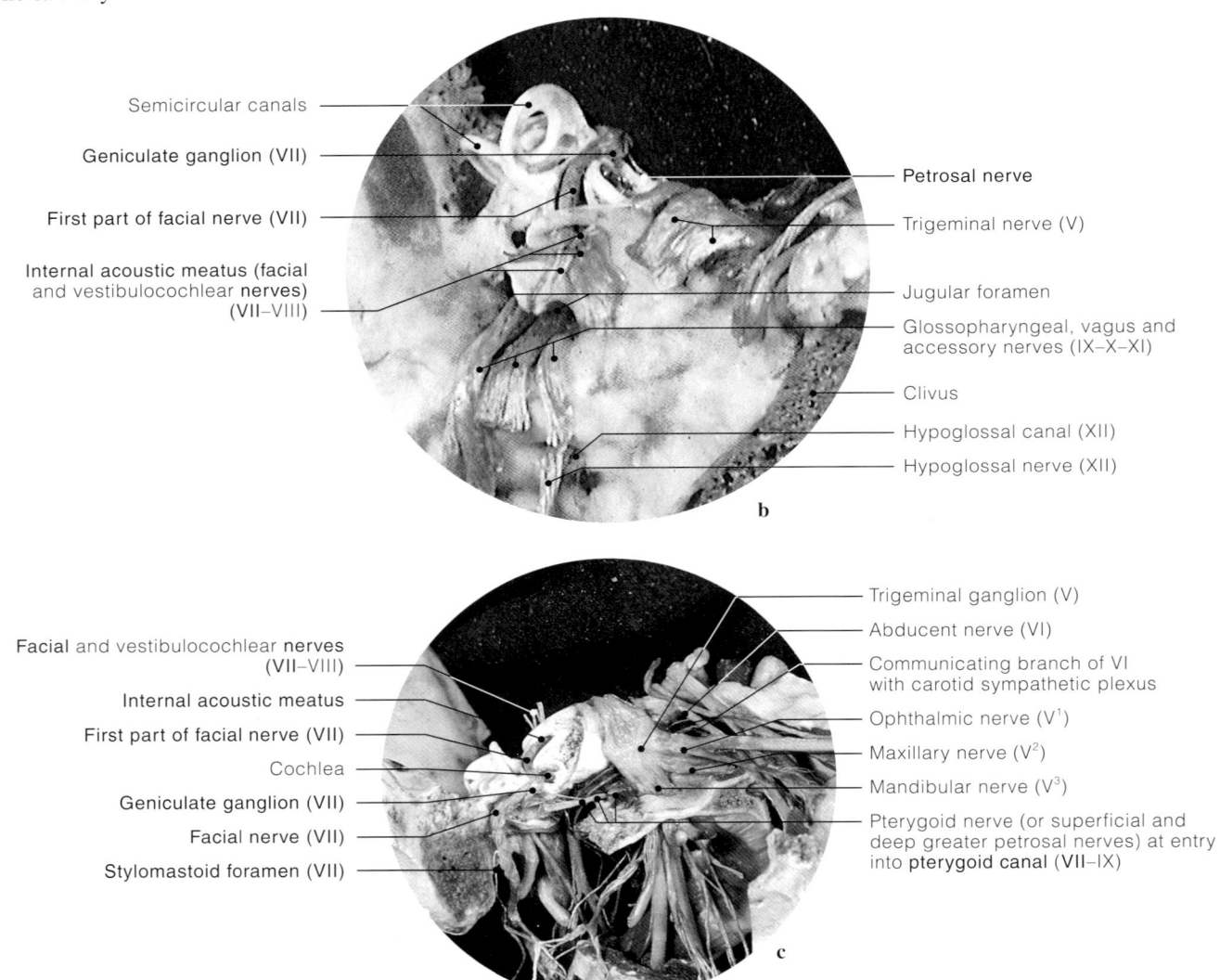

Fig. 7.2 b, c. Sagittal intracranial view of facial nerve at the internal acoustic meatus and first part of facial canal (**b**); right superolateral view showing intrapetrous course of facial nerve and communicating branches (**c**)

Cerebellopontine angle

Magnetic resonance imaging (MRI)

AXIAL AND FRONTAL VIEWS

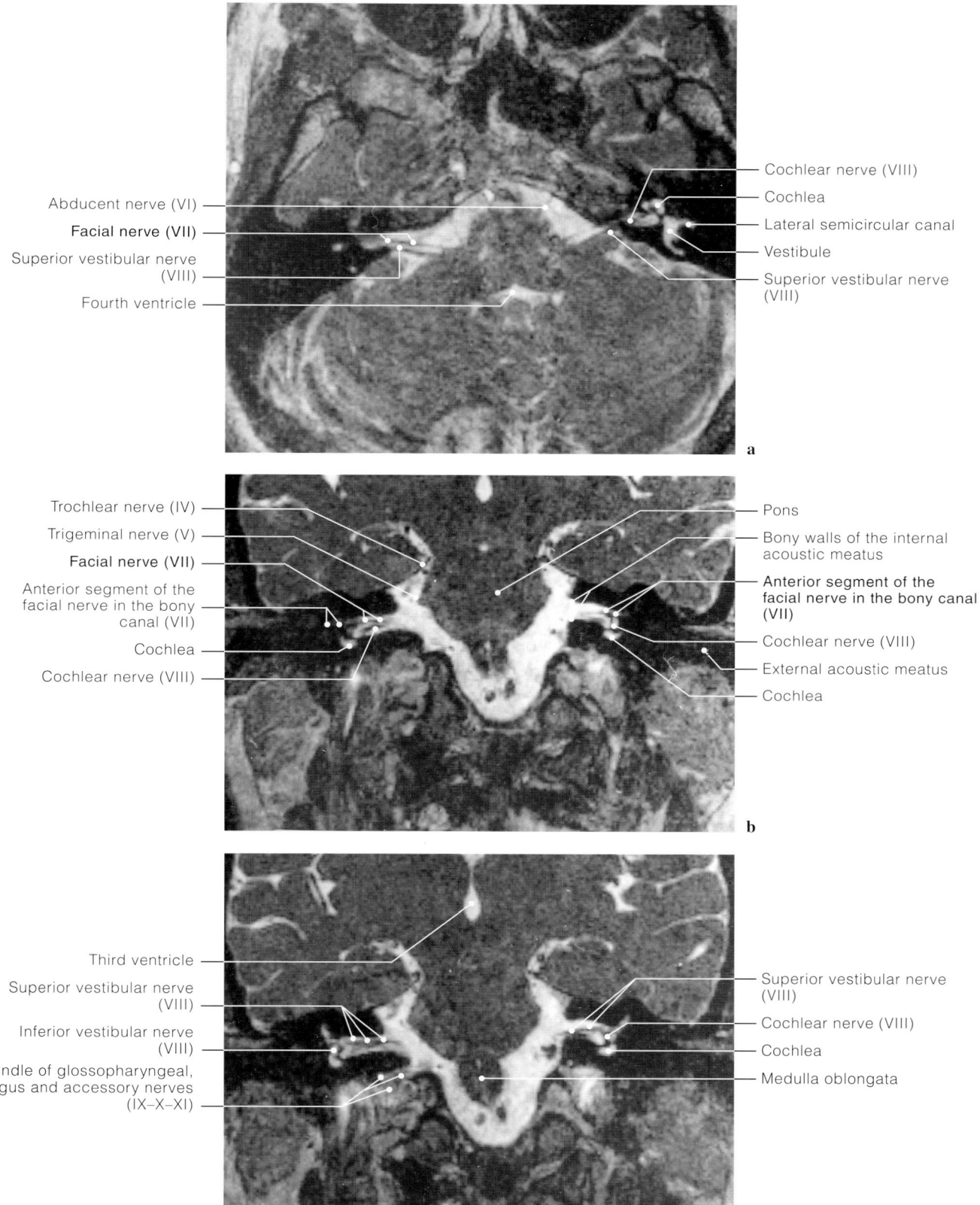

Fig. 7.3. a Axial magnetic resonance imaging (MRI) and **b, c** frontal views of the medullopontine sulcus for the facial nerves (VII). (MRI: Dr. J.W. Casselman, A.Z. St-Jan, Brugge)

178 Facial nerve (VII)

Cerebellopontine angle

Magnetic resonance imaging (MRI)

AXIAL VIEWS

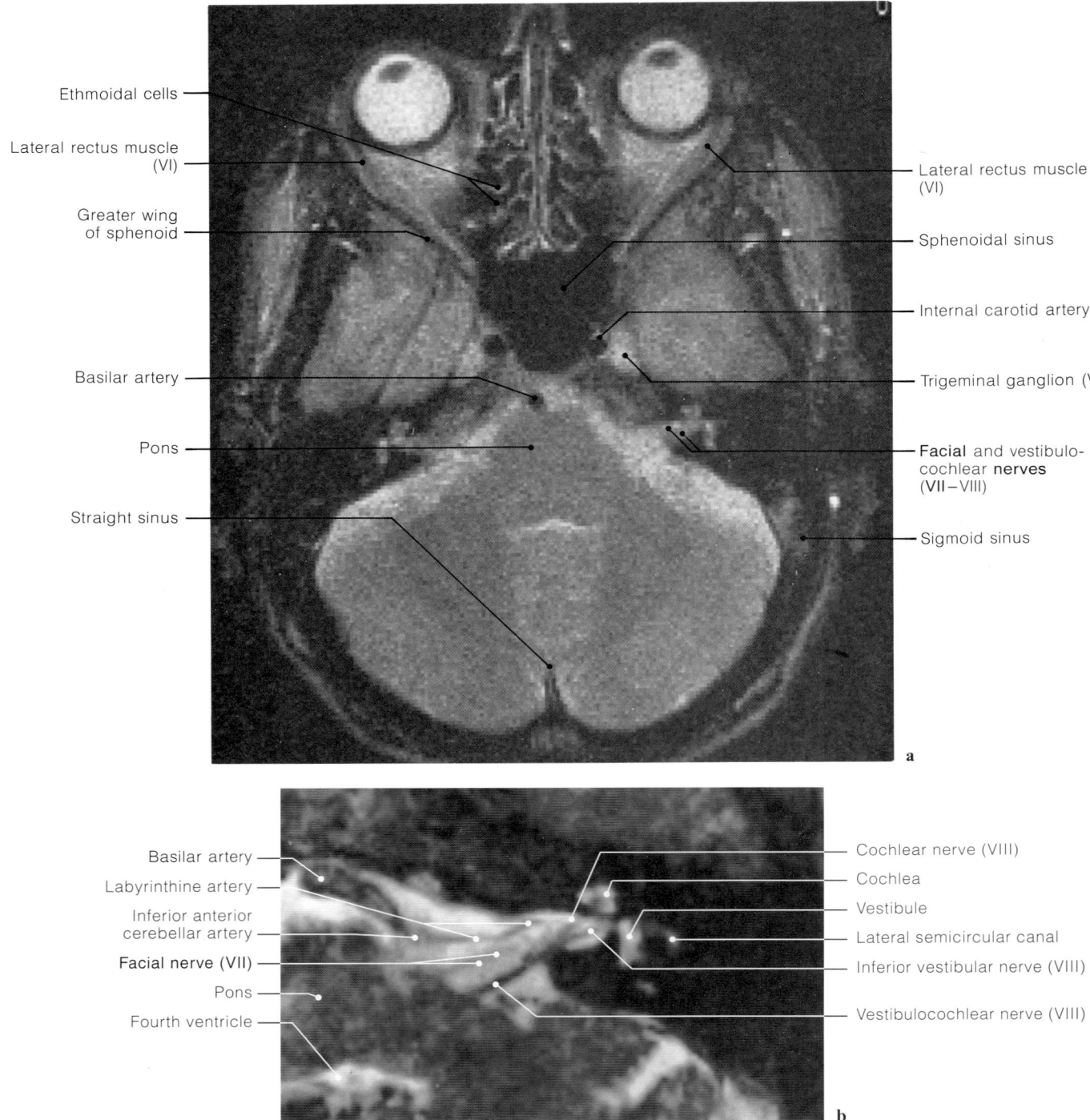

Fig. 7.4a, b. Axial magnetic resonance imaging (MRI) of cerebellopontine angle for apparent origin of the facial and vestibulocochlear nerves (VII–VIII). (MRI: b Dr. J.W. Casselman, A.Z. St-Jan, Brugge)

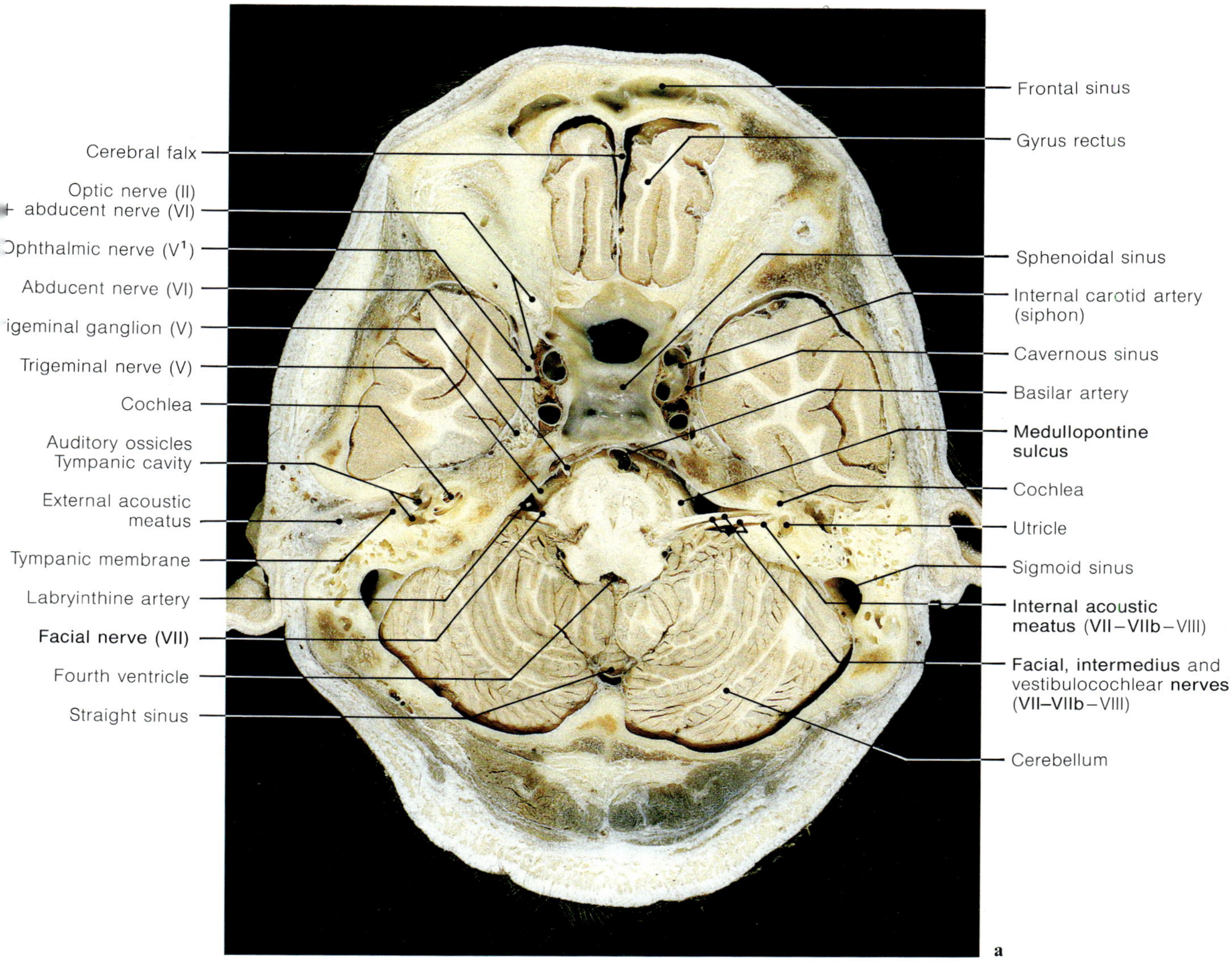

Facial nerve (VII) 179

Fig. 7.5a. Axial anatomic section at level of the vestibulocochlear and facial nerves (VII–VIIb–VIII) from apparent origin to the internal ear

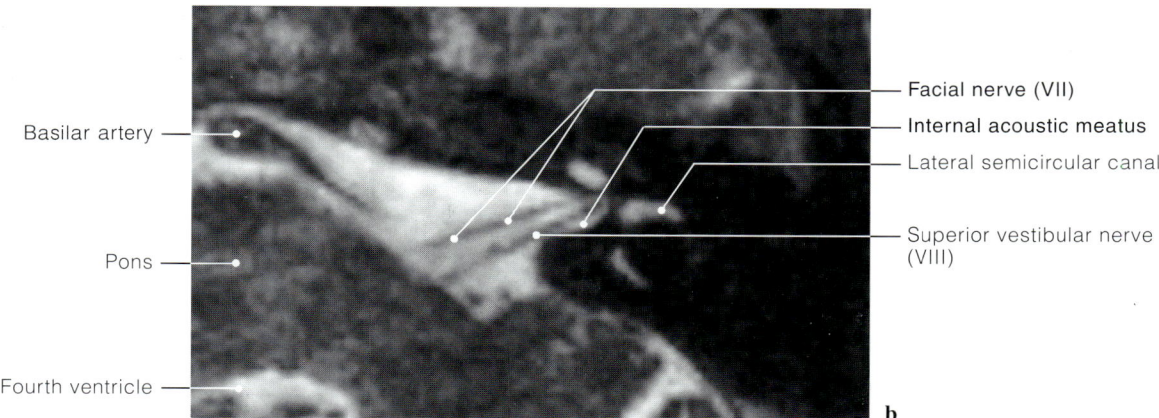

Fig. 7.5b. Axial magnetic resonance imaging (MRI) of the vestibulocochlear nerve (VIII). (MRI: Dr. J.W. Casselman, A.Z. St-Jan, Brugge)

Intrapetrous course and collaterals (anatomy, course, relations)

Intrapetrous course

The two roots of the facial nerve travel forwards and outwards from the medullopontine sulcus to reach the internal acoustic meatus (Fig. 7.1; 7.3–7.5; 7.14; 7.17).
Having reached the fundus of the acoustic meatus, the two roots enter the facial canal (Fig. 7.7; 7.17; 7.18; 7.34). The facial nerve and the facial canal exhibit three sections:

- The first or labyrinthine section begins at the fundus of the internal acoustic meatus and passes obliquely forwards and outwards, perpendicular to the petrous axis.
- The second or tympanic section passes obliquely outwards, posterior and slightly lower, and is situated in a vertical plane almost parallel to the long petrous axis.
- The third or mastoid section is vertical, commencing under the aditus ad antrum and ending at the stylomastoid foramen (Fig. 7.7; 7.34; 7.45).

At its exit from the petrous bone, the facial nerve enters the parotid gland, where it divides into its terminal branches (Fig. 7.8; 7.49).
After having emerged from the medullopontine sulcus, the facial nerve and the intermedius nerve (VÎI–VIIb) travel in the posterior fossa and traverse the cerebellopontine subarachnoid confluence.
The facial nerve is first in front of and then above the vestibulocochlear nerve (Fig. 7.1; 7.3–7.5); the intermedius nerve lies between the facial and vestibulocochlear nerves (Fig. 7.5).
In the internal acoustic meatus, the vestibulocochlear nerve assumes the shape of a grooved structure with an upper concavity, containing the facial and intermedius nerves (Fig. 7.4; 7.5; 7.7). These three nerves have a common dural sheath.
The internal auditory artery enters the internal acoustic meatus (Fig. 7.5).
In the first part of the facial canal, situated between the cochlea and the vestibule, the facial and intermedius nerves are still quite distinct. The facial nerve then takes another direction and continues in the second part of the canal. Here it forms the genu, opposite the hiatus of the greater petrosal nerve. At this first angle there is found the geniculate ganglion, which blends at its base with the nerve trunk.
The intermedius nerve enters the ganglion and, from here on, only a single nerve bundle exists (Fig. 7.7; 7.17; 7.29; 7.34).
In the second part of the facial canal, the facial nerve is situated within the tympanic cavity, above and behind the vestibular window (Fig. 7.7).
It descends behind the canal for the stapedius muscle in the bony wall that separates the tympanic cavity from the cells of the mastoid antrum. This section ends below the aditus at antrum at the bend where it joins the third, vertical, mastoid portion.
The facial nerve becomes almost vertical and slightly oblique downwards and outwards (Fig. 7.7; 7.29; 7.34).
Within the canal, the facial nerve is accompanied by a branch of the posterior auricular artery, the stylomastoid artery.
Emerging from the facial canal via the stylomastoid foramen, the facial nerve travels outwards, forwards and downwards, crosses the outer aspect of the styloid process and then enters the parotid compartment, passing between the stylohyoid and digastric muscles.

Collaterals

The facial nerve gives off:

- intrapetrous branches (Fig. 7.7; 7.29; 7.34; 7.37),
- extrapetrous branches (Fig. 7.8),
- terminal branches (Fig. 7.8; 7.94).

Intrapetrous collateral branches

These are six in number and arise from the facial nerve within the facial canal:

- the superficial greater petrosal nerve,
- the superficial lesser petrosal nerve (Fig. 7.28; 7.29; 7.37),
- the nerve to stapedius muscle (Fig. 7.7; 7.36),
- the chorda tympani (Fig. 7.37; 7.39),
- the sensory branch of the internal acoustic meatus (Fig. 7.7; 7.34),
- the communicating branch of the jugular fossa (vagal) (Fig. 7.2; 7.7; 7.37; 7.41; 7.44).

Superficial greater petrosal nerve: This separates from the geniculate ganglion, emerges from the petrous bone by the hiatus (Fig. 7.7; 7.17; 7.29) where it receives the anastomosis of the deep greater petrosal nerve (IX) (Fig. 7.29).
After leaving the hiatus, it glides in its sulcus (Fig. 7.21–7.23; 7.28) and passes under the trigeminal ganglion (V). After having received an anastomotic strand from the pericarotid plexus, it traverses the pterygoid canal (Fig. 7.24; 7.28), where it is known as the nerve of the pterygoid canal, and is distributed to the pterygopalatine ganglion. By way of this ganglion, it supplies the lacrimal gland and then the bucconasopharyngeal mucosa (Fig. 7.48).
Superficial lesser petrosal nerve: This also arises from the geniculate ganglion, traverses the accessory hiatus and receives the deep lesser petrosal nerve (IX) (Fig. 7.7; 7.29).
Emerging from the hiatus, it enters its groove (Fig. 7.8; 7.22–7.24), and is then joined by an anastomotic branch from the plexus around the middle meningeal artery. It traverses the skull base via the canal of the otic ganglion or the foramen lacerum, sometimes via the sphenopetrosal suture, to enter the otic ganglion (Fig. 7.29; 7.37c; 7.49).
Nerve to stapedius muscle: This arises from the vertical segment of the facial nerve. To reach the stapedius muscle, it

traverses the thin bony wall that separates this muscle from the facial canal (Fig. 7.7; 7.29; 7.36).

Chorda tympani: The chorda tympani separates from the facial nerve about 3 mm above the stylomastoid foramen. It follows a course passing outwards, upwards and slightly forwards and enters a bony channel, the posterior canal of the chorda (Fig. 7.37).

It then enters the tympanic cavity via an orifice situated on the posterior wall between the pyramid of stapedius muscle and the tympanic sulcus.

The chorda then travels in the anterior mallear folds, skirts the inner aspect of the neck of malleus (Fig. 7.7), passes in the sulcus of the pars tympanica of temporal bone and emerges from the petrous bone via the petrotympanosquamous fissure (Fig. 7.37–7.40).

The chorda then joins the lingual nerve (V^3) (Fig. 7.29; 7.37).

By way of this nerve, the fibers of the chorda tympani go to the sublingual and submandibular ganglia (Fig. 7.49).

Sensory branch of external acoustic meatus: This separates from the facial nerve at the level of, or a little behind, the stylomastoid foramen and immediately above the external acoustic meatus.

It skirts the anterior border of the mastoid process and then enters the posterior region of the external acoustic meatus, innervating this and also part of the tympanic membrane (Fig. 7.7; 7.34).

Anastomotic branch of jugular fossa (VII–X) (or auricular branch of vagus nerve): This branch arises above the stylomastoid foramen and enters a small intrapetrous bony canal to reach the upper wall of the jugular foramen, where it emerges at the ostium introitus (Fig. 7.41–7.44).

It joins the superior ganglion of the vagus nerve (X) (Fig. 7.41; 7.44).

Extrapetrous collateral branches

Beneath the petrous bone and at its exit from the stylomastoid foramen, the facial nerve gives off four branches:

- the anastomotic branch of the glossopharyngeal nerve,
- the posterior auricular branch,
- the branches to the digastric and stylohyoid muscles,
- the lingual branch (Fig. 7.8).

Anastomotic branch of the glossopharyngeal nerve (VII–IX) (or Haller's ansa): This arises from the facial nerve just below the stylomastoid foramen, crosses the internal jugular vein, and terminates in the petrosal fossula of the inferior ganglion (IX) (Fig. 7.2; 7.44).

Posterior auricular branch: This separates from the facial nerve below the stylomastoid foramen. It anastomoses with the auricular branch of the cervical plexus and then divides into two branches to supply the occipitalis muscle and the muscles of the inner aspect of the external ear (Fig. 7.8).

Branches to stylohyoid and to posterior belly of digastric muscles: These nerve bundles arise from the facial nerve a little below the former branch.

The digastric branch often anastomoses with the glossopharyngeal nerve, an anastomotic branch replacing the communicating branch with the glossopharyngeal nerve (Fig. 7.7; 7.8)

Lingual branch: This branch separates from the facial nerve near the origin of the preceding branches.

It is rarely present and probably substitutes for the anastomotic branch.

This inconstant anastomosis joins the digastric branch to the glossopharyngeal nerve (IX).

It skirts the styloglossus muscle, passes forward and downwards, and arrives at the base of the tongue, where it anastomoses with the glossopharyngeal nerve. Here, fibers arise destined for the mucosa of the tongue and for the styloglossus and palatoglossus muscles (Fig. 7.2).

Terminal branches

At its exit from the facial canal (stylomastoid foramen) the facial nerve divides into two terminal branches:

- the temporofacial branch,
- the cervicofacial branch (Fig. 7.8).

Temporofacial branch: This anastomoses with the auriculotemporal nerve (V^3) and then divides into several branches destined to the cutaneous muscles of the skull and face. The twigs of this branch first enter the parotid gland (Fig. 7.8; 7.49) where they are connected by communicating branches. The branches leave the parotid gland and reach their territories. From below upwards, there are:

- superior buccal branches for the buccinator and upper part of the orbicularis oris muscle (Fig. 7.8);
- infraorbital branches supplying the greater and lesser zygomatic muscles, levators of the upper lip and nasal ala, transverse and dilator nasal muscles;
- frontal and palpebral branches for the palpebral part of the orbicularis oculi and frontal part of the epicranius muscles (Fig. 7.8; 7.9);
- temporal branches to the tragicus muscle and the muscles of the outer aspect of the external ear (Fig. 7.8).

Cervicofacial branch: This anastomoses with the auricular branch of the cervical plexus, it divides into several branches in the region of the mandibular angle to reach the platysma muscles of the neck and face:

- inferior buccal branches for the lower half of the orbicularis oris muscle;
- a cervical branch supplying the platysma muscle (Fig. 7.9).

Anastomoses

The facial nerve exhibits numerous anastomoses:

- with the pterygopalatine and otic ganglia (V, VII, IX) via the superficial and deep greater and lesser petrosal nerves which, after leaving their hiatuses, enter the pterygoid canal and the canal of the otic ganglion (Fig. 7.28; 7.29; 7.37; 7.48; 7.49);
- with the glossopharyngeal nerve (IX) via the communicating branch (Fig. 7.7; 7.44);
- with the vagus nerve (X) via the ostium introitus (Fig. 7.7; 7.41);
- with the lingual nerve (V^3) (chorda tympani) via the petrotympanosquamous fissure (Fig. 7.37–7.40);
- with the auriculotemporal branch of the mandibular nerve (V^3) (Fig. 7.29; 7.39);
- with the vestibulocochlear nerve (VIII) by fibers derived from the intermedius nerve (VIIb) and geniculate ganglion;
- and with the trigeminal nerve (V) via the labial, palpebral and mental branches (Fig. 7.8; 7.9)

Intrapetrous course

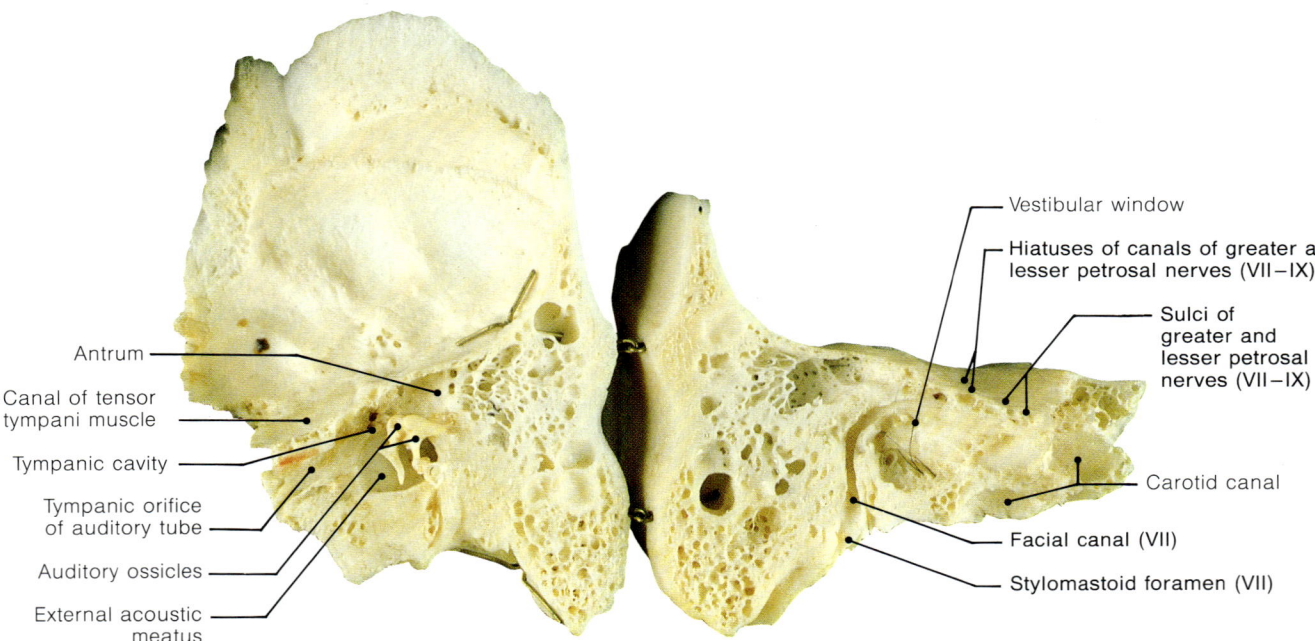

Fig. 7.6a. Section of petrous bone (dried bone) through intrapetrous course of VII

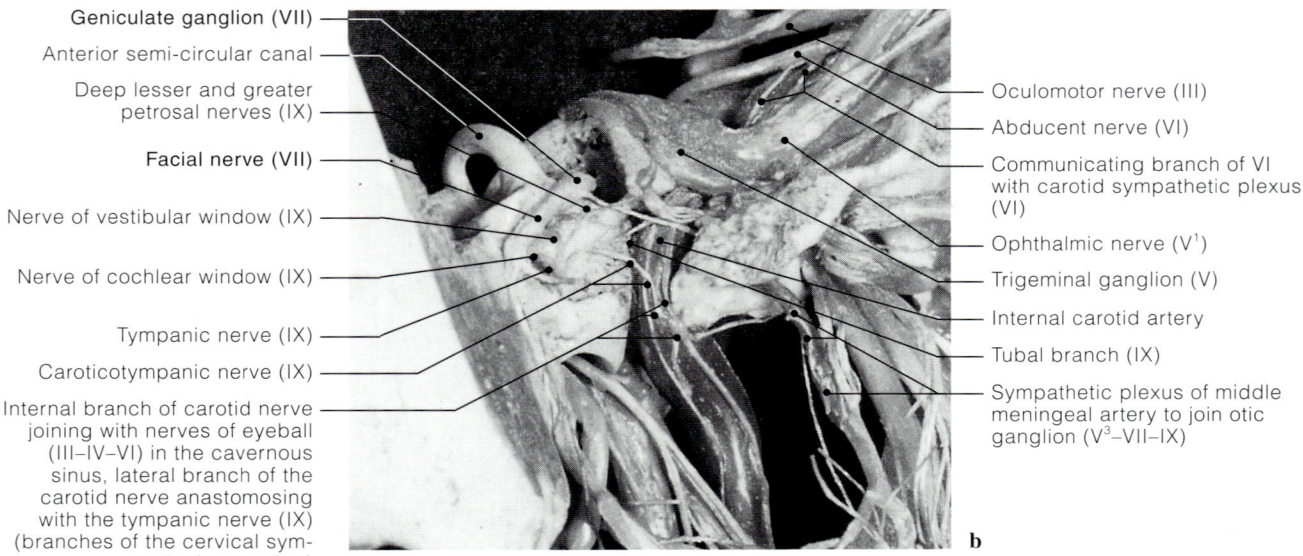

Fig. 7.6b. Anatomic dissection showing anastomotic relations of facial, trigeminal and glossopharyngeal nerves (VII–V–IX) with carotid sympathetic plexus

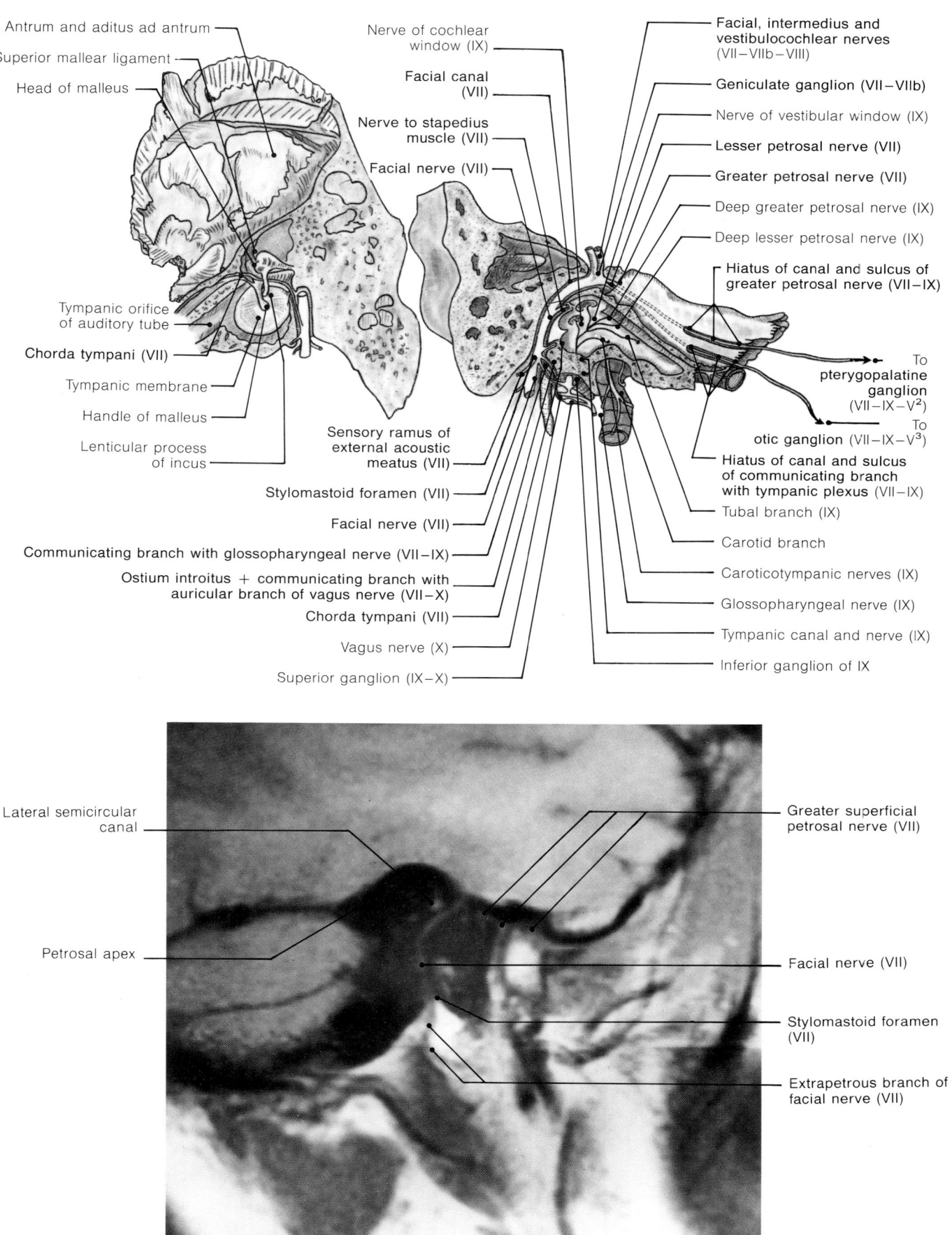

Fig. 7.7. a Anatomic section of Fig. 7.6 and diagram of facial nerve (VII) and its intrapetrous collaterals; **b** magnetic resonance imaging (MRI) of facial nerve (VII) in sagittal view

Extrapetrous course

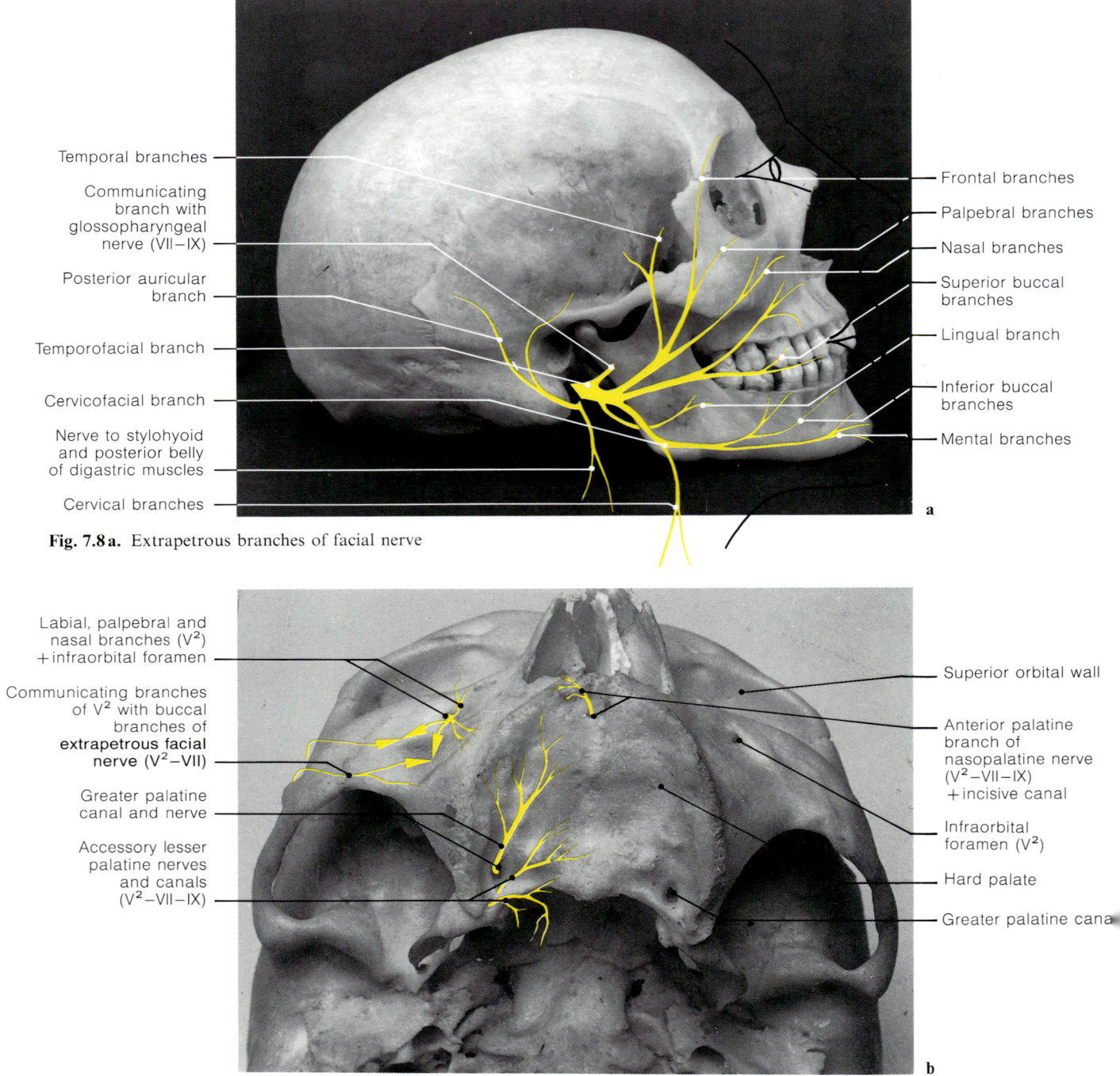

Fig. 7.8 a. Extrapetrous branches of facial nerve

Fig. 7.8 b. Diagram of anastomoses of extrapetrous facial nerve with infraorbital branches (V^2–VII)

Facial nerve and collaterals, facial canal and its orifices

Imaging (views required)

- **Comparative study of internal acoustic meatus in the oblique Chaussé IV view (Fig. 7.10; 7.11) and in sagittal view (Fig. 7.12).**

CLINICAL FEATURES

- Impaired acuity of hearing, tinnitus, headache, vertigo with falling to the side of the ear affected,
- Ménière's syndrome.

POSSIBLE CAUSES

- Acoustic neurinoma within the canal compressing the facial nerve,
- lesions of the vestibulocochlear/facial nerves within the canal due to disturbance of the labyrinthine circulation or to compression by tumor or hematoma (fracture).

- **Tomographic study of facial canal and compartment of geniculate ganglion, hiatuses of greater and lesser petrosal nerves and other collateral orifices in prestudied inclined sagittal view (Cornélis) (Fig. 7.17–7.19; 7.35; 7.41; 7.45).**

CLINICAL FEATURES

- Diminution of lacrimal and salivary secretion,
- peripheral facial palsy (Bell's sign), loss of taste sensation in anterior two-thirds of tongue with difficulty in swallowing,
- acute otitis media, diminished stapedius reflex, loss of taste, hyperacuity of hearing.

POSSIBLE CAUSES

- Fracture of skull base and petrous bone, tumor of auditory tube that may involve the hiatuses and damage the greater and lesser petrosal nerves,
- fracture of first or second part of the facial canal or canal of the nerve to stapedius muscle; antro-adito-attical cholesteatoma extending towards the intrapetrous course of VII which may damage the facial nerve, geniculate ganglion or nerve to stapedius muscle,
- otosclerosis of base of stapes, stage V, surrounding the second part of the facial canal, situated below the lateral semicircular canal.

- **Tomographic or computed tomographic (CT) study of sulci of superficial and deep greater and lesser petrosal nerves (anterior aspect of petrous apex) in unilateral oblique view in petrous axis (Fig. 7.20–7.23).**

CLINICAL FEATURES

- Disturbance of lacrimal secretion.

POSSIBLE CAUSES

- Gradenigo's syndrome (osteitis of petrous apex) extending towards anterior petrous region,
- aneurysm of internal carotid artery (siphon),
- fracture of greater wing of sphenoid extending towards the anterior petrous region.

- **Computed tomographic (CT) study of the pterygoid canals in symmetric frontal views (Fig. 7.24; 7.25), axial views (Fig. 7.27; 7.28), and unilateral sagittal view (Fig. 7.24; 7.26).**

CLINICAL FEATURES

- Disturbance of lacrimal secretion.

POSSIBLE CAUSES

- Tumor of sphenoidal sinus,
- tumor of cavum,
- tumor of pterygopalatine fossa,
- syndrome of pterygopalatine ganglion (Sluder),
- aneurysm of carotid siphon extending towards pterygoid canal,
- fracture of skull base extending towards sphenoidal sinus,
- fracture of upper region of pterygoid process.

- **Study of canal of otic ganglion in high oblique face view (Fig. 7.30; 7.32) and in tomographic section in Hirtz view (Fig. 7.27; 7.28).**

CLINICAL FEATURES

- As for the hiatus of the canal of superficial lesser petrosal nerve.

POSSIBLE CAUSES

- Neurinoma of the foramen ovale affecting the canal of the otic ganglion,
- aneurysm of the internal carotid artery (siphon),
- tumor of cavum, fracture of skull base.

- **Tomographic study of the petrotympanosquamous fissure, posterior orifice of chorda tympani and facial canal in sagittal views (Fig. 7.37; 7.39) and axial views (Fig. 7.38; 7.40).**

CLINICAL FEATURES

- Loss of taste sensation of the anterior two-thirds of the tongue with decrease of salivary secretion due to deficiency of the sublingual and submandibular glands,
- superficial anesthesia in the zone of Ramsay Hunt, of the hairy scalp and postauricular region, and peripheral facial palsy (Bell's sign).

POSSIBLE CAUSES

- Before emergence of chorda tympani: affection of facial nerve, either by a neurinoma, an antro-adito-attical cholesteatoma or a fracture involving the facial canal,
- after emergence of chorda tympani: affection of chorda tympani in its posterior canal or in the middle ear, either by a cholesteatoma of the aditus ad antrum or by a fracture or dislocation of the malleus,
- involvement of the chorda tympani at its exit at the petrotympanosquamous fissure by a fracture of the mandibular fossa of the temporal bone (or mandible) involving the petrotympanosquamous fissure.

- **Tomographic study of the ostium introitus (tegmen of jugular foramen) in prestudied inclined sagittal view (Cornélis) (Fig. 7.41).**

CLINICAL FEATURES

- Peripheral facial palsy (Bell's sign),
- loss of taste sensation in the posterior third of the tongue (IX),
- dysphagia,
- paralysis of trapezius and sternocleidomastoid muscles.

POSSIBLE CAUSES

- Syndrome of jugular foramen (Vernet's syndrome), associated with involvement of cranial nerves IX–X–XI, due to compression by a tumor of the glomus jugulare or an injury affecting the ostium introitus (and damaging the auricular branch of X) and the inferior portion of the third part of the facial canal.

- **Radiography and tomography of the stylomastoid foramen in axial views (Fig. 7.45b–d; 7.46; 7.47), frontal views and prestudied inclined sagittal view (Cornélis) (Fig. 7.45a).**

CLINICAL FEATURES

- Peripheral facial palsy (Bell's sign),
- lesion of external acoustic meatus and tympanic membrane,
- disturbed transmission,
- parotid gland deficiency,
- paralysis of the cutaneous muscles of the skull, face, neck and outer aspect of the external ear, with involvement of the parotid gland, orbicularis oris and greater and lesser zygomatic muscles, levators of upper lip and nasal ala, nasalis, palpebral, frontalis muscles, etc.

POSSIBLE CAUSES

- Tympanojugular paraganglioma extending outwards, or fracture of the petrous bone, posterior cranial fossa or occipitotemporal region extending to the stylomastoid foramen, possibly damaging the sensory branch of the external acoustic meatus (Fig. 7.7) and the communicating branch with the glossopharyngeal nerve (IX), and affecting the two terminal branches of the VIIth nerve extracranially in the parotid gland.

Imaging (views required)

Remarks: Before carrying out the special views listed previously, the petrous bone must be studied by the classical clarification views:

- frontal view (petrous bones projected in orbits),
- Worms-Bretton view (lower frontal),
- Hirtz view (Fig. 7.27a, b),
- comparative sagittal views,
- Stenvers-Schüller view,
- comparative oblique anteroposterior view (Meyer) (Fig. 7.20a, b).

These classical views allow approximate localization of the lesional zone (tumor or fracture) and indicate the special appropriate views required in terms of the lesion or the course of the fracture, taking the clinical picture into account.

Three cases may be cited:

- A temporal fracture (visible in the lateral radiograph) may extend towards the petrous bone and involve the facial canal or one of the collateral orifices: petrotympanosquamous fissure, orifice of nerve to stapedius muscle, etc. (peripheral facial Bell's palsy, loss of sensation of anterior two-thirds of tongue); it may also involve the auditory ossicles and produce displacement or dislocation of the incudomallear or incudostapedial joints (tinnitus, lessened hearing acuity or total hearing loss, otorrhagia, etc.).
- An occipitotemporal fracture disrupting the lambdoid suture (visible in the Meyer and lateral views) may sometimes take the form of a Y and follow two different directions:
  * one towards the postero-inferior region of the petrous bone and the third part of VII or the stylomastoid foramen (peripheral facial palsy, paralysis of cutaneous muscles, etc.),
  * the other towards the jugular fossa and running into the jugular foramen (IX–X–XI) or the hypoglossal canal (XII) [loss of taste sensation in the posterior third of the tongue (IX) or of the entire half of the tongue (VII b–IX) (posterior condylolacerate syndrome)].
- An antro-adito-attical cholesteatoma (visible in the views of Worms and Bretton and of Stenvers) may erode the auditory ossicles and involve the lateral semicircular canal, destroying the second part of the facial canal, and may extend towards the geniculate ganglion (vertigo, facial palsy, decreased lacrimal secretion, painful hyperacuity of hearing, risk of decreased taste sensation in the anterior two-thirds of the tongue).

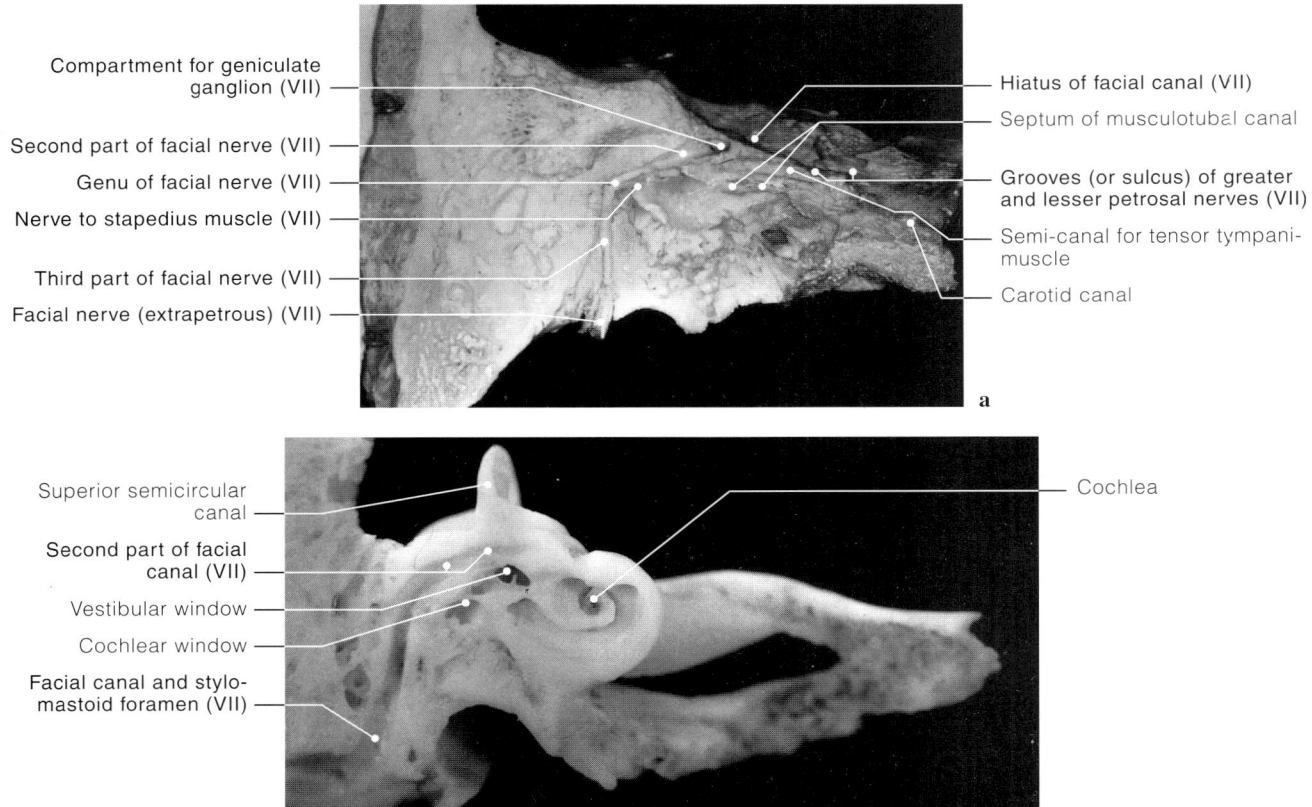

Fig. 7.9a, b. Sagittal anatomic sections at the level of facial nerve and canal (VII)

Intrapetrous course, internal acoustic meatus, facial nerve and intermedius nerve (VII–VIIb)

Imaging

TECHNIQUE (OBLIQUE VIEW)

Unilateral oblique tomographic study of internal acoustic meatus in varied Chaussé IV view:

- The subject is in dorsal decubitus, the head inclined by 50° to 60° in relation to the median sagittal plane towards the side opposite to that to be examined;
- the beam is centered at the level of the external acoustic meatus and 4 cm in front and is inclined by 5° to 10° to the orbitomeatal plane (OM);
- the sections are made starting from 2 cm below the meatus over a depth of 2 cm (Fig. 7.10).

Displayed: This view permits visualization of the internal acoustic meatus in its long axis, its transverse (or falciform) crest, the auditory ossicles and the antro-attical region.

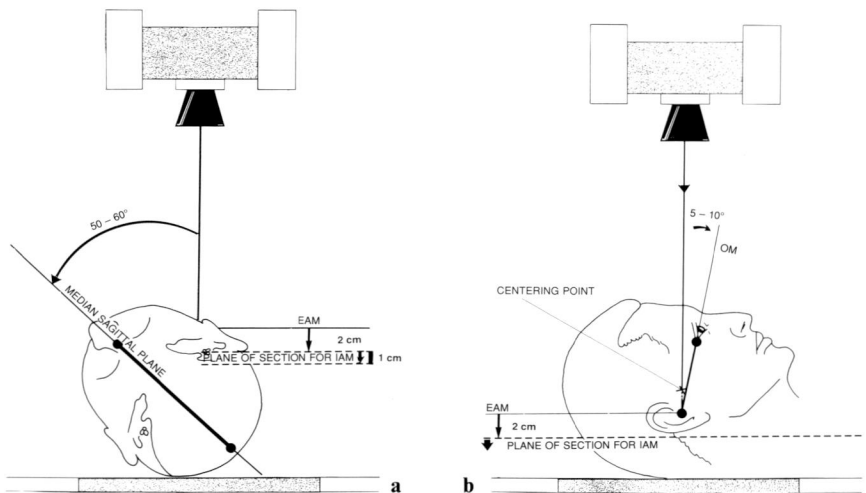

Fig. 7.10 a, b. Centering diagrams for radiography and tomography of the internal acoustic meatus in the varied Chaussé IV view

Facial nerve (VII) 189

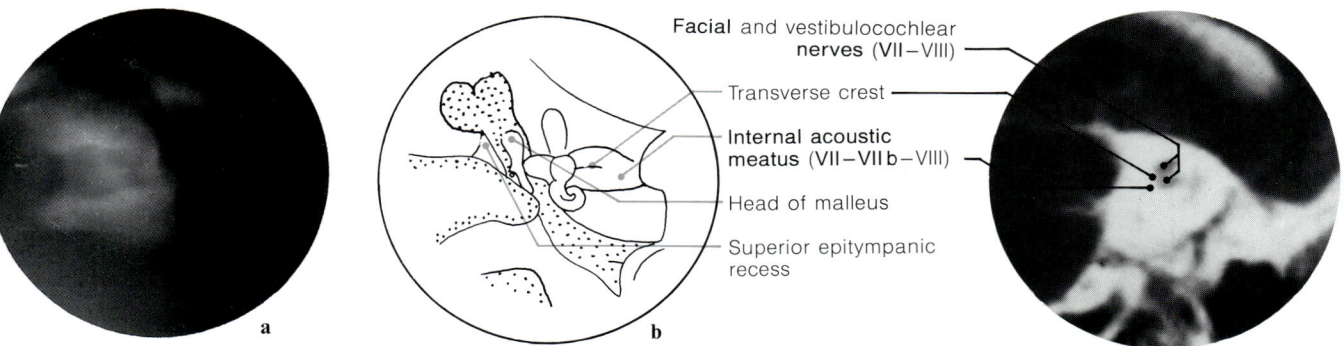

Fig. 7.11 a, b. Tomogram of internal acoustic meatus in Chaussé IV view

Fig. 7.12. Sagittal MRI of facial and vestibulocochlear nerves

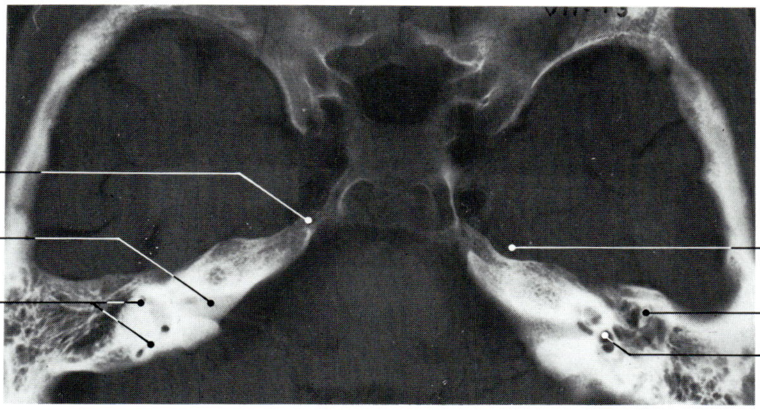

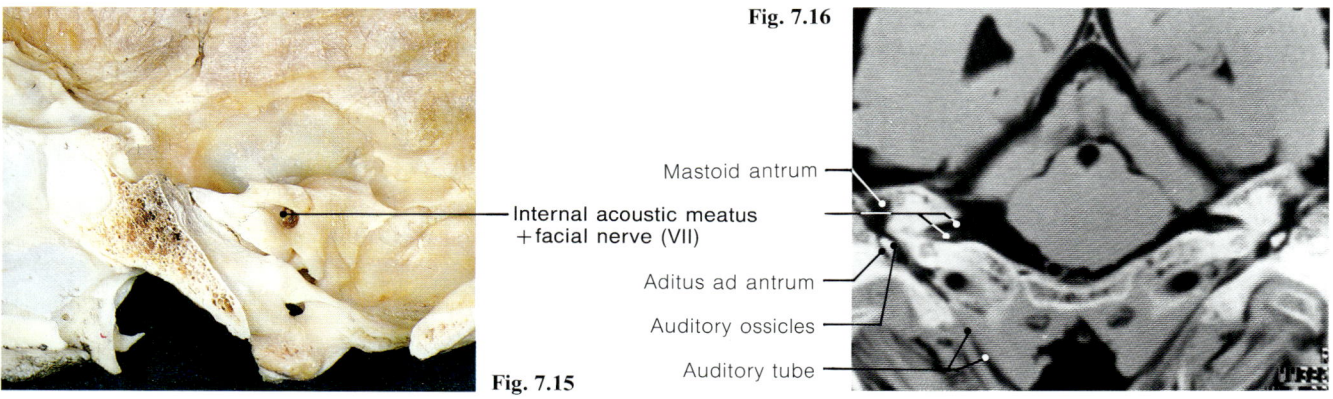

Fig. 7.13–7.16. Axial tomogram (**Fig. 7.13**) and anatomic view (**Fig. 7.14**), sagittal intracranial view of dried bone (**Fig. 7.15**); computed tomographic (CT) section (**Fig. 7.16**) of internal acoustic meatuses in Worms-Bretton view

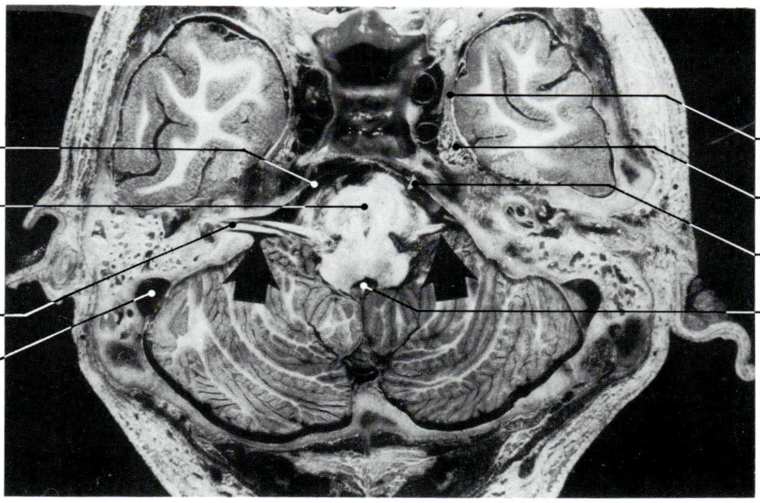

First part of facial canal, compartment of geniculate ganglion, hiatuses of canals, superficial greater and lesser petrosal nerves
Tomography and magnetic resonance imaging (MRI)
PRESTUDIED SAGITTAL VIEW (Fig. 7.19)

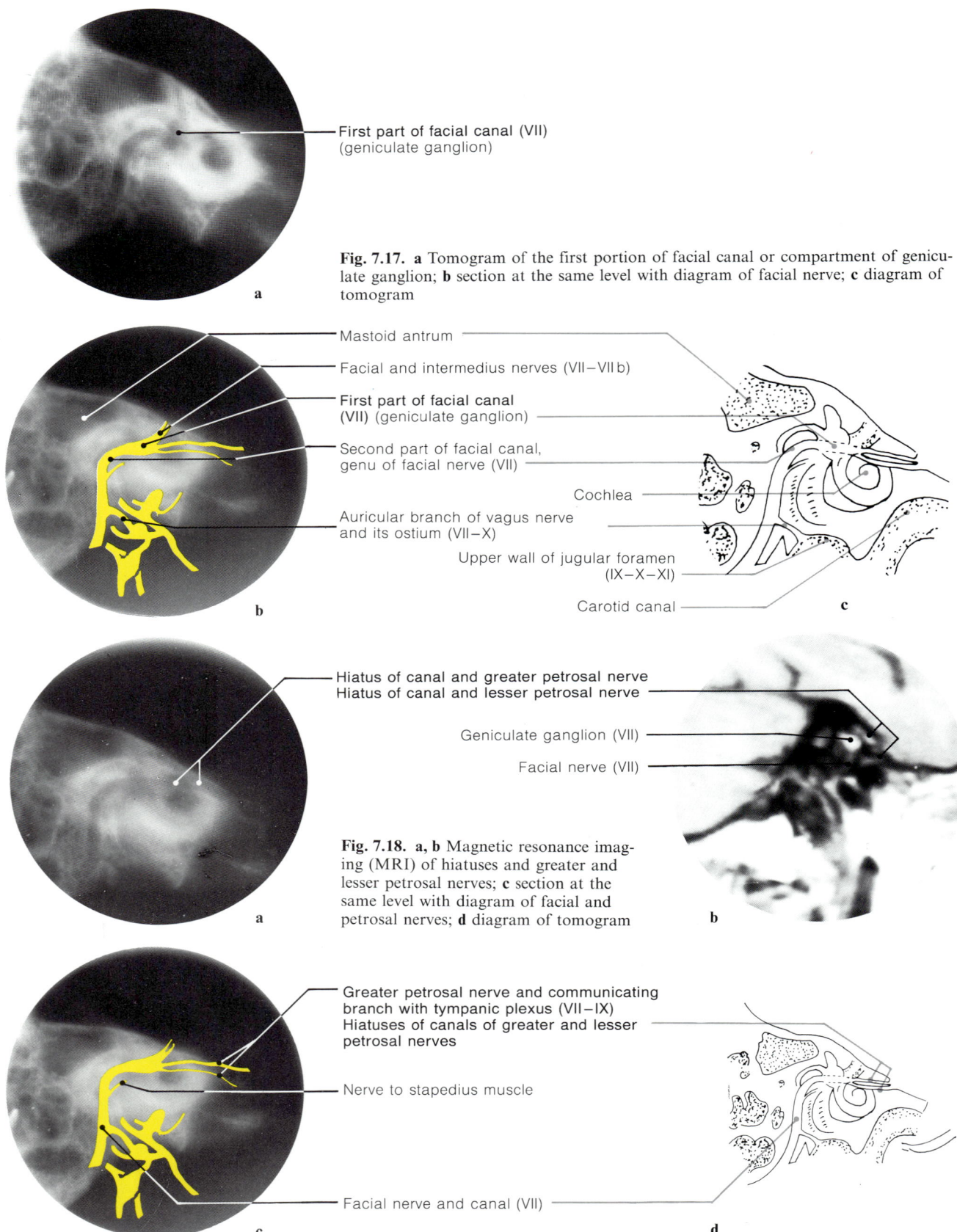

Fig. 7.17. a Tomogram of the first portion of facial canal or compartment of geniculate ganglion; **b** section at the same level with diagram of facial nerve; **c** diagram of tomogram

Fig. 7.18. a, b Magnetic resonance imaging (MRI) of hiatuses and greater and lesser petrosal nerves; **c** section at the same level with diagram of facial and petrosal nerves; **d** diagram of tomogram

Facial canal

Imaging

Technique

Tomographic study of the facial canal and its collateral orifices in prestudied varied inclined sagittal view (Cornélis):

- The subject is in lateral decubitus; the head in profile rests on the temporoparietal region, making an angle of 15° to 20° in relation to the median sagittal plane (Fig. 7.19);
- the centering point is situated at the level of the external acoustic meatus opposite to the table; the ear studied is that which is furthest from the table;
- it is initially necessary to make a tomographic series starting from the mastoid process every 0.5 mm as far as the petrous apex; after having identified the best planes for the facial canal, sections must be made every mm.

Displayed: This angled view allows successive study of:

- the facial canal,
- the stylomastoid foramen (Fig. 7.45),
- the ostium introitus (Fig. 7.41),
- the canal of stapedius muscle (Fig. 7.36),
- the compartment of the geniculate ganglion (Fig. 7.17),
- the posterior canal of chorda tympani (Fig. 7.37),
- the petrotympanosquamous fissure (exit of the chorda) (Fig. 7.37),
- the hiatuses of greater and lesser petrosal nerves (Fig. 7.18),
- the auditory ossicles with the base of stapes opposite the vestibular window,
- the antrum and aditus ad antrum,
- the jugular foramen,
- the petrosal fossula or compartment of the inferior ganglion (IX),
- the carotid canal,
- the vestibule and cochlea,
- the internal acoustic meatus.

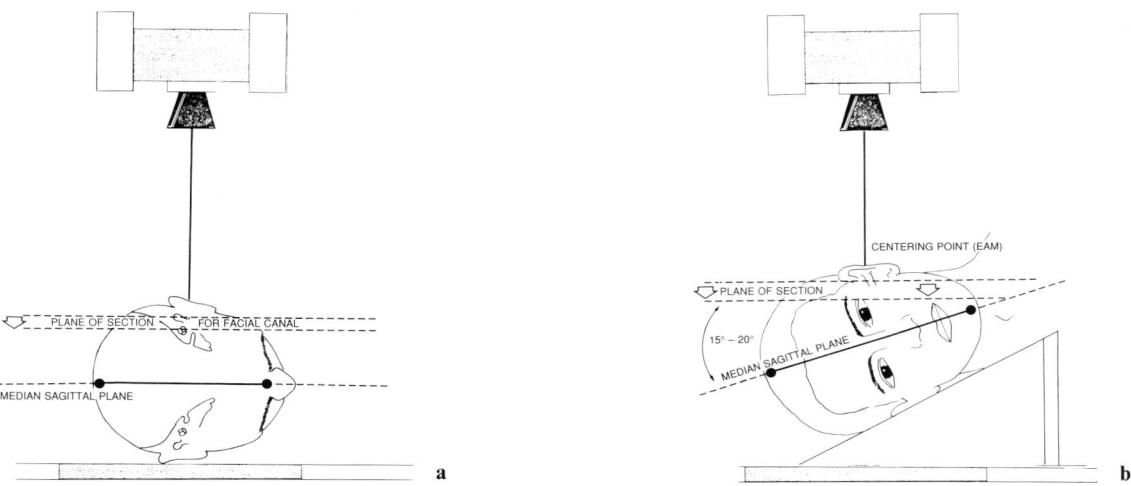

Fig. 7.19 a, b. Centering diagrams for tomographic study of the facial canal in prestudied varied inclined sagittal view

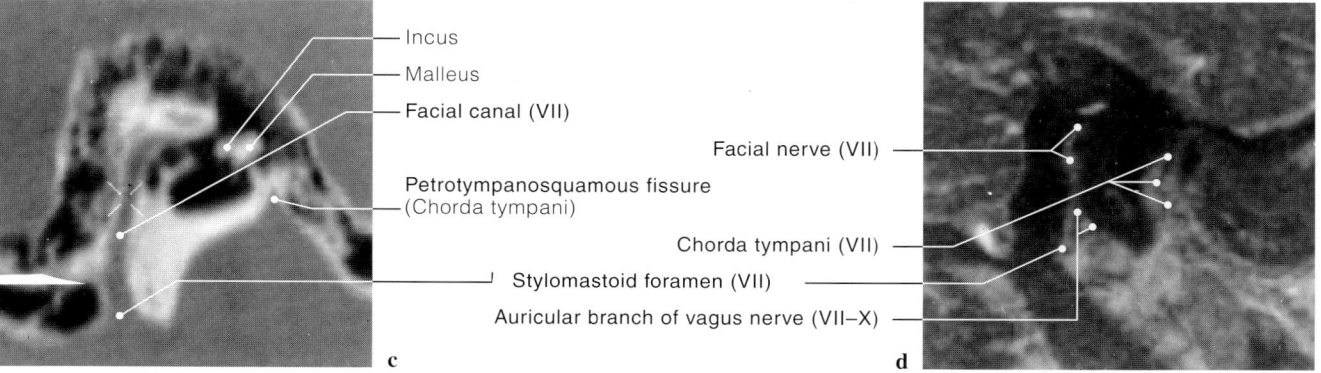

Fig. 7.19 c, d. Sagittal computed tomography (CT) of the facial canal (**c**); sagittal magnetic resonance imaging (MRI) of the facial nerve (VII) (**d**)

Sulci and course of superficial and deep greater and lesser petrosal nerves (VII–IX)

Imaging

TECHNIQUE (OBLIQUE VIEW)

Tomographic study of the antero-inferior aspect of the petrous bone for the sulci of the superficial and deep greater and lesser petrosal nerves, in the axis of the petrous pyramid in unilateral oblique view:

- The subject is in dorsal decubitus; the head is turned between 40° and 45° so as to place the anterior aspect of the petrous bone parallel to the plane of the table (Fig. 7.20) as it is this aspect that contains the sulci of the petrosal nerves;
- the incident vertical beam makes an angle of some 20°, open upwards, in relation to the orbitomeatal plane (OM) (Fig. 7.21);
- the centering point is situated two fingersbreadths above and lateral to the outer angle of the eye, opposite the external acoustic meatus;
- the tomographic plane is set to start from the anterior region of the external acoustic meatus, descending every 3 mm, then to start from the best plane every mm.

Displayed: This examination gives good definition of the sulcus of the superficial and deep lesser petrosal nerves up to the canal of the otic ganglion (Fig. 7.21), which they traverse. It visualizes the foramen lacerum, the carotid canal, the nasotubal orifice, the trigeminal impression, the sulcus of VI and the internal acoustic meatus.

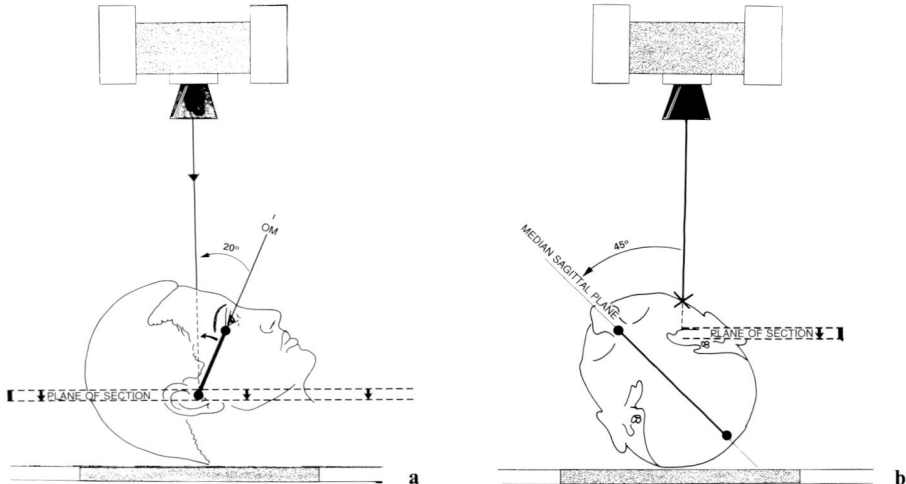

Fig. 7.20a, b. Centering diagrams for tomographic study of the sulci of the superficial and deep greater and lesser petrosal nerves

Facial nerve (VII) 193

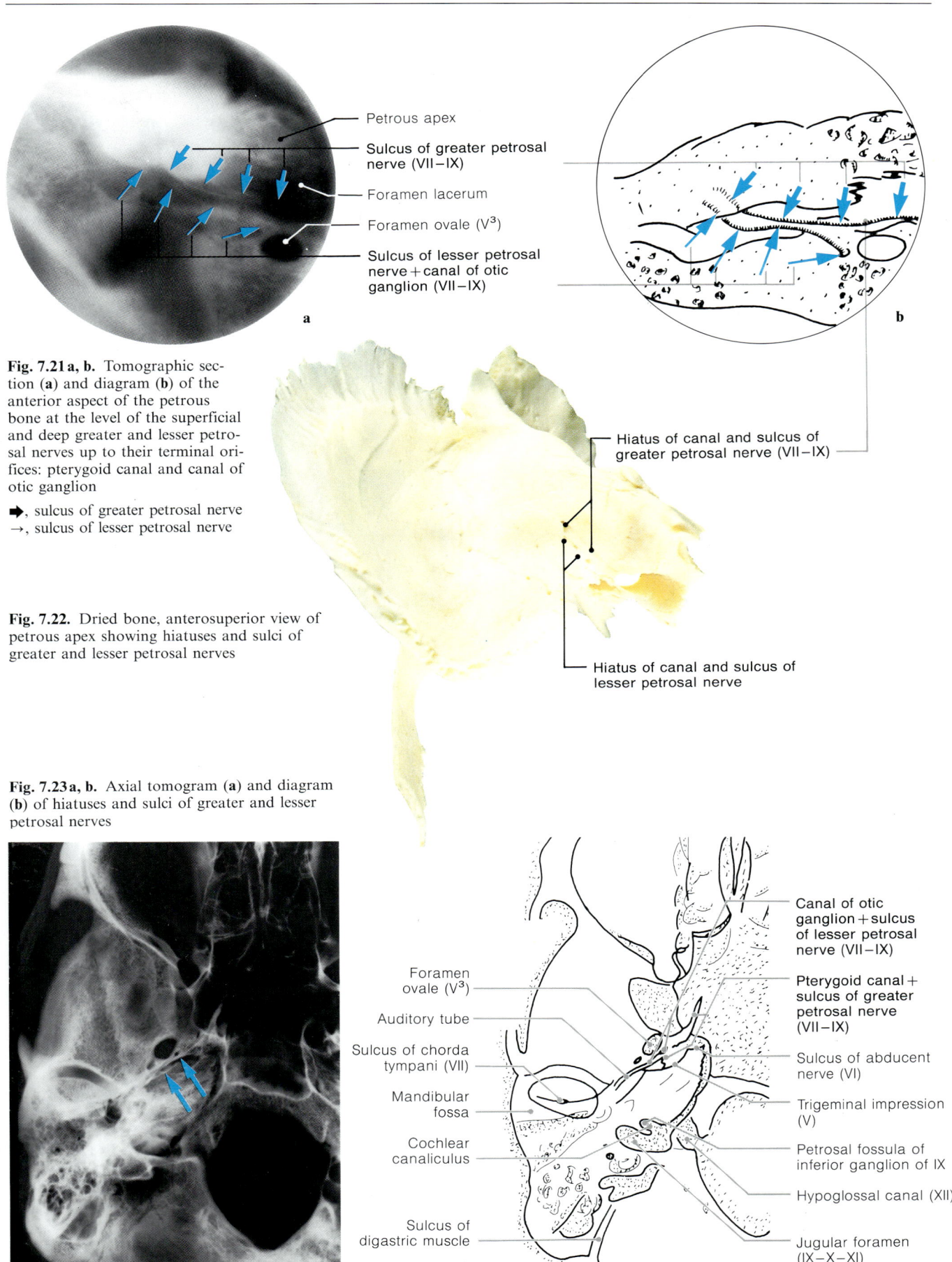

Fig. 7.21 a, b. Tomographic section (**a**) and diagram (**b**) of the anterior aspect of the petrous bone at the level of the superficial and deep greater and lesser petrosal nerves up to their terminal orifices: pterygoid canal and canal of otic ganglion

➡, sulcus of greater petrosal nerve
→, sulcus of lesser petrosal nerve

Fig. 7.22. Dried bone, anterosuperior view of petrous apex showing hiatuses and sulci of greater and lesser petrosal nerves

Fig. 7.23 a, b. Axial tomogram (**a**) and diagram (**b**) of hiatuses and sulci of greater and lesser petrosal nerves

Pterygoid canal, pterygoid nerve (VII–IX)
Magnetic resonance imaging (MRI) and computed tomography (CT)
FRONTAL AND SAGITTAL VIEWS (Fig. 5.71 d)

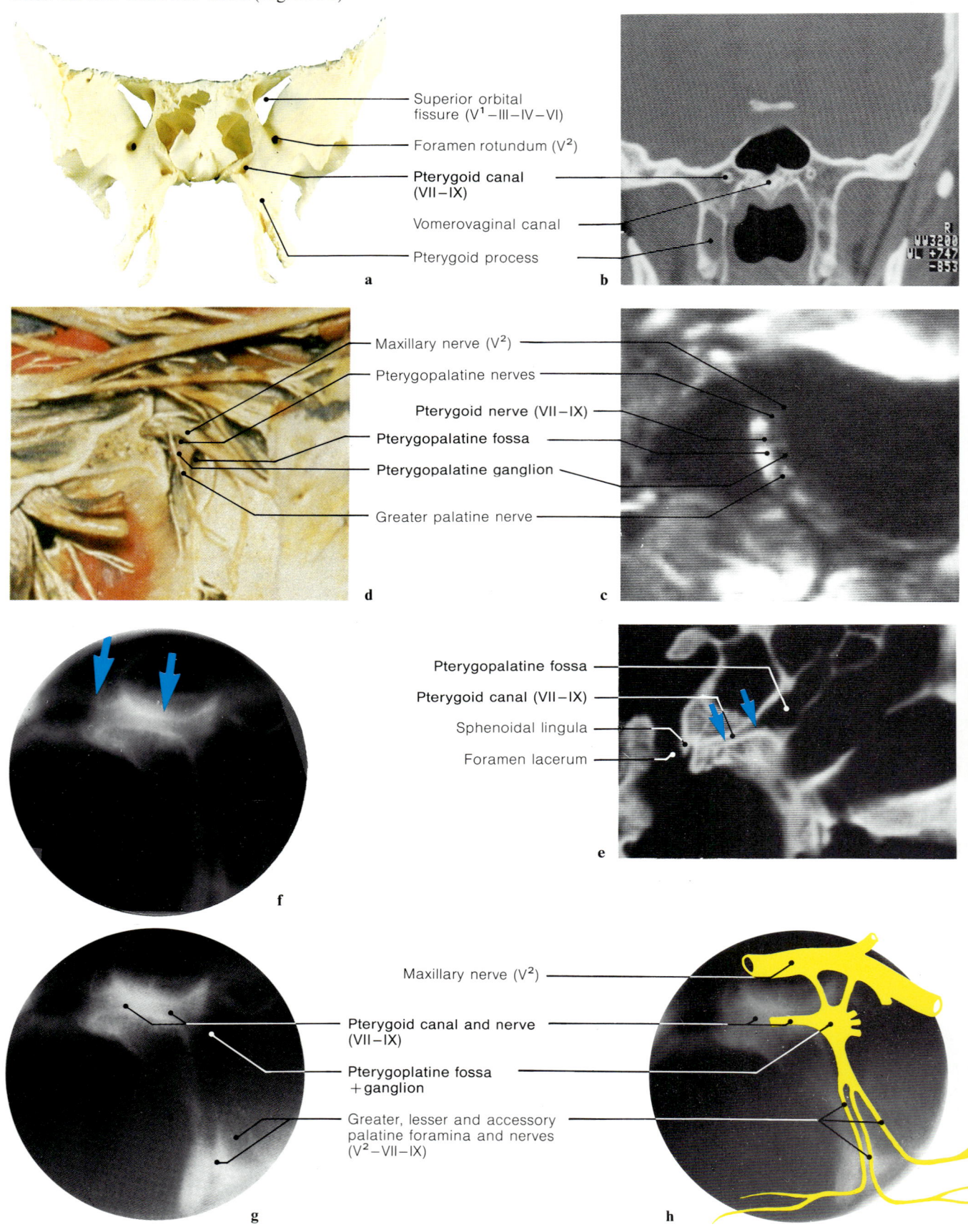

Pterygoid canal

Imaging

TECHNIQUE (FRONTAL VIEW)

Frontal and symmetric tomographic study of pterygoid canals:

- The subject is in dorsal decubitus, with the head facing strictly forwards supported by flour bags; the orbitomeatal plane (OM) is to be seen as perpendicular to the plane of the table (Fig. 7.25);
- the centering point is situated at the middle of the nose, at the level of the infraorbital margins;
- after having identified the inferolateral margin of the orbit, a point is marked 3.5 cm below, corresponding to the plane of section;
- the sections are performed starting from this point, every 3 mm, descending to the anterior region of the mandibular condyle (Fig. 7.25).

Displayed: superior orbital fissures, foramina rotunda, sphenoidal sinuses, pterygoid processes, vomerovaginal canal and palatovaginal canals, anterior and posterior clinoid processes, hypophyseal fossa and dorsum sellae (Fig. 7.24a, b).

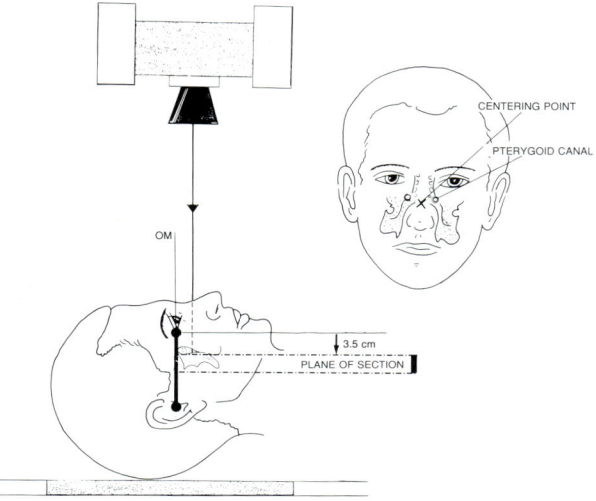

Fig. 7.25. Centering diagram for frontal and symmetric tomographic study of pterygoid canals

TECHNIQUE (SAGITTAL VIEW)

Sagittal tomographic study of pterygoid canal:

- The subject is in lateral decubitus in "gun-dog" position, the head strictly lateral resting on plastic cushions;
- after having located the orbitomeatal plane (OM), a point "A" is marked 3.5 cm from the external acoustic meatus towards the orbit, and then a point "B" 1 cm lower which is the centering point (Fig. 7.26);
- a point "C" is marked at 1 cm lateral to the median sagittal plane towards the side to be examined;
- sections are made from "C", centering on "B", every 2 mm travelling outwards over a depth of 1 cm on each side.

Displayed: pterygoid process, pterygopalatine fossa, greater and lesser palatine canals (Fig. 7.24 d, g, h).

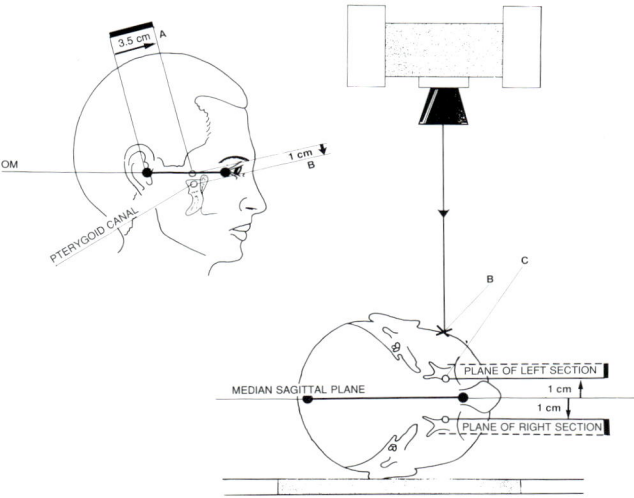

Fig. 7.26. Centering diagrams for sagittal tomographic study of pterygoid canal

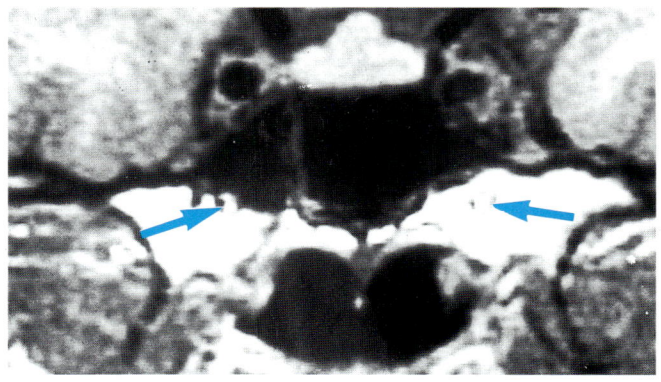

Fig. 7.24. a, b Frontal anatomic and computed tomographic (CT) view of pterygoid canals; **c, d** sagittal magnetic resonance imaging (MRI) and anatomic section for pterygoid nerve; **e–h** sagittal computed tomography (CT) and tomograms of pterygoid canal, with diagram of pterygoid nerve (VII–IX); **i** MRI frontal view of pterygoid nerves in their canals (arrows)

Pterygoid canal and canal of otic ganglion, superficial and deep greater and lesser petrosal nerves (VII–IX) (See vascular relations, p. 279)

Imaging

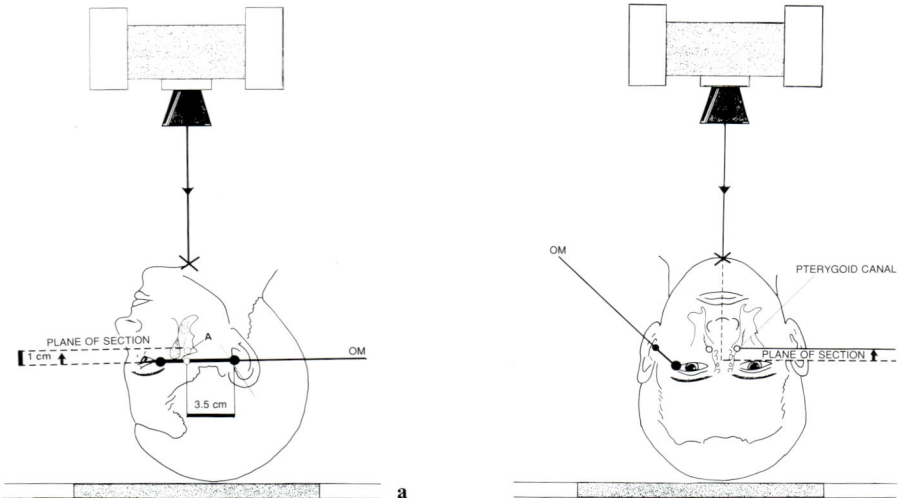

Fig. 7.27 a, b. Centering diagrams for axial symmetric tomographic study of pterygoid canals

TECHNIQUE (AXIAL VIEW)

Axial symmetric tomographic study of pterygoid canals:

- The subject is in dorsal decubitus, the back raised on cushions, the head extended in the Hirtz position, the orbitomeatal plane (OM) horizontal and parallel to the table (Fig. 7.27);
- the centering point is situated at the median line, 5 or 6 cm behind the mental symphysis;
- the planes of section are made every 2 mm starting from point "A" over 1 cm, descending towards the orbitomeatal plane (OM).

Displayed: This view visualizes the course of the superficial greater petrosal nerve from its hiatus, its sulcus up to the pterygoid canal and the pterygopalatine fossa, then the course of the superficial lesser petrosal nerve from its hiatus and its sulcus up to the canal of the otic ganglion (Fig. 7.28; 7.30 a). It also shows:

- the petrotympanosquamous fissures (Fig. 7.38–7.40),
- the foramina ovalia (Fig. 7.28; 7.30 a; 7.38),
- the foramina lacera (Fig. 7.28; 7.30 a),
- the carotid canals (Fig. 7.28),
- the auditory tubes up to the aditus ad antrum (Fig. 7.30 a),
- the inferior orbital fissures (Fig. 7.28 b),
- the vomerovaginal canal and the palatovaginal canals (Fig. 7.28 a, b).

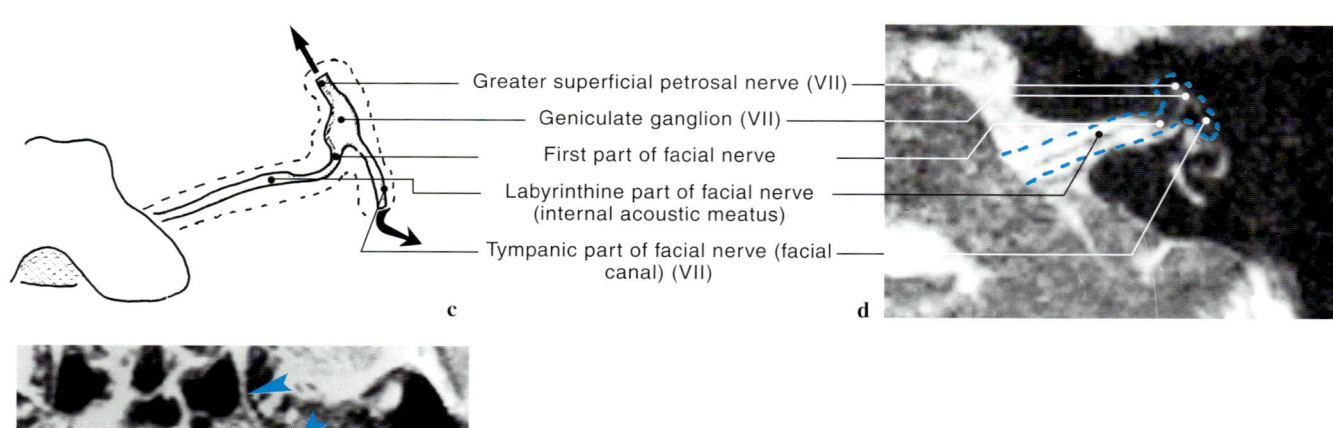

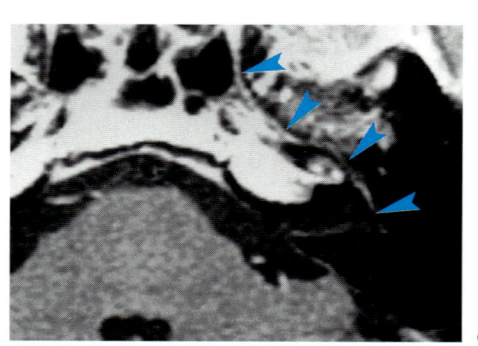

Fig. 7.27 c–e. Axial magnetic resonance imaging (MRI) and diagram clearly demonstrating the position of the facial nerve (VII) in its labyrinthine and tympanic segments. *Arrow*, pterygopalatine ganglion; *curved arrow*, facial canal; *arrowheads*, superficial greater petrosal nerve (**e**). (MRI: Dr. J.W. Casselman, A.Z. St-Jan, Brugge)

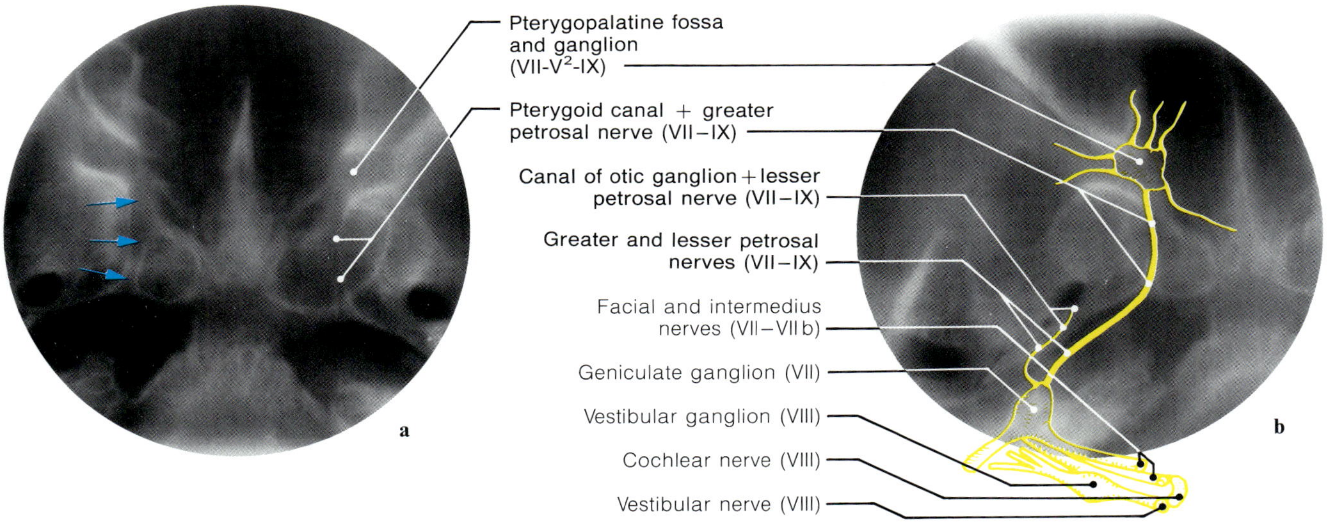

Facial nerve (VII) 197

Fig. 7.28. a, c Axial tomographic and computed tomographic (CT) sections of pterygoid canals; **b** same section, with diagram of petrosal nerves; **d** magnetic resonance imaging (MRI), axial view of pterygoid nerves (VII–IX) (arrows)

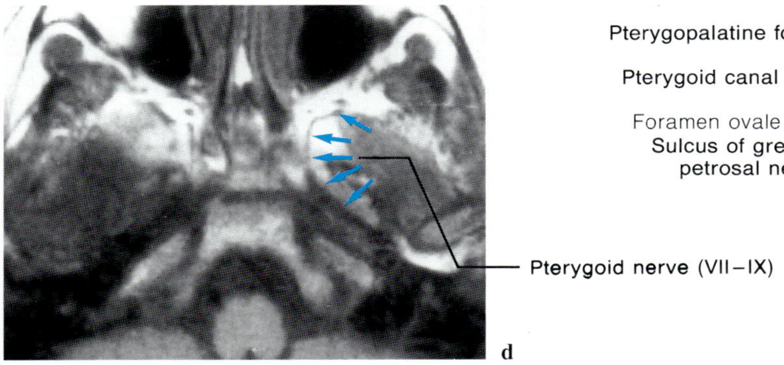

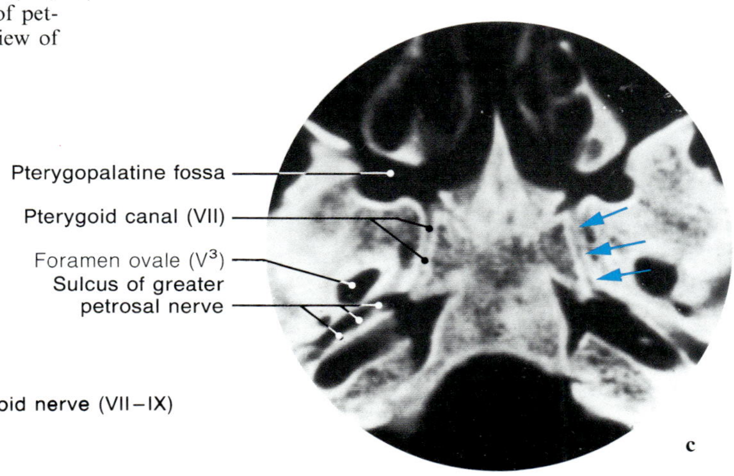

Fig. 7.29. Diagram of facial and trigeminal nerves showing relations between the greater and lesser petrosal nerves and the otic, pterygopalatine and inferior ganglia of IX (V–VII–IX)

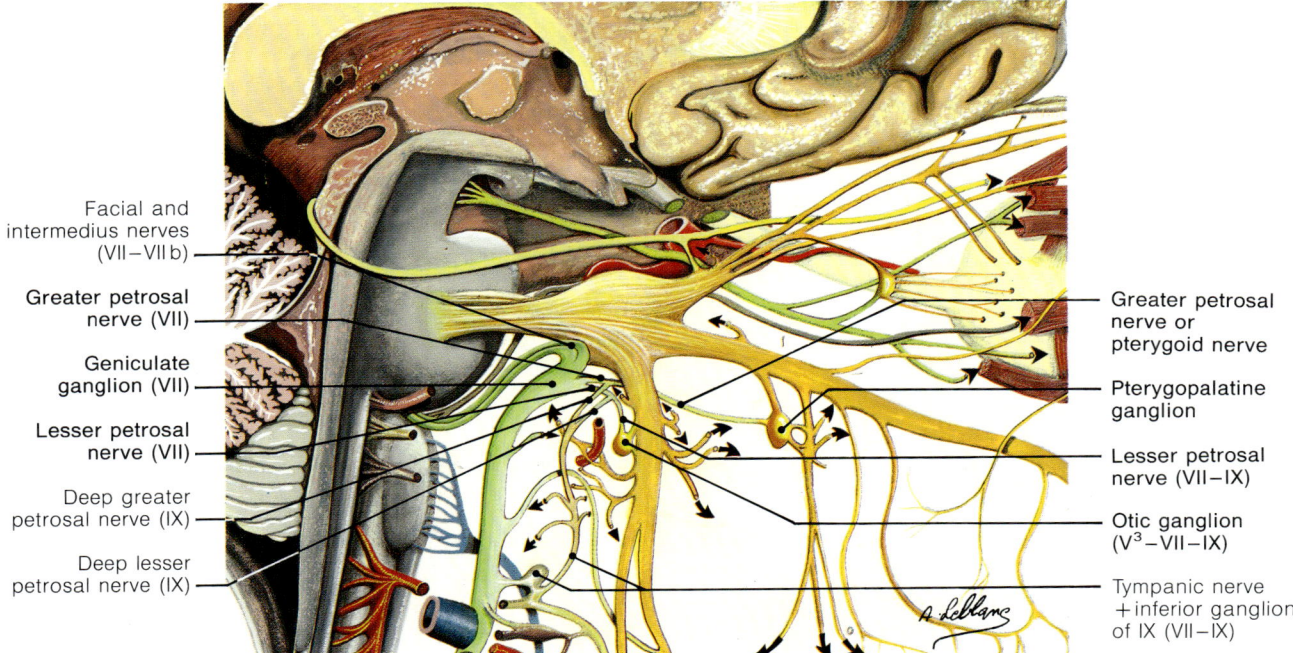

198 Facial nerve (VII)

Canal of otic ganglion, superficial and deep lesser petrosal nerves (VII–IX) (or communicating branch with tympanic plexus)
Radiology
OBLIQUE VIEW

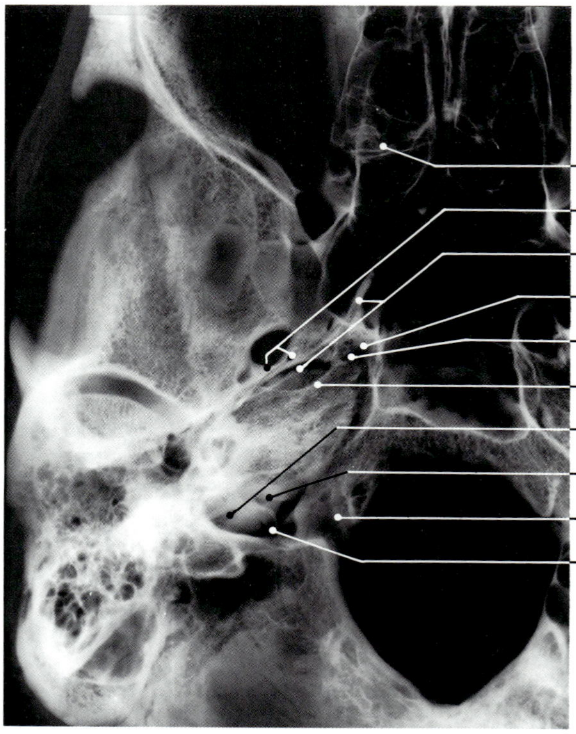

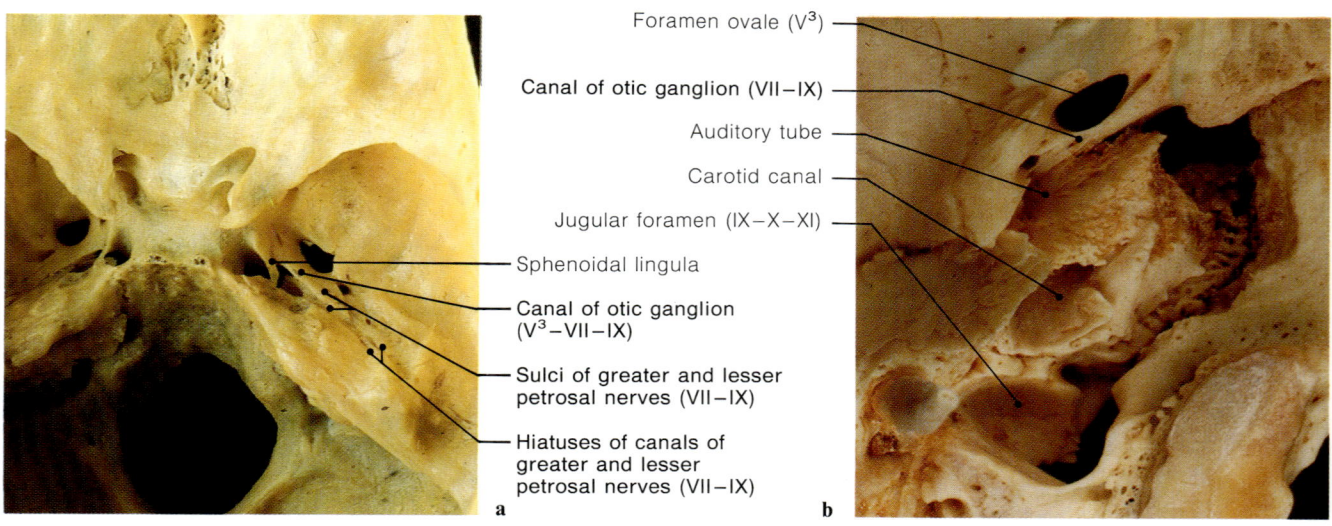

Fig. 7.30 a, b. Radiographs of subject (b) and of anatomic specimen (a)

Labels (a):
- Posterior ethmoidal foramen (V¹)
- Canal of otic ganglion and sulcus of lesser petrosal nerve (VII–IX)
- Pterygoid canal + sulcus of greater petrosal nerve (VII–IX)
- Foramen lacerum
- Sulcus of abducent nerve (VI)
- Trigeminal impression (V)
- Ostium of auricular branch of vagus nerve (VII–X)
- Petrosal fossula of inferior ganglion of IX
- Hypoglossal canal (XII)
- Jugular foramen

Labels (b):
- Coronoid process of mandible
- Foramen ovale (V³)
- Canal of otic ganglion (V³–VII–IX)
- Petrosal fossula of inferior ganglion of glossopharyngeal nerve (IX–VII)
- Dens of axis

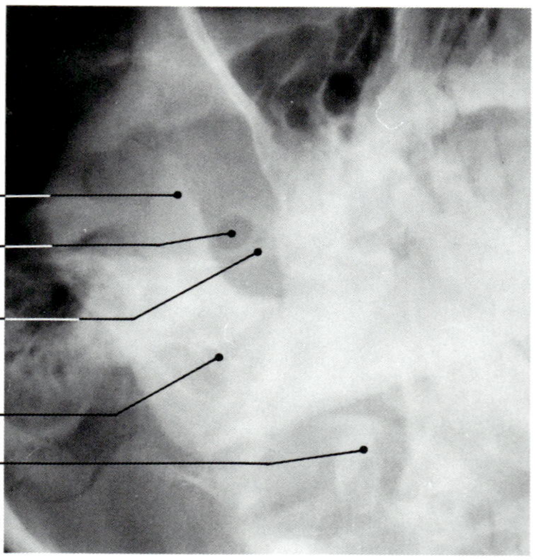

Fig. 7.31 a, b. Intracranial (a) and extracranial (b) views of canal of otic ganglion; sulcus of superficial and deep lesser petrosal nerves (or communicating branch with tympanic plexus)

Labels (a):
- Sphenoidal lingula
- Canal of otic ganglion (V³–VII–IX)
- Sulci of greater and lesser petrosal nerves (VII–IX)
- Hiatuses of canals of greater and lesser petrosal nerves (VII–IX)

Labels (b):
- Foramen ovale (V³)
- Canal of otic ganglion (VII–IX)
- Auditory tube
- Carotid canal
- Jugular foramen (IX–X–XI)

Canal of otic ganglion

Imaging

TECHNIQUE

Radiographic study of canal of otic ganglion in unilateral oblique view:

- The subject is in dorsal decubitus, the back raised on cushions, the head extended so that the vertical incident beam makes an angle of 50° to 55° to the orbitomeatal plane (OM) (Fig. 7.32);
- the head is then turned by 40° to 50° in relation to the median sagittal plane towards the side opposite to that to be examined (Fig. 7.32);
- the centering point is situated at about 1.5 cm from the mandibular angle. This view is largely identical with that for the foramen ovale.

Displayed:

- the foramen ovale (V^3),
- the trigeminal impression (V),
- the jugular foramen (IX–X–XI),
- the zygomatic arch and the coronoid process.

Reminder

Structural variant: As previously mentioned, when the canal of the otic ganglion (Fig. 7.30; 7.31) is nonexistent, the superficial and deep lesser petrosal nerves pass through the foramen lacerum or the sphenopetrosal suture before anastomosing with the otic ganglion (Fig. 7.29; 7.37c; 7.49).

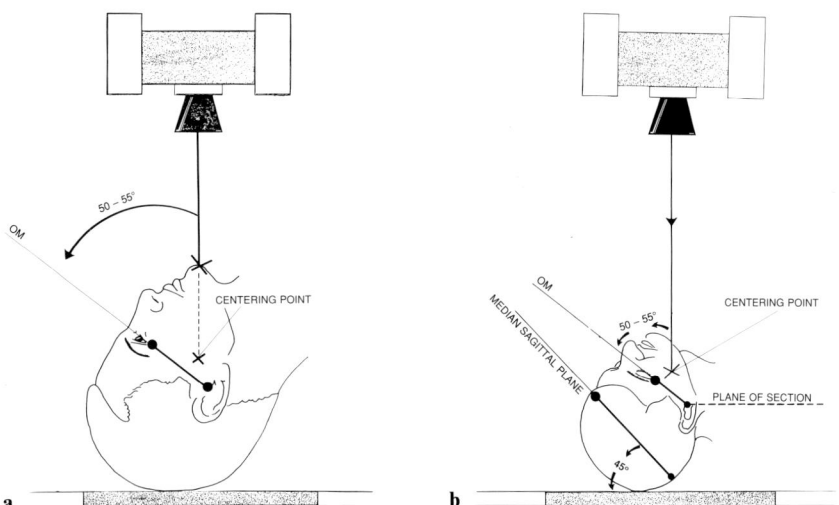

Fig. 7.32 a, b. Centering diagrams for radiographic study of canal of otic ganglion in unilateral oblique view

Facial canal and nerve

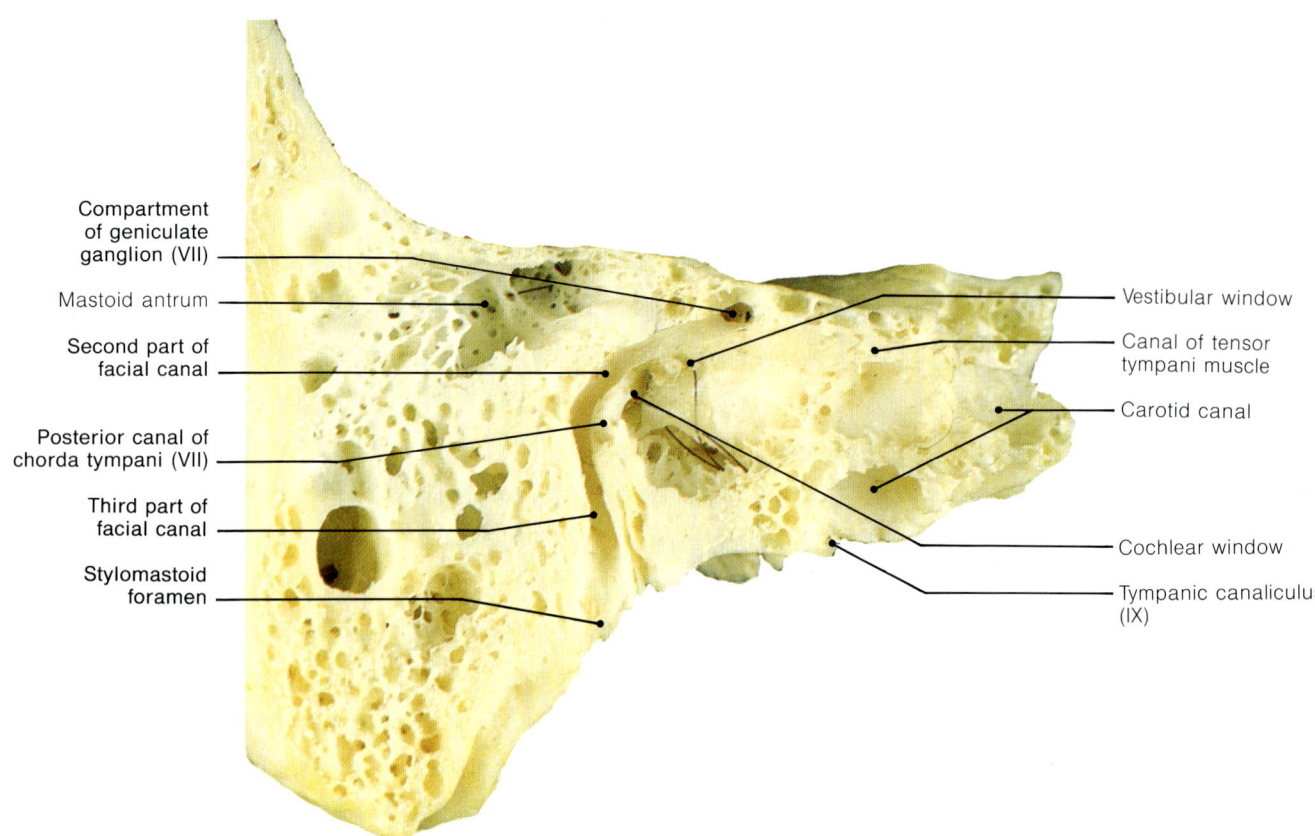

Fig. 7.33. Section of petrous bone along facial canal

Fig. 7.34. Dissection of facial, trigeminal and oculomotor nerves

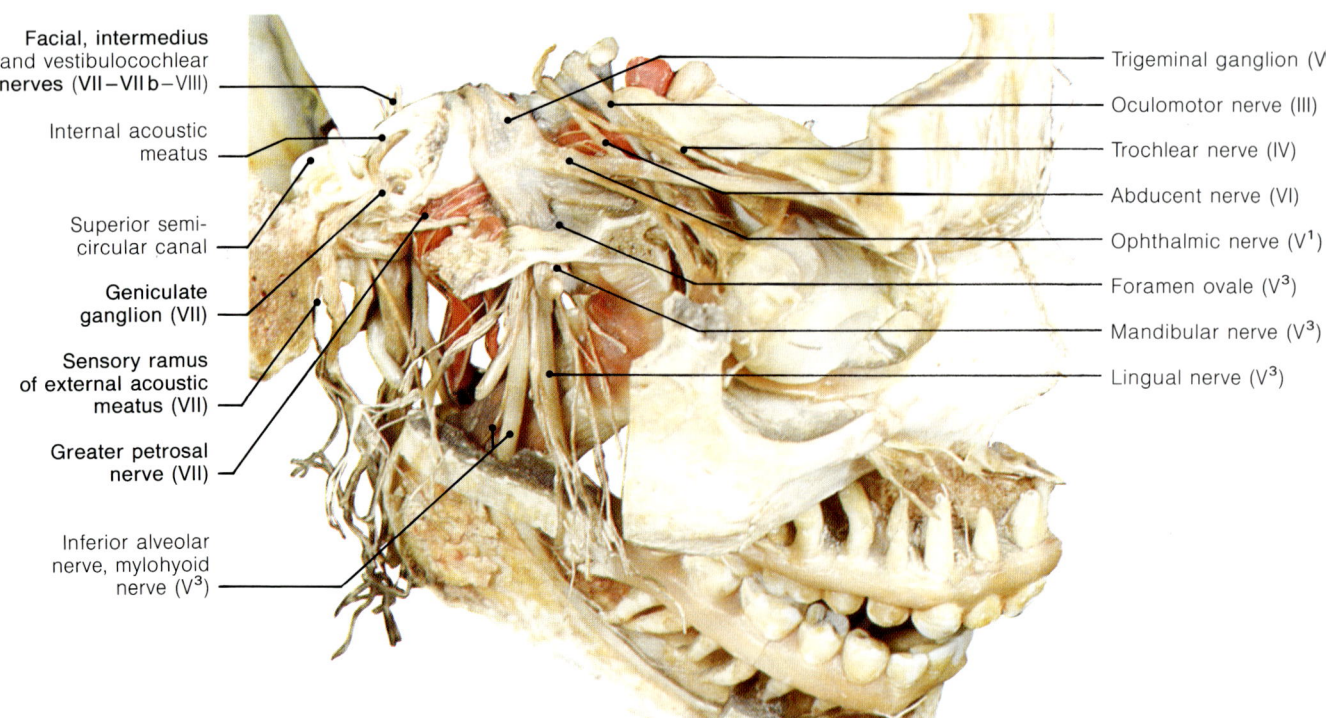

Second part of facial canal

Tomography

PRESTUDIED SAGITTAL AND GUILLEN VIEWS

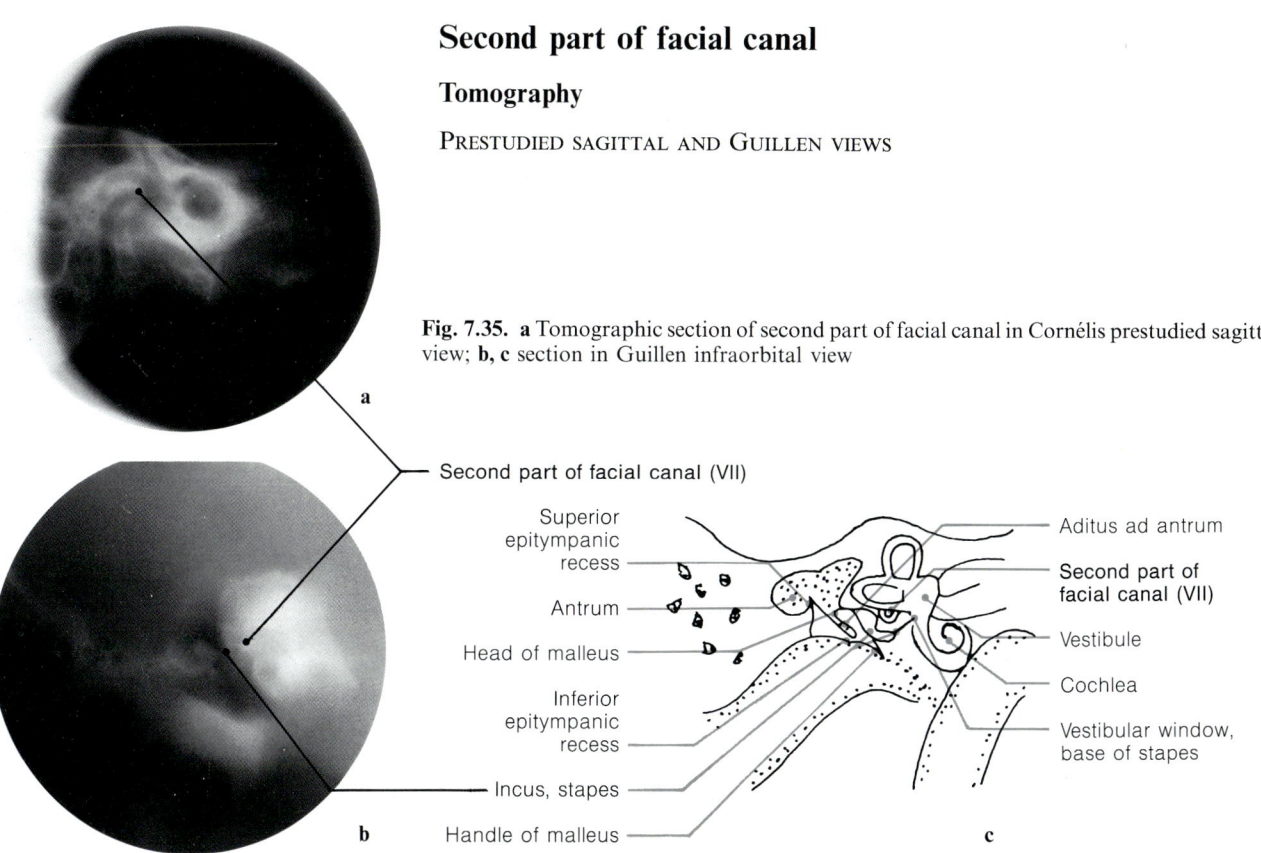

Fig. 7.35. a Tomographic section of second part of facial canal in Cornélis prestudied sagittal view; b, c section in Guillen infraorbital view

Orifice of nerve to stapedius muscle

Tomography and computed tomography (CT)

PRESTUDIED SAGITTAL VIEW (Fig. 7.19)

Fig. 7.36 a–d. Tomographic (a) and computed tomographic (CT) (b) sections in Cornélis prestudied inclined sagittal view of origin of nerve to stapedius muscle, with diagrams (d) and radiograph (c) of facial nerve

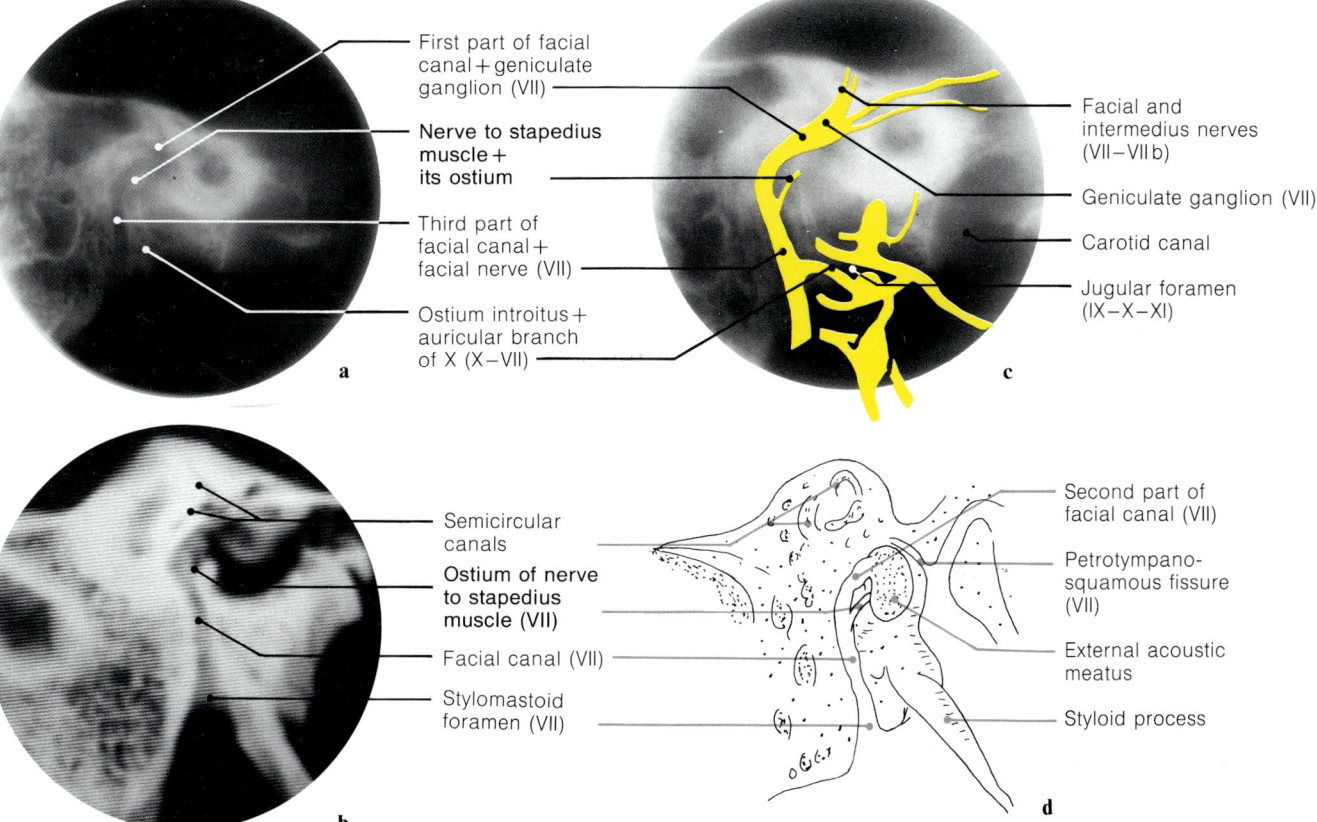

Petrotympanosquamous fissure, chorda tympani (VIIb)

Tomography

PRESTUDIED SAGITTAL VIEW (Fig. 7.19)

Fig. 7.37. a, b Sagittal tomogram and diagram of posterior canal of chorda tympani; **c** diagram showing relations of chorda tympani and lingual nerve; **d, e** sagittal tomograms of petrotympanosquamous fissure and sagittal anatomic section of chorda tympani

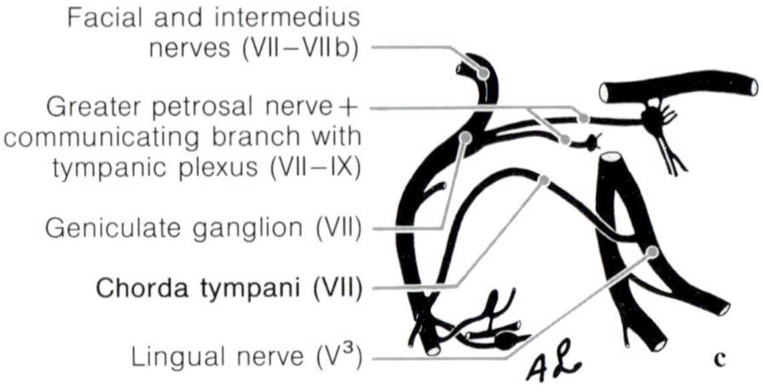

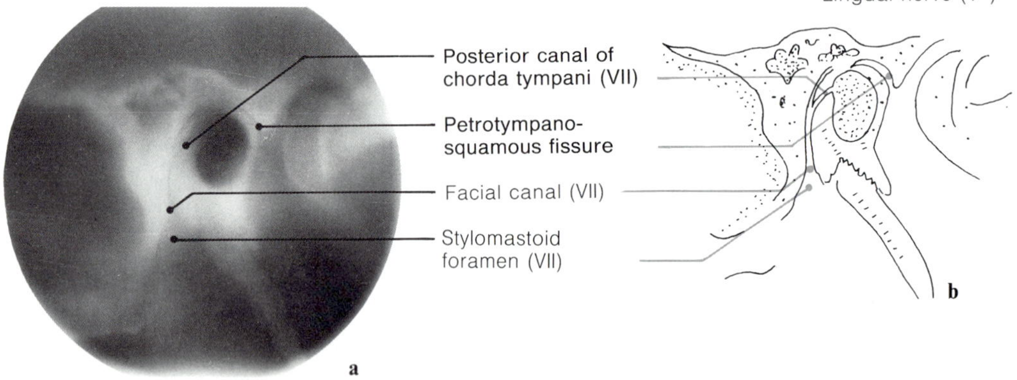

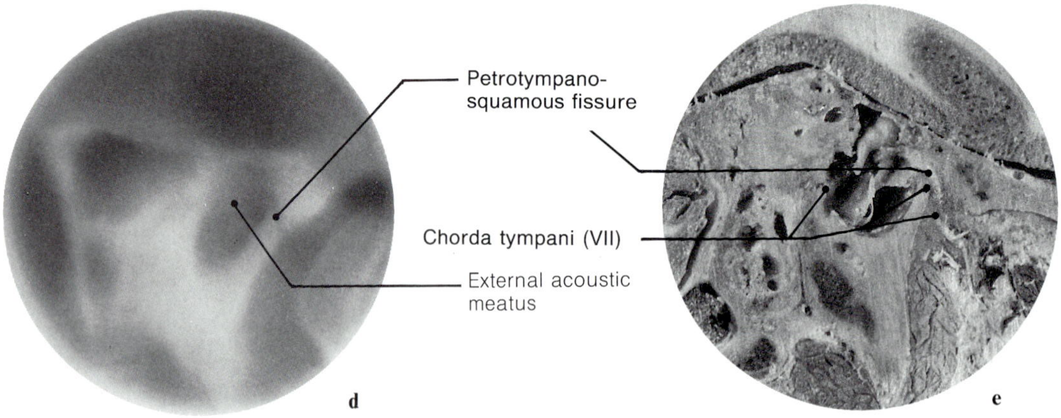

AXIAL VIEW

Fig. 7.38 a, b. Axial tomographic section of mandibular fossa of temporal bone to show petrotympanosquamous fissure

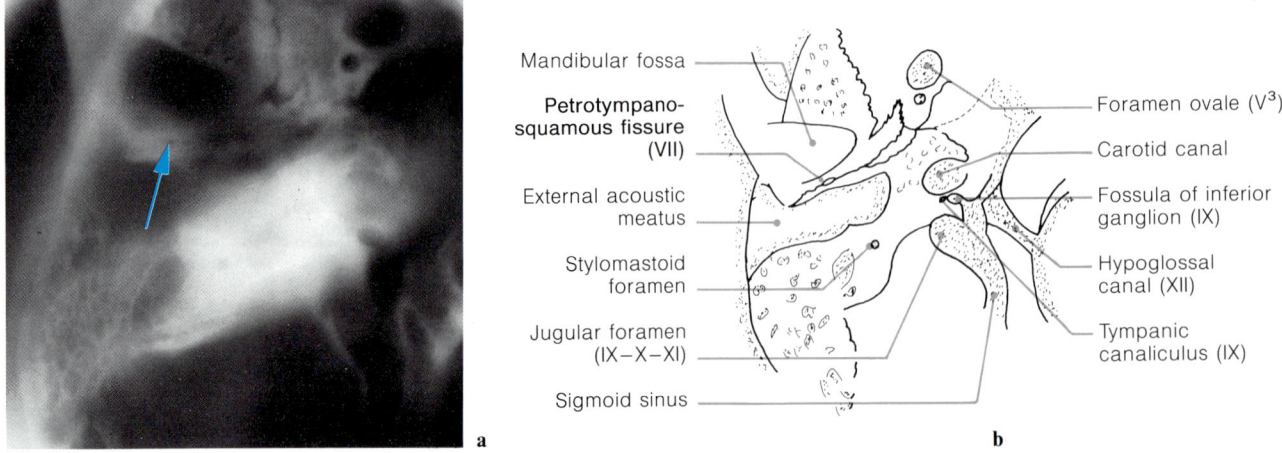

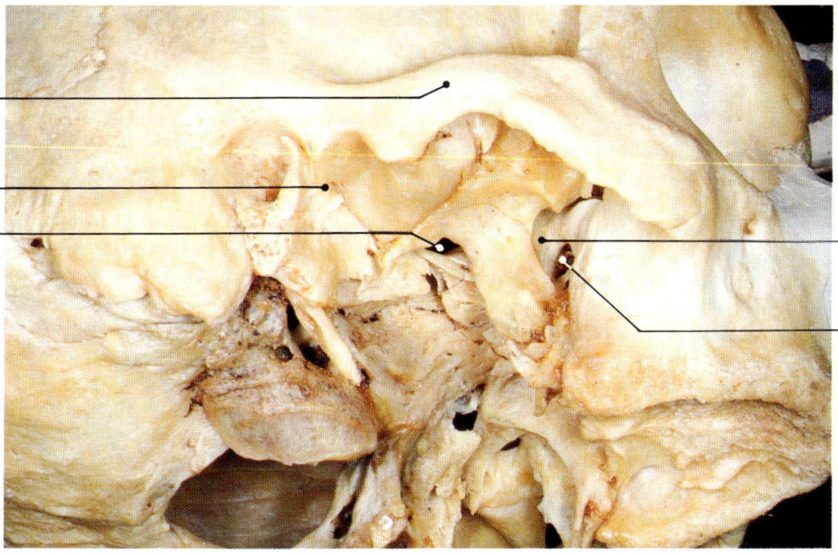

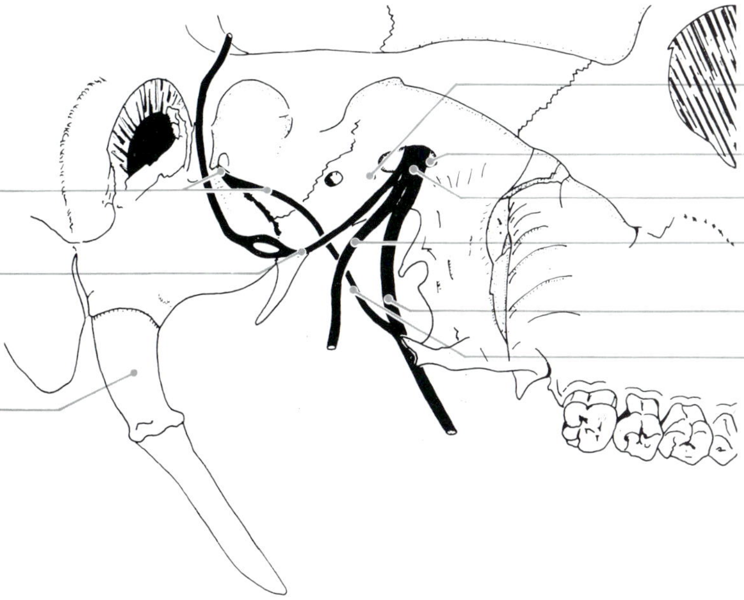

Facial nerve (VII) 203

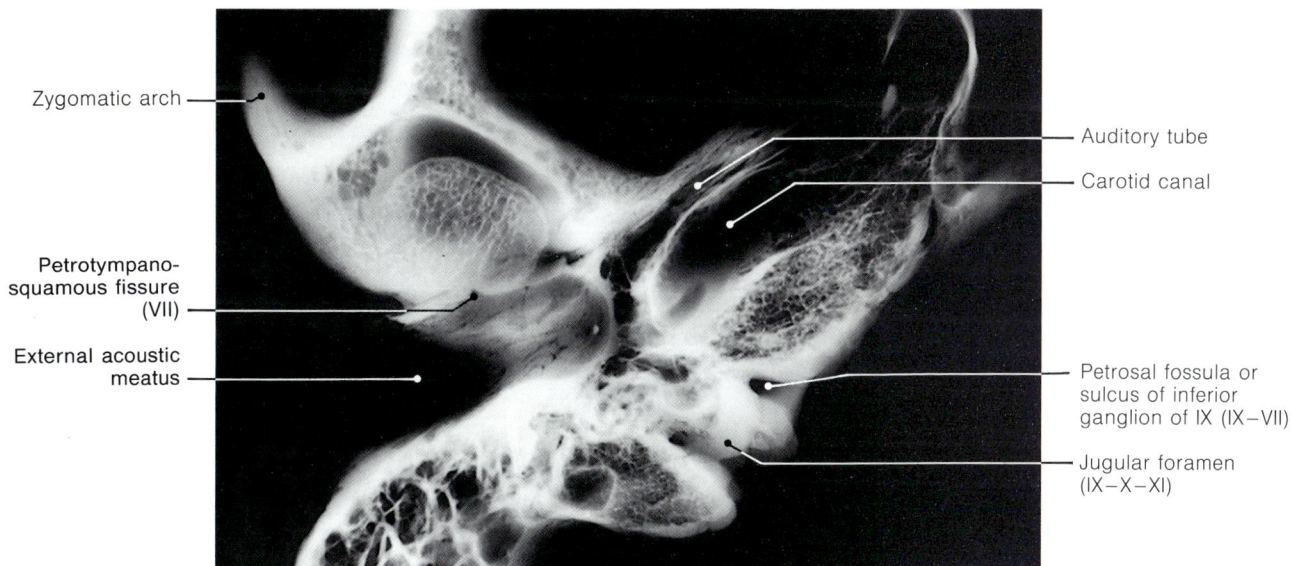

Fig. 7.39 a, b. Inferolateral view of mandibular fossa of temporal bone with petrotympanosquamous fissure transmitting chorda tympani (VII)

Fig. 7.40. Axial section of petrotympanosquamous fissure

204   Facial nerve (VII)

Ostium introitus, auricular branch of vagus nerve (VII–X)

Tomography

PRESTUDIED VARIED SAGITTAL VIEW (Fig. 7.19)

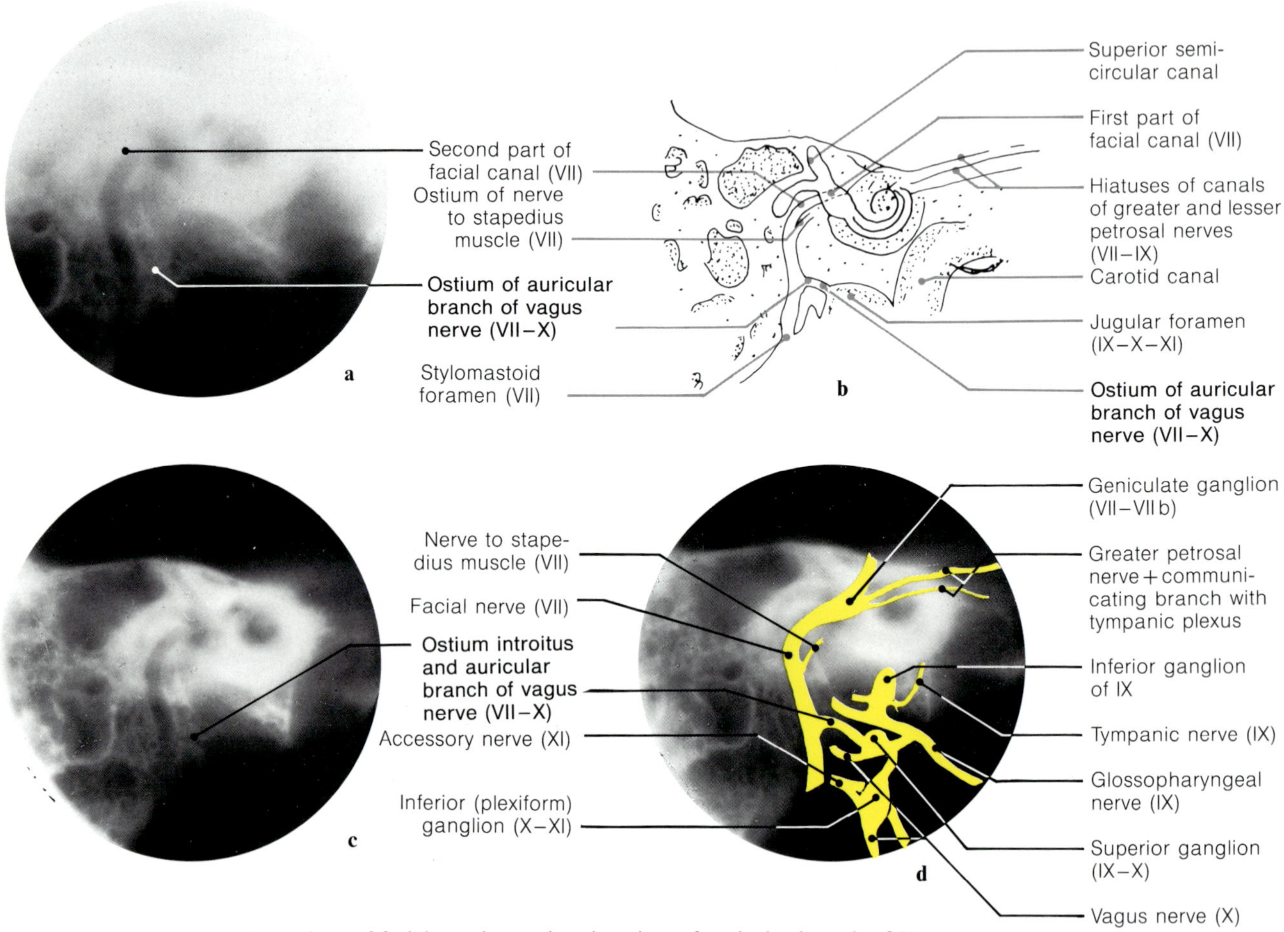

Fig. 7.41 a–d. Tomographic sections of facial canal at ostium introitus of auricular branch of X

Fig. 7.42 a, b. Extracranial view (a) of tegmen of jugular foramen showing ostium introitus and diagram (b) of anastomotic branch with vagus nerve

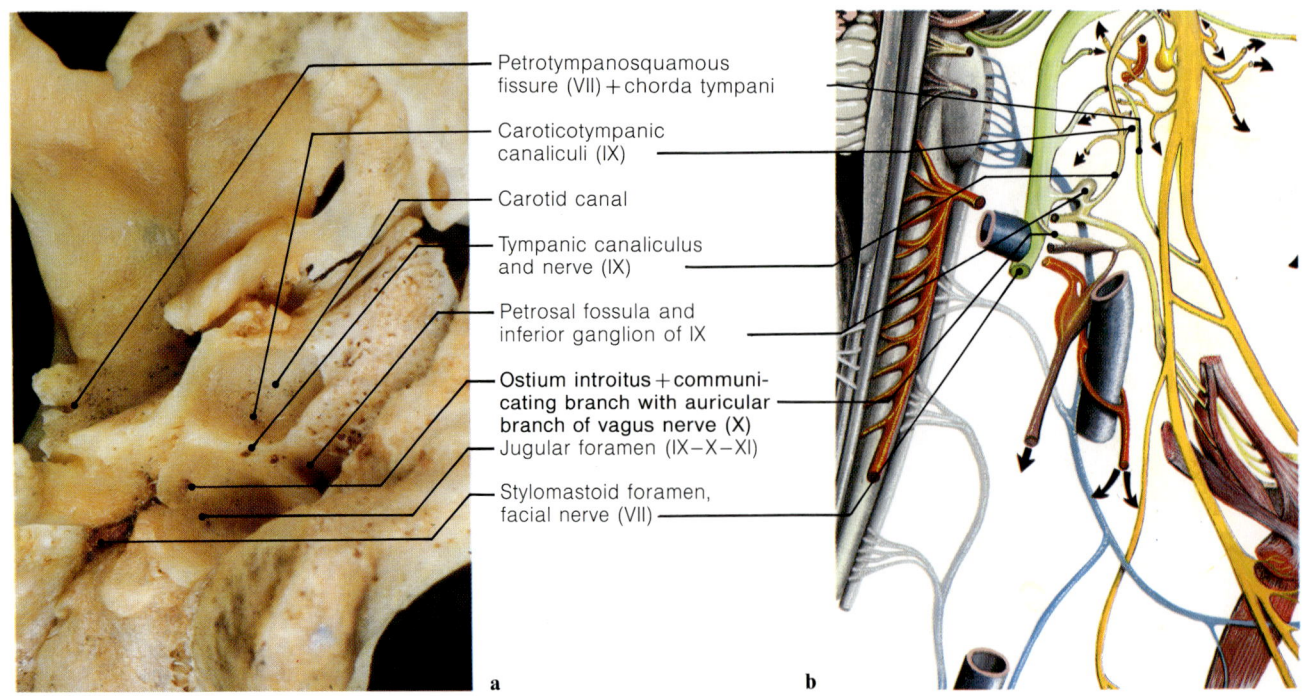

Sulci of auricular branch of vagus nerve (VII–X) and communicating branch with glossopharyngeal nerve (VII–IX)

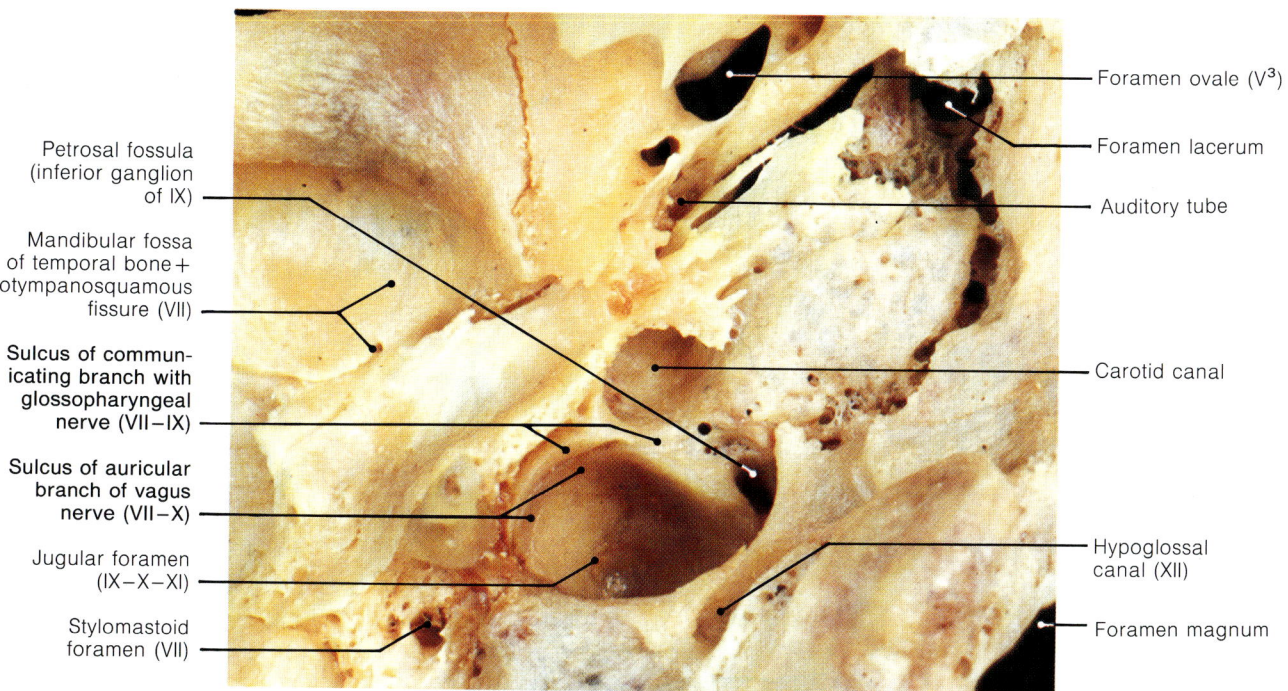

Fig. 7.43. Extracranial anatomic view of jugular foramen showing sulci of auricular branch of X and communicating branch of IX (Haller's ansa)

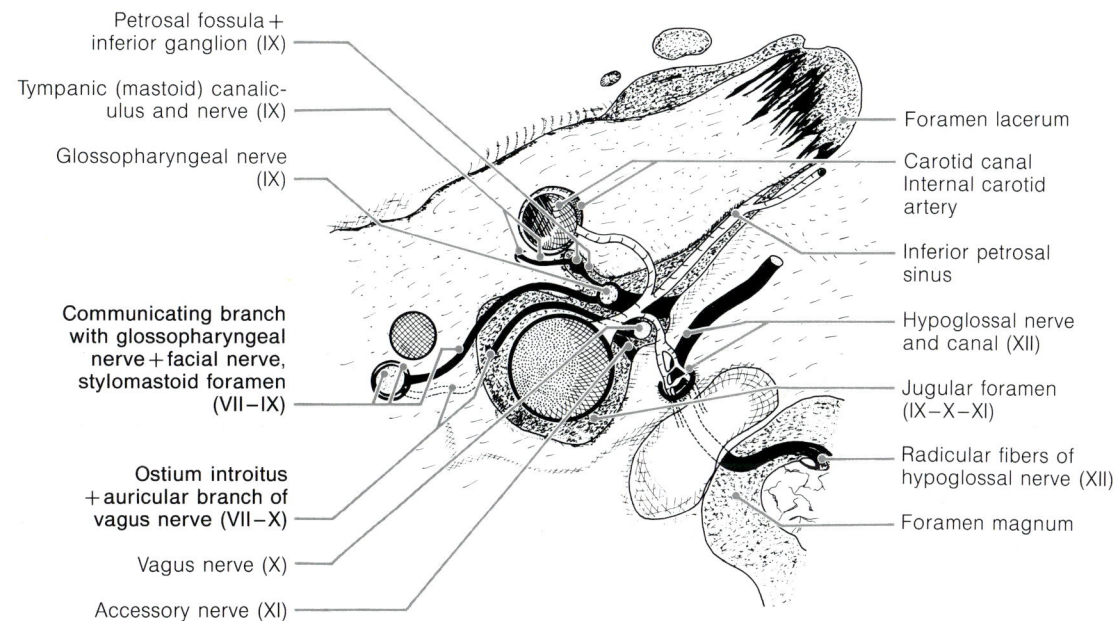

Fig. 7.44. Diagram of auricular branch (X) and communicating branch with glossopharyngeal nerve (IX), showing anastomotic relations of facial nerve with glossopharyngeal and vagus nerves (VII–IX–X)

206 Facial nerve (VII)

Stylomastoid foramen

Fig. 7.45 a–e. Sagittal (**a**) and axial (**b–d**) tomographic sections and diagram (**e**) of stylomastoid foramen

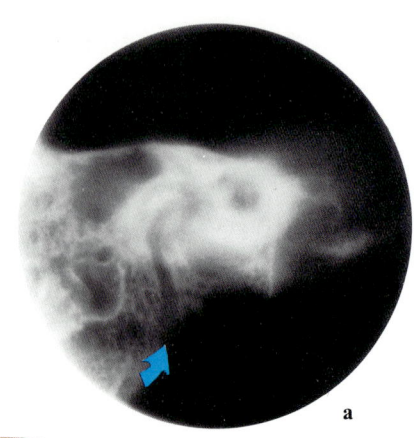

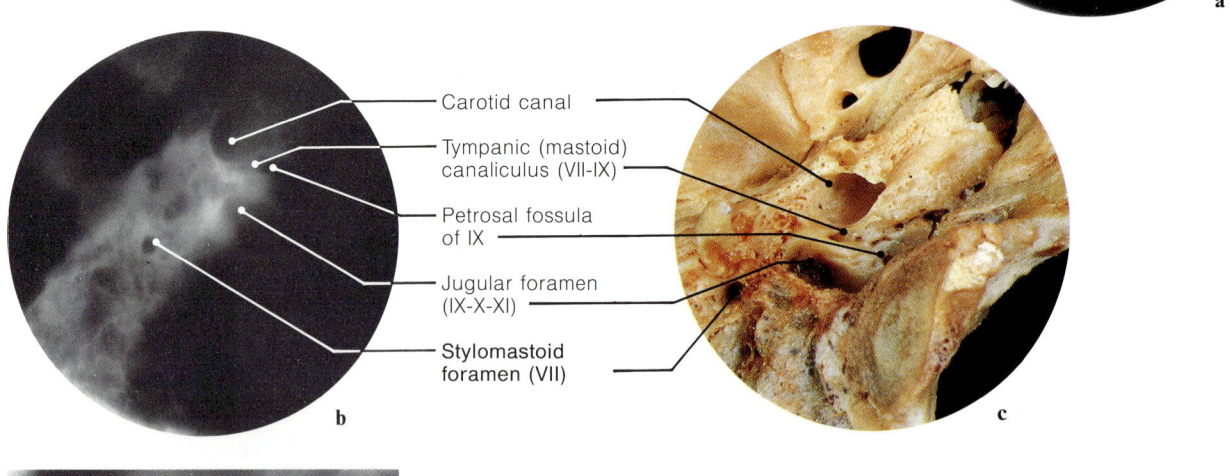

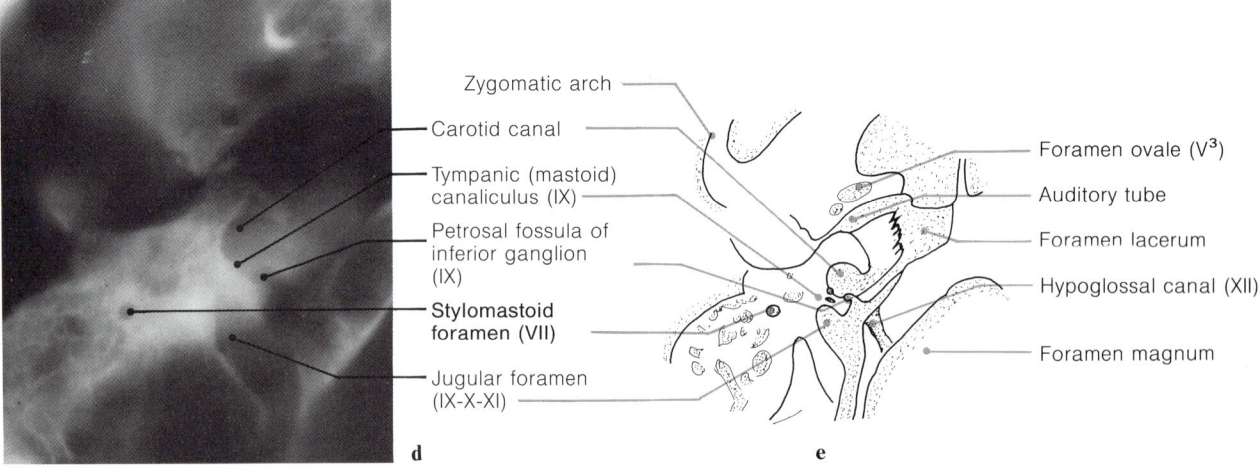

Fig. 7.46 a, b. Radiograph of stylomastoid foramina in Hirtz symmetric axial view

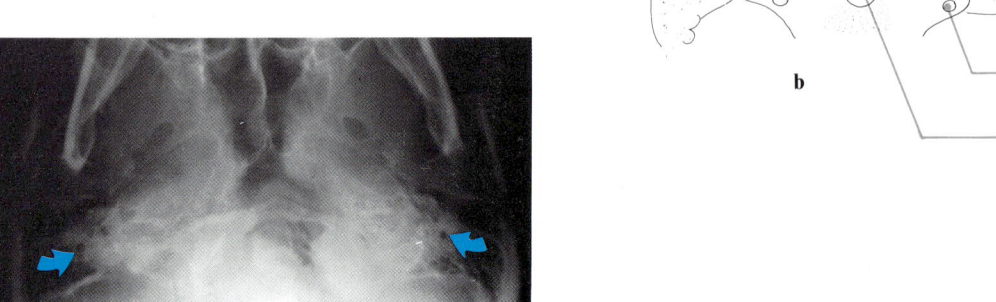

Stylomastoid foramen (See vascular relations, p. 286)

Imaging

TECHNIQUE

Radiographic and tomographic study of stylomastoid foramina in symmetric axial view:

- The subject is in dorsal decubitus, shoulders raised on cushions; the head facing strictly forward, resting on the vertex so that the orbitomeatal plane (OM) makes an angle of 10° with the horizontal, open towards the facial massif (Fig. 7.47);
- the centering point is situated four fingersbreadths behind the mental symphysis.

A standard radiograph is made, and four tomographic sections starting from 1 cm above the external acoustic meatus and descending; after having defined the best plane for the diseased or suspect zone, sections must be made every 2 mm starting from this plane.

Displayed: This tomographic examination shows successively:

- the stylomastoid foramen (VII),
- the facial canal (VII),
- the jugular foramen (IX–X–XI),
- the hypoglossal canal (XII),
- the petrotympanosquamous fissure,
- the auditory tube, aditus ad antrum, mastoid antrum, auditory ossicles,
- the petrosal fossula of the inferior ganglion (IX),
- the foramen ovale (V^3),
- the foramen lacerum,
- the hiatuses of the greater and lesser petrosal nerves (VII–IX),
- the sulci of the greater and lesser petrosal nerves up to the pterygoid canals and otic ganglion (VII–IX),
- the pterygopalatine fossa (V^2–VII–IX),
- the notch of the abducent nerve (VI) (petrous apex),
- the hypophyseal fossa,
- the sulcus of the oculomotor nerve (III) (dorsum sellae),
- the carotid canal,
- the trigeminal impression (V).

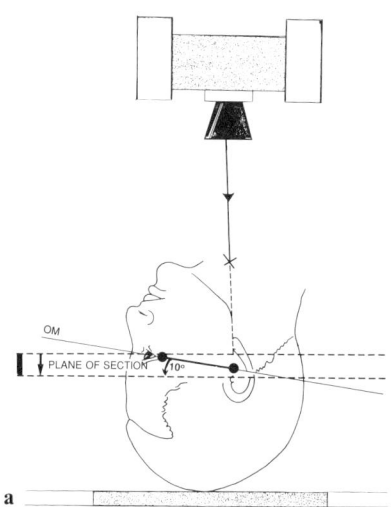

Fig. 7.47a. Centering diagram for symmetric radiographic and tomographic studies of stylomastoid foramina in axial view

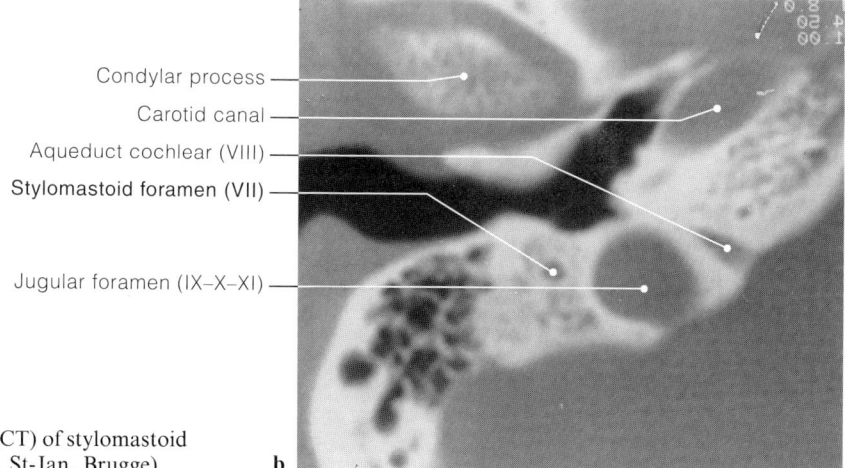

Fig. 7.47b. Axial view computed tomography (CT) of stylomastoid foramen (VII). (CT: Dr. J.W. Casselman, A.Z. St-Jan, Brugge)

Anatomic and physiologic review (motor and sensory components)

Motor component: the facial nerve (VII)
As previously indicated, the radicular fibers have a complex course within the pons. The facial nerve is initially intracranial and travels upwards, outwards and forwards. It then enters the internal acoustic meatus to follow an intrapetrous course within the facial canal. Here, it has three segments:

- labyrinthine,
- tympanic,
- mastoid.

It leaves the skull via the stylomastoid foramen, enters the parotid gland and gives off two terminal branches destined for the muscles of the face.

Sensory component: intermedius nerve (VII b)
Its true origin lies in the geniculate ganglion, which is applied to the intrapetrous genu of the facial nerve, between the tympanic and labyrinthine portions. The afferent fibers are formed by the dendrites of sensory cells; they derive either from the zone of Ramsay Hunt and the postauricular hairy scalp via the sensory branch of the external acoustic meatus and the posterior auricular branch (Fig. 7.7; 7.8; 7.34), or from the anterior two-thirds of the tongue (taste sensation) via the lingual nerve and then the chorda tympani (Fig. 7.2; 7.37 c; 7.45; 7.49). The efferent fibers make up the intermedius nerve, which, in contraflow, enters the pons via the medullopontine sulcus and terminates in the upper part of the salivary nucleus.

The autonomic component, part of the cranial parasympathetic, has its origin in two nuclei:

- the lacrimomuconasal nucleus, which gives origin to fibers that follow the motor root and traverse the geniculate ganglion and travel with the superficial greater petrosal nerve and the pterygoid nerve to terminate in the pterygopalatine ganglion (Fig. 7.24 g; 7.28 b; 7.29; 7.37 c) where the fibers arise that innervate the lacrimal gland (Fig. 7.48).
- the superior salivary nucleus, which gives origin to fibers that follow VII b as far as the geniculate ganglion, then the chorda tympani and the lingual nerve (Fig. 7.29; 7.37 c; 7.39 b) to reach the submandibular and sublingual ganglia, the origin of postganglionic fibers destined for the salivary glands (Fig. 7.49).

Thus the facial nerve has a threefold function:
1) a motor function, since it innervates the muscles of the face, the muscles of expression;
2) a sensory function: It transmits taste sensation from the anterior two-thirds of the tongue and superficial sensation from the cutaneous territory of Ramsay Hunt, which includes in part the tympanum, the auditory meatus, the tragus, antitragus, fossa of the antihelix, walls of the external acoustic meatus and the concha;
3) an autonomic function, through innervation of the lacrimal and salivary glands.

Salivary (V^3–VII–IX) and lacrimomuconasal (V^2–VII–IX) secretory pathways

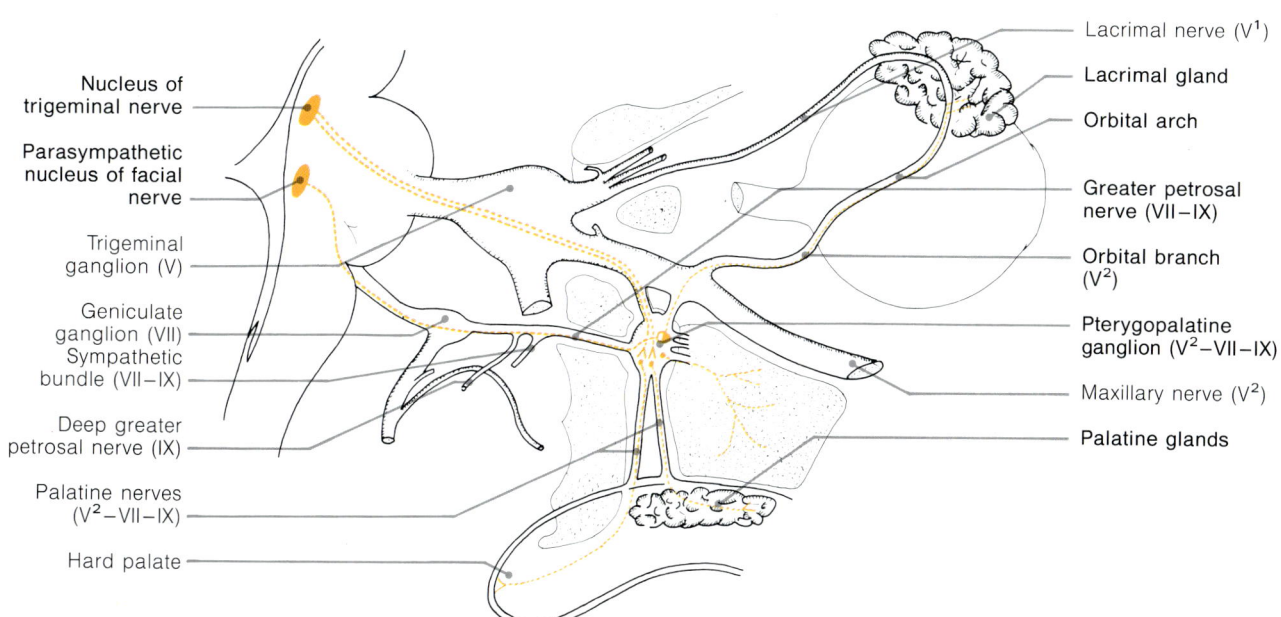

Fig. 7.48. Lacrimomuconasal secretory pathways (V^2–VII–IX)

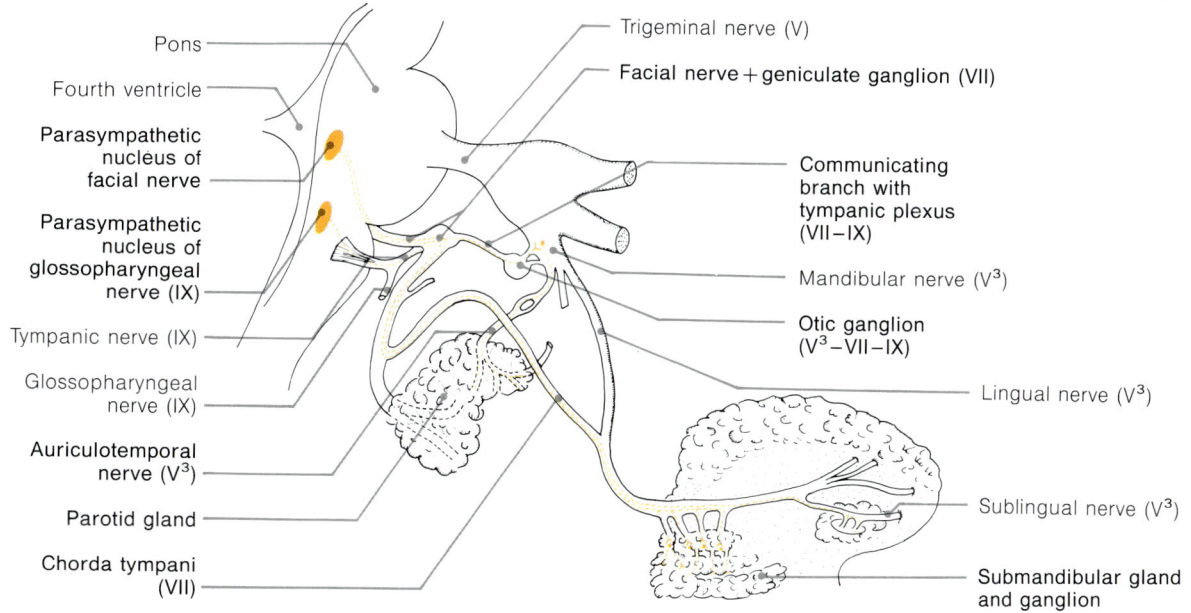

Fig. 7.49. Salivary secretory pathways (V^3–VII–IX)

Carotid sympathetic plexus (anastomotic branches)

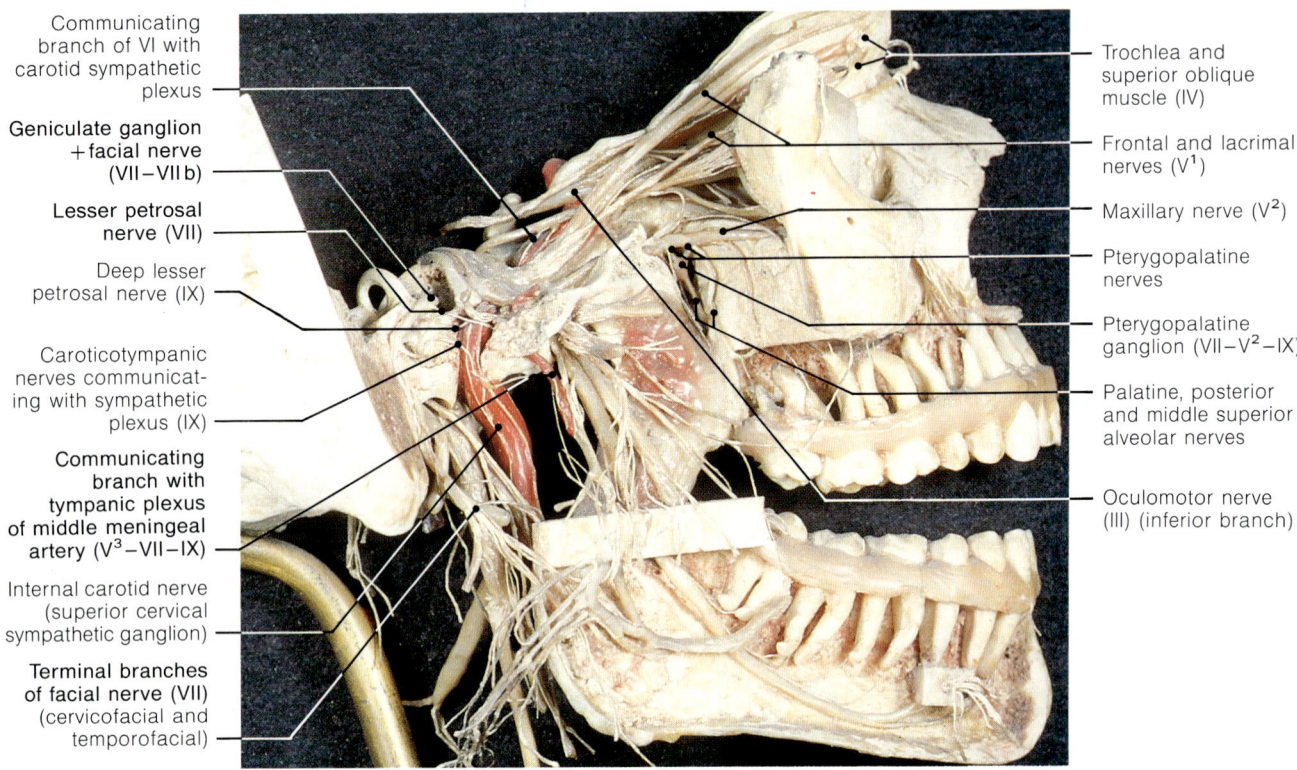

Fig. 7.50. Dissection of facial, trigeminal and oculomotor nerves (VII–V–III–IV–VI), sagittal view

Fig. 7.51. Right superolateral view

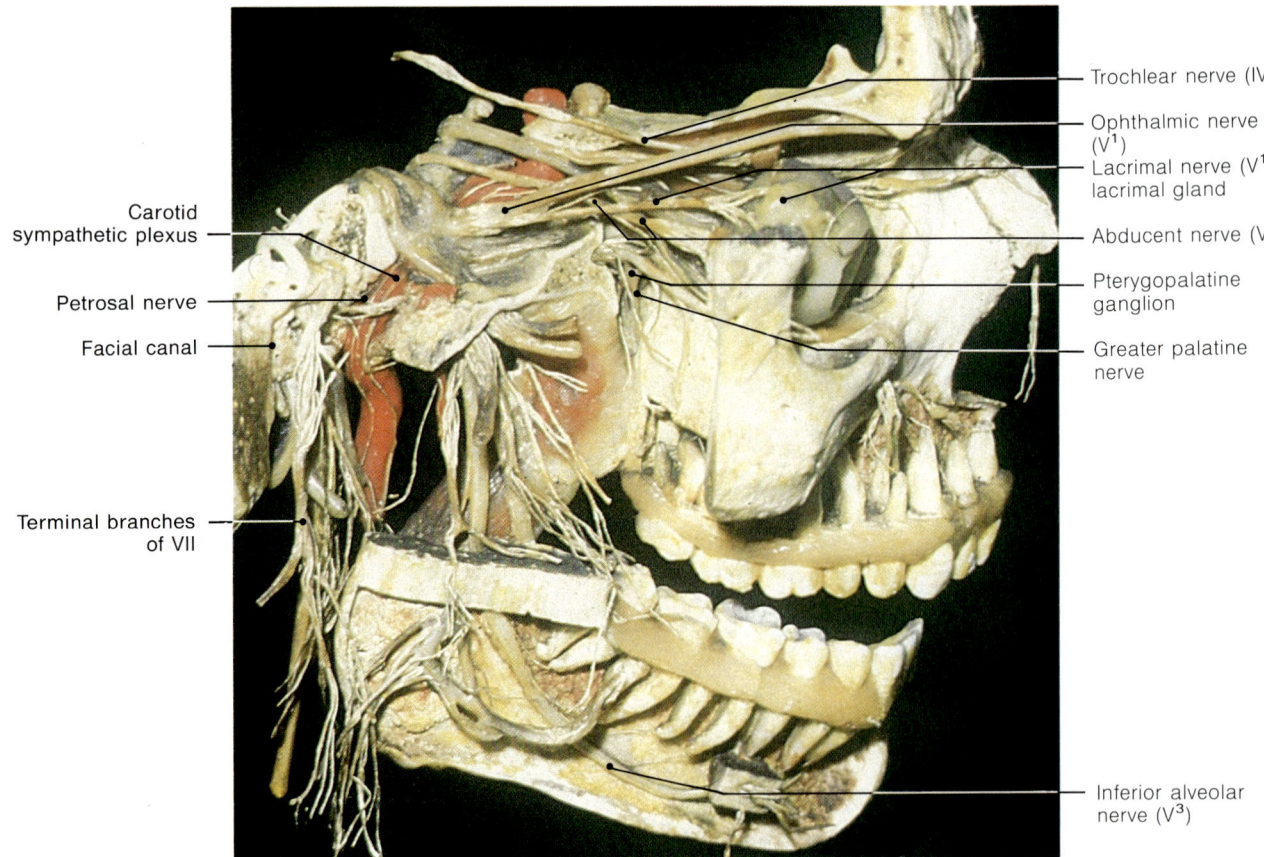

Vestibulocochlear nerve (VIII)

Anatomy (course–terminals–collaterals) 213
Imaging (regions examined) 213
Pathology 213
Apparent origin of vestibulocochlear nerve,
medullopontine sulcus, cerebellopontine angle
    Anatomy and imaging (examination) 215
    Axial views (MRI, CT) 215
Internal acoustic meatus, cavity of the internal ear
    Anatomy and imaging (examination) 216
    Anatomic, MRI and tomographic sections 216
Internal ear
    Tomographic and anatomic sections 218
Middle ear (cavity, auditory ossicles, auditory tube)
    Anatomy and imaging (examination) 219
    Varied views (radiology, CT) 221
    Frontal, oblique and axial views (CT) 224
Cavities of the external ear (external acoustic meatus)
    Anatomy and imaging (examination) 225
Vestibulocochlear nerve and pathways
    Frontal, axial, and oblique views (MRI) 226

Vascular relations:
Labyrinthine artery,
inferior anterior cerebellar artery 212, 215, 226

The vestibulocochlear nerve is a sensory nerve. It consists of two parts: the cochlear nerve and the vestibular nerve. The nerve enters the pons at the lateral extremity of the medullopontine sulcus, lateral to the facial nerve and a little above and in front of the glossopharyngeal nerve.

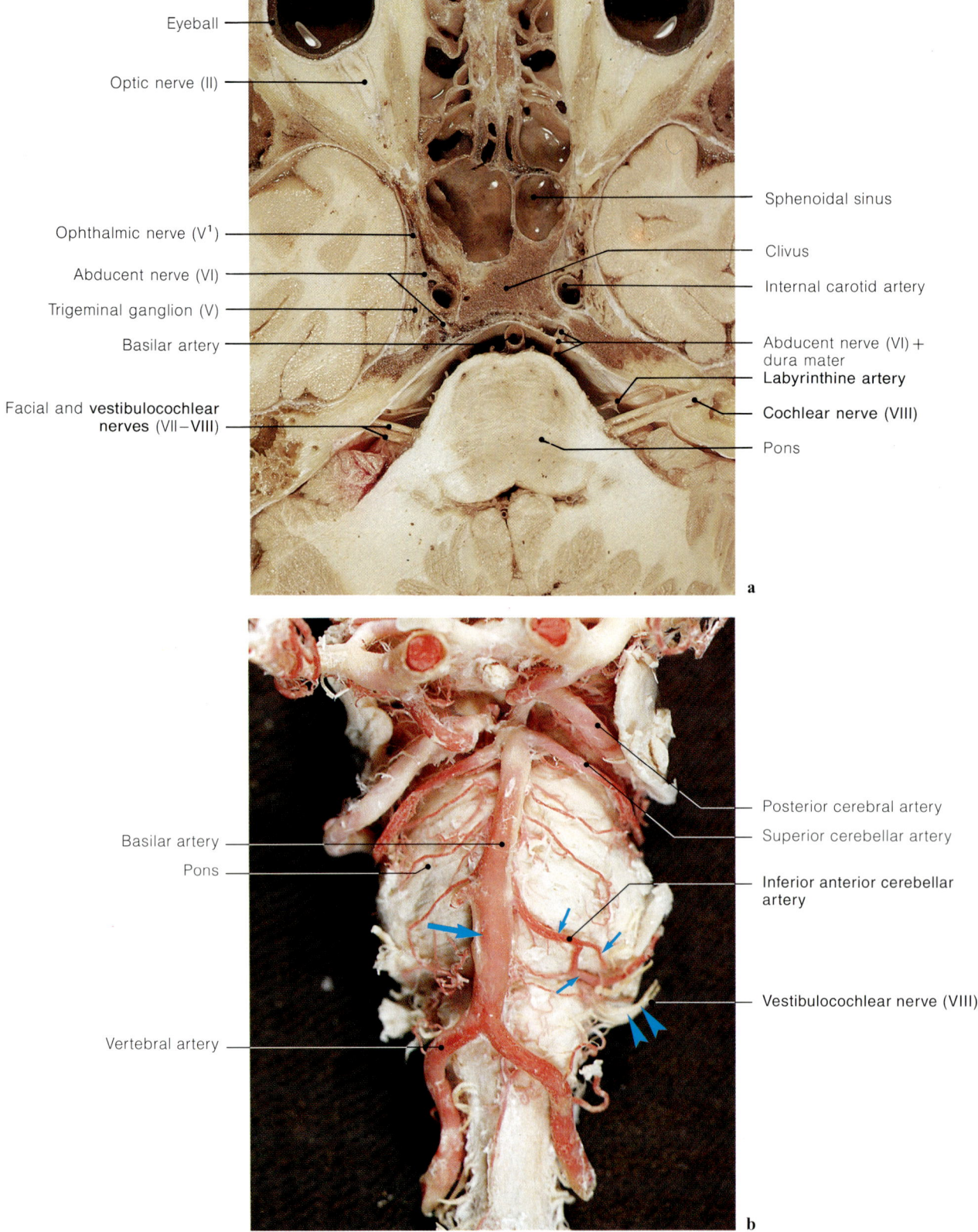

Fig. 8.1a–f. Axial section of brainstem at level of the vestibulocochlear nerve (VIII) and labyrinthine artery in the internal acoustic meatus (**a**), dissection of brainstem to show inferior anterior cerebellar artery (**b**), axial anatomic section (**c**), axial magnetic resonance imaging (MRI) view (**d**) and diagrams (**e, f**) showing vascular relations of vestibular, facial and intermedius nerves (VIII–VII–VIIb). (Anatomic dissection: Pr. J.P. Francke, Faculty of Medicine, Lille; diagrams: Pr. Y. Guerrier, *Anatomie chirurgicale de l'os temporal de l'oreille et de la base du crâne*, Vol. 1. La Simarre, 1988)

Facial nerve (VII)

Anatomy

COURSE – TERMINALS – COLLATERALS

Apparent origin and intracranial course

Intracanalicular course, compartment of vestibular ganglion (fundus of internal acoustic meatus)

Ganglion of cochlear nerve (spiral ganglion)

Auditory ossicles

Middle ear – Auditory tube

Imaging

REGIONS EXAMINED

Medullopontine sulcus
Study of cerebellopontine angle

Examination of internal acoustic meatus and semicircular canals

Study of internal ear showing cochlea

Imaging of incudostapedial and incudomallear joints (auditory ossicles)

Study of mastoid antrum, aditus ad antrum, bony and pharyngeal orifices of auditory tube, pharyngeal recess

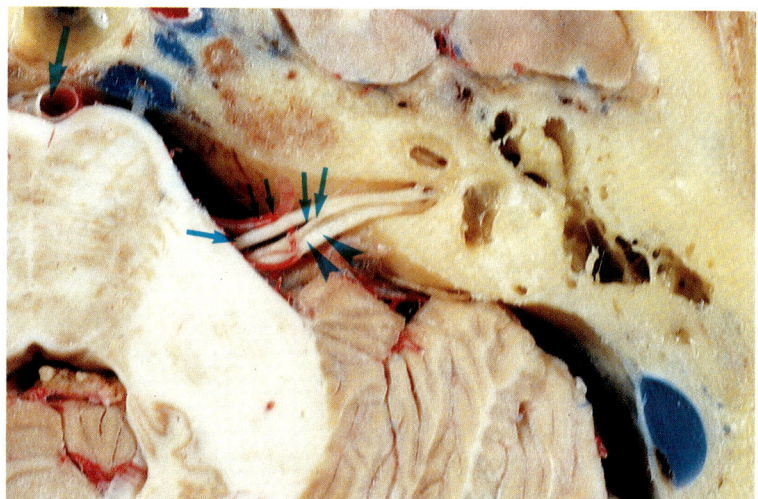
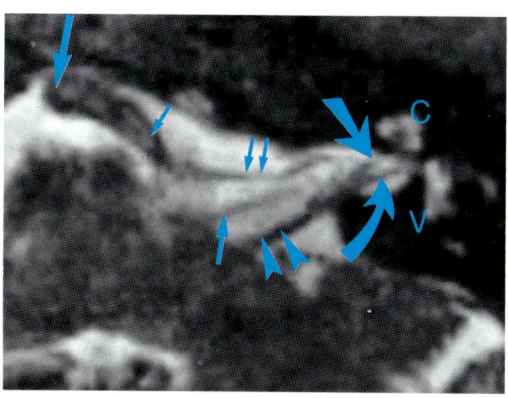
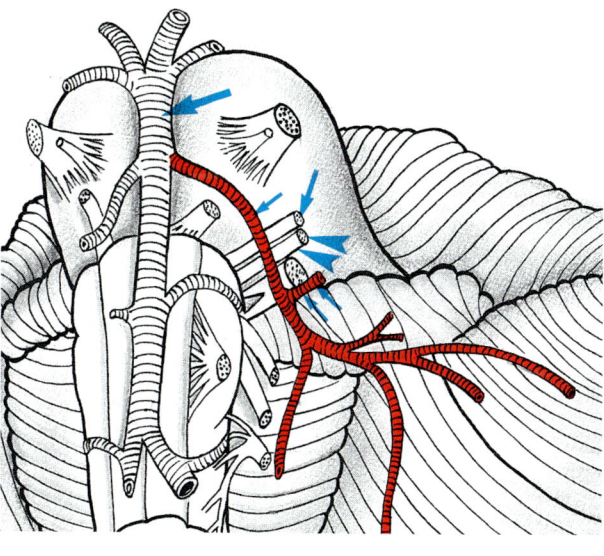
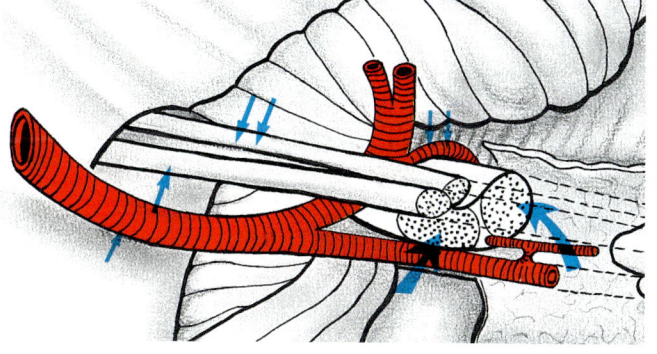

Basilar artery (*large, straight arrow*)
labyrinthine artery (*small, double arrows*)
inferior anterior cerebellar artery (*small arrow*)
facial nerve (VII) (*medium, straight arrow*)
nervus intermedius (VIIb) (*double, medium arrows*)
vestibulocochlear nerve (VIII) (*double arrowheads*)
inferior vestibular nerve (VIII) (*curved arrow*)
cochlear nerve (VIII) (*large arrow*)
cochlea (*c*); vestibule (*v*)

Vestibulocochlear nerve (VIII)

Topography

Apparent origin of vestibulocochlear nerve (VIII)
- Medullopontine sulcus
- Cerebellopontine angle

Vestibular nerve, vestibular ganglion
- Internal acoustic meatus
- Cavities of internal ear

Cochlear nerve, spiral ganglion
- Cochlea

Internal ear

Middle ear
- Tympanic cavity
- Chain of ossicles
- Auditory tube
- Cavum

External ear
- External acoustic meatus

Pathology

Apparent origin:
- Syndrome of inferior protuberance (Foville's syndrome),
- neurinoma of cerebellopontine angle.

Internal ear:
- Ménière's disease,
- syndrome of internal acoustic meatus,
- intracanalicular acousticofacial neurinoma,
- otosclerosis of base of stapes, stage 4 or 5, extending towards ossicles.

Middle ear:
- Fracture of wall of attic obstructing aditus ad antrum,
- fractures and dislocations of chain of ossicles, incudomallear and incudostapedial luxations,
- antro-attical cholesteatoma destroying chain of ossicles,
- tumor of cavum obstructing auditory tube,
- tympanojugular tumor.

External ear:
- Temporal fracture,
- tympanosclerosis demineralizing the walls of the external acoustic meatus.

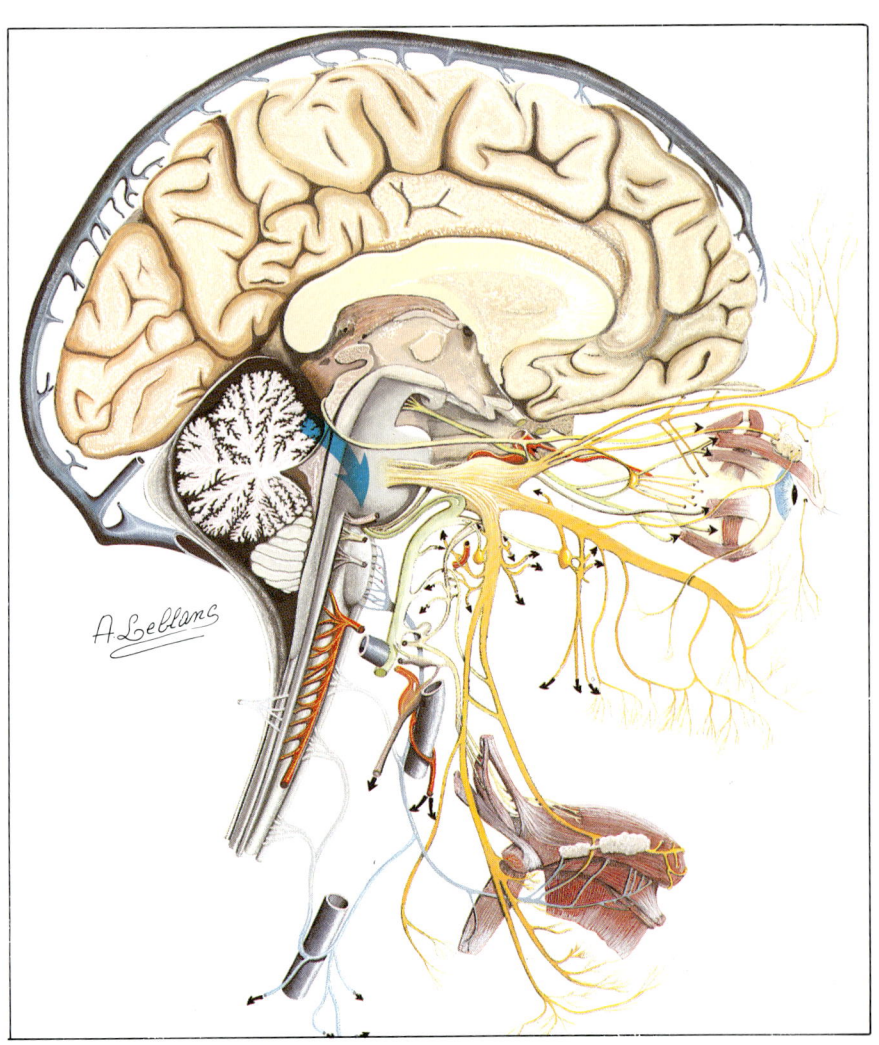

Fig. 8.2

Apparent origin of vestibulocochlear nerve, medullopontine sulcus, cerebellopontine angle

Anatomy

The **vestibulocochlear nerve** is a sensory nerve and consists of two parts: the cochlear nerve (auditory nerve) and the vestibular nerve (nerve of equilibration).

The **cochlear nerve** joins with the vestibular nerve, traverses the internal acoustic meatus, becomes intracranial and then enters the neuraxis via the lateral part of the medullopontine sulcus. It terminates in the cochlear nuclei at the lower part of the pons: the anterior nucleus and the dorsal nucleus.

The **vestibular nerve** gathers the auditory impressions in the internal ear and then transmits these centrally.

Imaging

CLINIQUE: Paralysis of lateral ocular movements, paralysis of the abducent nerve (VI) and peripheral paralysis on the side of the lesion and hemiplegia involving the face on the side opposite to the lesion, vertigo, diminished hearing acuity, headache, nystagmus (horizontal-rotary).

POSSIBLE CAUSES: Inferior protuberantial syndrome (Foville's syndrome), acousticofacial neurinoma (VII–VIIb–VIII) at the level of the cerebellopontine angle, lesions of the pons and the medulla oblongata.

EXAMINATION: Study by magnetic resonance imaging (MRI) or computed tomography (CT) of the cerebellopontine angle of the medullopontine sulcus, so as to visualize the apparent origin of the vestibulocochlear nerve (VIII) in sagittal and axial views and the Worms-Bretton semiaxial view.

The sections in the Worms-Bretton view are made starting from the level of the sella turcica up to below the external acoustic meatus. The technique of examination is identical to that used for the apparent origin of the facial nerve (VII).

Note: In order to eliminate any possibility of an intracanalicular lesion (ballooning of the internal acoustic meatus), it is necessary to make a comparative study of the internal acoustic meatuses using the intraorbital survey view before embarking on this study.

Cerebellopontine angle

Magnetic resonance imaging (MRI) and CT

AXIAL VIEWS

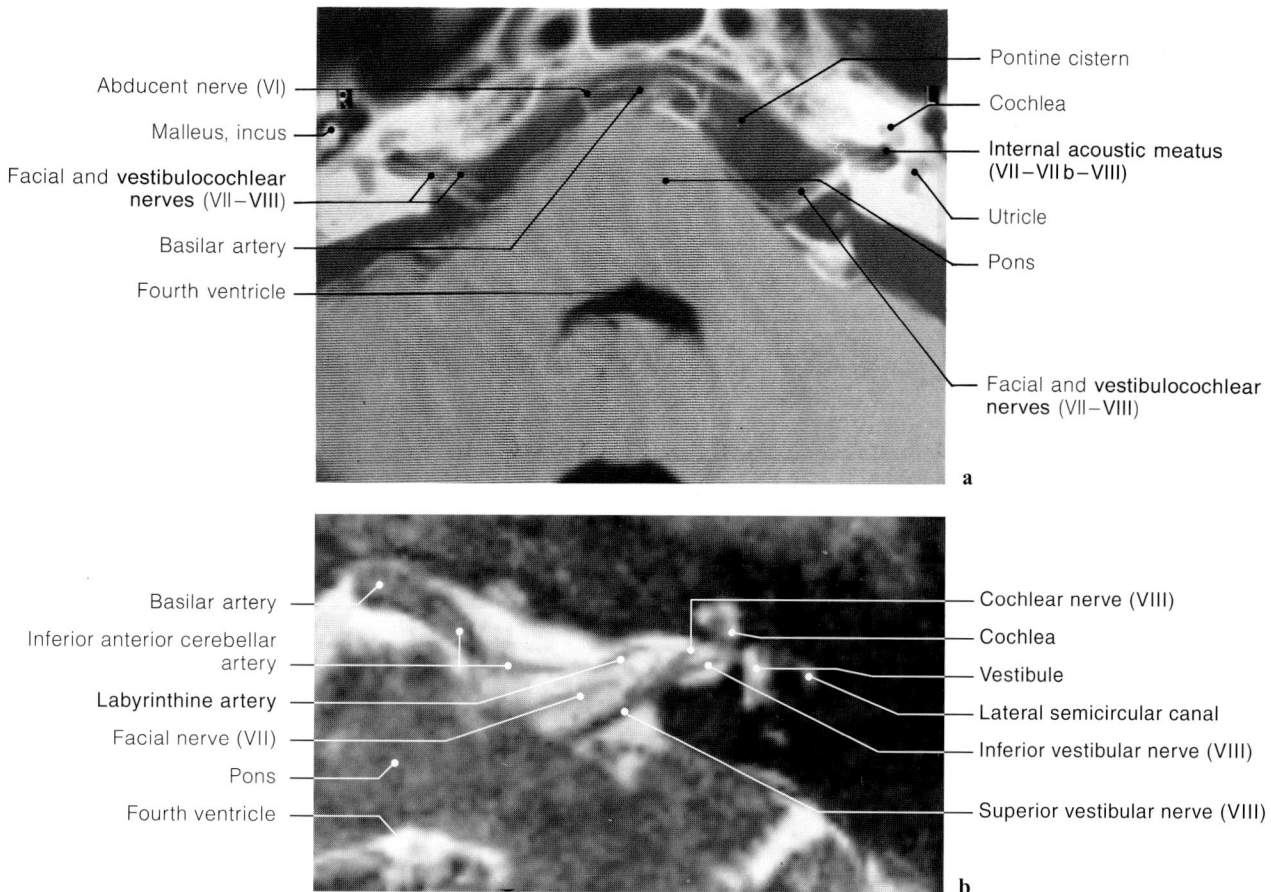

Fig. 8.3 a, b. Axial views computed tomography (CT; **a**) and magnetic resonance imaging (MRI; **b**) of vestibulocochlear nerves (VIII)

Internal acoustic meatus, cavities of the internal ear

Anatomy

COURSE – RELATIONS

The *cochlear ganglion* occupies the extent of the spiral cochlear canal.

The ramifications of origin of the vestibulocochlear nerve join the cochlear ganglion via the canaliculi of the secondary spiral lamina (Fig. 8.4f–h).

The axons of the cells of the cochlear ganglion constitute the fibers of the cochlear nerve. This nerve reaches the pons in the lateral part of the medullopontine sulcus. It ends in the ventral and dorsal cochlear nuclei.

The *ganglion of the vestibular nerve* is situated in the fundus of the internal acoustic meatus (Fig. 8.4f–h). The axonal prolongations of its cells conduct sensations arising in the saccule, utricle and the ampullae of the semicircular canals. These axons form the fibers of the vestibular nerve, which enters the pons at the same site as the cochlear nerve and medial to it. It terminates in the nuclei of the vestibular region of the floor of the fourth ventricle.

Imaging

CLINICAL FEATURES

- Ménière's disease,
- diminished hearing acuity, tinnitus, headache, vertigo with falling away from the side of the lesion.

POSSIBLE CAUSES

- Acoustic neurinoma,
- extensive cholesteatoma of the antro-adito-attical region expanding inwards and capable of damaging either the vestibule or the cochlear region,
- otosclerosis of the base of stapes, stage 5, penetrating the vestibule and the first turn of the cochlear spiral,
- fracture of the bony labyrinth, especially of the internal acoustic meatus,
- spreading fracture with disjunction of the lambdoid suture.

EXAMINATION

- Radiologic and computed tomographic (CT) studies of the internal acoustic meatuses in symmetric, intraorbital, frontal survey view,
- radiographic or CT study of the internal acoustic meatus in the long axis of the petrous bone in unilateral Chaussé IV view (Fig. 7.10),
- study of the internal acoustic meatus in Pöschl-Meyer view,
- radiography in Stenvers view,
- study in 40° opposed transorbital view of François and Barrois,
- tomographic study in prestudied inclined sagittal view of Cornélis.

These views display the internal acoustic meatus, its transverse (or falciform) crest, the cochlea, vestibule, semicircular canals, chain of ossicles and the antro-adito-attical region (Fig. 8.4a, c, e; 8.5c, d; 8.6a; 8.9a, b).

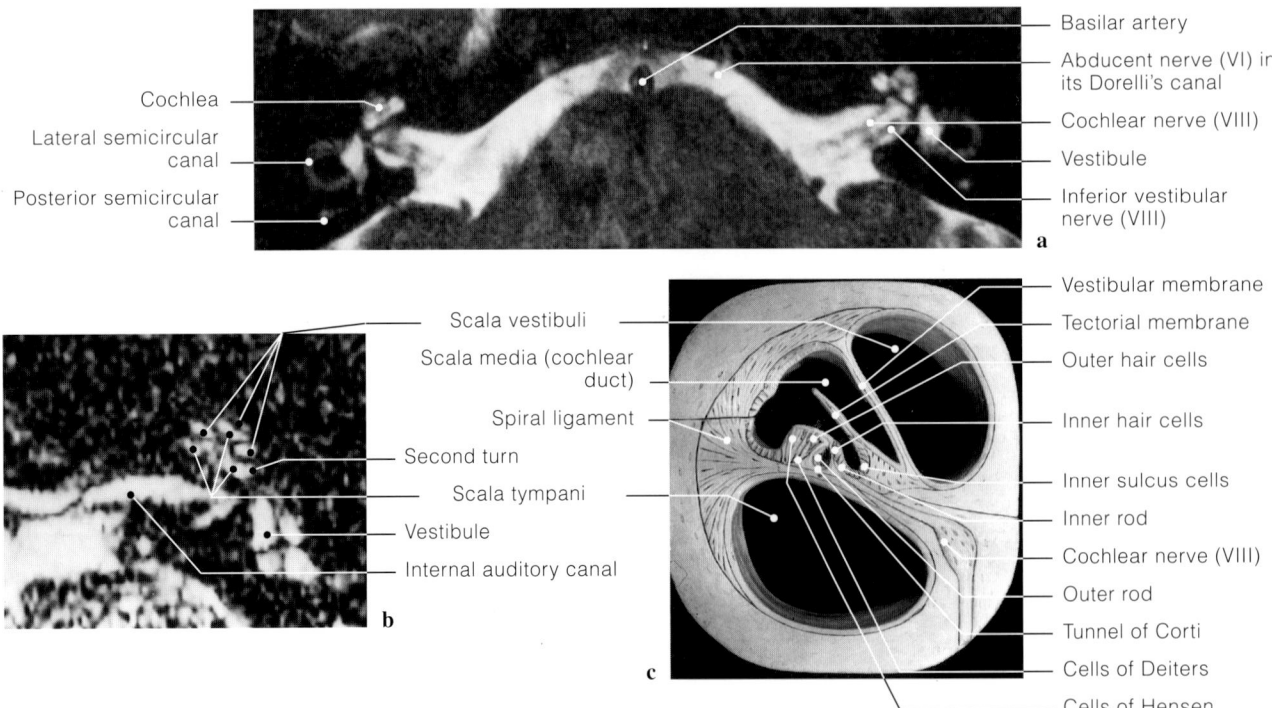

Fig. 8.4a–j. Magnetic resonance imaging (MRI) view and section through the cochlea showing the detail of spiral organ of Corti (**a–c**); diagrams, tomography, MRI, computed tomography (CT) and anatomic sections showing the vestibulocochlear nerve and the cavities of the internal ear (**d–j**). (MRI: Dr. J.W. Casselman, A.Z. St-Jan, Brugge)

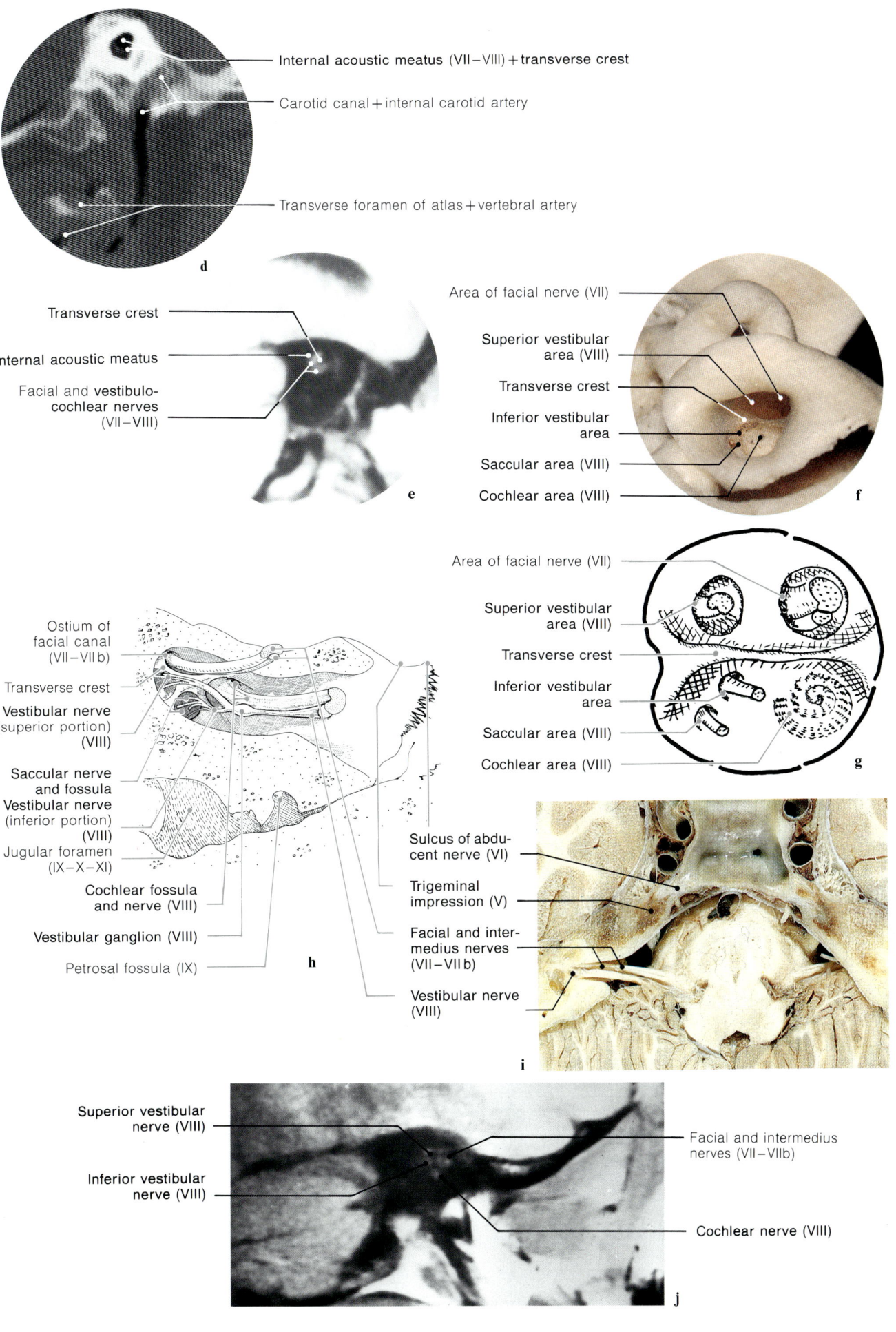

Internal ear

Anatomy

The internal ear comprises the *bony labyrinth* and the *membranous labyrinth*.
The vestibular and acoustic nerve pathways arise from the membranous labyrinth.

The bony labyrinth consists of three parts:

– middle, the vestibule,
– posterior, the semicircular canals,
– anterior, the cochlea.

The internal acoustic meatus also forms part of the bony labyrinth (Fig. 8.4f; 8.5b).

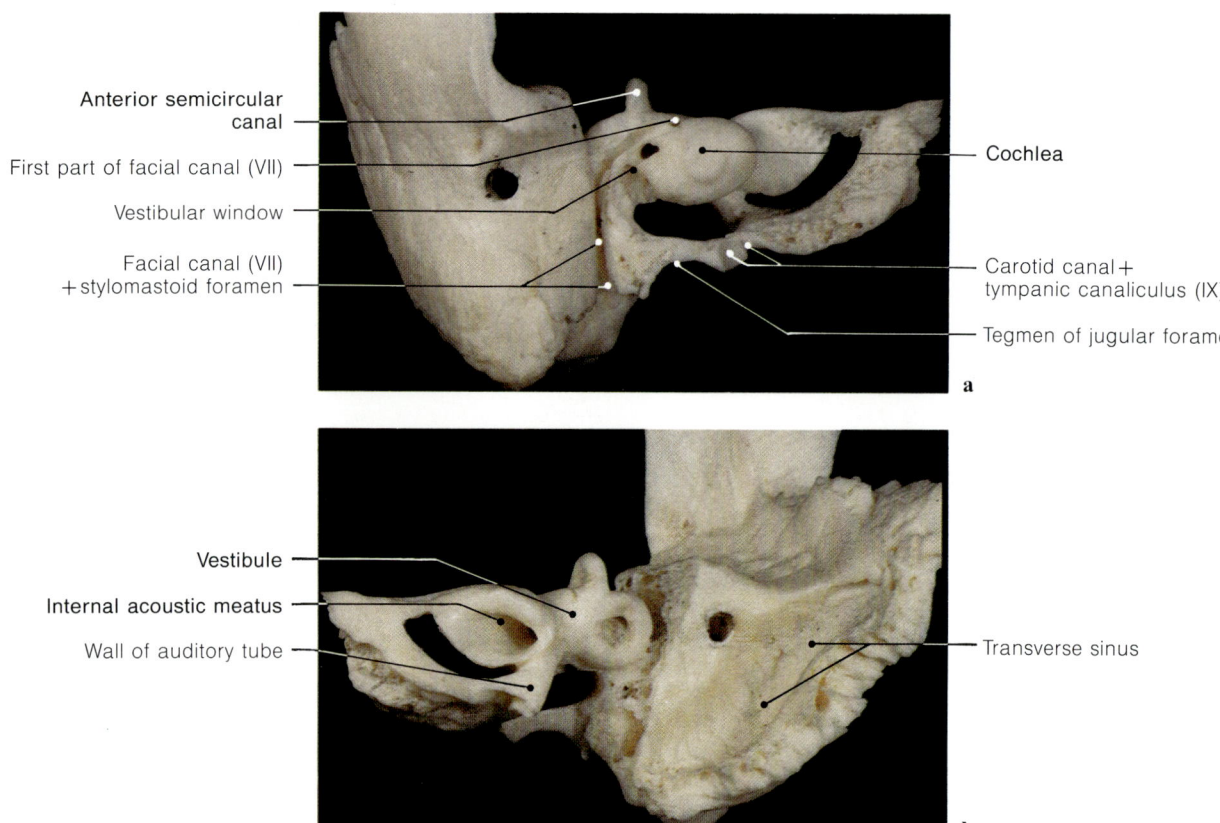

Fig. 8.5 a, b. Anterior (a) and posterior (b) views of bony labyrinth

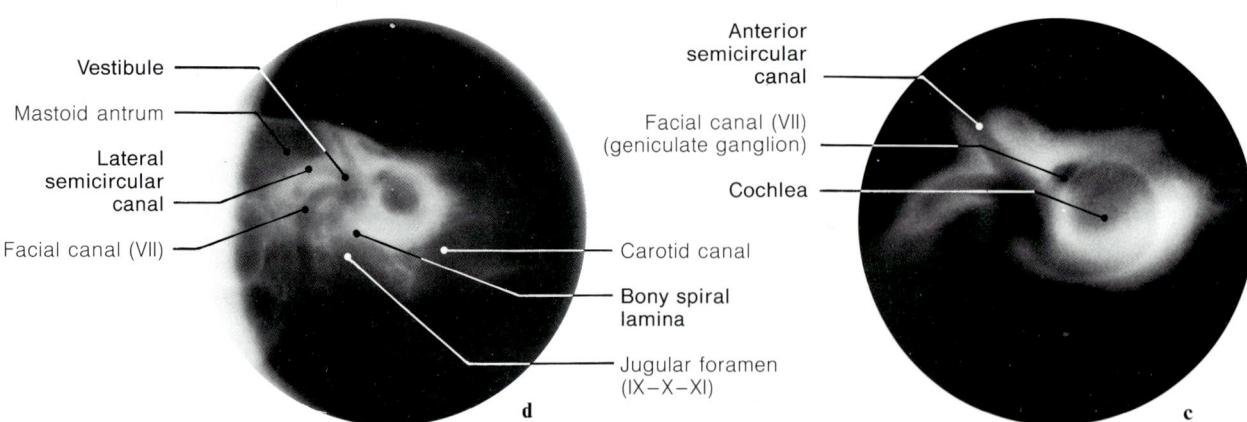

Fig. 8.5 c, d. Tomograms of semicircular canals, vestibule and facial canal (anatomic specimen)

Middle ear (organ of transmission)

Anatomy

The **middle ear** is a long cavity containing air and formed of three parts:

- the tympanic compartment,
- the auditory tube,
- the mastoid cavities.

The tympanic compartment, hollowed out in the temporal bone, is separated from the external ear by the tympanic membrane and from the internal ear by

- the vestibular window above, corresponding to the vestibule,
- the cochlear window below, corresponding to the scala tympani of the cochlea.

The middle ear communicates with the rhinopharynx via the auditory tube. It is occupied by the chain of auditory ossicles – the malleus, incus and stapes – which connect the tympanum with the vestibular window (Fig. 8.6a, b).
The **malleus** has a head, a neck, a handle and two processes, one anterior and one lateral (Fig. 8.8a, b). The head of the malleus is joined to the body of the incus at the incudomallear articulation.

The **incus** is situated behind the malleus and has a body and two limbs, long and short. It is situated in the attic and its body is flattened lateromedially, its articular surface is adapted to the articular surface of the head of the malleus.
The *short (upper or horizontal) limb* is squat, thick and of a flattened cone shape; its posterior end rests against the notch situated at the antero-inferior angle of the ostium of the *aditus ad antrum*.
The *long (lower) limb* is more slender and longer than the former and initially descends almost vertically behind and medial to the handle of the malleus. Its lower end bends inwards to terminate in a rounded tubercle: the *lenticular process* which articulates with the stapes.
The **stapes** is situated medial to the incus and extends almost horizontally from the lenticular process to the vestibular (oval) window.
It has a head, a platelike base and two limbs. Laterally, the head is hollowed by a glenoid cavity which articulates with the lenticular process of the incus (Fig. 8.8a, b). The stapes is an oval membrane connected with the vestibular window (Fig. 8.6a, b; 8.10e).
The limbs of the stapes are two: anterior and posterior.
Connexions of the ossicles: The ossicles are interconnected by two articulations: the incudomallear and incudostapedial joints.
The **motor muscles of the ossicles** are two in number: the stapedius and the tensor tympani (Fig. 8.6b).

Fig. 8.6a, b. Computed tomography (CT) of the antro-adito-attical passage and of the incus and base of the stapes; diagram of the middle ear with the incudomallear and incudostapedial articulations

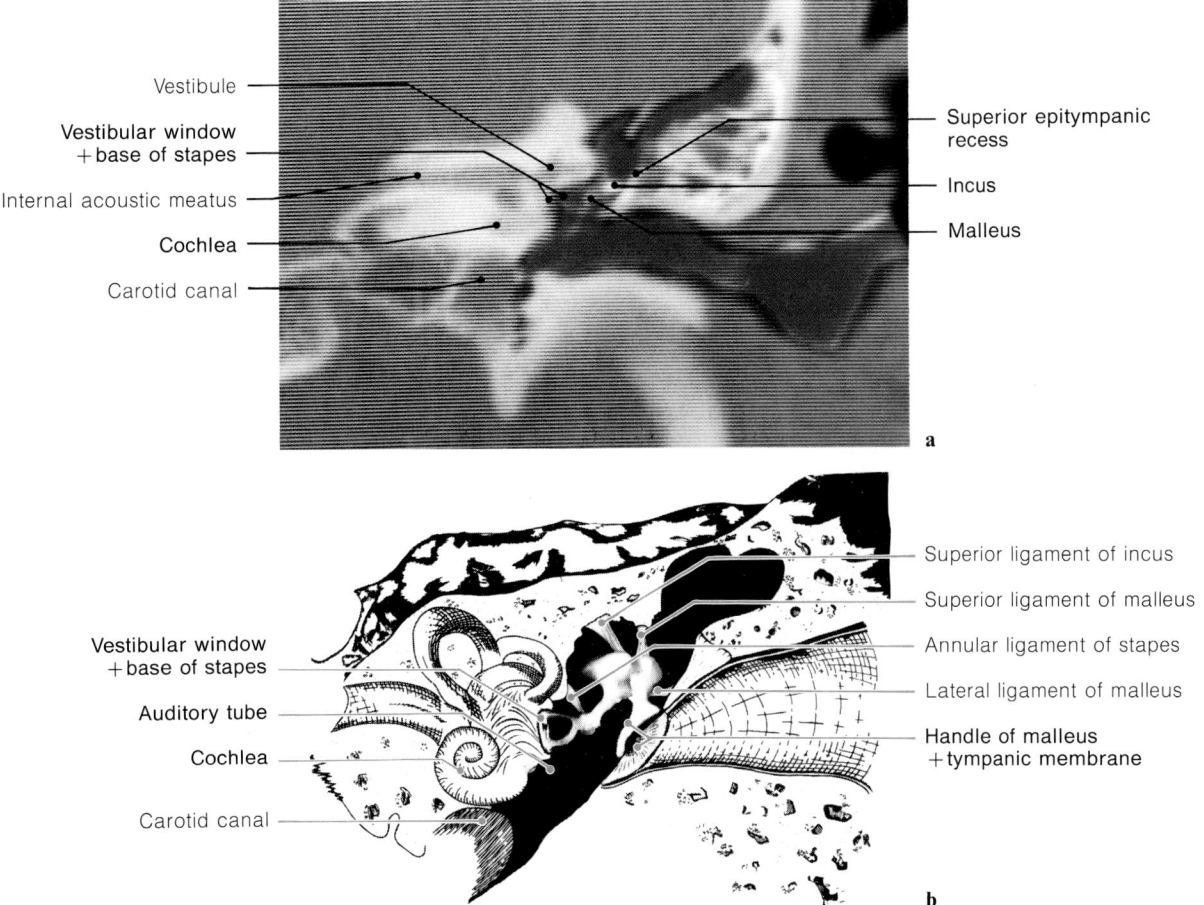

The *stapedius muscle* occupies a bony canal hollowed in the thickness of the posterior wall of the tympanic box. This stapedial canal is situated in front of the upper part of the facial canal. The muscle is inserted at the posterior side of the head of the stapes (Fig. 8.6 b).

The *tensor tympani muscle* is contained within the bony canal situated at the upper wall of the bony orifice of the auditory tube (Fig. 7.6; 7.7; 7.33); it is inserted at the upper end of the handle of the malleus.

Imaging

Clinical variants

Whatever the clinical types of affection of the petrous bone, before carrying out special views it is essential to examine the petrous bone by the classic survey views:

- frontal, with projection of the petrous bones into the orbits,
- sagittal (comparative) view,
- Stenvers-Schüller view,
- Worms-Bretton view,
- Meyer view,
- Hirtz view (Fig. 7.27).

These radiographs must be made symmetrically or comparably, save when investigating for fractures. After assessment of the abnormal or suspect zones in these films and of the clinical picture, special and more appropriate views may be used.

These views will depend on the clinical picture:

1) Otosclerosis of the base of the stapes or tympanosclerosis of the external ear:
Radiographic, tomographic and computed tomographic (CT) studies:

- in Guillen transorbital view,
- in Pöschl-Meyer view,
- in symmetric transorbital frontal view.

These display the antro-adito-attical passage, the whole of the auditory ossicles and the space between the base of the stapes and the vestibular (oval) window (Fig. 7.35 b).

2) Antral or antro-adito-attical cholesteatoma:
Radiographic and computed tomographic (CT) study of the middle ear, the auditory tube from the aditus ad antrum up to the antrum with the tegmen tympani and the tegmen of the external acoustic meatus to display any possible destruction:

- in Stenvers view,
- in Chaussé III view,
- in Guillen view,
- in Pöschl-Meyer view,
- in the 40° opposed transorbital view of François and Barrois.

These views are also advisable to complete examination of the superior bulb of the jugular vein when there is a fracture or a tumor of the glomus jugulare that may have affected or destroyed the roof of the jugular foramen.

3) Intracanalicular acoustic neurinoma or fracture of internal ear:
Tomographic study of internal acoustic meatus:

- in Chaussé IV (50° to 60°) view,
- in Stenvers view,
- in Guillen view,
- in Hirtz view,
- in symmetric frontal view (petrous bones projected in orbits),
- in the prestudied inclined sagittal view of Cornélis and Vignaud.

4) Fracture or dislocation of the ossicles or posttraumatic incudomallear or incudostapedial luxation, or ossicular destruction (antro-adito-attical cholesteatoma):
Radiographic study with tomographic and computed tomographic (CT) sections of ossicles:

- in Pöschl-Meyer view,
- in symmetric frontal view with projection of petrous bones into orbits,
- in Guillen comparative view,
- in the prestudied inclined sagittal view of Cornélis and Vignaud (Fig. 8.7a, b).

Technique

Tomographic study of the auditory ossicles and middle ear in prestudied inclined sagittal view:

- The subject is in lateral decubitus, with the head in profile resting on the temporoparietal region and making an angle of 30° to 40° in relation to the median sagittal plane (Fig. 8.7);
- the centering point is situated at the level of the external acoustic meatus to be examined, which is the furthest from the table (Fig. 8.7);
- a tomographic series is to be made starting from the mastoid process, every 5 mm up to the petrous apex; after having identified the best planes for the ossicles several sections are made at 1 mm intervals.

Displayed: This prestudied view allows display of the chain of ossicles along its longest axis and of all its bony components (Fig. 8.8 a, b) as well as the stapes and its base opposite the vestibular (oval) window and the lenticular process of the incus. It makes it possible to study: the carotid canal, the jugular foramen, the ostium introitus, the semicircular canals, the vestibule and cochlea, the facial canal and the sulcus of the chorda tympani, the geniculate ganglion, the hiatuses of the greater and lesser petrosal nerves, the antrum, aditus and external acoustic meatus.

Middle ear, auditory ossicles

Tomography and computed tomography (CT)

INCLINED AND VARIED SAGITTAL VIEWS OF GUILLEN AND STENVERS

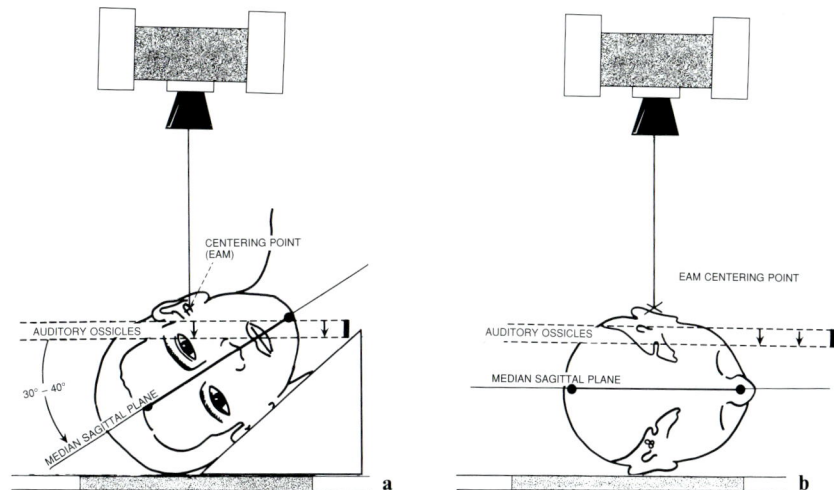

Fig. 8.7a, b. Centering diagrams for tomographic study of ossicles in prestudied inclined sagittal view of Cornélis and Vignaud

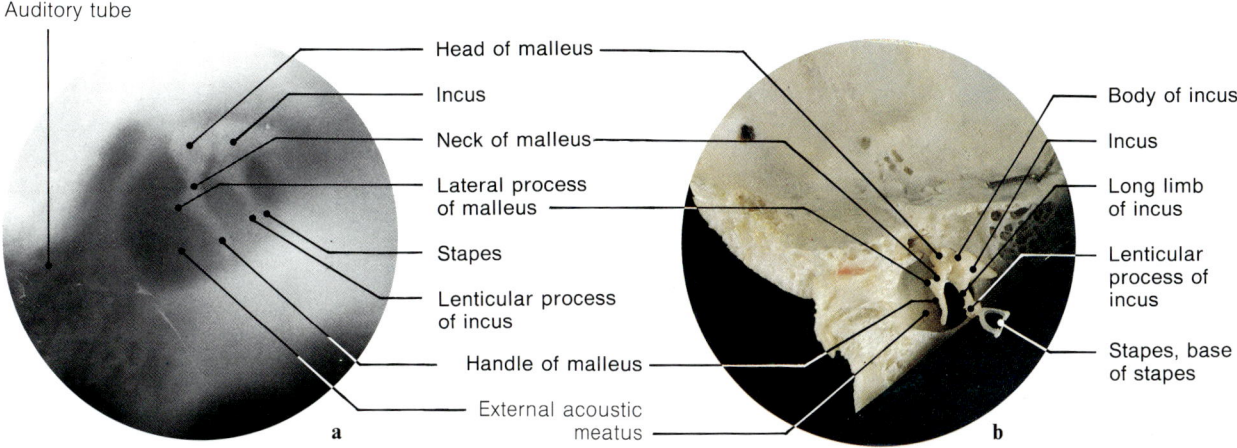

Fig. 8.8. a Tomographic study of anatomic specimen; b view of chain of ossicles in dried bone (sagittal views)

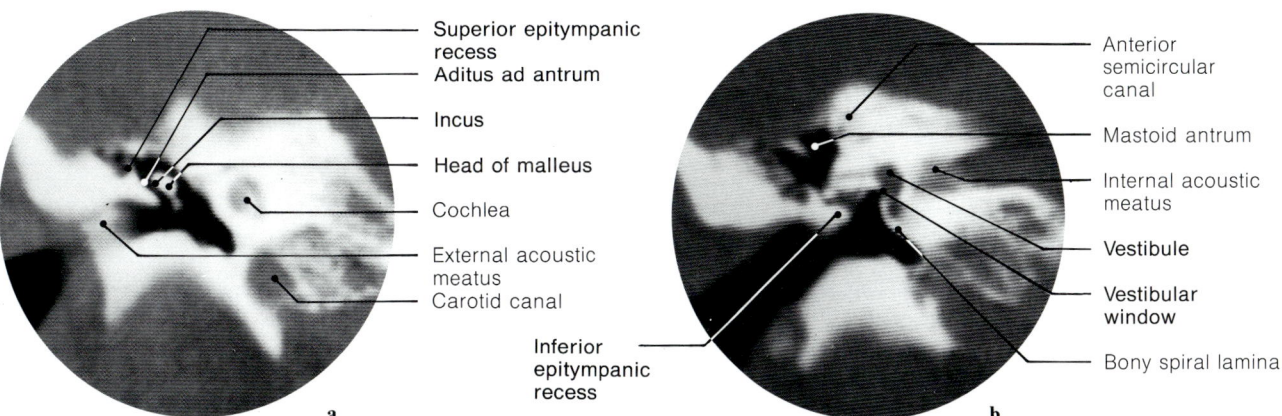

Fig. 8.9a, b. CT in varied views of Guillen and Stenvers; a antro-adito-attical passage; b vestibular window

Middle ear, chain of ossicles

Computed tomography (CT) and tomography

VARIED VIEWS

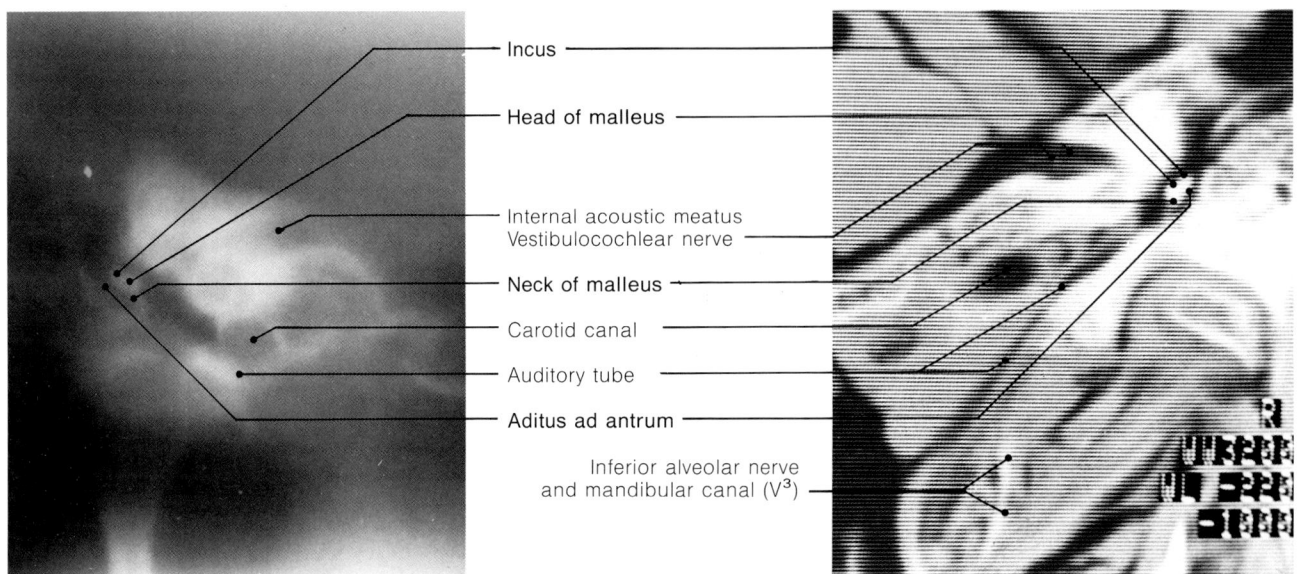

Fig. 8.10 a. Tomographic Guillen view

Fig. 8.10 b. Computed tomographic (CT) Worms-Bretton view

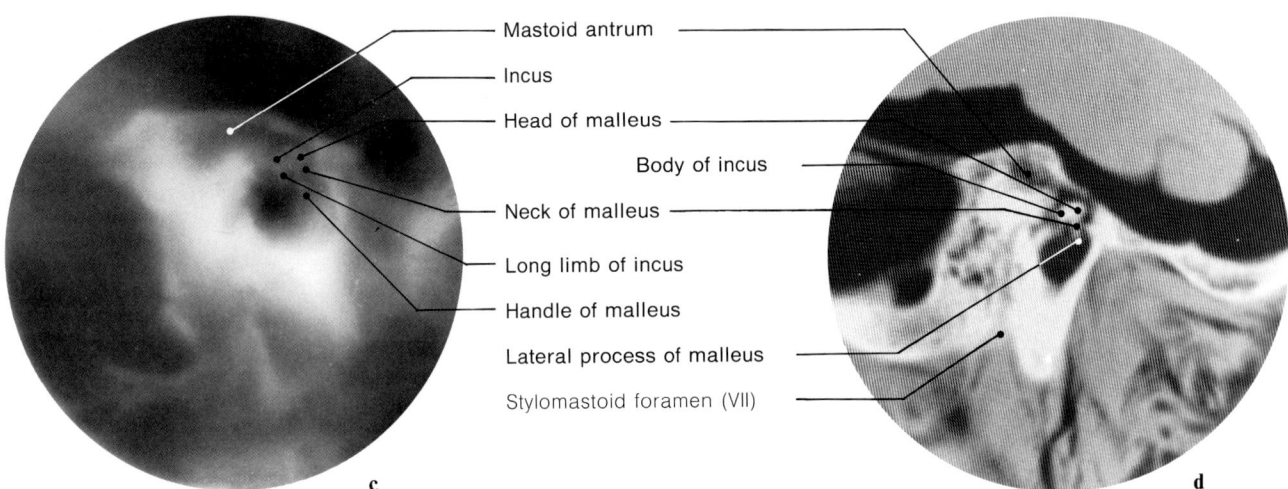

Fig. 8.10 c, d. Tomography and computed tomography (CT) in prestudied inclined sagittal view

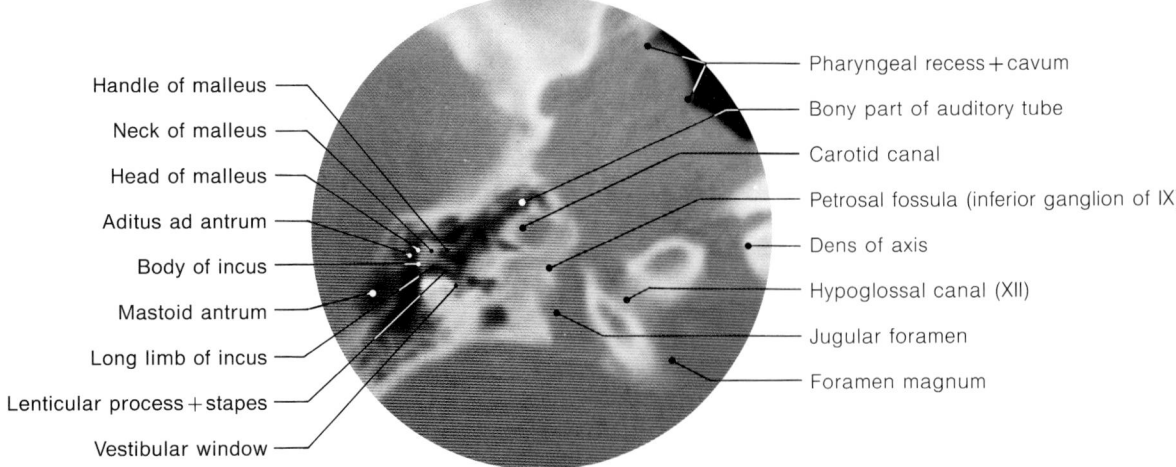

Fig. 8.10 e. Computed tomography (CT) in oblique axial view

Middle ear, auditory tube (or eustachian tube)

Anatomy

The auditory tube is the channel for aeration of the middle ear. It connects the tympanic cavity with the rhinopharynx, from which air enters at every swallowing movement to maintain the balance of pressure in the various part of the tympanic cavity.
The auditory tube lies in front of the cavum, aditus and mastoid antrum (Fig. 8.10a, b, e; 8.12a–c). It travels obliquely forwards, downwards and inwards.
The auditory tube consists of two parts, bony behind and fibrocartilaginous in front. It is lined by a mucous membrane.

Imaging

CLINICAL FEATURES

When the canal is obstructed, either by a sarcoma or by tumors of cavum, rhinopharynx, jugular glomus or of the pharyngeal recess, this causes displacement of the tympanic membrane towards the interior of the cavity. The equilibrium on both sides of the membrane no longer exists and the stapes becomes embedded in the vestibular window, so producing diminished hearing acuity, vertigo and severe continuous tinnitus. Investigation of the auditory tube then becomes necessary.

EXAMINATION

– Tomographic or computed tomographic (CT) study of the auditory tube and pharyngeal recess in symmetric axial view,
– radiography with tomographic or computed tomographic (CT) study in symmetric view, with display in the same axis of the auditory tube, the antro-adito-attical passage, the antrum and the chain of ossicles in the varied Worms-Bretton view (Fig. 8.11),
– tomographic study of the internal acoustic meatus, the bony nasotubal orifice of the auditory tube, the antro-adito-attical passage and the ossicles of the ear in Guillen view (Fig. 8.9a, 8.13).

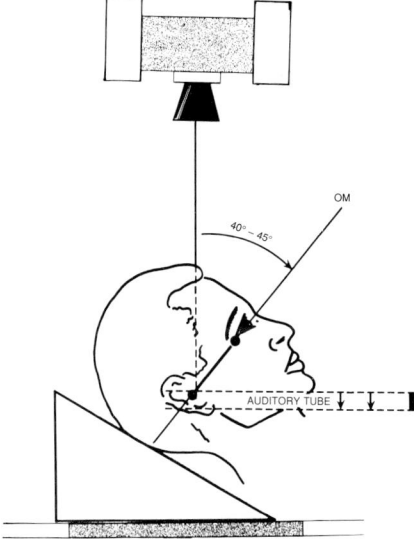

Fig. 8.11. Centering diagram for tomographic and computed tomographic (CT) study of auditory tube, varied Worms-Bretton view

Middle ear, auditory tube (or eustachian tube)

Computed tomography (CT)

FRONTAL, OBLIQUE AND AXIAL VIEWS

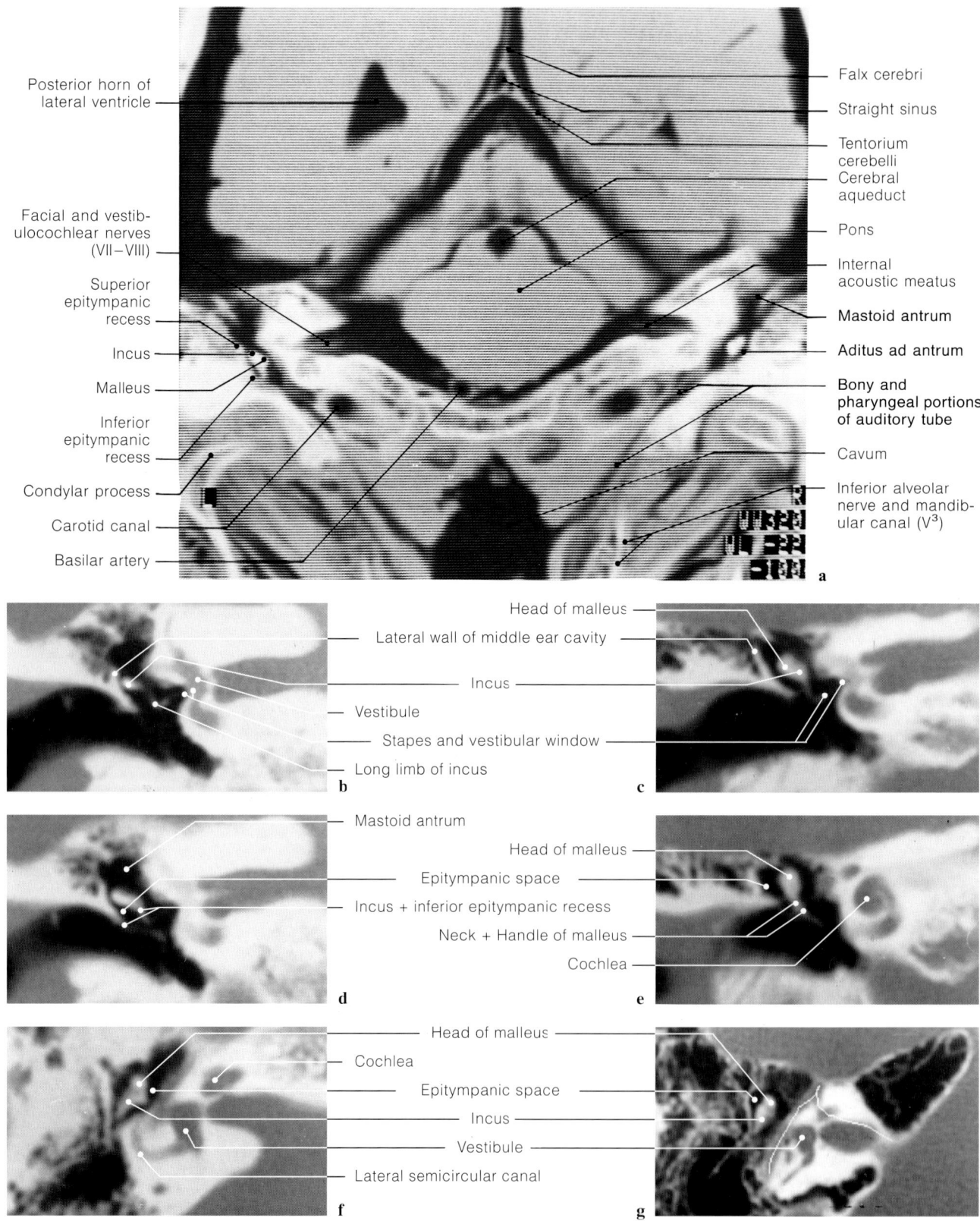

Fig. 8.12a–g. Computed tomography (CT) frontal view (**a**) of auditory tubes in the varied Worms-Bretton view; oblique views in the Guillen view (**b–e**) and axial views (**f, g**) of antro-adito-attical passages and of the ossicles and vestibulocochlear pathways. (CT: Dr. J.W. Casselman, A.Z. St-Jan, Brugge)

Cavities of the external ear, external acoustic meatus (sound-receptor organ)

Anatomy

The external ear is formed of two segments: the auricle and the external acoustic meatus.
The external acoustic meatus is a canal extending from the concha to the tympanic membrane.
The wall of the meatus is cartilaginous and is covered throughout the extent of its internal surface by a skin lining continuous with the skin of the external ear.
The external ear, thanks to its shape and immediate relations, is the receptor organ for sound, which plays a very minimal part in man.

Imaging

CLINICAL FEATURES – INVESTIGATION

In cases of temporal fracture, and if the patient exhibits otorrhagia accompanied by tinnitus with blunted hearing, radiologic examination of the external acoustic meatus is necessary.
It is possible for a temporal fracture to extend into the walls of the external acoustic meatus, involve and displace the inferior epitympanic recess (or wall of the compartment) and produce obstruction of the aditus ad antrum. This fracture may also extend as far as the chain of ossicles and produce incudomallear or incudostapedial dislocation; the stapes may be embedded in the vestibular window, producing continuous tinnitus.

Other pathologic conditions of the external acoustic meatus:
– tympanosclerosis,
– an antral and antro-adito-attical cholesteatoma expanding upwards and inferolaterally may, after having destroyed the tegmen tympani, erode the roof of the external acoustic meatus.

EXAMINATION

– View of Stenvers and Schüller,
– tomographic study in Guillen view,
– prestudied inclined sagittal tomographic study of external acoustic meatus of Cornélis and Vignaud,
– radiography with tomographic and computed tomographic (CT) studies using the varied Worms-Bretton view (Fig. 8.11; 8.12 a–c).

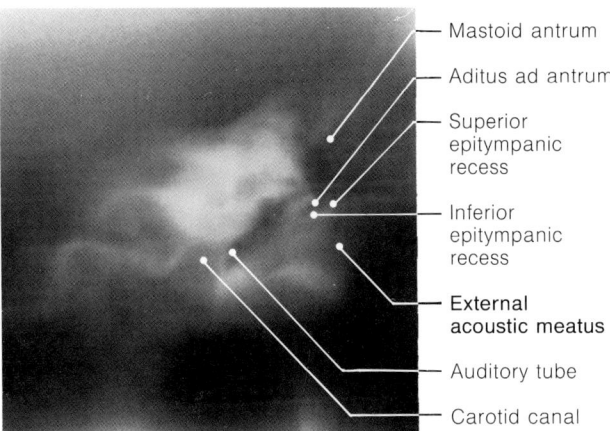

Fig. 8.13. Tomogram of external acoustic meatus in Guillen view

Vestibulocochlear nerves and pathways
Magnetic resonance imaging (MRI)
FRONTAL, AXIAL AND OBLIQUE VIEWS

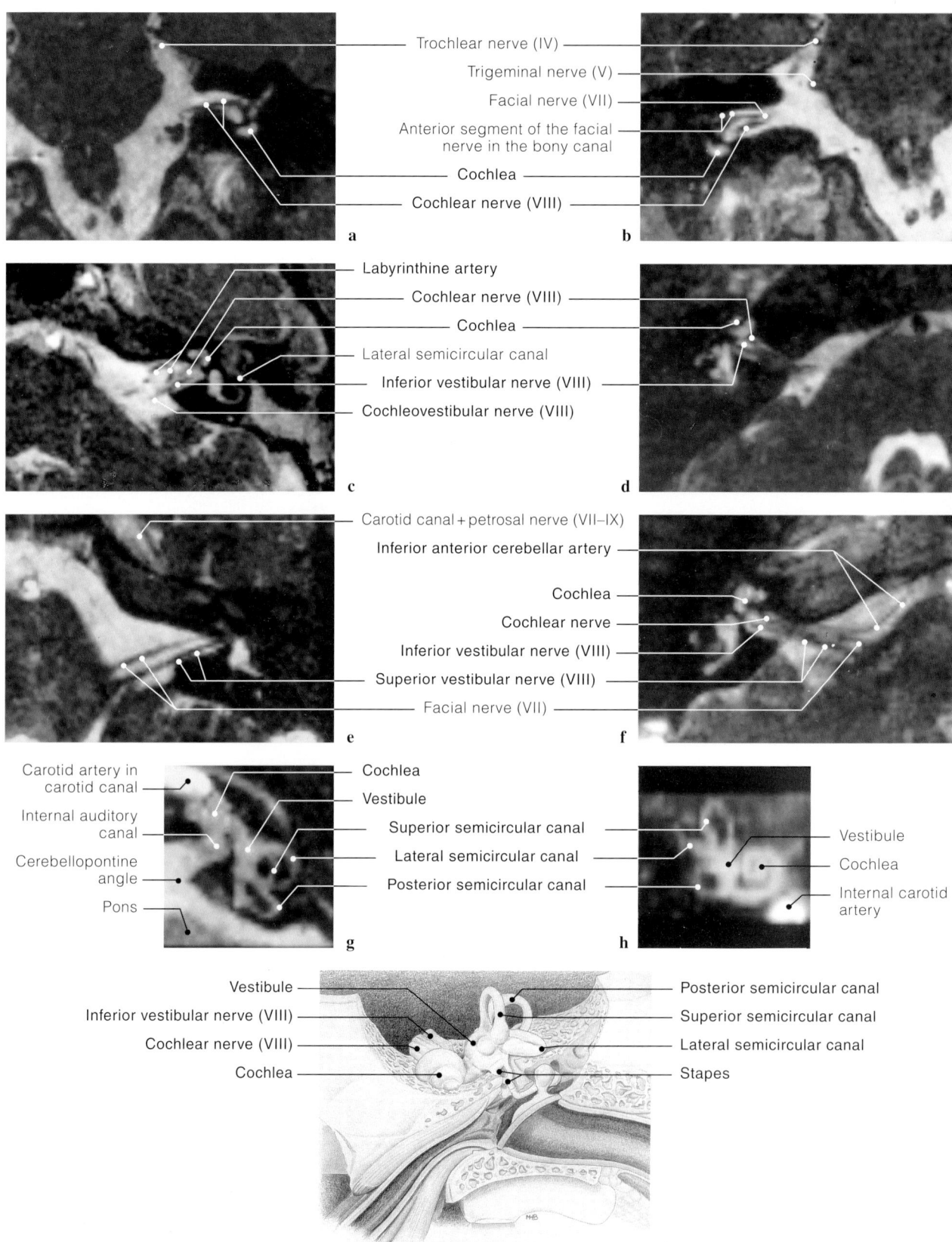

Fig. 8.14a–i. Frontal magnetic resonance imaging (MRI) views of the vestibulocochlear nerves (**a, b**); axial views (**c–f**); study of vestibulocochlear pathways (**g–i**) of antro-adito-attical passages and of the ossicles and vestibulocochlear pathways. (MRI: Dr. J.W. Casselman, A.Z. St-Jan, Brugge)

Glossopharyngeal nerve (IX)

Anatomy (course–terminals–collaterals) 229
Imaging (regions examined) 229
Pathology 229
Apparent origin of glossopharyngeal nerve,
posterior lateral sulcus of medulla oblongata
cerebellopontine angle
    Anatomy and imaging (examination) 231
    Frontal and sagittal views (MRI) 231
    Axial view (CT) 232
Jugular foramen
    Anatomy and imaging (examination) 233
Petrosal fossula or sulcus of inferior ganglion
    Anatomy and imaging (examination) 234
    Extracranial, intracranial views of petrosal fossula
    and diagram of inferior ganglion 235
Tympanic nerve, tympanic canaliculus
    Anatomy and imaging (examination) 236
    Axial view 237
    Diagram of glossopharyngeal nerve and of
    communicating branches 238
Glossopharyngeal nerve
    Axial views (MRI) 240

Vascular relations:
Internal jugular vein (jugular foramen) 238, 249, 258
Jugular branch of the ascending pharyngeal
artery 276, 277
Inferior tympanic artery 286

The glossopharyngeal is a mixed nerve and has a triple function:

– a motor function, for the muscles of the pharynx and some of the tongue muscles,
– a sensory function, for the mucous membrane of the pharynx and the posterior third of the tongue,
– an autonomic function, for the parotid gland.

The glossopharyngeal or IXth cranial nerve arises in the medulla and terminates under the mucosa of the base of the tongue, after having followed, first an intracranial, and then an extracranial course.

228 Glossopharyngeal nerve (IX)

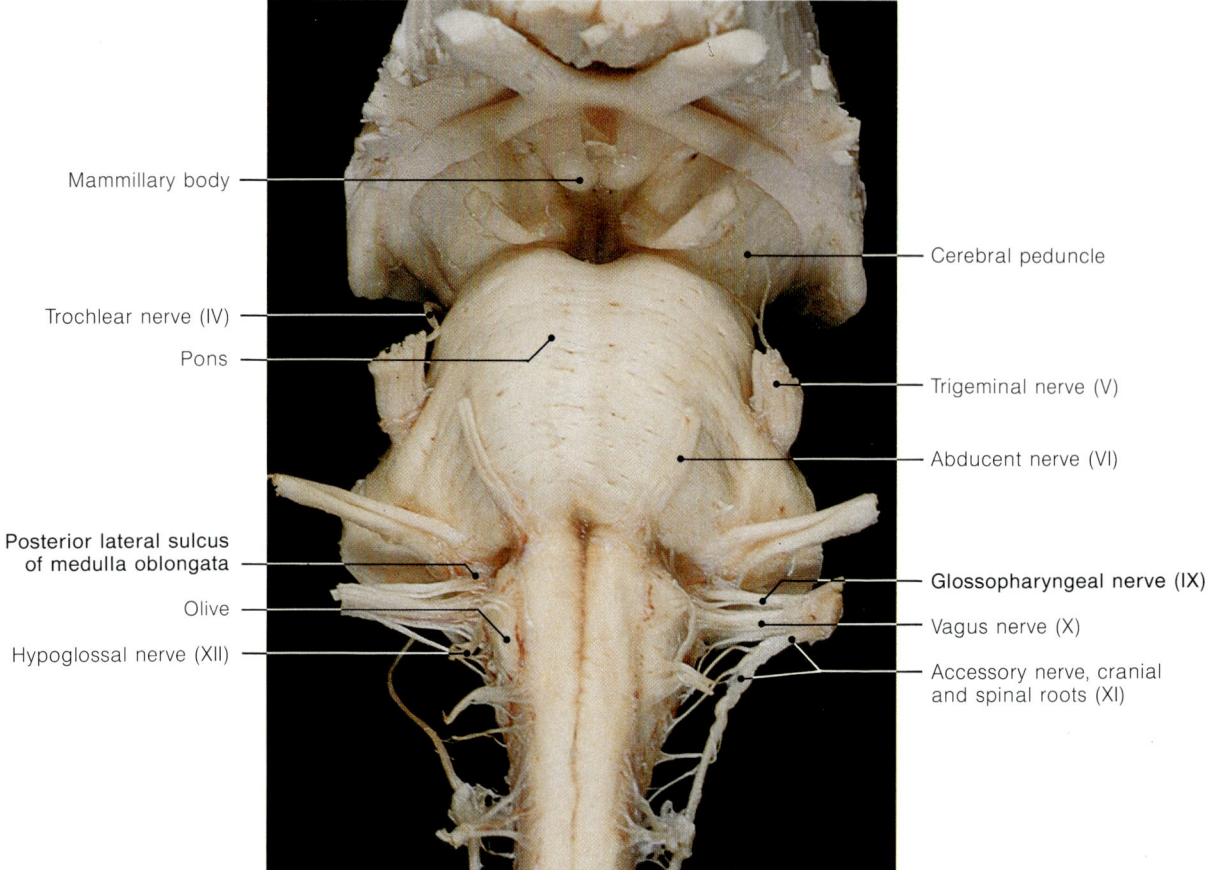

Fig. 9.1. Apparent origin of glossopharyngeal nerve in anterior frontal view of the brain-stem

Fig. 9.2. Frontal section of brain-stem at level of glossopharyngeal nerve (IX)

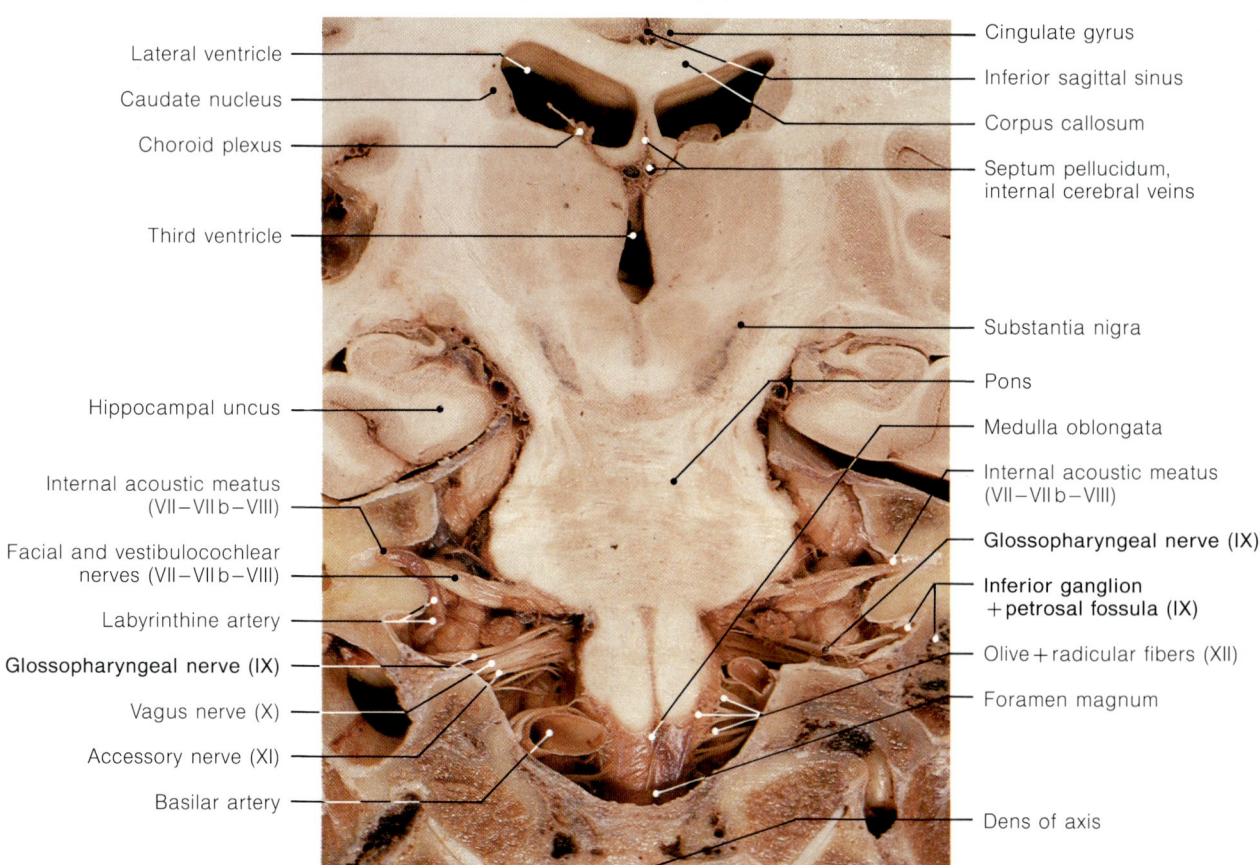

Anatomy

COURSE – TERMINALS – COLLATERALS

Apparent origin in posterior lateral sulcus of medulla oblongata or sulcus of mixed nerves, and intracranial course

Intracanalicular course of glossopharyngeal nerve and orifice of its anastomotic branch (Haller's ansa) with the facial nerve (IX–VII)

Inferior and superior ganglia of glossopharyngeal nerve (IX) (or Andersch's and Ehrenritter's ganglia), anastomotic branches of facial, glossopharyngeal and tympanic nerves (IX–VII)

Tympanic nerve (or Jacobson's nerve)

Imaging

REGIONS EXAMINED

Posterior lateral sulcus of medulla oblongata

Study of cerebellopontine angle

Study of jugular foramen (IX–X–XI) and stylomastoid foramen (VII)

Study of petrosal fossula (sulcus of inferior ganglion of IX) and of jugular foramen (IX–X–XI)

Imaging of tympanic canaliculus (IX)

Pathology

Apparent origin:
- Tumor of cerebellopontine angle,
- medullary syndromes,
- acousticofacial neurinoma.

Jugular foramen and petrosal fossula:
- Tumor of jugular glomus,
- major cholesteatoma of middle ear,
- syndrome of posterior condylolacerate junction (Collet-Sicard syndrome),
- fractures,
- tumors of cavum and pharynx.

Tympanic canaliculus:
- Syndrome of tympanic canaliculus,
- aneurysm of internal carotid artery in the carotid canal (extracranial).

Glossopharyngeal nerve (IX)

Topography

Apparent origin of glossopharyngeal nerve (IX)
- Posterior lateral sulcus of medulla oblongata

Intracanalicular course
- Jugular foramen (IX–X–XI)

Inferior and superior ganglia (IX)
- Petrosal fossula or sulcus of inferior ganglion of IX

Tympanic nerve (Jacobson's nerve)
- Tympanic canaliculus

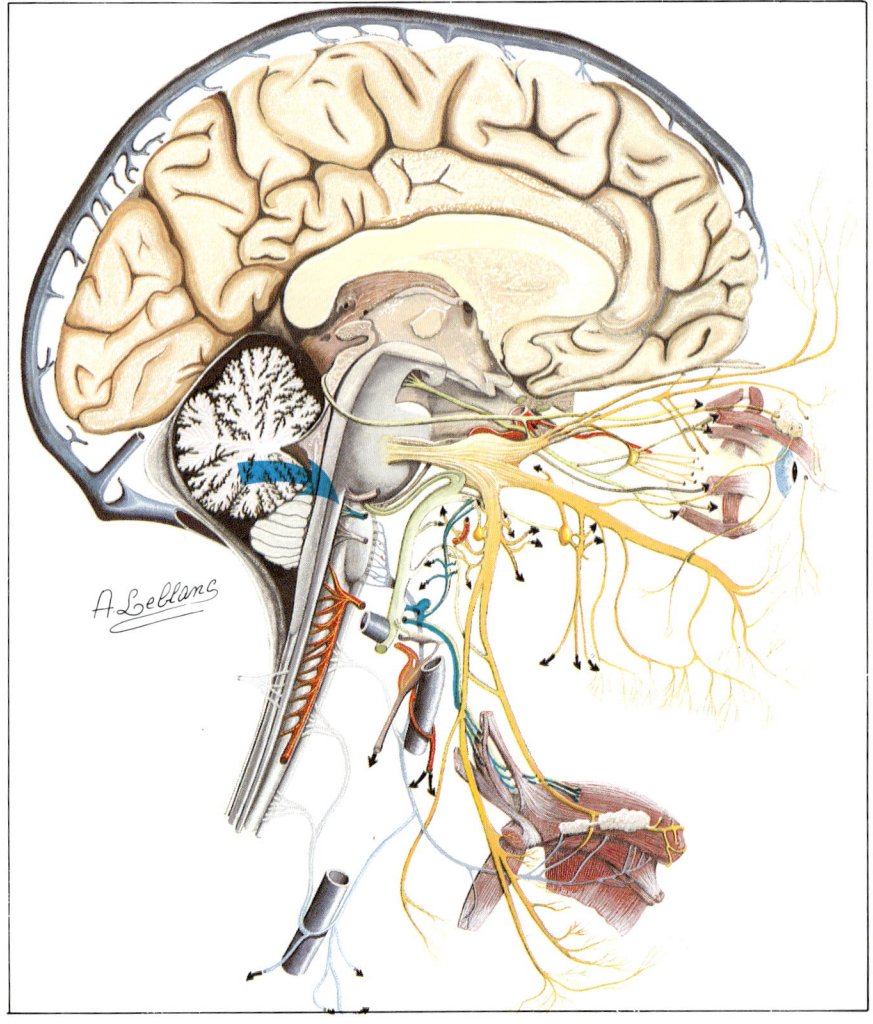

Fig. 9.3

Apparent origin of glossopharyngeal nerve, posterior lateral sulcus of medulla oblongata

Anatomy

The glossopharyngeal nerve leaves the neuraxis via the posterior lateral sulcus of the medulla oblongata. It consists of five superimposed bundles which are situated:

- at the superolateral aspect of the medulla oblongata,
- at the upper part of the posterior lateral sulcus,
- above the lateral fossula,
- behind and below the vestibulocochlear nerve,
- above the vagus nerve (X) and the accessory nerve (XI).

The *motor nucleus* is situated in the bulbar triangle of the floor of the fourth ventricle.

The *motor fibers* first travel backwards, inwards and downwards towards the floor of the fourth ventricle and then bend at an acute angle and travel forwards and outwards towards the posterior lateral sulcus of the medulla oblongata.

The *sensory fibers* arise in the inferior and superior ganglia (IX), situated at the level of the jugular foramen, or more precisely in the petrosal fossula (Fig. 9.7; 9.13).

The central fibers arising in the middle portion of the solitary tract follow the lemniscus as far as the thalamus and the terminal neurones link up with the cortical gustatory center.

Imaging

Clinical features

- Involvement of the glossopharyngeal nerve by a vascular or tumoral lesion,
- abolition of sensation of the posterior third of the tongue,
- dysphagia,
- paralysis of superior pharyngeal constrictor muscle,
- bulbar syndromes,
- lateral syndrome of medulla oblongata (Wallenberg's syndrome).

Possible causes

- Tumor of cerebellopontine angle,
- acousticofacial neurinoma (expanding towards the posterior lateral sulcus) damaging the IXth, Xth and XIth cranial nerves.

Examination

- Study of magnetic resonance (MRI) or computed tomographic (CT) images of the cerebellopontine angle for the posterior lateral sulcus of the medulla oblongata in sagittal, axial and frontal views and in the Worms-Bretton view (Fig. 9.4a, b; 9.5a, b).

Technique

- The technique is essentially identical with that used for the study by MRI of the apparent origin of the facial and vestibulocochlear nerves; the sections are made at virtually the same level.

Cerebellopontine angle

Magnetic resonance imaging (MRI)

Frontal and sagittal views

Fig. 9.4a, b. MRI of cerebellopontine angle for the apparent origin of the glossopharyngeal nerve; **a** frontal view, **b** sagittal view

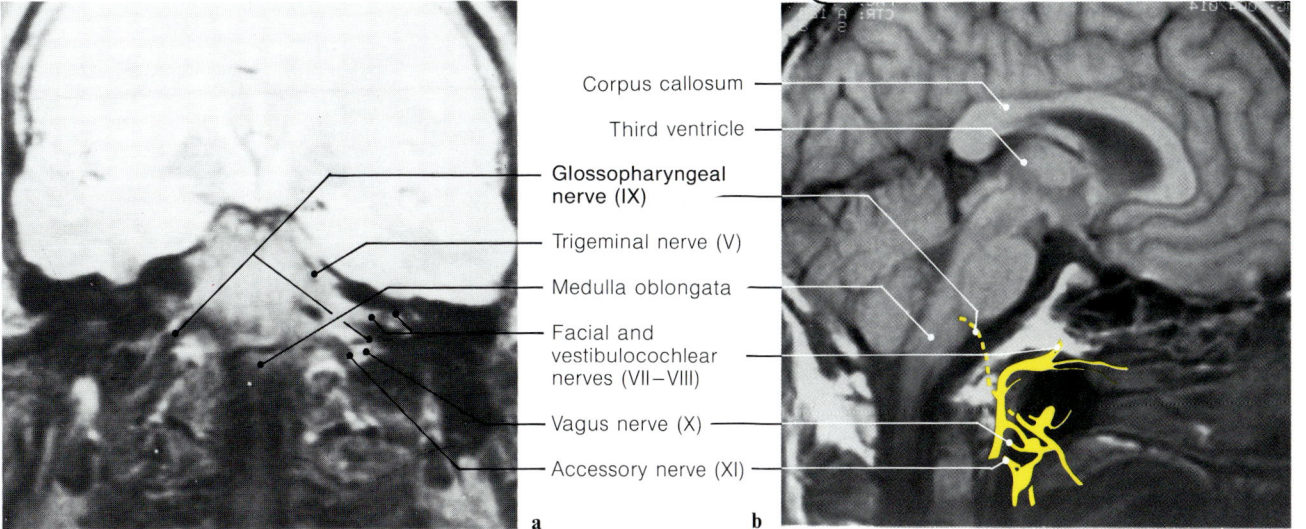

Cerebellopontine angle

Computed tomography (CT)

AXIAL VIEW

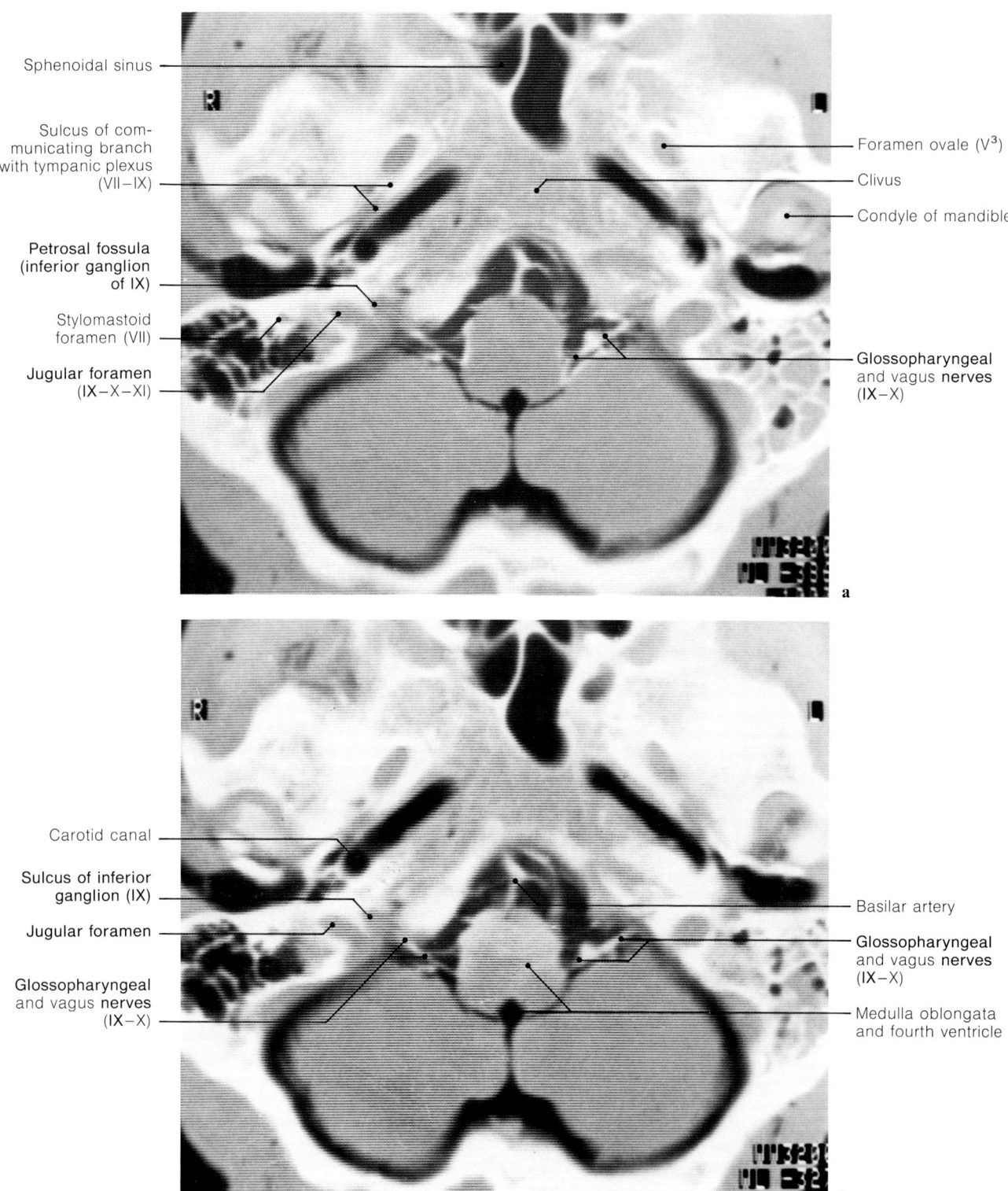

Fig. 9.5a, b. Axial CT sections at the level of the posterior lateral sulcus of the medulla oblongata for the apparent origin of the glossopharyngeal nerve (IX)

Jugular foramen

Anatomy

Course – relations

From the medulla oblongata the glossopharyngeal nerve travels forwards and outwards and leaves the skull via the jugular foramen (Fig. 9.5a). It then bends at a right angle and descends forming a curve concave forwards and upwards and ends at the base of the tongue (Fig. 9.3; 9.14).
In the posterior cranial fossa the nerve travels behind the bundle of the vestibulocochlear and facial nerves (VII–VIII), in front of the flocculus of the cerebellum and the vagus (X) and accessory (XI) nerves, and above the hypoglossal nerve (XII) which passes towards the hypoglossal canal.
The glossopharyngeal nerve occupies the anterior part of the jugular foramen.
The nerve lies lateral to and then behind the petrosal sinus (Fig. 10.8b, c). It is separated from the vagus and accessory nerves (X–XI) by a fibrous septum.
Collateral branches: The glossopharyngeal nerve gives off: the anastomotic branch with the facial nerve, the tympanic nerve, the carotid branches, the nerve to the stylopharyngeus muscle, the nerve to the styloglossus muslce and the tonsillar branches (Fig. 9.8c; 9.14).

Imaging

Clinical features

– Dysphagia,
– loss of sensation of posterior third of tongue,
– jugular foramen syndrome,
– posterior condylolacerate syndrome.

Possible causes

– Tumors of jugular glomus,
– tumors of cavum,
– major cholesteatoma of middle ear extending towards the jugular bulb,
– fractures.

Examination

– Survey radiographs using the Hirtz, Blondeau and Vatters views,
– tomographic study of the jugular foramen in the Chaussé II view,
– radiographic or computed tomographic study in unilateral oblique view.

Technique

Radiographic and computed tomographic (CT) studies of the jugular foramen in unilateral oblique view:

– The subject is in dorsal decubitus, the back raised on pillows, the head extended so that the incident beam makes an angle of 30° in relation to the orbitomeatal plane (OM) (Fig. 9.6b);
– the head is then turned to the side opposite to that to be examined by 30° to 35° in relation to the median sagittal plane (Fig. 9.6a);
– the centering point is situated 2 cm above the mandibular angle.

The sections start 1.5 cm beneath the external acoustic meatus and travel downwards for 2 cm.

Note: This view provides a good image of the entire jugular foramen and displays the sigmoid sinus, the fossula of the inferior ganglion (or petrosal fossula). The "open mouth" Chaussé II view gives a good survey image, but the superomedial region of the jugular foramen is often concealed by the teeth. It is possible that the patient's condition may not permit opening of the mouth.

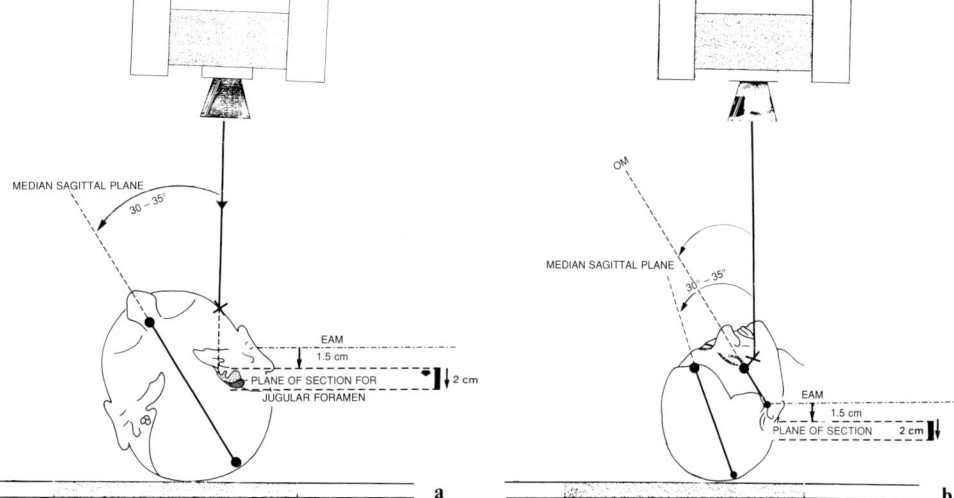

Fig. 9.6 a, b. Centering diagrams for radiographic and tomographic study of the jugular foramen in unilateral oblique view

Petrosal fossula or sulcus of inferior ganglion of glossopharyngeal nerve (or Andersch's ganglion)

Anatomy

In the jugular foramen the glossopharyngeal nerve exhibits ganglionic swellings, of which the inferior (or petrosal) ganglion is the most obvious. It is embedded in the petrosal fossula, hollowed in the postero-inferior aspect of the petrous bone (Fig. 9.8a–c; 9.14).

Beneath the skull the glossopharyngeal nerve is situated behind the internal carotid artery; it then crosses the outer aspect of the stylopharyngeus muscle and is applied to the superior pharyngeal constrictor muscle. Remaining in contact with this muscle, it reaches the base of the tongue and then the deep aspect of the styloglossus muscle. It crosses both the ascending palatine artery and the lower part of the tonsil.

The glossopharyngeal nerve also exhibits an inconstant ganglion, the superior ganglion situated above the inferior ganglion.

Imaging

Examination

- Tomographic study of the petrosal fossula in unilateral oblique view,
- frontal tomographic or computed tomographic (CT) study in symmetric view,
- axial computed tomographic (CT) study of petrosal fossula.

Technique

Axial tomographic study of petrosal fossula of inferior ganglion:

- The subject is in dorsal decubitus, the back raised on pillows, the head strictly frontal and resting on the vertex so that the orbitomeatal plane (OM) is parallel to that of the table;
- the centering point is median on the line joining the internal acoustic meatuses;
- the planes of section start from the orbitomeatal plane (OM) every 3 mm for 2 cm ascending towards the chin (Fig. 9.11; 9.12).

Fig. 9.7a–c. Tomograms of petrosal fossula or sulcus of inferior ganglion; **a** varied symmetric view of Blondeau, **b** unilateral oblique view, **c** axial view

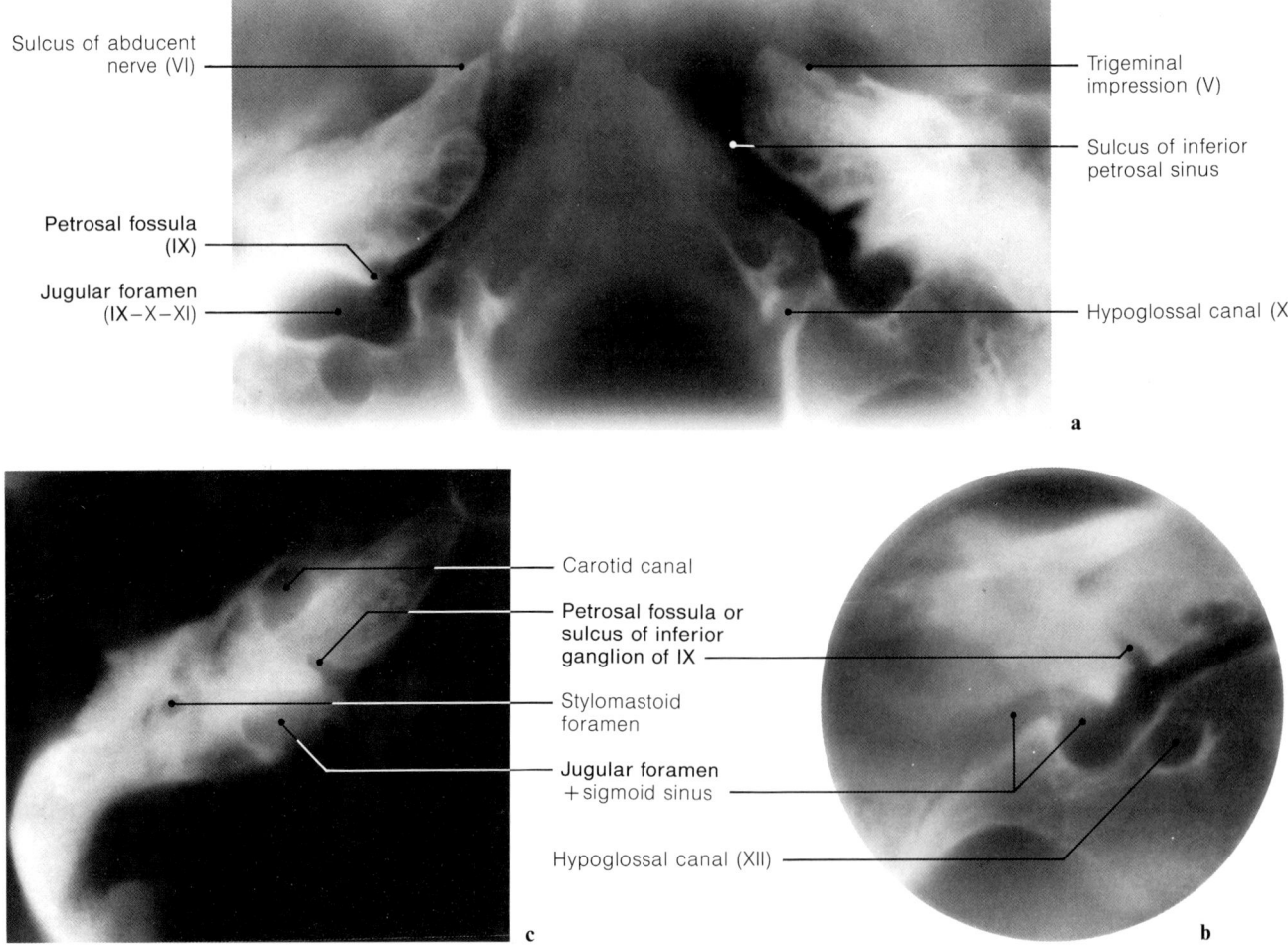

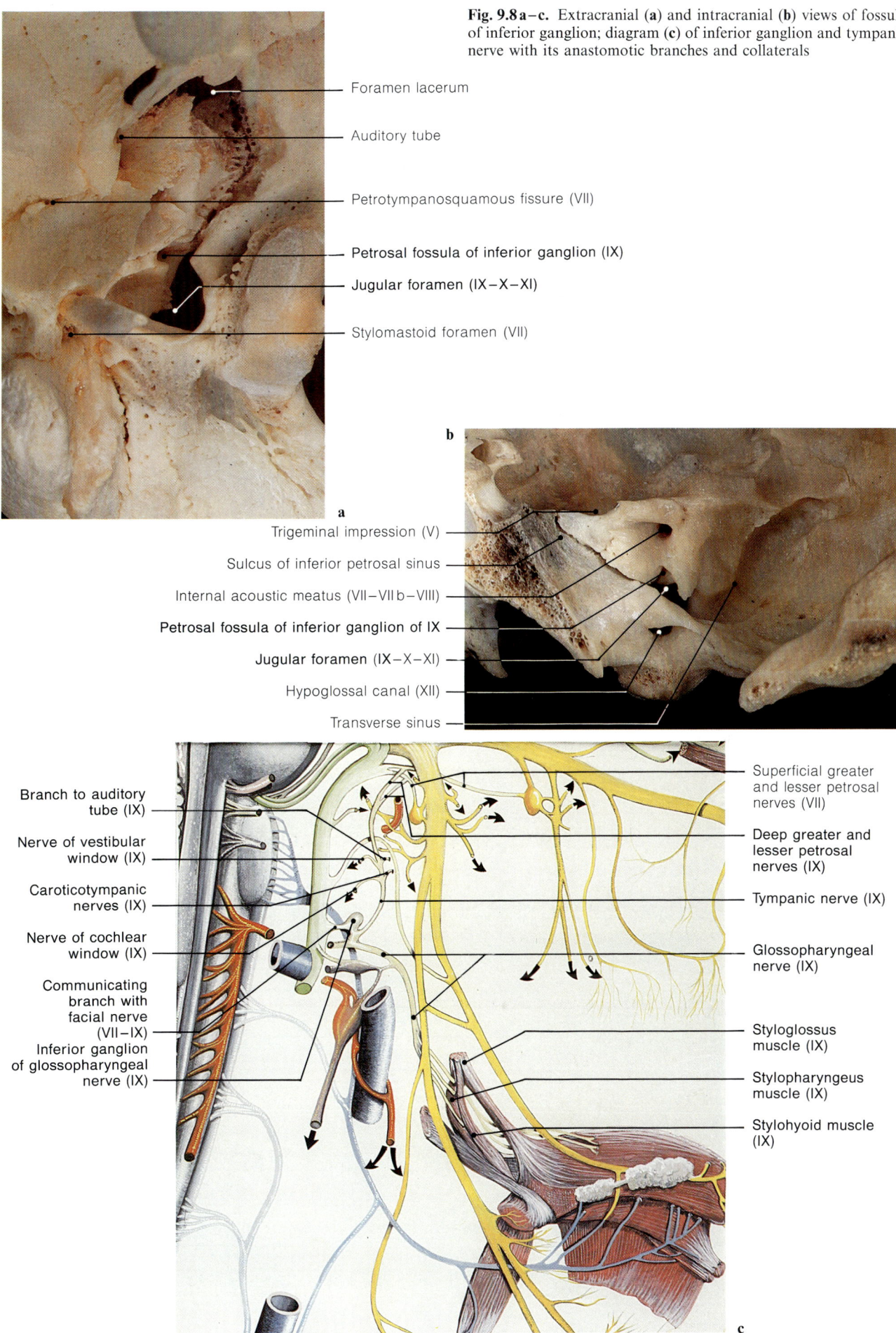

Fig. 9.8 a–c. Extracranial (**a**) and intracranial (**b**) views of fossula of inferior ganglion; diagram (**c**) of inferior ganglion and tympanic nerve with its anastomotic branches and collaterals

Tympanic nerve (Jacobson's nerve), tympanic canaliculus

Anatomy

The **tympanic nerve** arises at the upper and outer part of the inferior ganglion and initially travels outwards, towards the crest that separates the jugular fossa from the carotid canal (Fig. 9.9a, b). At the outer end of this sulcus, the tympanic nerve enters the tympanic canal and then exits via the upper orifice of this canal into the tympanic box. The nerve ascends towards the prominence of the promontory, where it creates a narrow groove and divides into six branches (Fig. 9.8):

- two posterior branches for the mucous membrane surrounding the vestibular (oval) and cochlear (round) windows;
- two anterior branches: the caroticotympanic nerve, which reaches the carotid canal (Fig. 9.9; 9.13), to anastomose with the pericarotid sympathetic plexus (Fig. 9.15), and a tubal branch to the mucosa of the auditory tube;
- two superior branches, the deep greater and lesser petrosal nerves (Fig. 9.14). These two terminal branches enter the superior wall of the tympanic box.

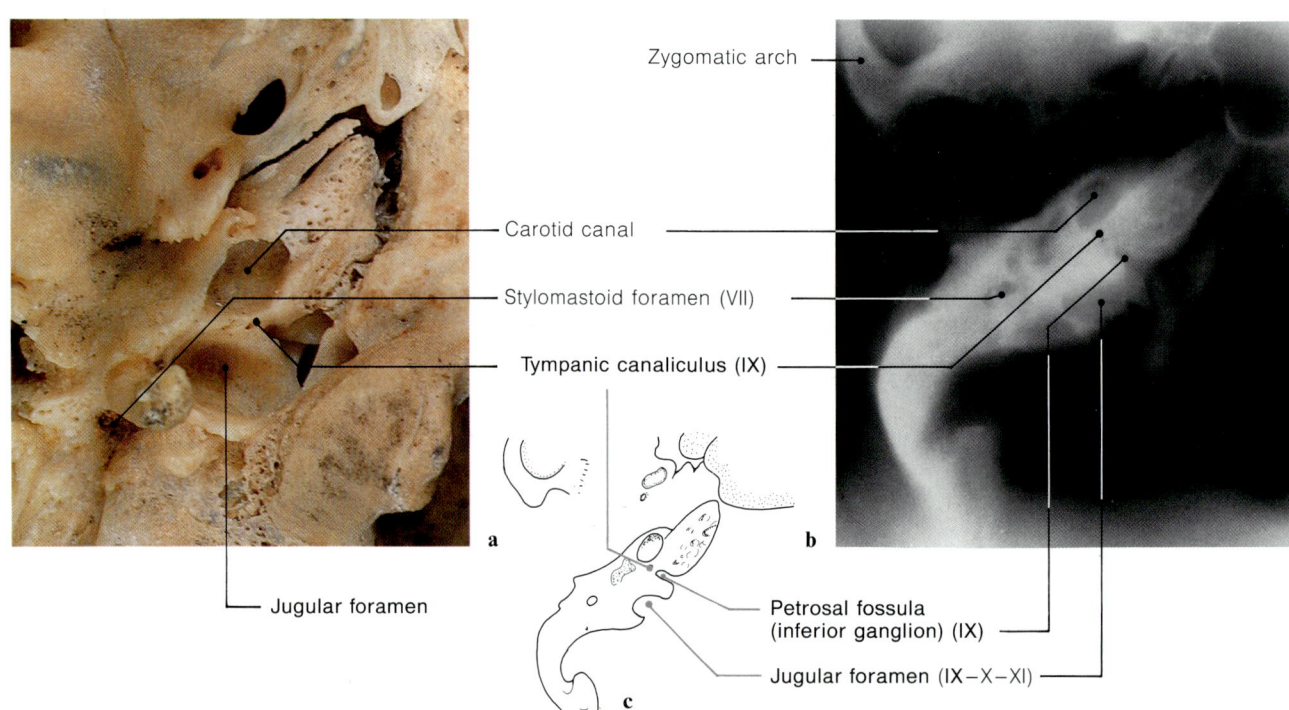

Fig. 9.9 a–c. Anatomic extracranial view (**a**), axial tomographic section (**b**) and diagram (**c**) of tympanic canaliculus

Fig. 9.10. Extracranial view of carotid canal showing caroticotympanic canaliculus (IX–VII)

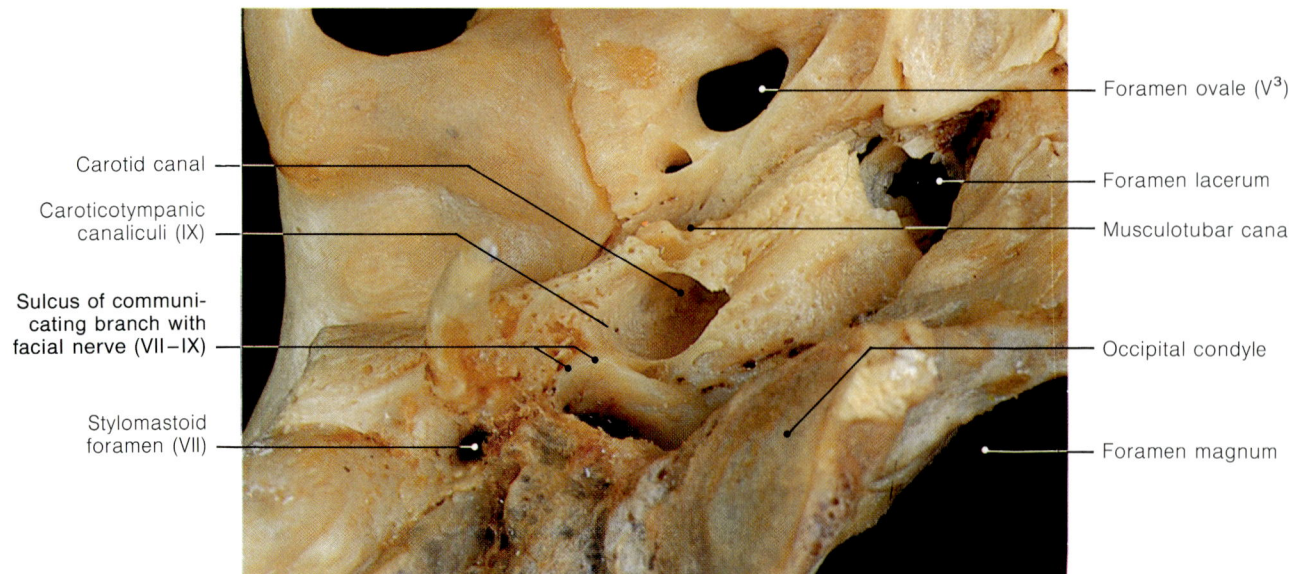

The *deep greater petrosal nerve* anastomoses with the superficial greater petrosal nerve to form the pterygoid nerve, which joins the *pterygopalatine ganglion* (Fig. 7.24; 7.28). The *deep lesser petrosal nerve* anastomoses with the superficial lesser petrosal nerve and then enters the *otic ganglion* ($IX-VII-V^3$) (Fig. 9.15).
The secretory stimuli transmitted by the superficial and deep lesser petrosal nerves are conducted to the parotid gland by the efferent rami of the otic ganglion within the auriculotemporal nerve.

The tympanic canaliculus is situated behind the carotid canal, in front of the jugular canal and to the outer side of the petrosal fossula of the inferior ganglion (Fig. 9.9–9.12). It may therefore be affected by a tympanojugular paraganglioma, a tumor of the pharynx or tongue, or by a spreading fracture of the petrous bone or the skull base.

Imaging

Examination

– Axial tomographic or computed tomographic (CT) studies of the tympanic canaliculus.

Technique

– For imaging technique, see p. 234; the centering diagram and film obtained are shown in Figs. 9.9b; 9.11. The imaging technique is similar to the technique used in axial tomographic study of the petrosal fossula.

Anatomic and physiologic review

The glossopharyngeal nerve has a threefold function:

– *a motor function*, i.e., innervation of the stylopharyngeus muscle, the superior pharyngeal constrictor muscle in association with branches of the vagus nerve (X), and the styloglossus muscle.

– *a sensory function*, relating to general sensation of the posterior third of the tongue and of the pharynx, transmission of taste sensation from the posterior third of the tongue (Fig. 9.14) behind the territory of the lingual nerve (V^3), while sensation of the anterior two-thirds is effected by the chorda tympani (Fig. 7.49; 9.14; 9.8 c).
– *an autonomic function*, since the tympanic nerve (IX) innervates the parotid gland to stimulate salivary secretion (Fig. 7.49).

Clinical types

Loss of sensation of the posterior third of the tongue is seen in glossopharyngeal paralysis (IX). Mainly affected is the capacity to taste bitter substances, associated with unilateral lingual anesthesia.
Loss of taste sensation of all of one side of the tongue is seen when the two pathways of the intermedius (VII b) and glossopharyngeal (IX) nerves are simultaneously affected.

Tympanic canaliculus

Tomographic imaging

Axial view

Fig. 9.11. Centering diagram for tomographic study of tympanic canaliculus and petrosal fossula of inferior ganglion

Fig. 9.12. Axial tomogram of tympanic canaliculus (IX)

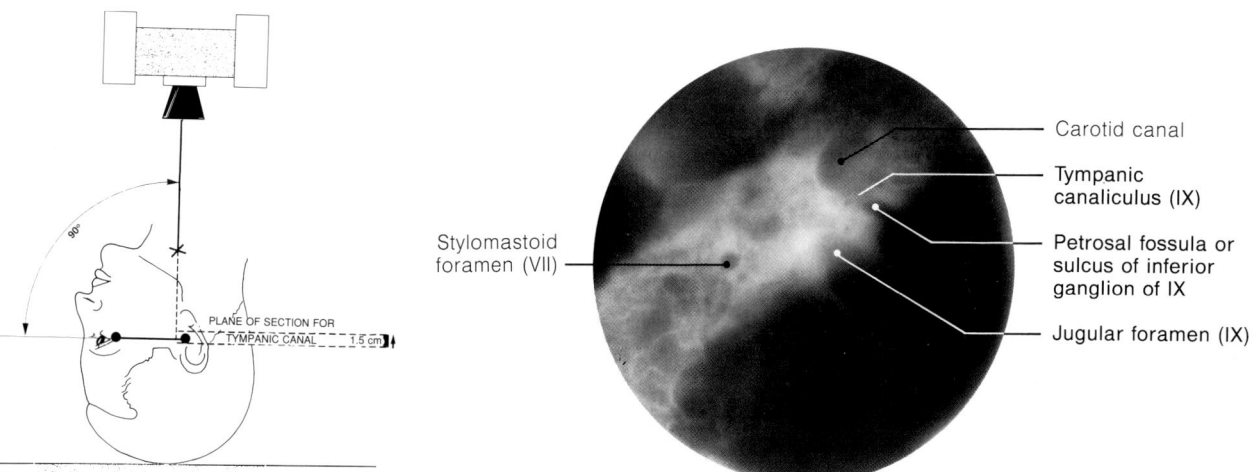

Glossopharyngeal nerve, tympanic nerve

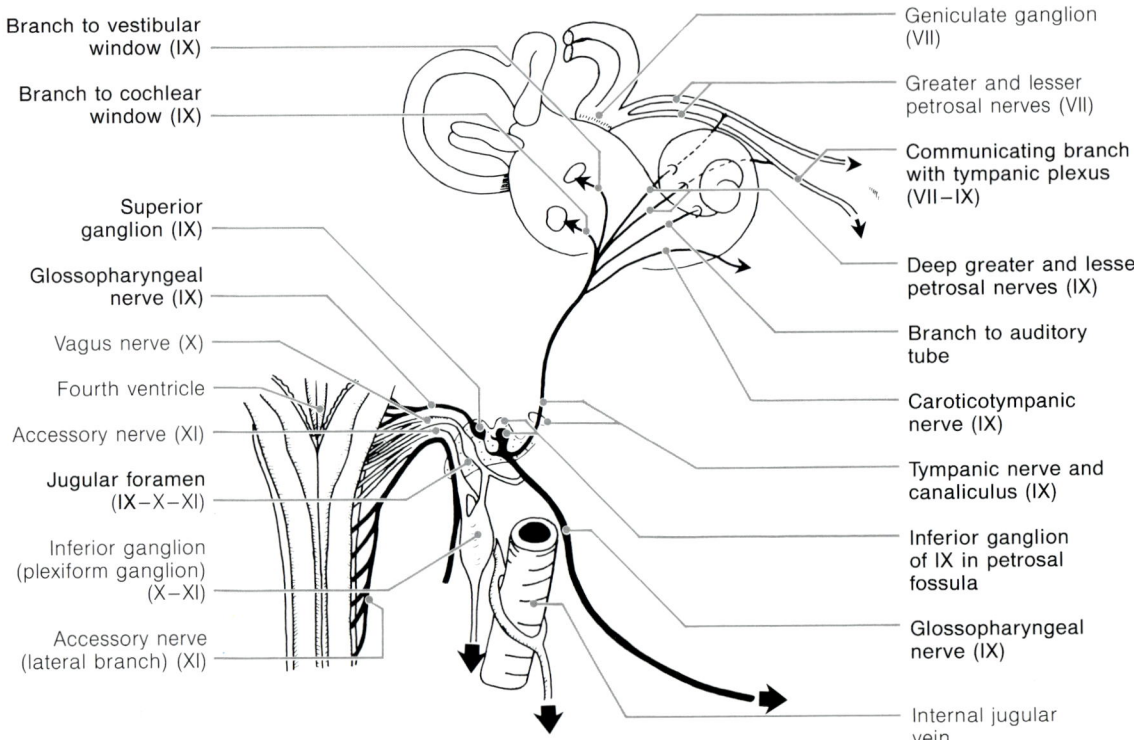

Fig. 9.13. Diagram of glossopharyngeal nerve to show tympanic nerve and its anastomotic branches (IX–VII)

Fig. 9.14. Diagram of glossopharyngeal nerve (IX); large dots: territory of innervation by glossopharyngeal nerve (IX); small dots: territory of innervation by lingual nerve (VII b–V^3)

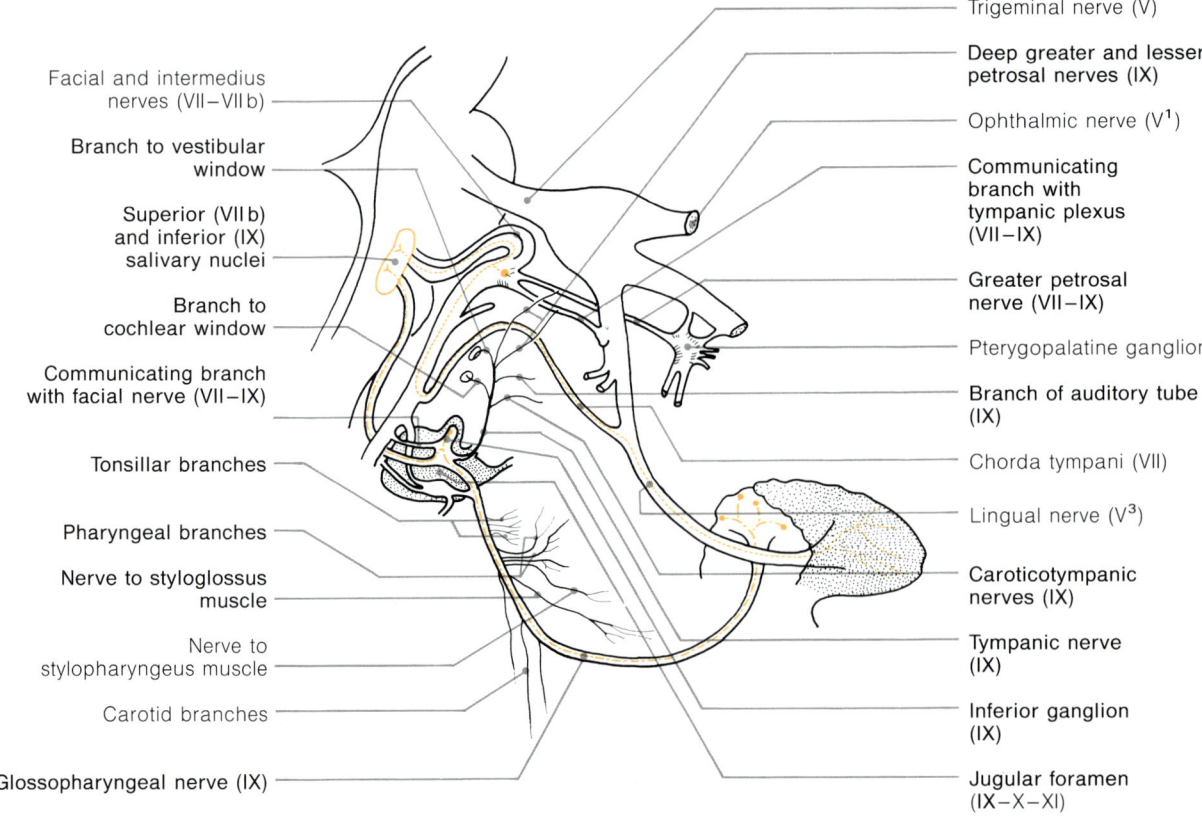

Glossopharyngeal nerve, tympanic nerve, cervical carotid sympathetic plexus

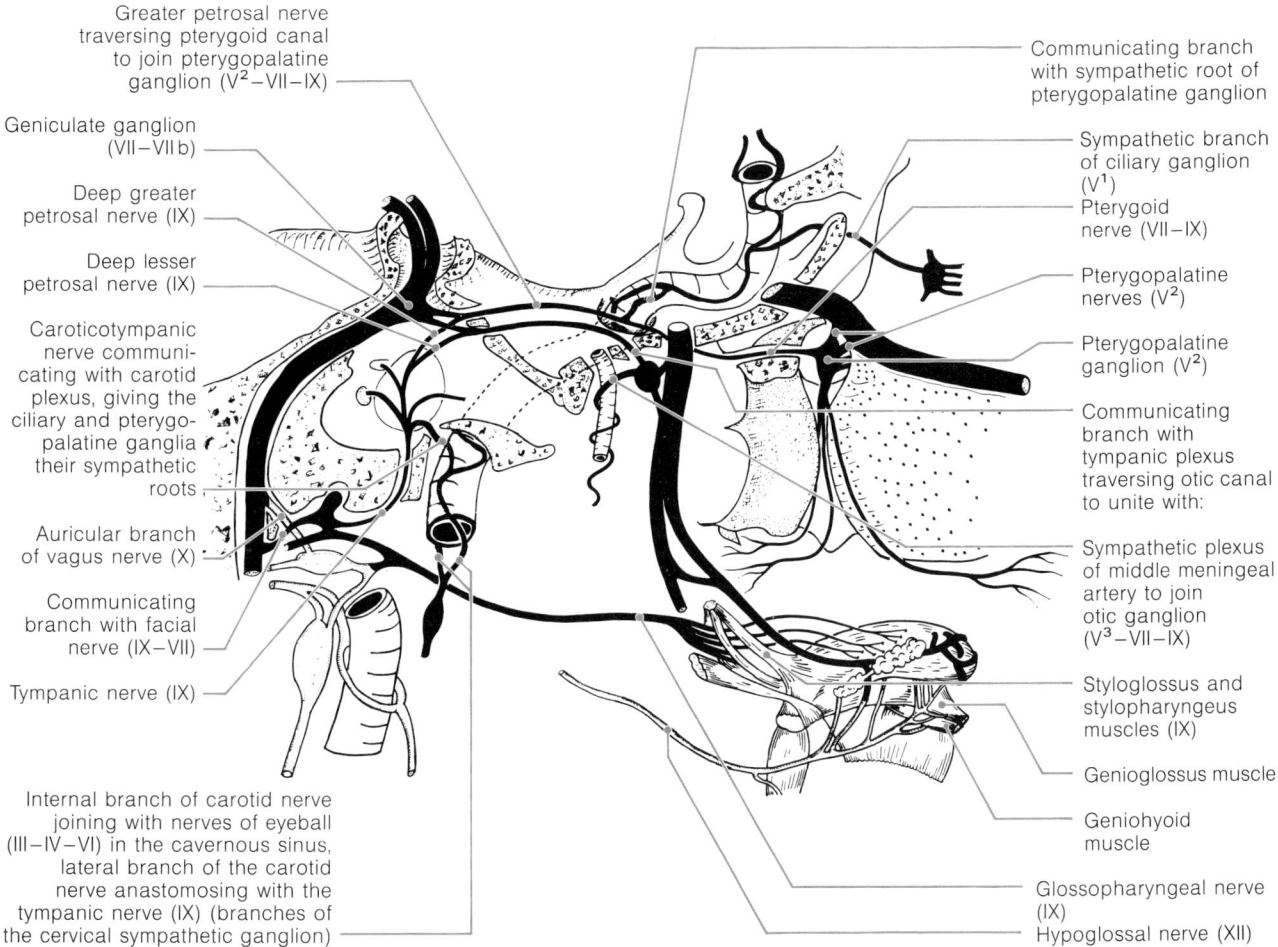

Fig. 9.15. Diagram showing anastomotic relations of glossopharyngeal, facial and trigeminal nerves (IX–VII–V) with carotid sympathetic plexus

Glossopharyngeal nerve (IX) (See vascular relations, p. 286)

Magnetic resonance imaging (MRI)

AXIAL VIEWS

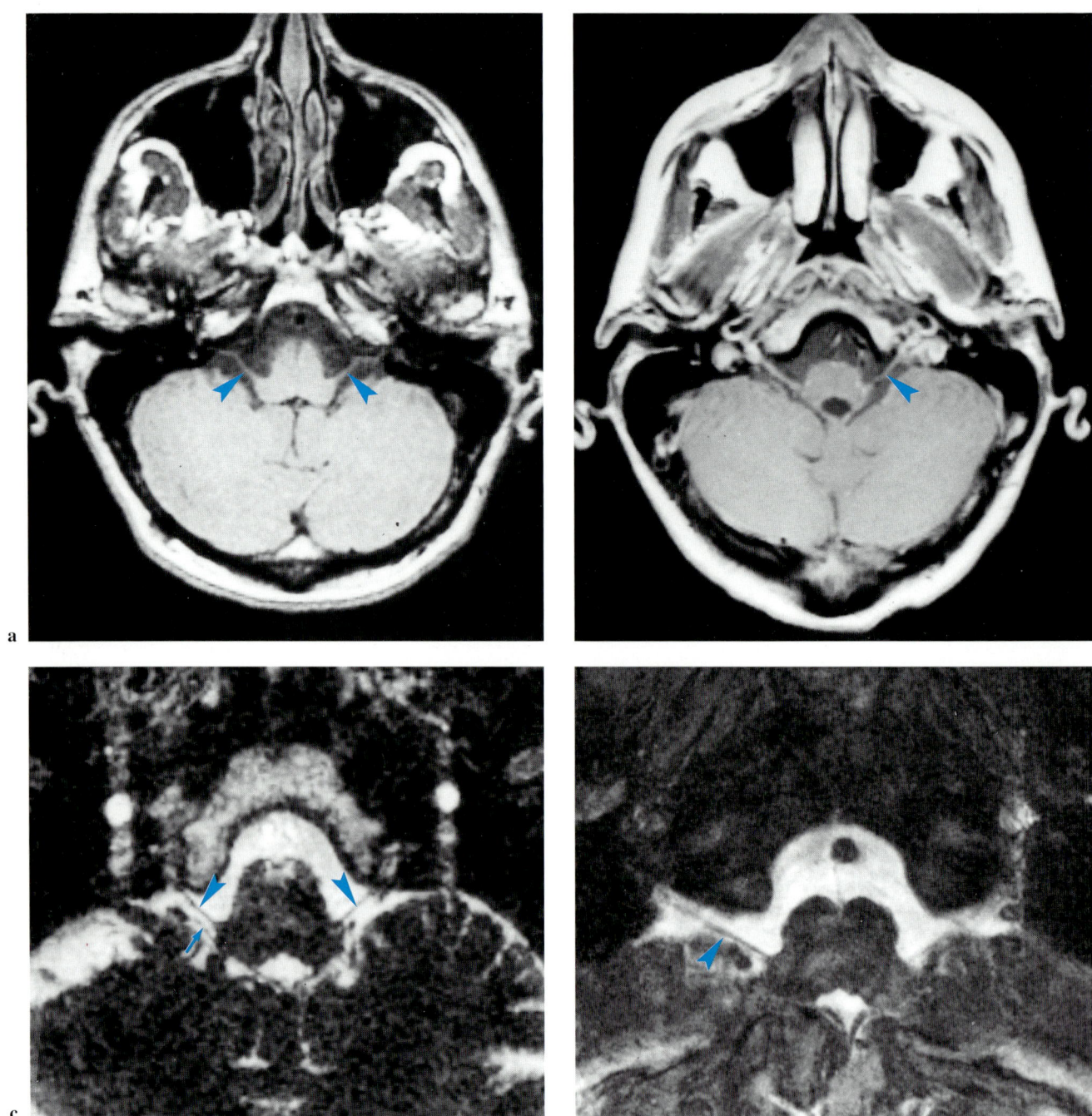

Fig. 9.16a–d. Magnetic resonance imaging (MRI): axial views of glossopharyngeal nerve (IX) (*arrowheads*), vagus nerve (X) (*small arrow*). (CT: Pr. Doyon, Hospital Kremlin Bicêtre, Paris; MRI: Dr. J.W. Casselman, A.Z. St-Jan, Brugge)

Vagus nerve (X)
(or pneumogastric nerve)

Anatomy (course–terminals–collaterals) 243
Imaging (regions examined) 243
Pathology 243
    Axial views (MRI, CT) 243
Apparent origin of vagus nerve, posterior lateral sulcus of medulla oblongata, cerebellopontine angle
    Anatomy and imaging (examination) 245
    Axial views (CT, MRI) 245
Jugular foramen
    Anatomy and imaging (examination) 246
    Oblique view (MRI) 246
    Anteroposterior view, symmetric view (radiology) . 247
    Saggittal view (MRI) 247
Ostium introitus, auricular branch of vagus nerve (X–VII)
    Anatomy and imaging (examination) 248
    Sagittal view 249
    Varied anatomic views 249
Functions of vagus nerve
    Diagram 250

Vascular relations:
Internal jugular vein (jugular foramen) 238, 249, 258
Jugular branch of the ascending pharyngeal artery 276, 277

The vagus is a mixed nerve with particularly important functions and a very extensive distribution extending to the organs of the neck, thorax and abdomen.

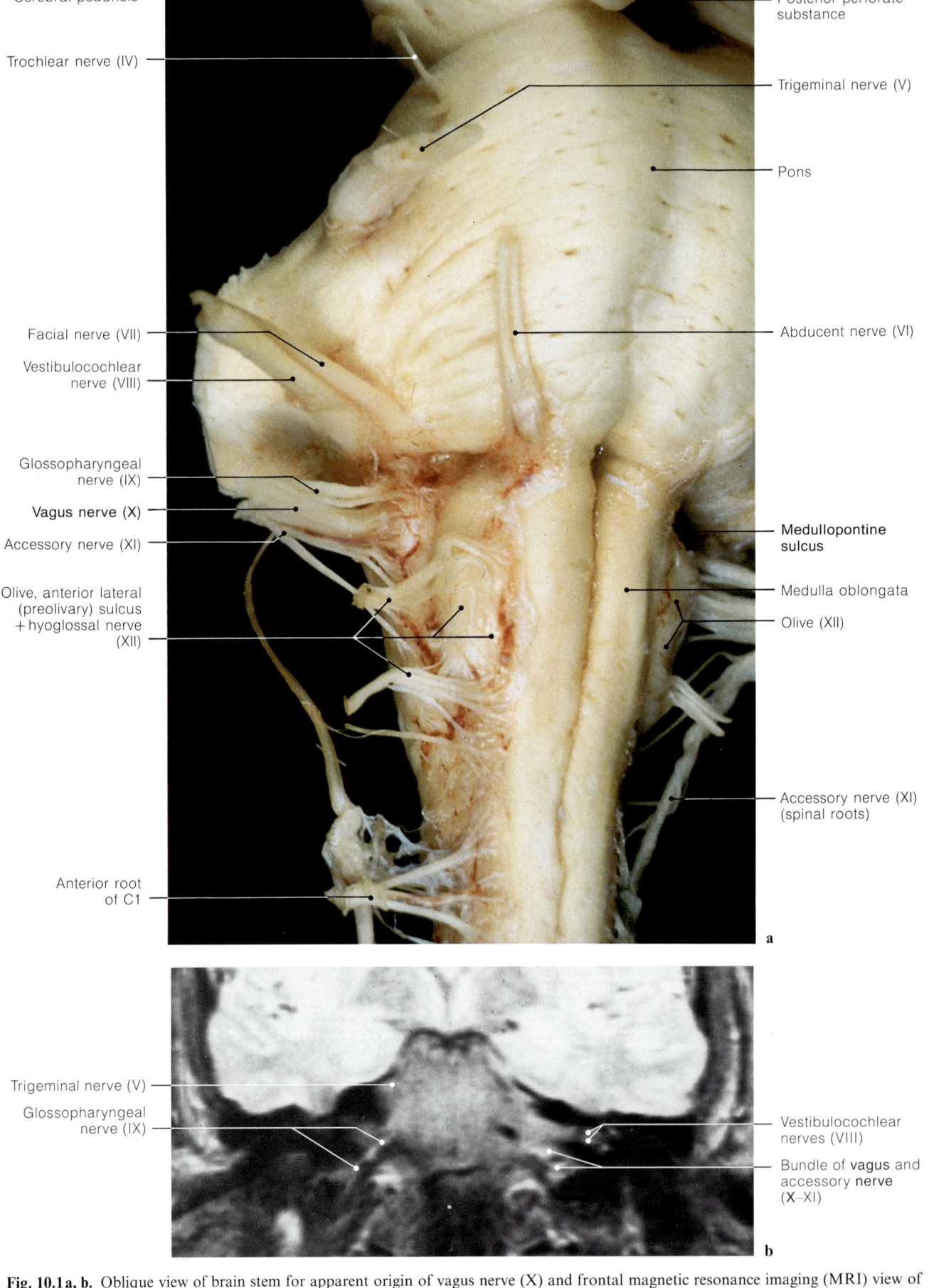

Fig. 10.1 a, b. Oblique view of brain stem for apparent origin of vagus nerve (X) and frontal magnetic resonance imaging (MRI) view of the bundle of glossopharyngeal, vagus and accessory nerve (IX–X–XI). (MRI: Pr. Doyon, Hospital Kremlin Bicêtre, Paris)

Anatomy

COURSE–TERMINALS–COLLATERALS

Apparent origin and intracranial course

Intracanalicular course

Orifice of auricular branch of vagus nerve (anastomotic branch with facial nerve (VII–IX))

Imaging

REGIONS EXAMINED

Posterior lateral sulcus of medulla oblongata
Study of cerebellopontine cistern

Comparative study of jugular foramina

Examination of third part of facial canal and tegmen of jugular foramen to display the ostium introitus and sulcus of the vagus nerve (VII–X)

Pathology

Apparent origin:
– Syndrome of medulla oblongata with paralysis of sternocleidomastoid and trapezius muscles,
– syndrome of medulla oblongata,
– Jackson's syndrome.

Jugular foramen and ostium introitus of auricular branch:
– Jugular foramen syndrome (Vernet's syndrome),
– posterior condylolacerate junction syndrome (Collet-Sicard syndrome),
– syndrome of the posterior retroparotid space, with paralysis of the last four pairs of cranial nerves and of the cervical sympathetic plexus (Villaret's syndrome),
– paralysis of the dilator muscles of the glottis (Gerhardt's syndrome),
– large cholesteatoma of middle ear extending towards jugular bulb.

Author's note: This study of the vagus nerve is restricted to examination of the proximal segment as far as its entry into the retrostyloid space.

Vagus nerve (X)

Magnetic resonance imaging (MRI) and computed tomography (CT)

AXIAL VIEWS

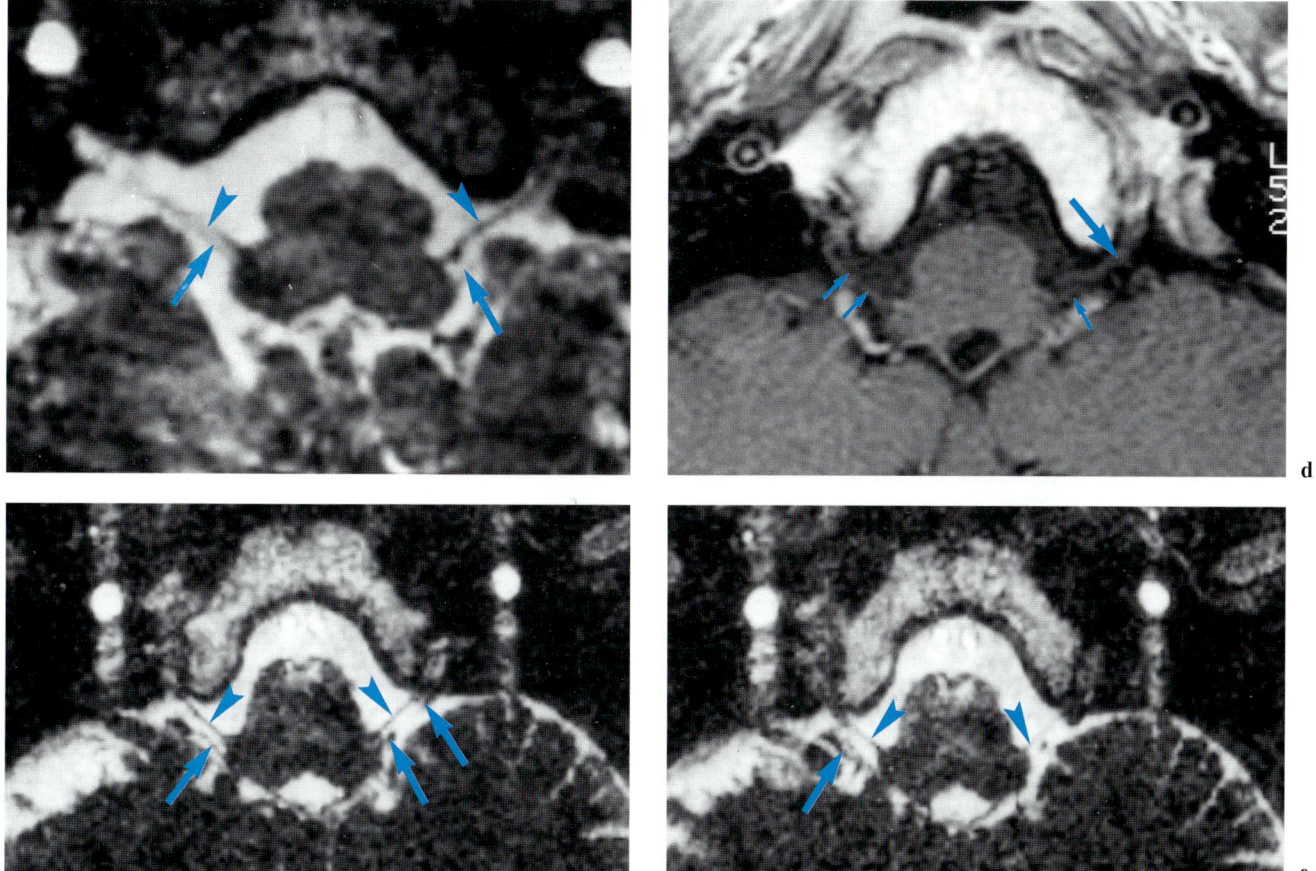

Fig. 10.1c–f. Axial magnetic resonance imaging (MRI) of the vagus nerve (X) (*arrow*), accessory nerve (XI) (*small arrows*), glossopharyngeal nerve (IX) (*arrowhead*). (MRI: **e, f** Neuroradiology A.Z. St-Jan, Brugge; **c, d** Radiology Hospital Kremlin Bicêtre, Paris)

Topography

Apparent origin of vagus nerve (X)
– Posterior lateral sulcus of medulla oblongata

Intracanalicular course
– Jugular foramen (IX–X–XI)

Auricular branch of vagus nerve (X)
– Ostium introitus of auricular branch and sulcus of vagus nerve (X)

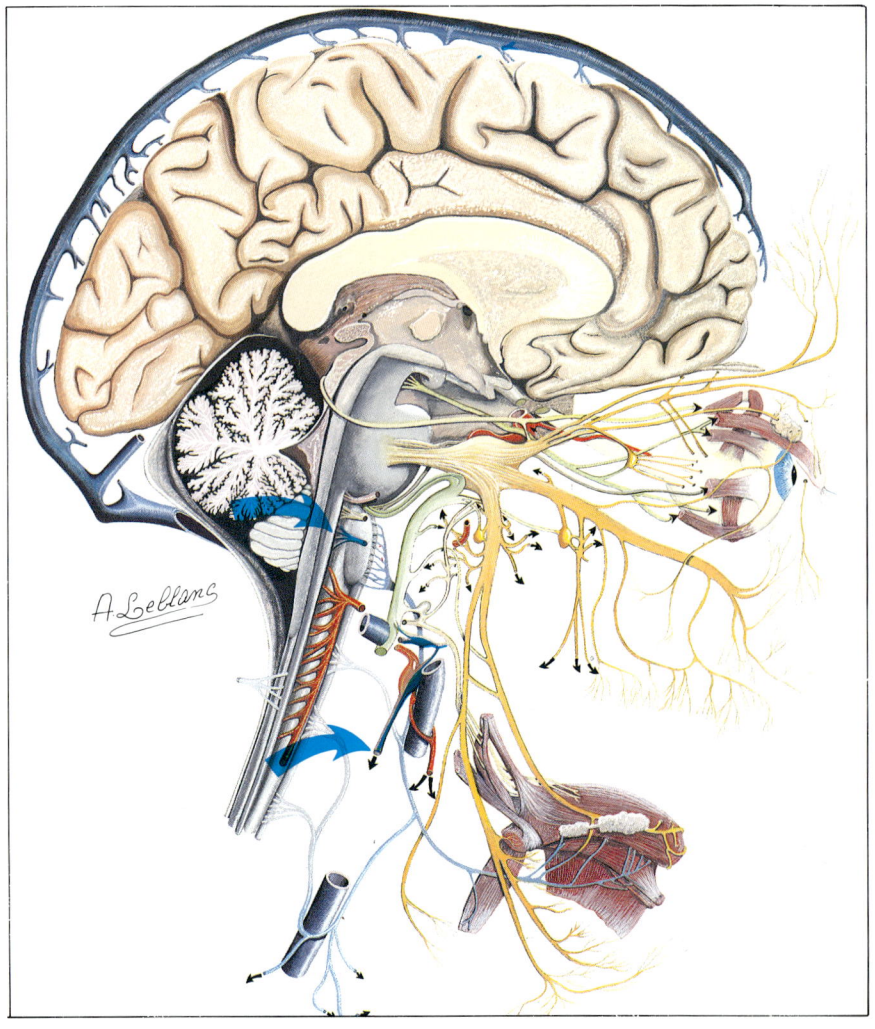

Fig. 10.2

Apparent origin of vagus nerve, posterior lateral sulcus of medulla oblongata

Anatomy

The vagus nerve (X) consists of autonomic, sensory and motor fibers. It emerges by six to eight roots which leave the neuraxis via the posterior lateral sulcus of the medulla oblongata (Fig. 10.1; 10.2).
The radicular bundles join to form a single nerve trunk.
The somatosensory fibers arise in the *superior* (or jugular) *ganglion* and enter the medulla oblongata in counterflow to the motor fibers.
The viscerosensory fibers arise in the *inferior* (or plexiform) *ganglion* (Fig. 10.6c, d; 10.7b).

Imaging

CLINICAL FEATURES

- Paralysis of soft palate and larynx,
- syndrome of medulla oblongata,
- syndrome of medulla oblongata with paralysis of sternocleidomastoid and trapezius muscles.

POSSIBLE CAUSES

- Tympanojugular paraganglioma,
- vascular lesion or root lesion at the medulla oblongata.

EXAMINATION

- Magnetic resonance imaging (MRI) or computed tomography (CT) of the cerebellopontine angle to show the posterior lateral sulcus of the medulla oblongata in sagittal, axial and frontal Worms-Bretton views (Fig. 9.4; 10.3; 10.4).

Note: The vagus nerve (X) emerges at much the same level and traverses the same orifice as the glossopharyngeal nerve. The technical procedures for the apparent origin and for imaging of the jugular foramen are therefore identical.

Cerebellopontine angle

Computed tomography (CT) and magnetic resonance imaging (MRI)

AXIAL VIEWS

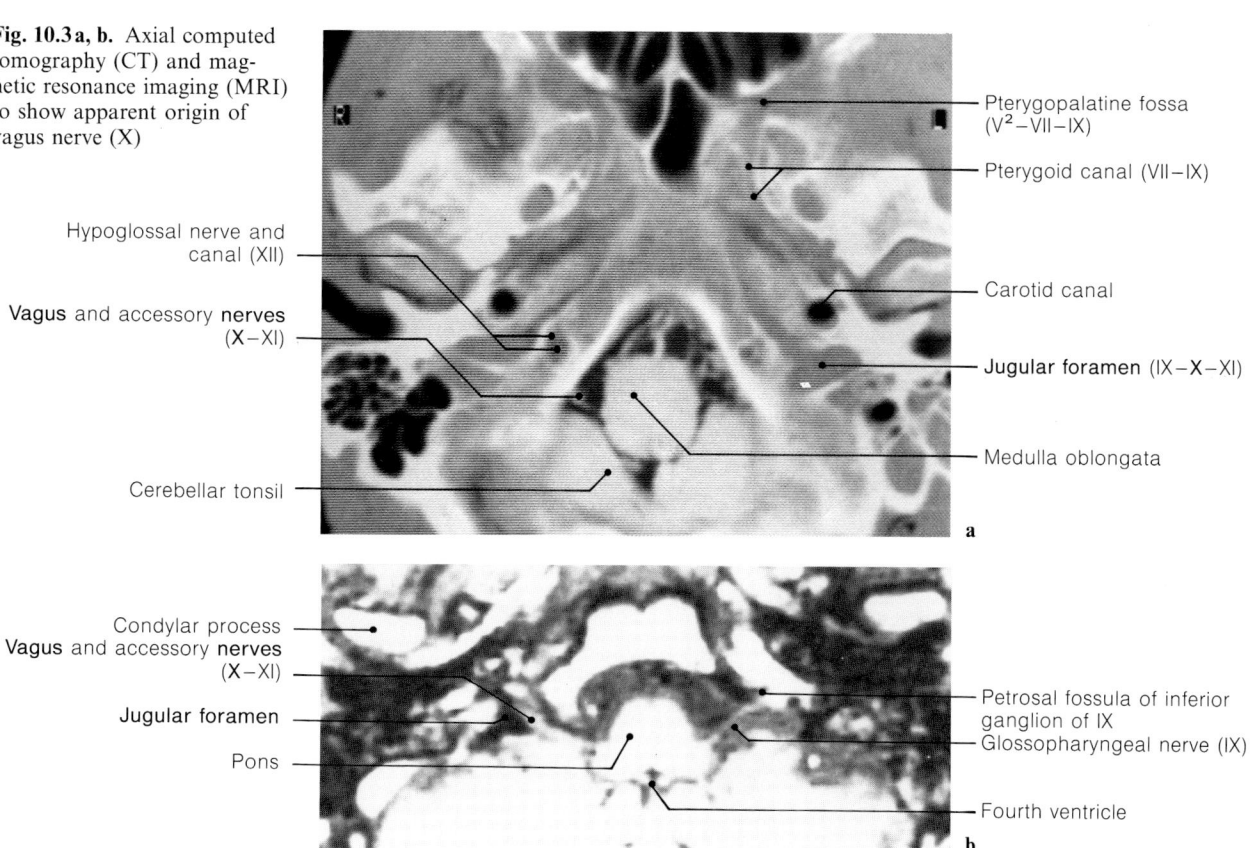

Fig. 10.3a, b. Axial computed tomography (CT) and magnetic resonance imaging (MRI) to show apparent origin of vagus nerve (X)

Jugular foramen

Anatomy

Course – relations

In its initial intracranial course, the vagus nerve (X) is situated in the posterior cranial fossa where it travels outwards, forwards and slightly upwards.

It then traverses the jugular foramen, where it exhibits the superior (or jugular) ganglion. Here, it occupies the intermediate compartment next to the accessory nerve (XI), the posterior meningeal artery, a sympathetic branch and a meningeal arterial branch. The posterior compartment contains the superior bulb of the internal jugular vein, and the anterior compartment is traversed by the glossopharyngeal nerve and the inferior petrosal sinus (Fig. 11.7c).

Once extracranial, the nerve has a long vertical course, traversing the retrostyloid space and carotid region in the neck, while in the *thorax* the right vagus nerve (X) passes behind the right main bronchus to reach the posterior aspect of the esophagus.

The left vagus nerve (X) passes in front of the aortic arch, gives off the left recurrent laryngeal nerve, and then passes at the back of the left main bronchus before reaching the anterior aspect of the esophagus.

Passage through the diaphragm occurs via the esophageal hiatus, and the nerve then spreads out into the posterior compartment of the abdomen. It exhibits long anastomoses constituting a periesophageal plexus. The *collateral branches* of the vagus nerve are numerous.

Imaging

Clinical features

- Lesions of the last four cranial nerves: glossopharyngeal (IX), vagus (X), accessory (XI) and hypoglossal (XII),
- lesions of the cranial nerves IX, X and XI,
- jugular foramen syndrome (Vernet's syndrome) or posterior condylolacerate junction syndrome (Collet-Sicart),
- paralysis of the dilator muscles of the glottis (Gerhardt's syndrome),
- lingual paralysis associated with otalgia.

Possible causes

- Jugular glomus tumor (paraganglioma) or traumatic lesions compressing cranial nerves IX, X, XI and XII,
- bulky cholesteatoma of the middle ear extending towards the jugular foramen,
- fractures of the petrous and occipital bones with disjunction of the lambdoid suture extending towards the posterior condylolacerate junction.

Examination

- This is identical with the methods given for study of the glossopharyngeal nerve (IX).

Vagus nerve (X)

Magnetic resonance imaging (MRI)

Oblique view

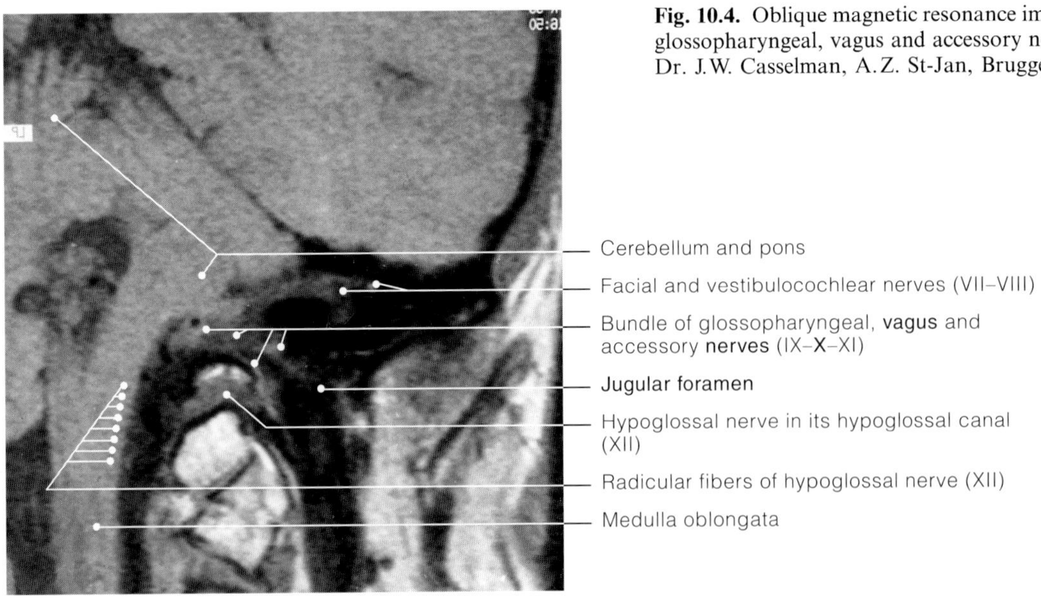

Fig. 10.4. Oblique magnetic resonance imaging (MRI) of bundle of glossopharyngeal, vagus and accessory nerves (IX–X–XI). (MRI: Dr. J.W. Casselman, A.Z. St-Jan, Brugge)

- Cerebellum and pons
- Facial and vestibulocochlear nerves (VII–VIII)
- Bundle of glossopharyngeal, **vagus** and accessory **nerves** (IX–**X**–XI)
- Jugular foramen
- Hypoglossal nerve in its hypoglossal canal (XII)
- Radicular fibers of hypoglossal nerve (XII)
- Medulla oblongata

Vagus nerve (X) 247

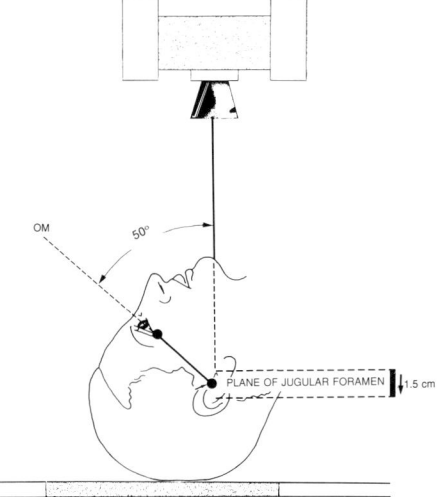

Fig. 10.5. Centering diagram for radiographic and tomographic study of the jugular foramina in symmetric view

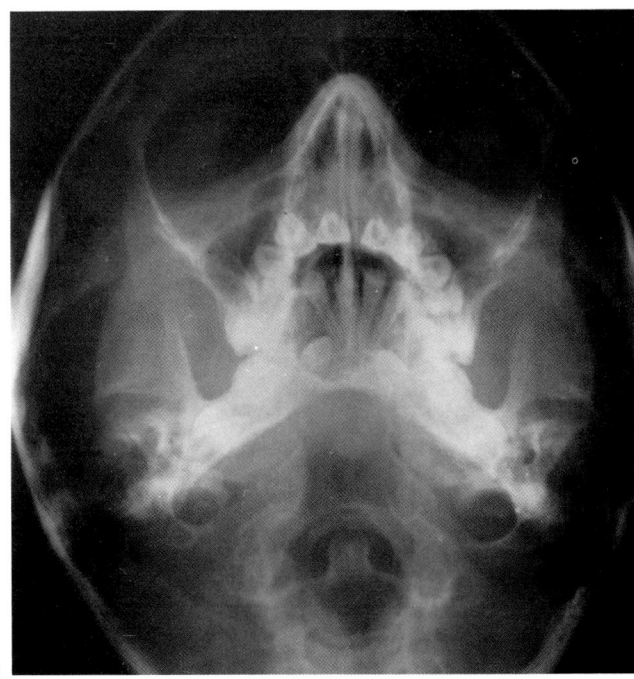

Fig. 10.6 a–d. Radiograph (**a**) and tomography (**b**) of jugular foramina in symmetric views; MRI (**c**) and diagram (**d**) of jugular foramen in sagittal views showing cranial nerves IX, X, XI and the inferior (or plexiform) ganglion

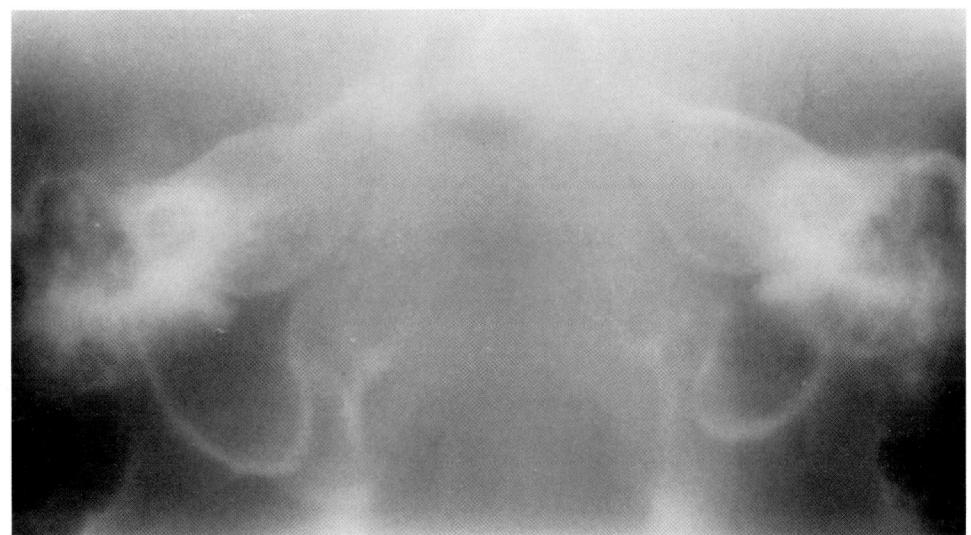

Sagittal jugular foramen and its nervous content

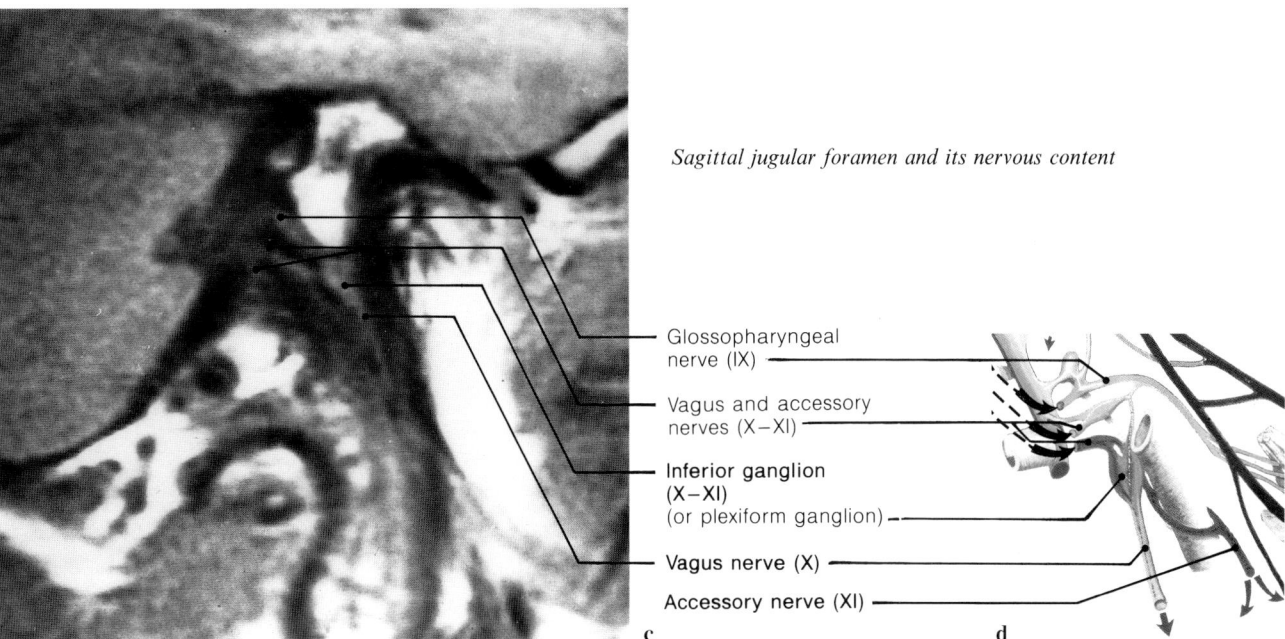

Glossopharyngeal nerve (IX)

Vagus and accessory nerves (X–XI)

Inferior ganglion (X–XI) (or plexiform ganglion)

Vagus nerve (X)

Accessory nerve (XI)

Ostium introitus, auricular branch of vagus nerve (anastomotic branch of X and VII)

Anatomy

The auricular branch emerges from the superior ganglion (Fig. 9.8c; 10.7b), enters its groove (Fig. 10.8b, c), skirts the anterolateral aspect of the jugular foramen and then enters its bony canal via the ostium introitus (Fig. 10.7b; 10.8b). Here, it travels into the facial canal to join the facial nerve (Fig. 10.7b; 10.8b).

Imaging

CLINICAL FEATURES

- Autonomic disturbances,
- jugular foramen syndromes, especially,
- Vernet's syndrome (involvement of cranial nerves IX, X and XI).

POSSIBLE CAUSES

- Jugular glomus tumor (paraganglioma),
- fractures of the skull base involving the ostium introitus and the sulcus of X (damaging the auricular branch) and the third part of the facial canal.

EXAMINATION

- Tomographic study of the third part of the facial canal and of the tegmen of the jugular foramen in the varied inclined sagittal view of Cornélis and Vignaud,
- radiographic and computed tomographic (CT) studies of the jugular foramen in sagittal, axial and oblique views and also, if possible, in discontinuous scanning so as to visualize the walls of this very sinuous foramen.

Ostium introitus and sulcus of auricular branch of vagus nerve

Fig. 10.7 a–c. Sagittal tomographic section (**a**) of ostium introitus, same section with diagram (**b**) of auricular branch of X, diagram (**c**) of the radiograph

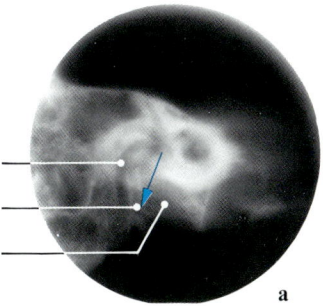

Fig. 10.8 a–c. Extracranial views of the jugular foramen in the dried bone showing ostium introitus (**a**), the sulcus of the auricular branch of X (**c**) and a diagram (**b**) of the jugular foramen to show the relations of cranial nerves IX, X and XI and the position of the auricular branch of X

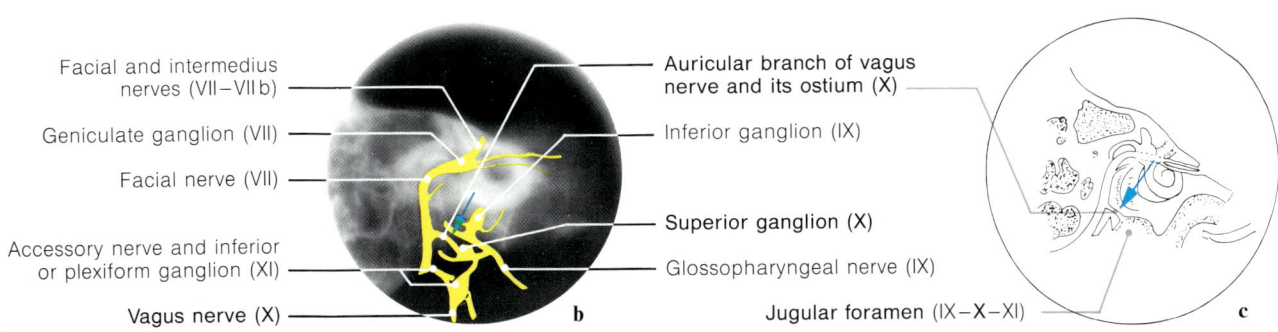

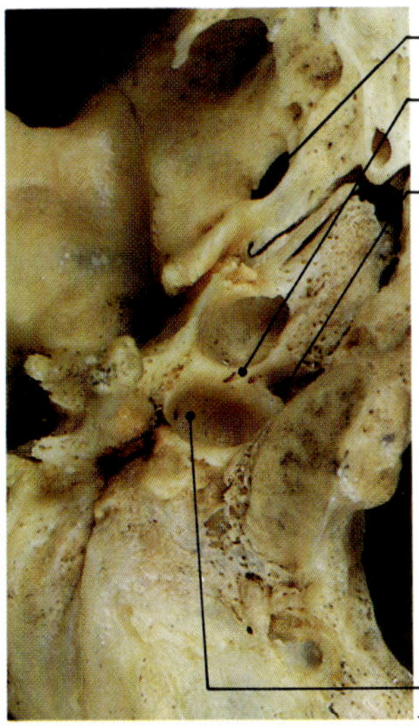

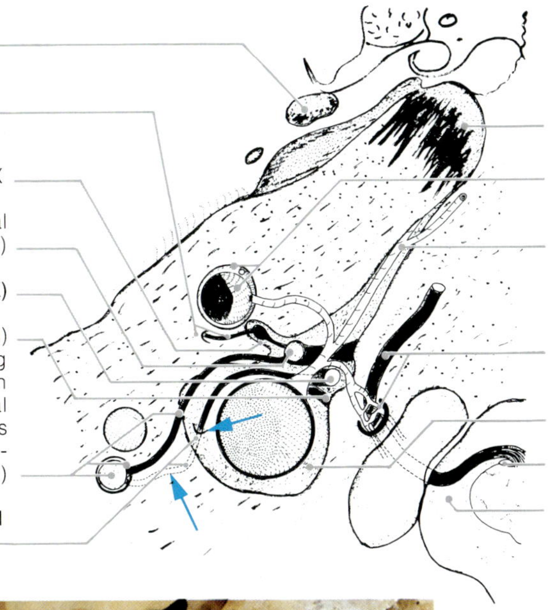

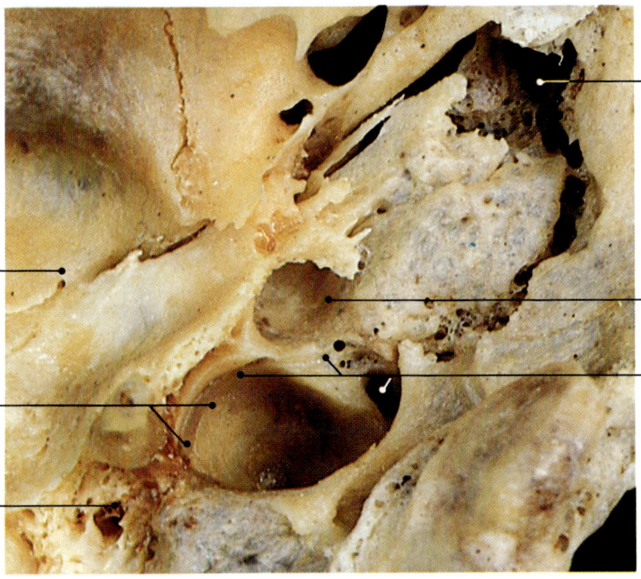

Functions of vagus nerve

Motor functions
are effected by innervation of the muscles of:
- the soft palate,
- the pharynx,
- the larynx.

Sensory functions
include:
- transmission of sensation from the larynx;
- and, together with IX, from the larynx, epiglottis, soft palate and part of the base of the tongue (Fig. 10.9; 9.14);
- it also innervates via the auricular branch a territory in the concha of the auricle and of the posterior wall of the external acoustic meatus, this territory usually being ascribed to the intermedius nerve (VII b).

The autonomic functions include innervation of the musculature of the cardiovascular, tracheobronchopulmonary and alimentary systems and of certain endocrine glands: thyroid, suprarenals and pancreas.

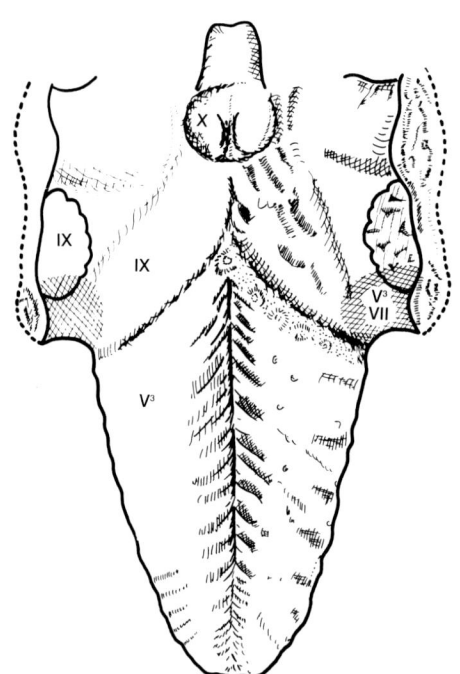

Fig. 10.9. V^3 territory of lingual nerve; V^3, VII territory of lingual branch of facial nerve; IX territory of glossopharyngeal nerve; X territory of vagus nerve (superior laryngeal nerve)

Accessory nerve (XI)
(or spinal nerve)

Anatomy (course – terminals – collaterals) 253
Imaging (regions examined) 253
Pathology 253
Axial and frontal oblique views (MRI) 253
Apparent origin of accessory nerve, posterior lateral sulcus of medulla oblongata
    Anatomy and imaging (examination) 255
    Frontal and sagittal views (MRI, CT) 255
    Axial view (CT) 256
Jugular foramen
    Anatomy and imaging 257
    Discontinuous scanning 257
    Axial view (CT) 258
    Anatomy (diagrams) 258

Vascular relations:
Internal jugular vein (jugular foramen) 238, 249, 258
Trunk in its lateral medullary portion 255, 289, 291
Jugular branch of the ascending pharyngeal
artery 276, 277
Lateral spinal artery 276, 277

The accessory nerve is a purely motor nerve. It ends partly in the vagus nerve, these fibers being destined for innervation of the pharynx and larynx, and partly in the sternocleidomastoid and trapezius muscles.
The accessory nerve arises in the spinal cord and medulla oblongata (bulb). It travels initially within the craniospinal cavity and then traverses the jugular foramen. Subsequently, it has a short extracranial course and rapidly divides into its terminal branches: the lateral and medial branches.

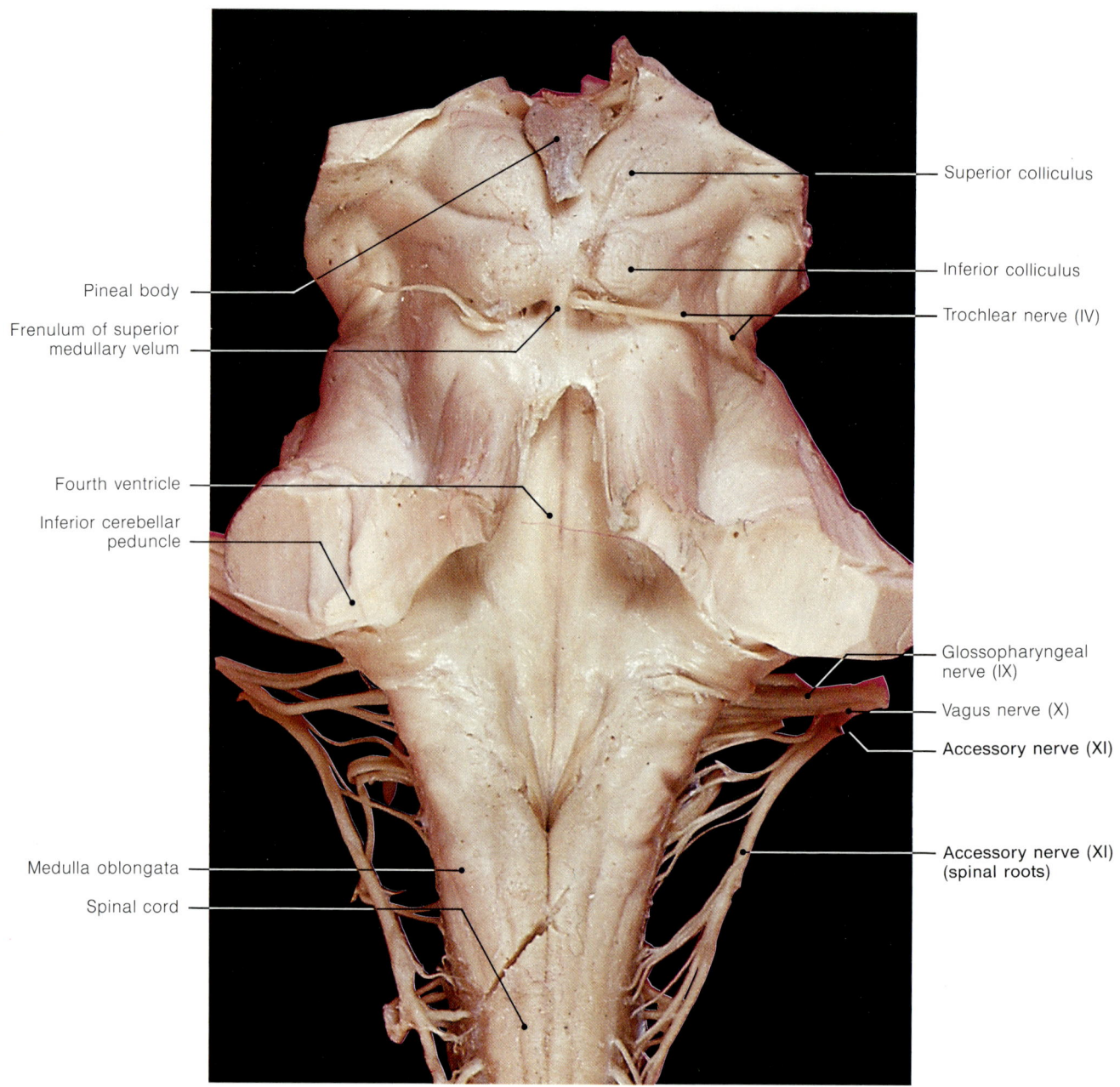

Fig. 11.1. Posterior anatomic view of brain-stem showing the apparent origin of the accessory nerve (XI)

Anatomy

COURSE – TERMINALS – COLLATERALS

Apparent origins of cranial and spinal roots

Intracanalicular course

Imaging

REGIONS EXAMINED

Posterior lateral sulcus and lateral cord of medulla oblongata

Study of cerebellopontine angle and medulla oblongata

Study of jugular foramen

Pathology

Apparent origin

Spinal cord:
- Basilar impression,
- Arnold-Chiari syndrome,
- cervical fractures, cervical spondylosis.

Medulla oblongata:
- Radicular involvement (vascular lesion) and cervical fractures,
- syndrome of medulla oblongata with paralysis of sternocleidomastoid and trapezius muscles (Avellis's syndrome),
- complete paralysis of the accessory and hypoglossal nerves (Jackson's syndrome).

Jugular foramen:
- Jugular foramen syndrome (Vernet's syndrome),
- posterior condylolacerate junction syndrome (Collet-Sicard syndrome),
- syndrome of the posterior retroparotid space, with paralysis of the last four pairs of cranial nerves and of the cervical sympathetic plexus (Villaret's syndrome),
- fractures.

Accessory nerve (IX) (See vascular relations, pp. 289, 291)

Magnetic resonance imaging (MRI)

AXIAL AND FRONTAL OBLIQUE VIEWS

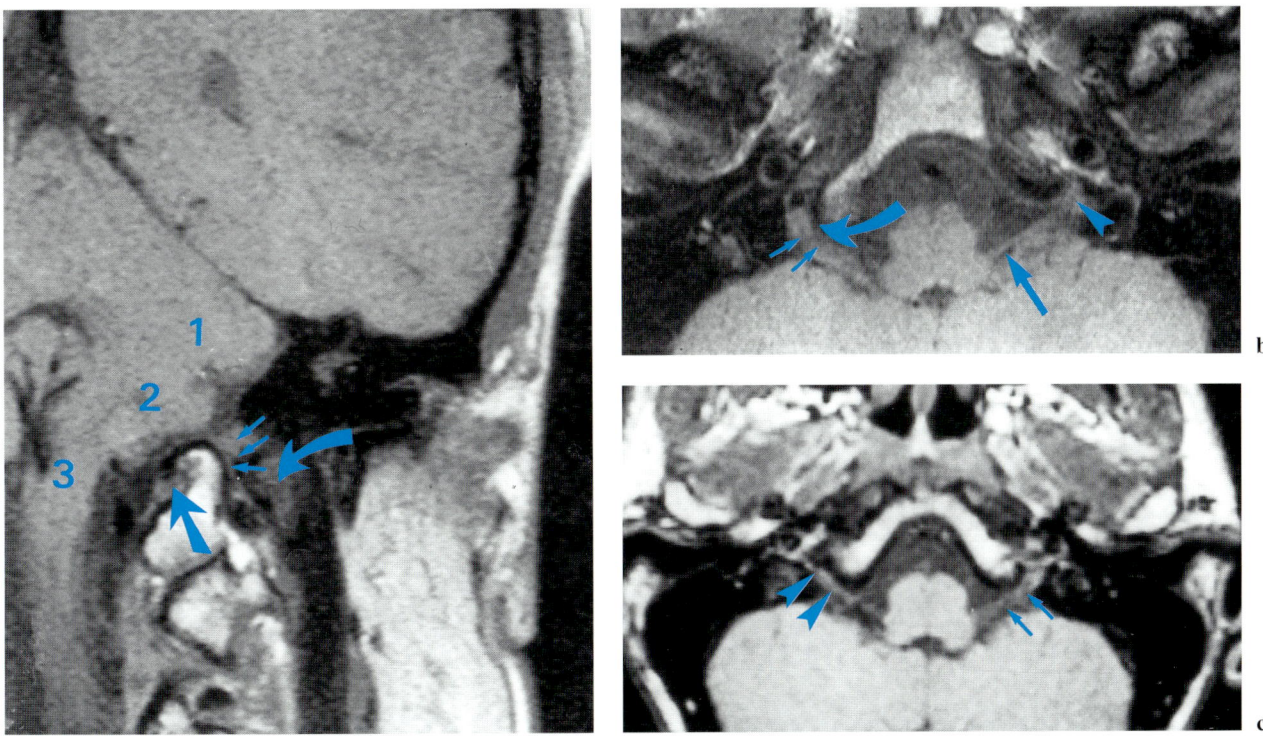

Fig. 11.1a–c. Axial and frontal oblique magnetic resonance imaging (MRI) showing mixed nerves: vagus and accessory nerves (X–XI) (*double, small arrows*), glossopharyngeal nerve (*large, straight arrow*), glossopharyngeal nerve entering petrosal fossula (*arrowhead*), glossopharyngeal and vagus nerves (IX–X) (*double arrowheads*), bundle of glossopharyngeal, vagus and accessory nerves (IX–X–XI) (*triple, small arrows*), hypoglossal nerve (XII) (*large arrow*), jugular foramen (*curved arrow*). *1*, cerebral peduncle; *2*, pons; *3*, medulla oblongata. (MRI: Dr. J.W. Casselman, A.Z. St-Jan, Brugge)

Accessory nerve (XI)

Topography

Apparent origins of cranial and spinal roots of accessory nerve (XI)
- Posterior lateral sulcus and lateral cord of medulla oblongata

Intracanalicular course
- Jugular foramen (IX–X–XI)

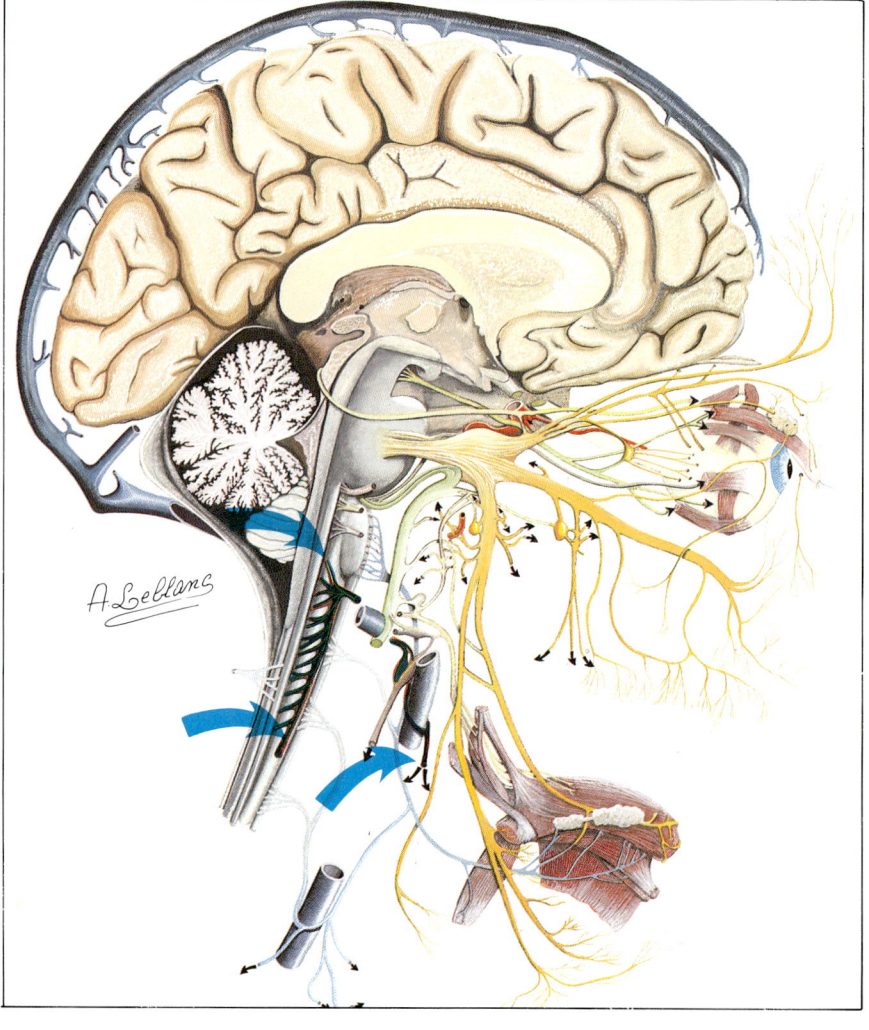

Fig. 11.3 a–c. Frontal MRI (**c**) showing the cranial nerves IX, X and XI at their encephalic origins; sagittal computed tomographic (CT) (**a**) and anatomic section (**b**) of the lateral region of the cord to show the cranial and spinal roots of the accessory nerve (XI)

Fig. 11.2

Apparent origin of accessory nerve, posterior lateral sulcus of medulla oblongata

Anatomy

The origin of the accessory nerve is double: cranial (bulbar) and spinal.
The **spinal root** arises in the spinal cord from C1 to C6 (Fig. 11.1; 11.2).
The radicular fibers travel backwards and then transversely outwards. They emerge in front of the posterior cervical roots towards the front of the posterior lateral sulcus as six or seven strands which come together: The spinal root ascends vertically within the spinal canal between the posterior roots behind and the denticulate ligament in front, traverses the foramen magnum and then, once intracranial, travels obliquely outwards and upwards in the posterior cranial fossa.
The **cranial root**: The radicular fibers travel outwards and forward to reach the posterior lateral sulcus of medulla oblongata. The apparent origin consists of four to five roots which unite in a trunk applied to the spinal root.

Imaging

Clinical features

- Paralysis of the sternocleidomastoid and trapezius muscles,
- limitation of movement of the neck, accompanied by occipital headache and vertigo,
- cervical fractures.

Possible causes in the spinal cord

- Compression produced during processes deforming the atlanto-occipital joint (basilar impression) or by tumoral lesions. Further, the lateral branch of XI may be damaged in the neck by injury or by compression due to adenopathy.

Possible causes in the medulla oblongata

- Radicular involvement associated with a vascular or tumoral lesion or with polyencephalitis,
- Avellis's syndrome, etc.

Examination

- Computed tomography (CT) of the cerebellopontine angle to show the posterior lateral sulcus of medulla oblongata in axial and sagittal views and the frontal Worms-Bretton view.
It is additionally necessary to make lateralized sagittal sections of the cord in order to display the spinal roots of the accessory nerve (XI) (Fig. 11.3).

Note: The technical performance of this examination is virtually identical with that for the origins of the glossopharyngeal (IX) and vagus (X) nerves.

Magnetic resonance imaging (MRI) and computed tomography (CT)

Sagittal and frontal views

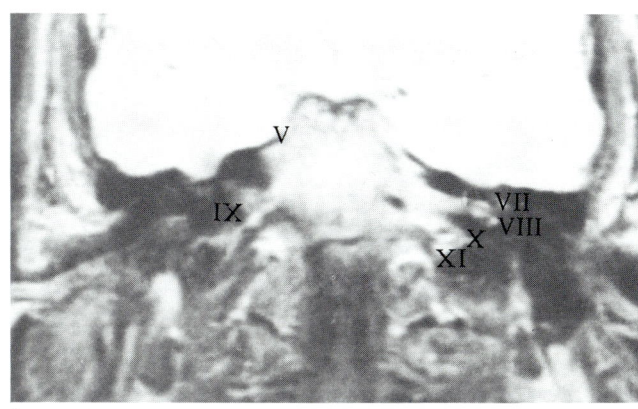

c

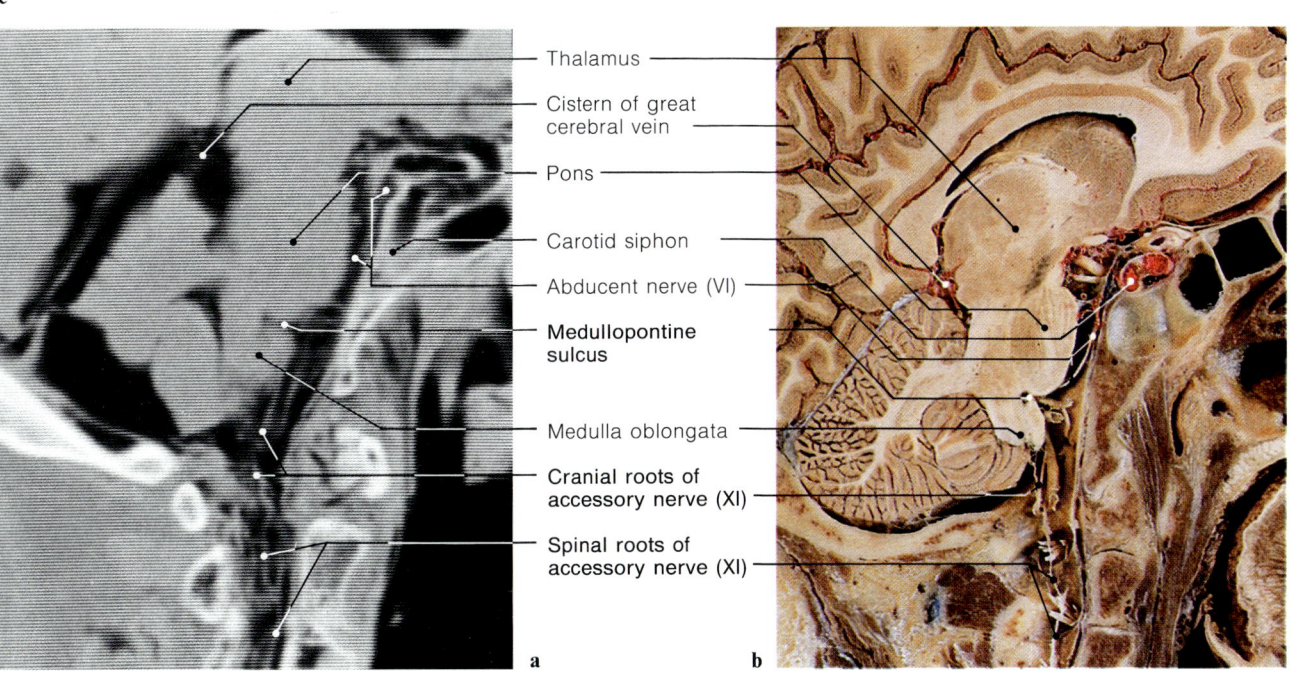

- Thalamus
- Cistern of great cerebral vein
- Pons
- Carotid siphon
- Abducent nerve (VI)
- Medullopontine sulcus
- Medulla oblongata
- Cranial roots of accessory nerve (XI)
- Spinal roots of accessory nerve (XI)

a   b

Computed tomography (CT)

AXIAL VIEW

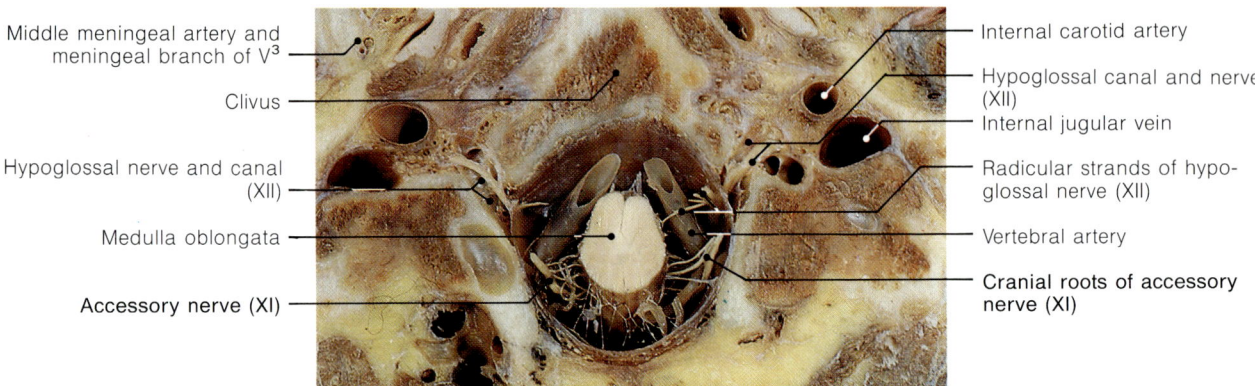

Fig. 11.4. Axial anatomic section of cranial roots of the accessory nerve (XI)

Fig. 11.5 a, b. Computed tomography (CT) of spinal cord and medulla oblongata, visualizing the accessory nerve and its spinal and cranial roots in semiaxial and axial views

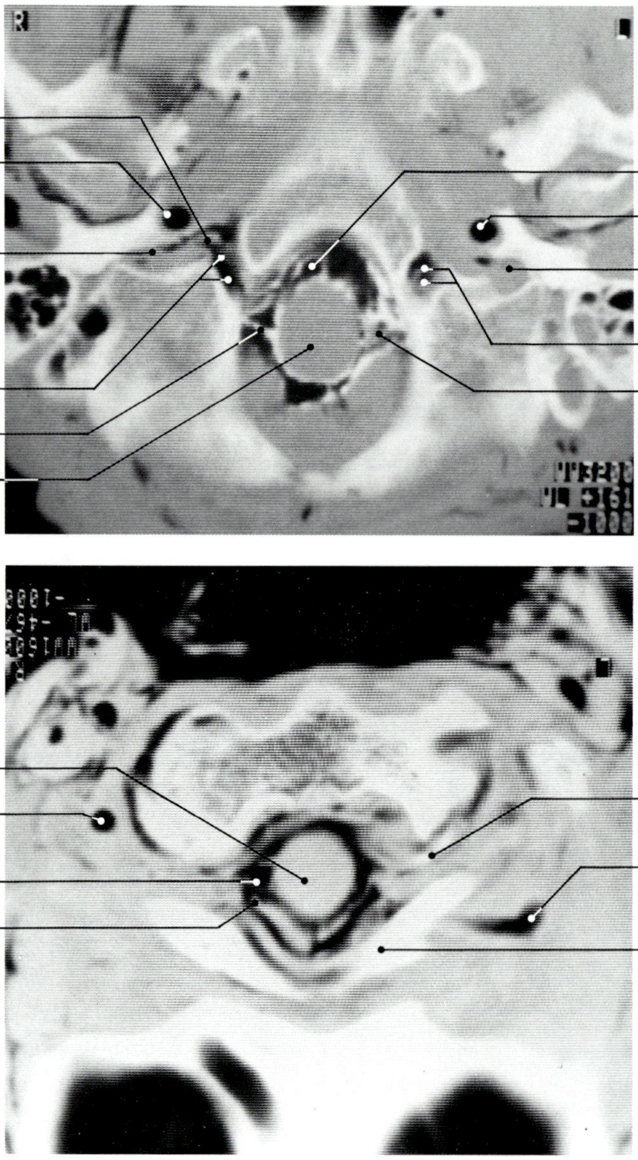

Jugular foramen

Anatomy

The accessory nerve (XI) traverses the jugular foramen, occupying the intermediate compartment together with the vagus nerve (X), the posterior meningeal artery and a sympathetic branch (Fig. 11.7c).
The anterior compartment is traversed by the glossopharyngeal nerve (IX) and the inferior petrosal sinus. The bulb of the internal jugular vein is situated in the posterior compartment.

Terminal branches

1) The *lateral branch* consists of nerve strands derived from the spinal root. It travels outwards and downwards in the posterior subparotid space and emerges to cross the inferior border of the digastric muscle to reach the deep aspect of the sternocleidomastoid muscle. Some fibers of the lateral branch of XI receive an anastomosis from the anterior branch of C3 cervical nerve; after having received an anastomosis from branches of C3, 4 and 5 cervical nerves, it ends by supplying the trapezius muscle.
2) The *medial branch* is formed of fibers derived from the cranial root. It is slender and short and proceeds rapidly to the upper end of the inferior (plexiform) ganglion, bringing to the vagus nerve (X) fibers destined for the larynx.

The accessory nerve (XI) thus gives fibers:
– to the pharyngeal plexus, which supplies all the muscles of the soft palate,
– to the superior laryngeal nerve, which goes to the cricothyroid muscle,
– to the recurrent nerve, which supplies the other laryngeal muscles. The accessory nerve (XI) takes the same orificial pathway as the glossopharyngeal (IX) and vagus (X) nerves.

Imaging

The syndromes and intracanalicular vulnerable points, as also the imaging, are identical with those cited previously for the jugular foramen. On this occasion the "discontinuous scanning" technique is cited.

Technique

– Radiologic study of jugular foramen by *"discontinuous scanning"*: The view and centering point are identical with those employed for imaging of the jugular foramen in unilateral oblique view (Fig. 9.6a, b). The patient's head remains in the same position and only the angle of the tube varies. After having taken a film of the jugular foramen in its axis, the tube is inclined by 5° to 7° in relation to the centering point, and then a successive series of four films is made during rotation of the tube (Fig. 11.6a).

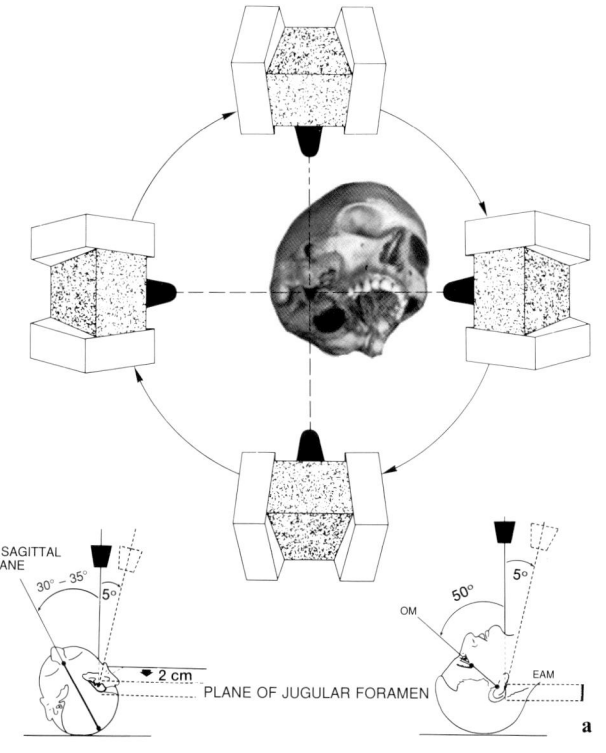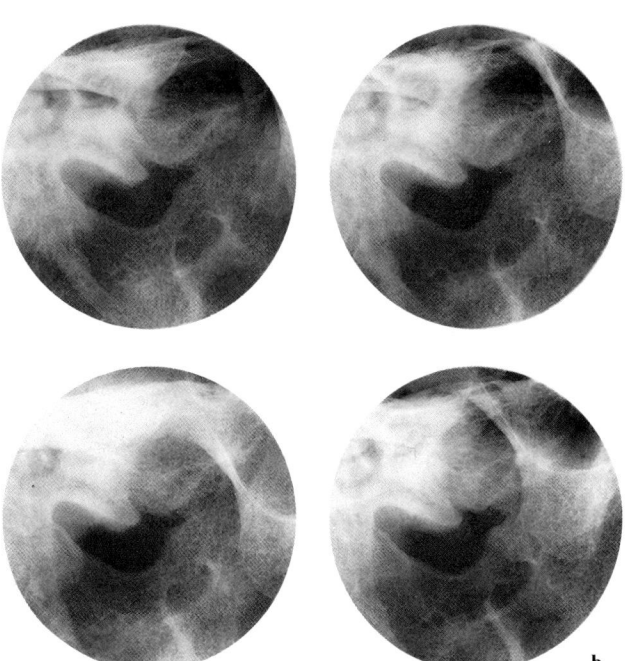

Fig. 11.6. **a** Centering diagram for imaging of the jugular foramen by "discontinuous scanning"; **b** films obtained

Jugular foramen

Computed tomography (CT)

AXIAL VIEW

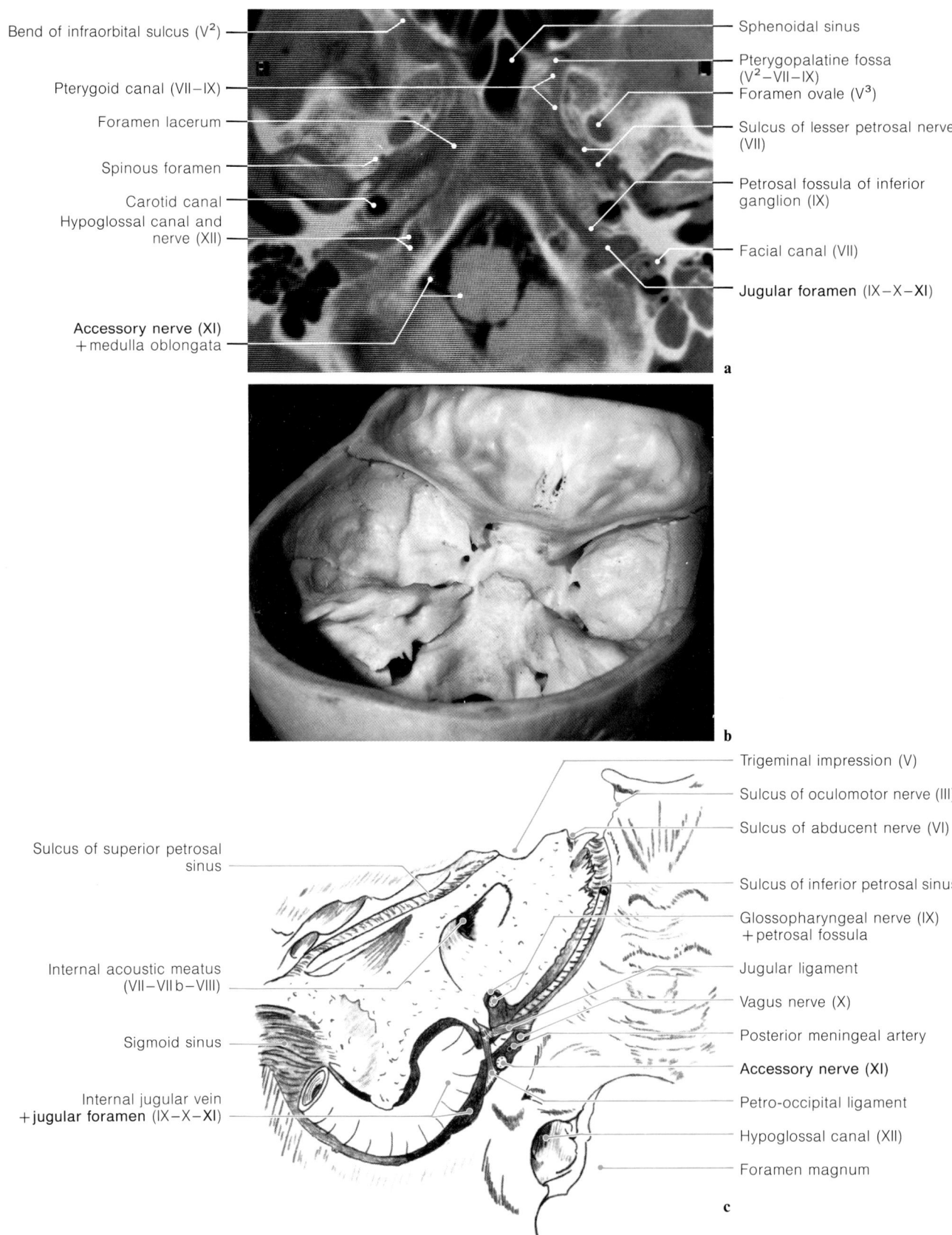

Fig. 11.7a–c. Axial computed tomographic (CT) section (**a**) of jugular foramina; dried bone (**b**) with diagram (**c**) showing arrangement of neurovascular structures of the jugular foramen – intracranial view

Hypoglossal nerve (XII)

Anatomy (course–terminals–collaterals) 261
Imaging (regions examined) 261
Pathology 261
Apparent origin of hypoglossal nerve,
anterior lateral medullary (preolivary) sulcus
of medulla oblongata
    Anatomy and imaging (examination) 263
      Cerebellopontine angle, prepontine cistern
        Sagittal view (MRI) 263
      Cerebellopontine angle
        Axial view (MRI, CT) 264
        Frontal view (CT) 266
Hypoglossal canal
    Anatomy and imaging (examination) 267
    Oblique view (radiology, tomography) 268
    Oblique, axial, semiaxial and sagittal views
    (radiology, tomography, MRI) 269
    Oblique view (discontinuous scanning) 270
    Oblique axial view (CT) 270
Hypoglossal nerve and canal
    Frontal, axial, sagittal, and oblique views (MRI) .. 271
Communicating and terminal branches
    Anatomy (diagram) 272

Vascular relations:
Vertebral artery 265
Hypoglossal vein,
hypoglossal branch of the ascending pharyngeal
artery 276, 277
Hypoglossal artery 292

The hypoglossal nerve provides the motor innervation of the tongue. The radicular strands leave the medulla oblongata via the preolivary sulcus and join to form two nerve trunks which reach the hypoglossal canal.
It then successively traverses the retrostyloid, carotid and submandibular and sublingual regions to end at the outer aspect of the genioglossus muscle.
Hypoglossal paralysis is indicated by loss or impairment of movement of the tongue; the lesion may affect the central or the peripheral neurone and may assume different clinical aspects.

260 Hypoglossal nerve (XII)

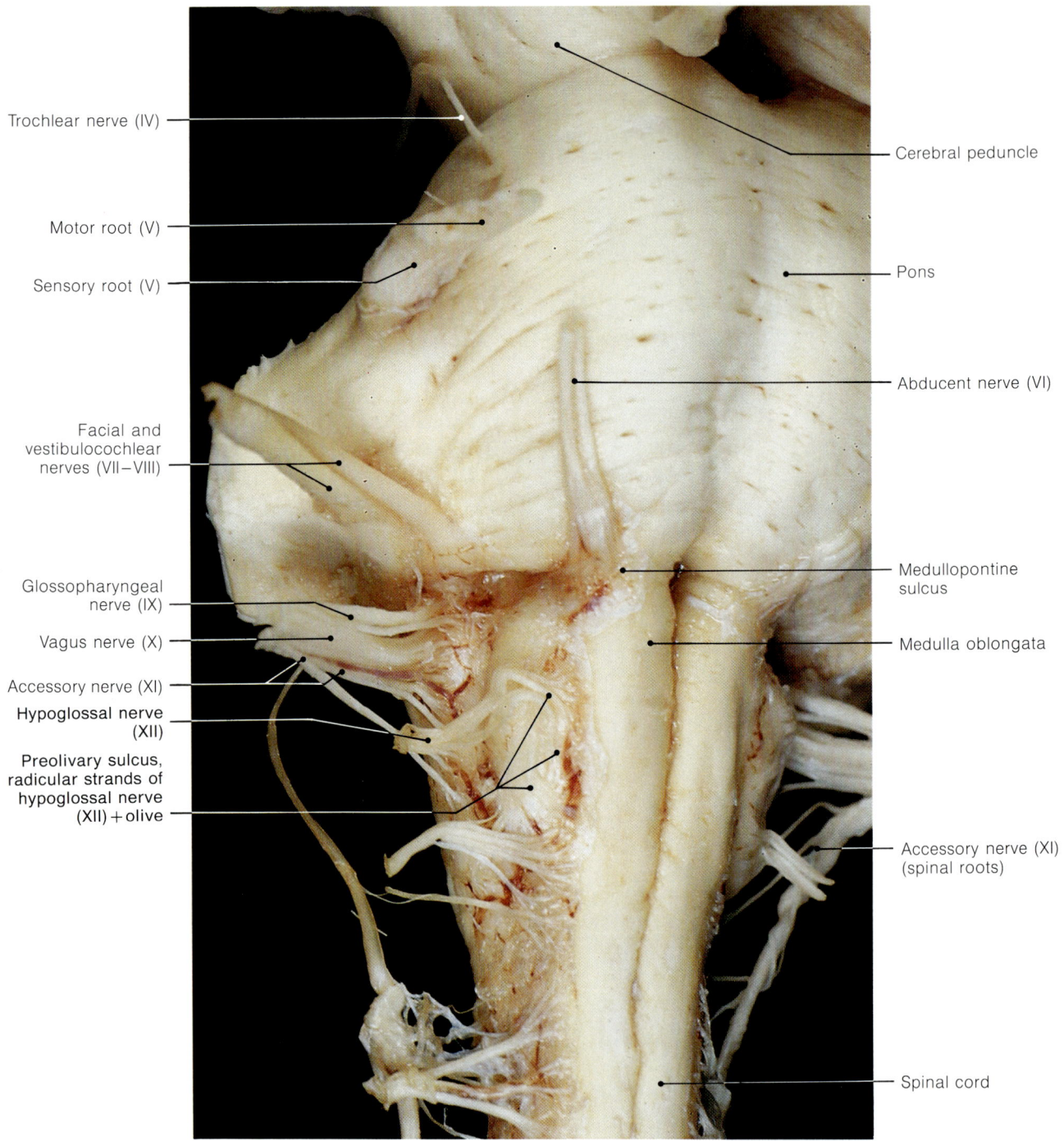

Fig. 12.1. Oblique view of brain-stem to show apparent origin of hypoglossal nerve (XII) at anterior lateral (preolivary) sulcus

Anatomy

COURSE – TERMINALS – COLLATERALS

Apparent origin

Intracanalicular course

Imaging

REGIONS EXAMINED

Anterior lateral (or preolivary) sulcus
Study of prepontine cistern and cerebellopontine angle

Study of hypoglossal canal

Pathology

Medulla oblongata:
– Complete paralysis of the accessory and hypoglossal nerves (XI and XII) (Jackson's syndrome).

Hypoglossal canal:
– Fracture,
– neurinoma,
– jugular glomus tumor (paraganglioma).

Periphery:
– Tumors of skull base,
– amygdaloid tumors, parotid tumors, neoplastic lymphadenopathies of buccorhinopharyngeal origin,
– bony compressions: malformations of the atlanto-occipital joint (basilar impression), suboccipital spinal tuberculosis,
– injury: section of the hypoglossal nerve by deep neck wounds.

Hypoglossal nerve (XII)

Topography

Apparent origin of hypoglossal nerve (XII)
– Anterior lateral (preolivary) sulcus of medulla oblongata

Hypoglossal canal (anterior condylar canal)
– Hypoglossal nerve

Communicating and terminal branches

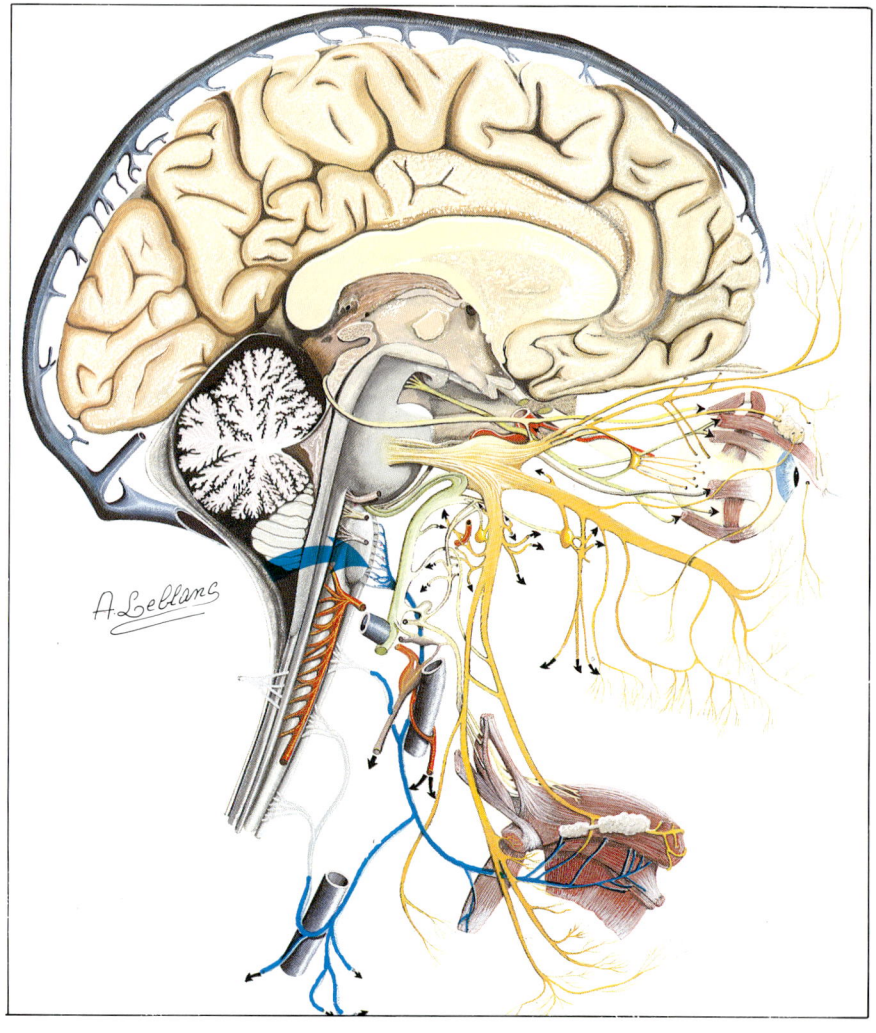

Fig. 12.2

Apparent origin of hypoglossal nerve, anterior lateral (preolivary) sulcus of medulla oblongata

Anatomy

The *nucleus of origin* extends throughout almost the entire length of the medulla oblongata (bulb) and projects into the hypoglossal trigone of the floor of the fourth ventricle (Fig. 11.1).

The *hypoglossal nucleus* receives fibers derived from the cortical center for lingual movements.

The *radicular fibers* of the hypoglossal nerve travel forward and then outwards, and pass between the median longitudinal fascicle, medial lemniscus, accessory olivary nucleus and pyramidal tract medially and the olive laterally.

These roots, to the number of 10 to 12, emerge from the neuraxis via the preolivary sulcus (Fig. 12.1–12.3; 12.12), and then, surrounded by a sheath, travel within the posterior cranial fossa obliquely outwards and forward towards the hypoglossal canal (Fig. 12.4a; 12.5a; 12.6a, b; 12.8). Inferiorly, the nerve is related to the vertebral artery, which passes under its lower roots.

Imaging

The hypoglossal nerve may be damaged at any point in its course.

CLINICAL FEATURES
- Bulbar syndrome,
- Jackson's syndrome (lesion of cranial nerves XI and XII, unilateral paralysis of vocal cord, soft palate, trapezius and sternocleidomastoid muscles plus hemiparalysis of tongue).

POSSIBLE CAUSES
- Vertebrobasilar aneurysm,
- fracture or impression of basilary region (compression of inferior olivary roots)

VIEWS REQUIRED
- Magnetic resonance imaging (MRI) and computed tomography (CT) of cerebellopontine angle and prepontine cistern to show anterior lateral (preolivary) sulcus of medulla oblongata in sagittal (Fig. 12.3), axial (Fig. 12.4) and frontal views (Fig. 12.6).

The techniques to be employed here are very much the same as those for examination of cranial nerves IX, X and XI, except that the hypoglossal nerve (XII) emerges slightly below and in front (Fig. 9.1; 12.1; 12.2).

Sagittal view (MRI)

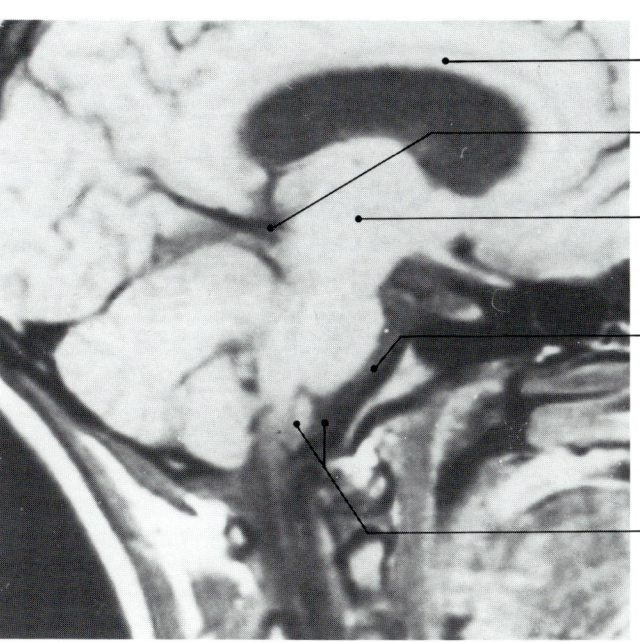

Fig. 12.3a, b. Sagittal magnetic resonance imaging (MRI) of preolivary sulcus of medulla oblongata to show apparent origin of hypoglossal nerve (XII). Cerebellopontine angle, prepontine cistern

Magnetic resonance imaging (MRI) and computed tomography (CT)

CEREBELLOPONTINE ANGLE

Axial view

Fig. 12.4a–c. Axial cisternal computed tomograms (CT) showing course of hypoglossal nerve from its origin to the hypoglossal canal (XII)

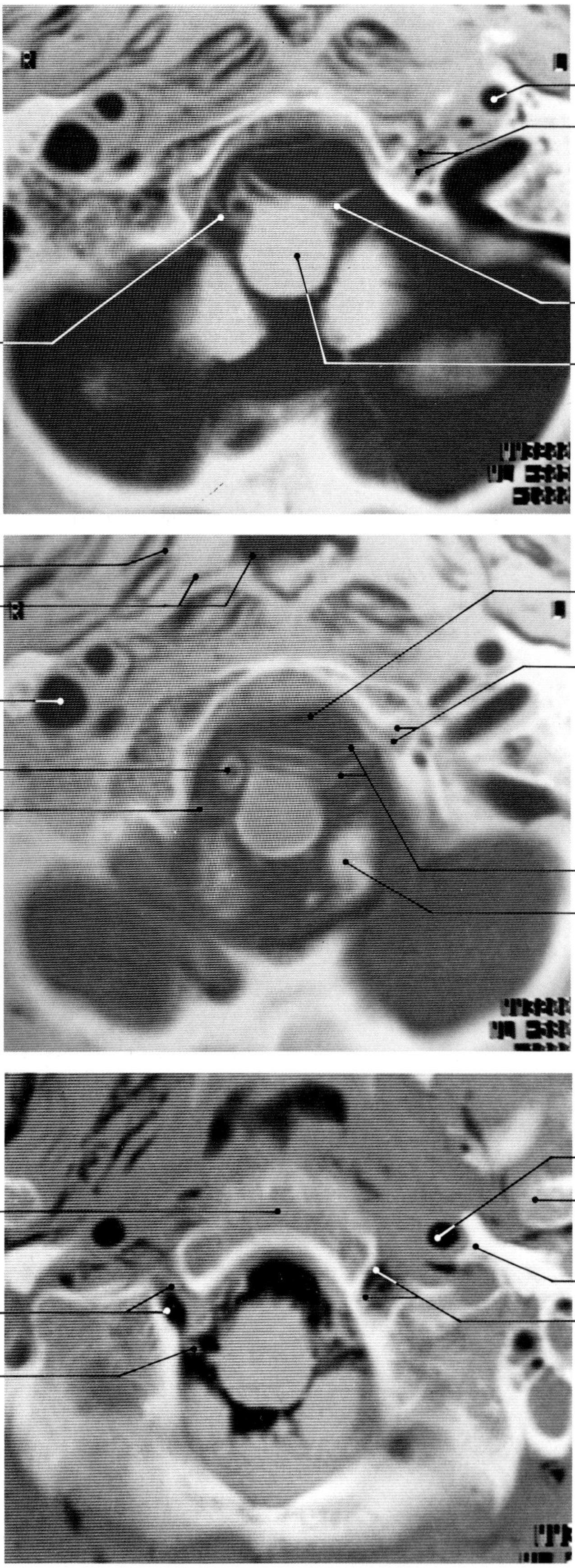

Radicular fibers of hypoglossal nerve (XII)

Internal carotid artery

Hypoglossal canal and nerve (XII)

Hypoglossal nerve (XII) (emergence)

Medulla oblongata

Auditory tube

Cavum + pharyngeal recess

Internal jugular vein

Vertebral artery
Vagus and accessory nerves (X–XII)

Foramen magnum

Hypoglossal canal and nerve (XII)

Radicular fibers of hypoglossal nerve (XII)

Cerebellar tonsil

Clivus

Hypoglossal canal and nerve (XII)

Accessory nerve (XI)

Internal carotid artery

Condylar process

Petrous apex

Hypoglossal canal and nerve (XII)

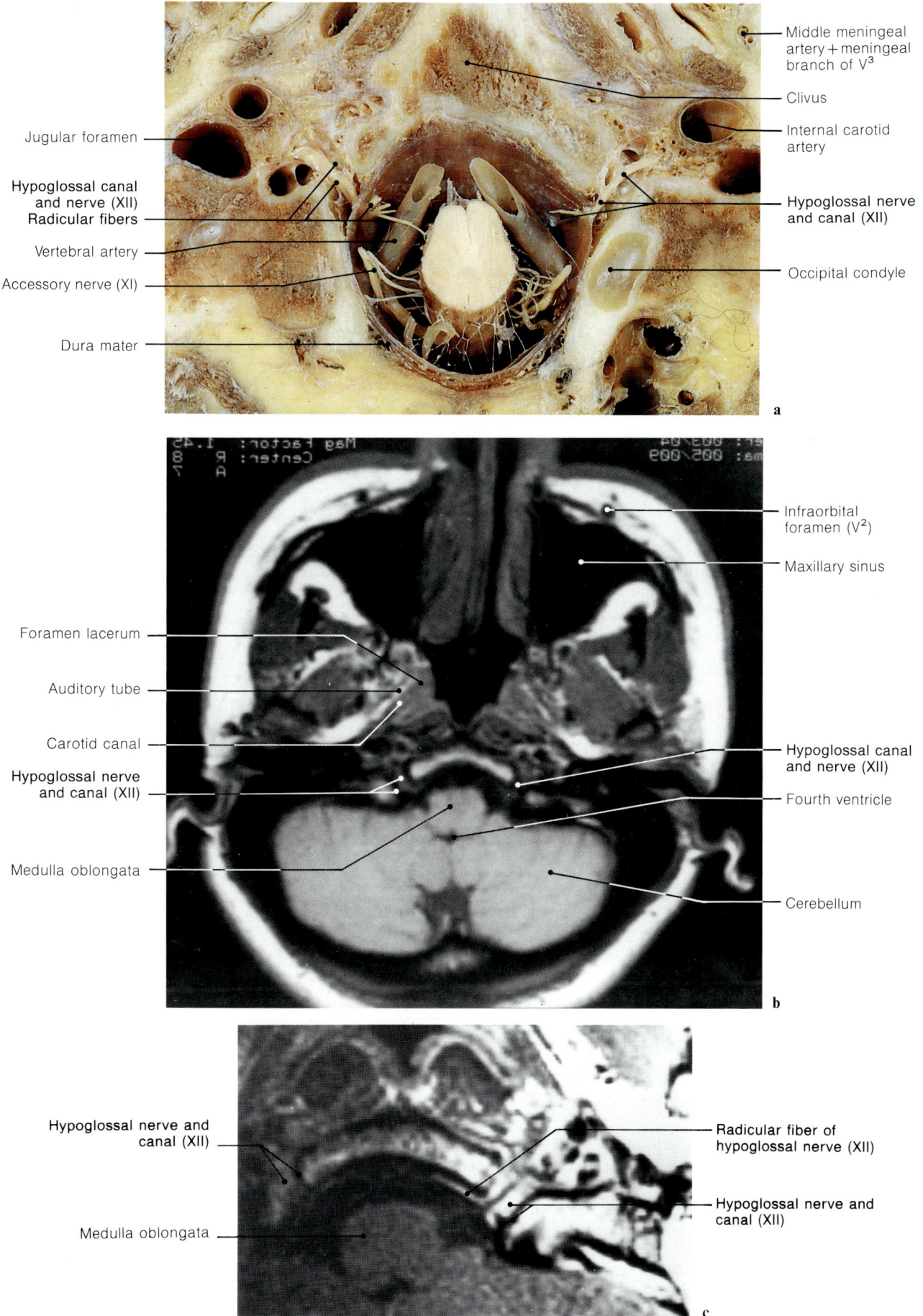

Fig. 12.5a–c. Anatomic section (**a**) and magnetic resonance imaging (**b, c**) axial views at apparent origin of hypoglossal nerve and its passage through the hypoglossal canal (XII). (MRI: Radiologie, Hospital Kremlin Bicêtre, Paris)

Computed tomography (CT)

CEREBELLOPONTINE ANGLE

Frontal view

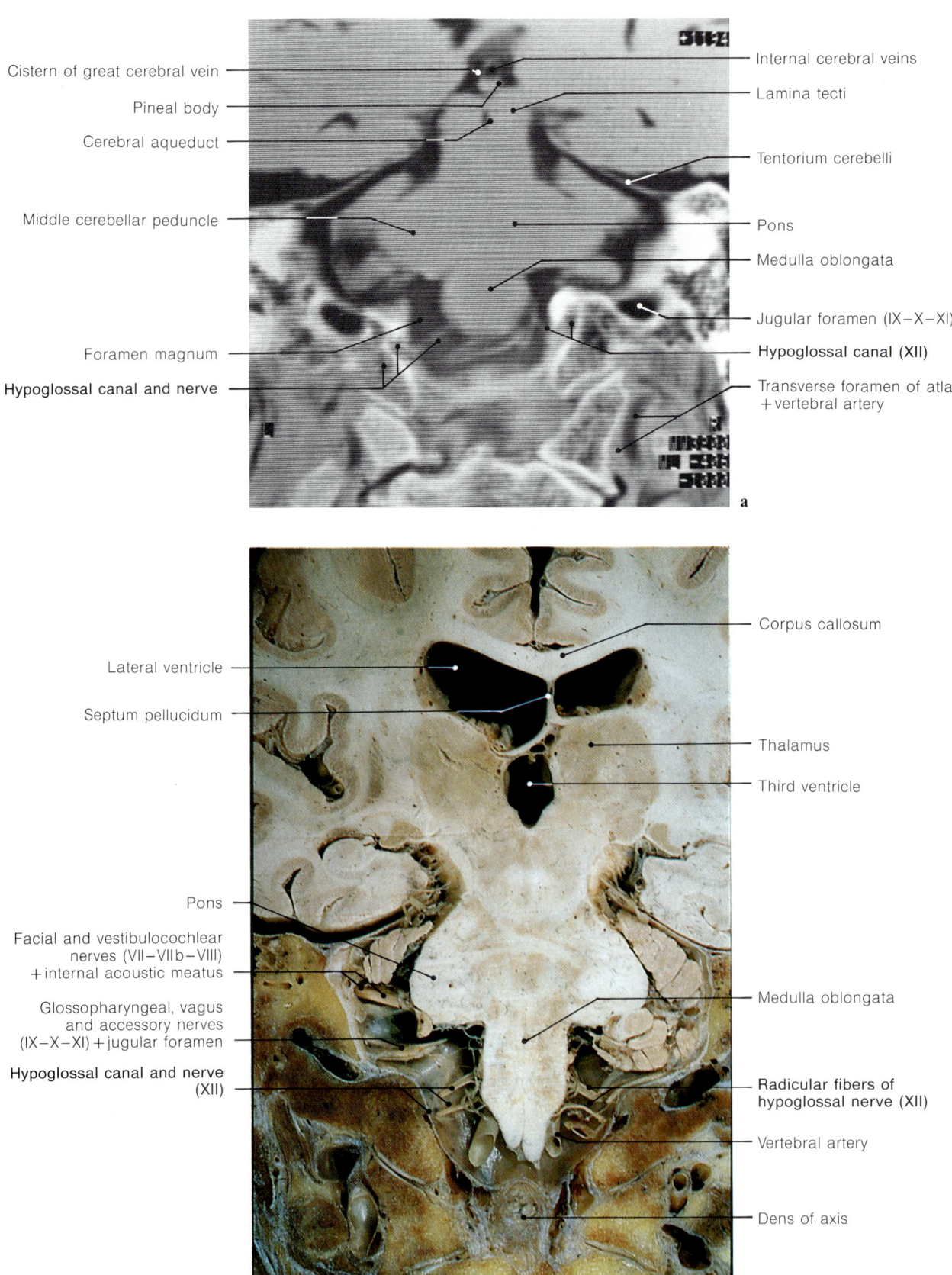

Fig. 12.6 a, b. Cisternal computed tomographic (CT) (**a**) and anatomic (**b**) frontal sections showing the hypoglossal nerve and its canal (XII)

Hypoglossal canal

Anatomy

The roots join into one or two trunks which perforate the dura mater. The trunk of the hypoglossal nerve runs obliquely outwards and forward to the lateral mass of the occipital bone (Fig. 12.4a, b; 12.5a; 12.6a, b; 12.8b–d). The hypoglossal nerve becomes extracranial and describes a large curve with anterosuperior concavity, traversing successively:

- the posterior subparotid or retrostyloid space, passing between the internal jugular vein laterally and the vagus nerve medially (Fig. 12.2),
- the carotid bifurcation region,
- the hyocarotid region,
- the submandibular region,
- the sublingual region, where it terminates.

During its course, the hypoglossal nerve gives off various collateral branches:

- a meningeal branch,
- anastomoses with the superior cervical sympathetic ganglion, the cervical plexus and the inferior (plexiform) ganglion of vagus nerve,
- a vascular branch to the internal carotid artery,
- a descending branch derived from the anastomosis with C1 and C2 cervical nerves (Fig. 12.12), which innervates the omohyoid, sternothyroid and sternocleidohyoid muscles,
- nerves to the thyrohyoid, hyoglossus, styloglossus and geniohyoid muscles,
- the anastomosis with the lingual nerve (V^3) (Fig. 12.12).

The function of the hypoglossal nerve is to provide motor innervation of the tongue. It therefore participates in swallowing, mastication and phonation.

Imaging

Clinical features

– Impaired posttraumatic motility of the tongue, either isolated or associated with lesions of cranial nerves VII and IX.

Possible causes

– Fracture of hypoglossal canal,
– fracture with separation of lambdoid suture extending to the walls of the hypoglossal canal, with hematoma compressing XII,
– neurinoma,
– tympanojugular tumor extending towards the inferolateral region of jugular foramen.

Views required

– Tomographic study of hypoglossal canal in its axis in unilateral oblique view (Fig. 12.7a, b; 12.8a, b),
– tomographic study in symmetric and axial views (Fig. 12.9b),
– tomographic study, Blondeau view (Fig. 12.9c),
– study of hypoglossal canal in oblique view by "discontinuous scanning" (Fig. 12.10a, b),
– tomographic study in the Cornélis prestudied varied sagittal view.

Technique

Radiologic and tomographic study of hypoglossal canal in its axis in oblique view:

– The subject is in dorsal decubitus, the head turned so that the incident beam makes an angle, open upwards, of 7° to 10° with the orbitomeatal plane (OM);
– the head is turned to the side opposite to that to be examined by 45° to 55° to the median sagittal plane, so as to free the hypoglossal canal from any superimposition (Fig. 12.7a, b);
– the centering point is at 1 cm towards the outside of the zygoma and 1 cm beneath the zygomatic process;
– the planes of section start at 2 or 2.5 cm below the external acoustic meatus, descending over a depth of around 1 cm thickness.

Hypoglossal canal

Radiograph and tomogram

OBLIQUE VIEW

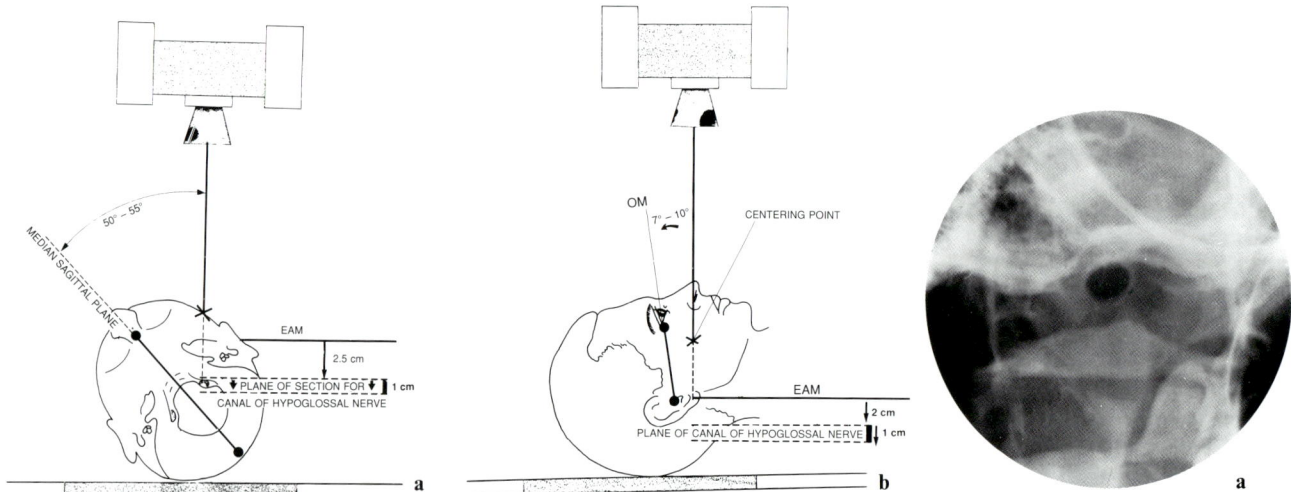

Fig. 12.7 a, b. Centering diagram for radiography and tomography of hypoglossal canal in its axis

Fig. 12.8 a, b. Radiograph (**a**) and tomogram (**b**) of hypoglossal canal

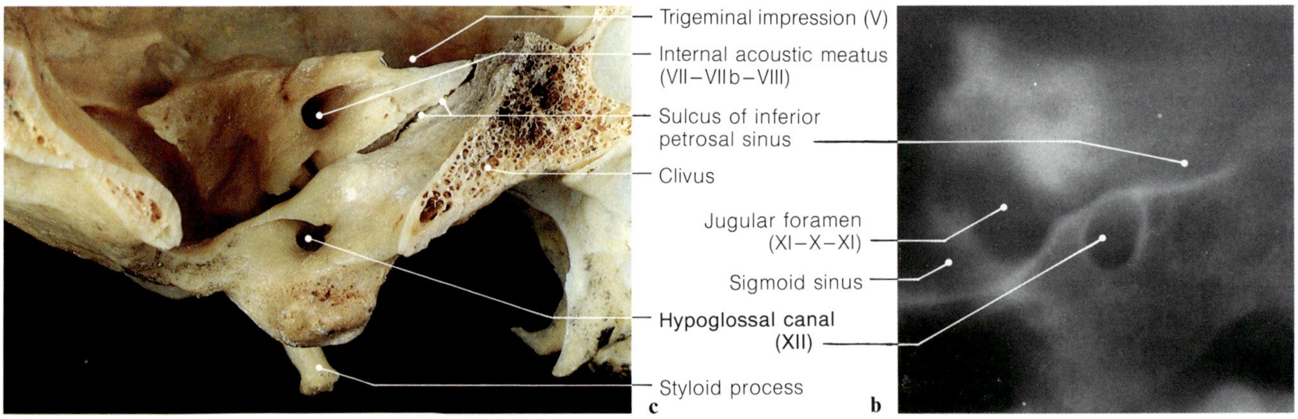

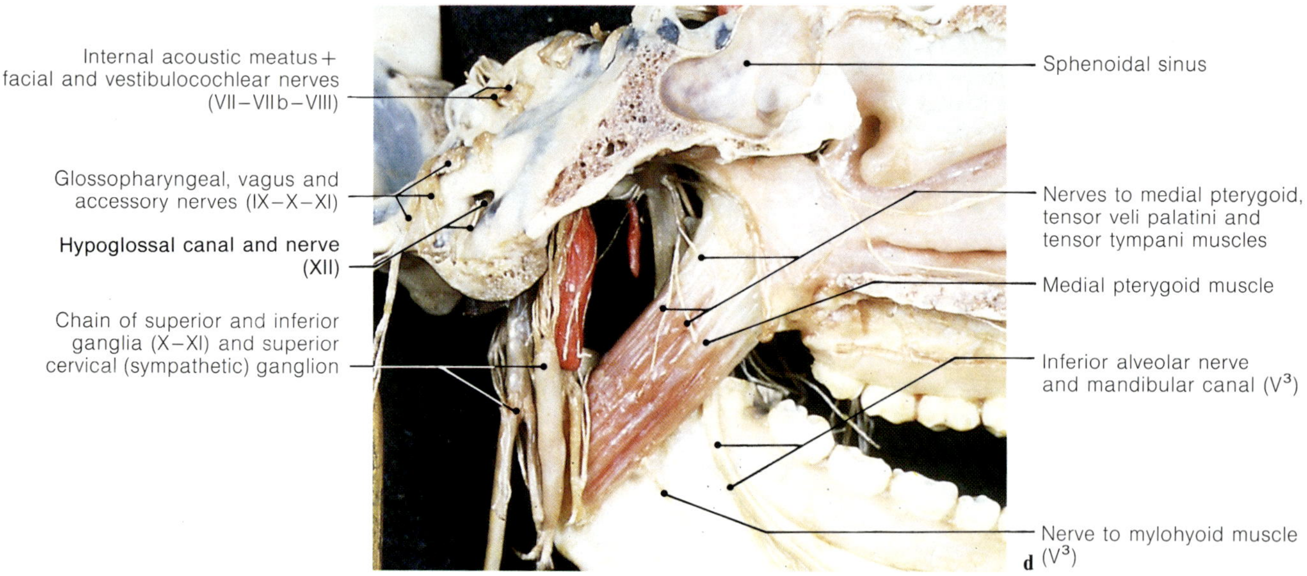

Fig. 12.8 c, d. Anatomic views of hypoglossal canal and nerve (XII)

Hypoglossal canal and nerve
Radiograph, tomogram and magnetic resonance imaging (MRI)
OBLIQUE, AXIAL, SEMIAXIAL AND SAGITTAL VIEWS

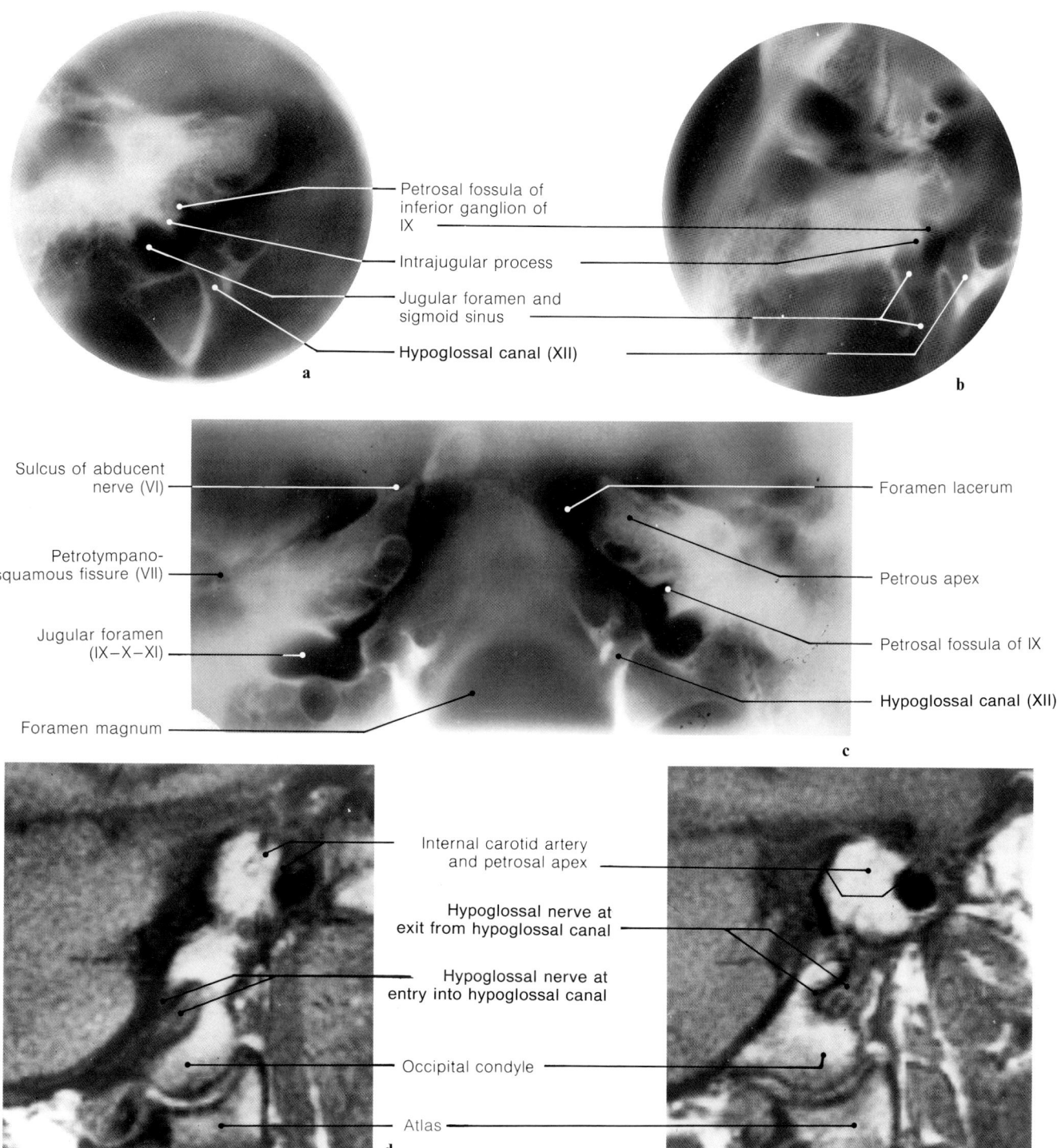

Fig. 12.9 a–e. Tomographic and MRI sections of hypoglossal canal in oblique (a), axial (b), semiaxial (c) and sagittal (d, e) views of hypoglossal nerve and its passage through the hypoglossal canal (XII). d: entry of XII; e: exit of XII

Hypoglossal canal

Discontinuous scanning

OBLIQUE VIEW

This view and the centering and reference points are identical with those of Fig. 12.7; after having centered the canal in its axis, the tube is then inclined by 5° to 8°.
A successive series of four films is made during rotation of the tube (Fig. 12.10a).

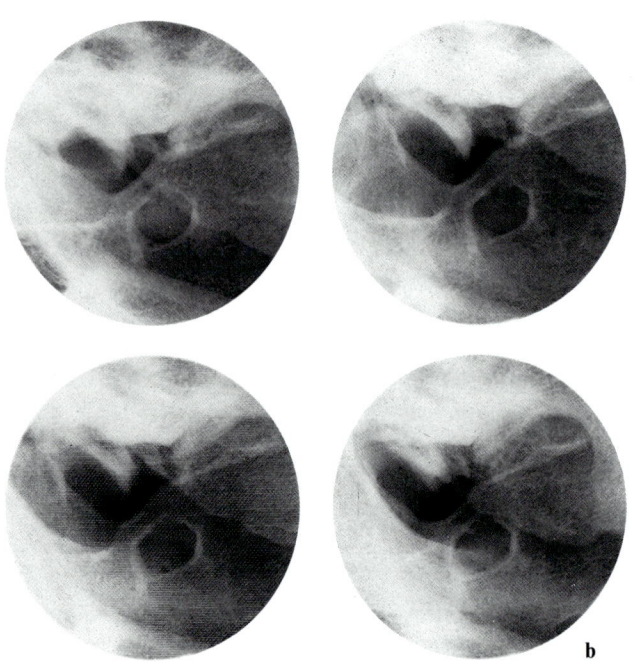

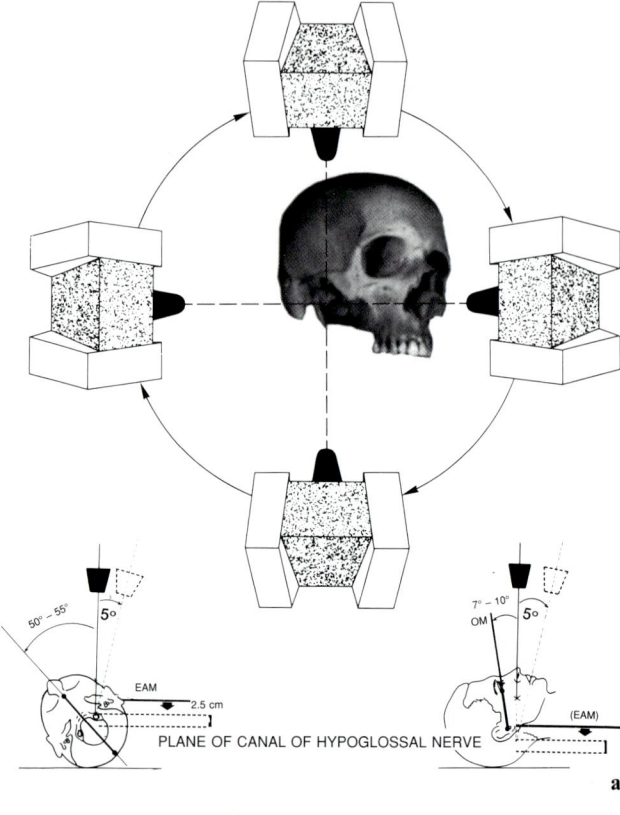

Fig. 12.10. a Centering diagram of hypoglossal canal in "discontinuous scanning"; b resulting radiograph

Computed tomography (CT)

OBLIQUE AXIAL VIEW

Fig. 12.11. Computed tomography (CT) of hypoglossal canal (XII)

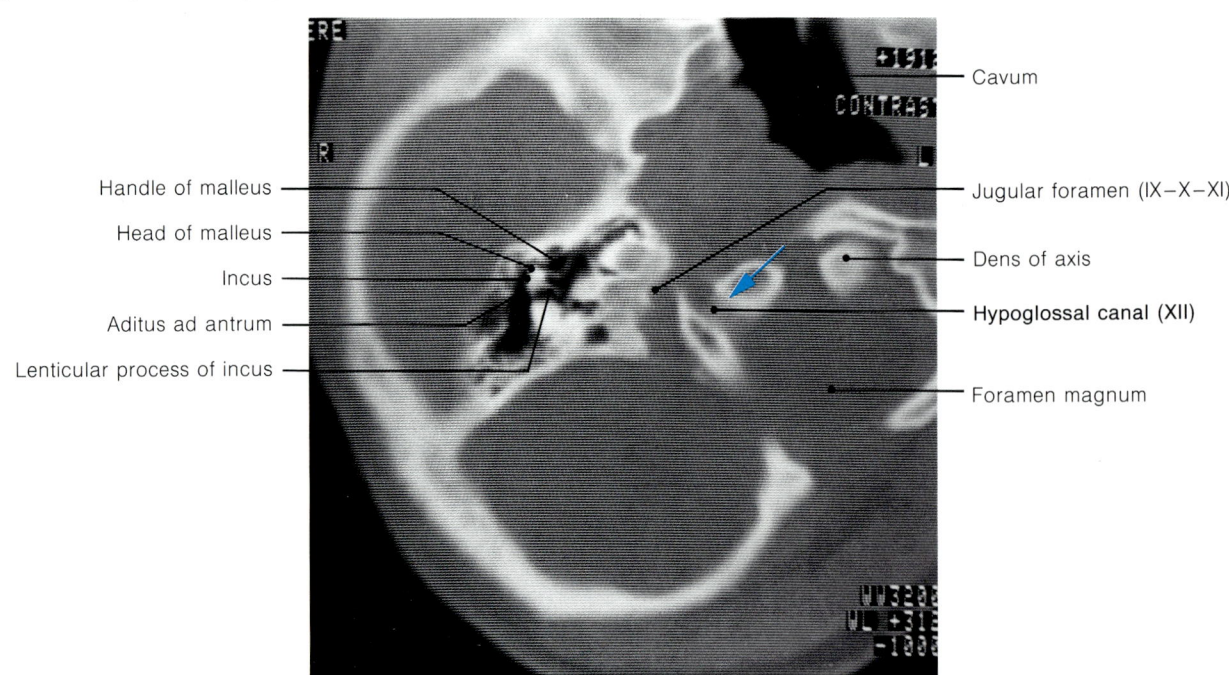

Hypoglossal nerve and canal (See vascular relations, p. 292)
Magnetic resonance imaging (MRI)
FRONTAL, AXIAL, SAGITTAL AND OBLIQUE VIEWS

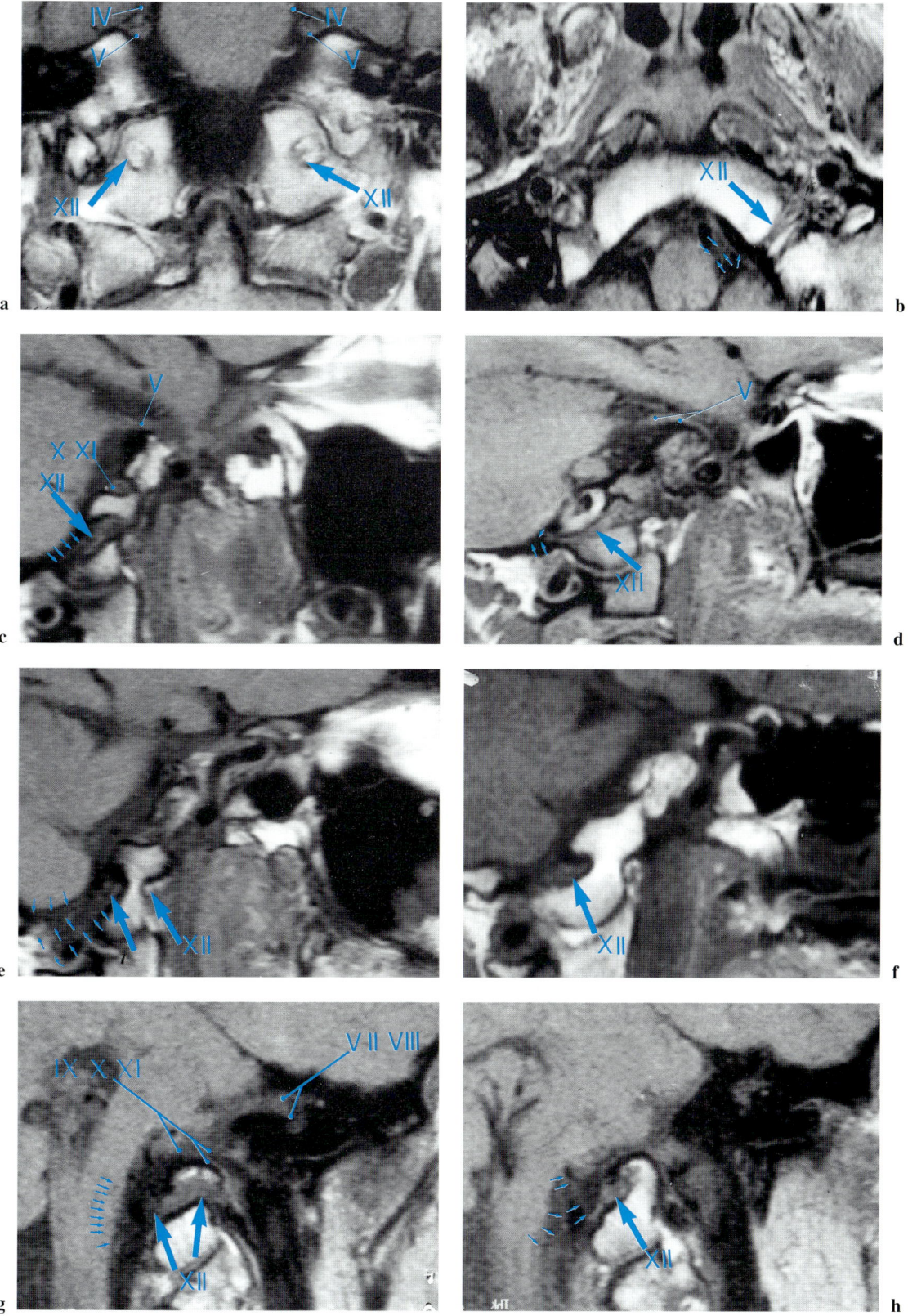

Fig. 12.12 a–h. Magnetic resonance imaging (MRI): frontal, axial, sagittal, oblique views of hypoglossal nerve and its passage through the hypoglossal canal (XII); hypoglossal nerve (*arrows*), radicular fibers of hypoglossal nerve (*small arrows*). (MRI: Dr. J.W. Casselman, A.Z. St-Jan, Brugge)

Communicating and terminal branches

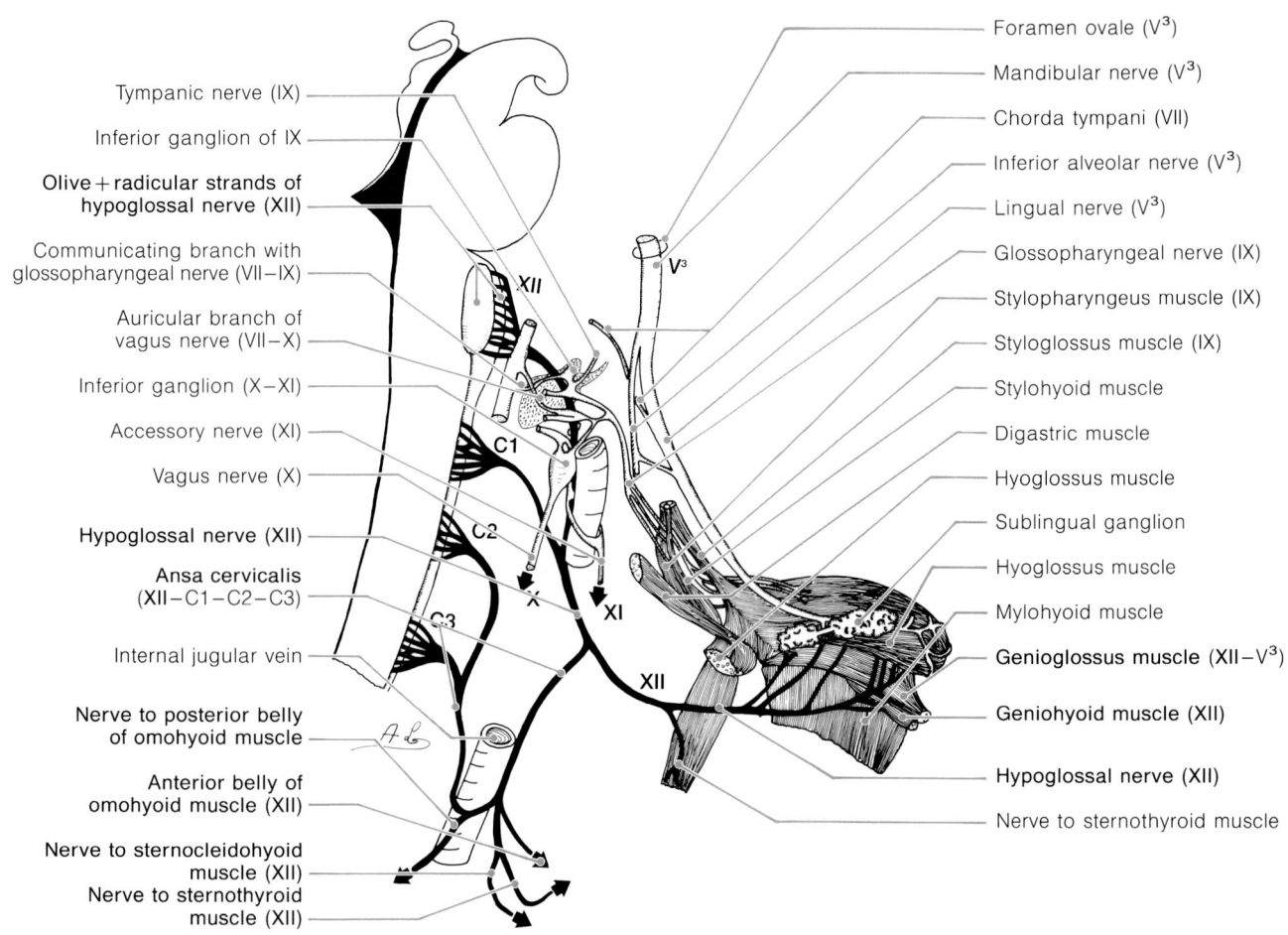

Fig. 12.13. Branches of hypoglossal nerve (XII)

The twelve pairs of cranial nerves

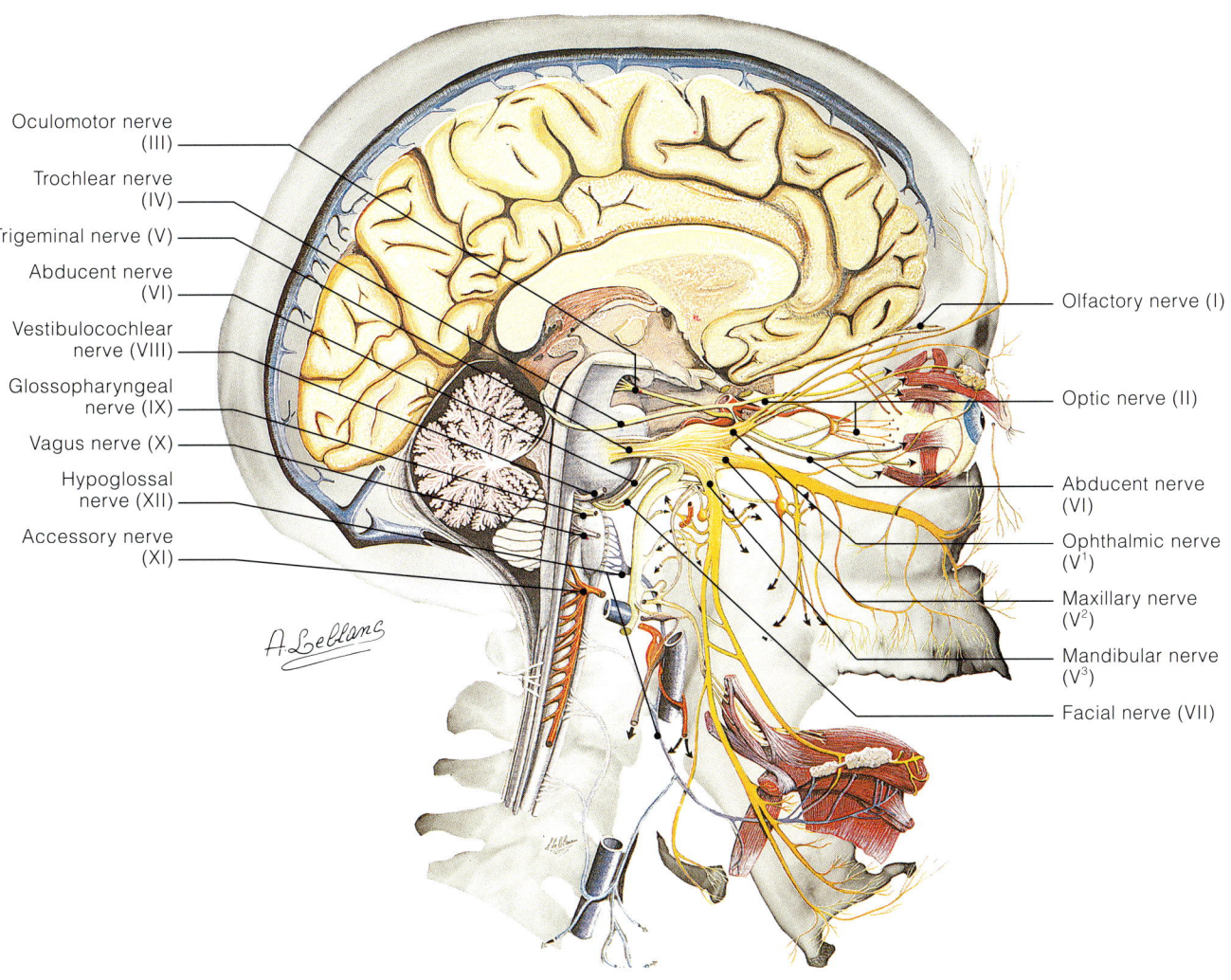

Fig. 12.14. Sagittal diagram showing apparent origins and courses of the cranial nerves

Vascular relations: Craniofacial arteries

Arteries of the skull base 276
Craniofacial arteries, courses, and orifices
    of the skull base 277
Ophthalmic artery, anterior ethmoidal artery, nasal
    and frontal terminal branches of the ophthalmic
    artery, and anterior ciliary arteries 278
Artery of the foramen rotundum, infraorbital artery,
    vidian artery, pterygovaginal artery 279
Superior alveolar and infraorbital arteries, greater
    palatine artery, arterial pedicles to the soft palate,
    and facial arteries 280
Infraorbital artery: labial, palpebral, and
    nasal branches 281
Facial artery, and submental artery 282
Lingual branch, submental branch, submental artery,
    and medial mandibular branch 283
Inferior labial artery, and facial artery 284
Inferior alveolar artery, and mandibular canal 285
Arterial system of the facial nerve and the
    stylomastoid foramen, inferior tympanic artery,
    chorda tympani, and posterior auricular artery ... 286
Artery of the submandibular gland, greater palatine
    artery, and pterygovaginal artery 287
Palatine branch of the accessory meningeal artery,
    and masseteric arteries 288
Ascending pharyngeal artery, hypoglossal branch,
    accessory artery, mastoid branch
    of the occipital artery, and emissary vein
    of the inferior petrosal sinus 289
Cavernous sinus – venous drainage
    at the skull base 290
Trigeminal artery, trunk in its lateral medullary
    portion 291
Hypoglossal branch 292

Arteries of the skull base

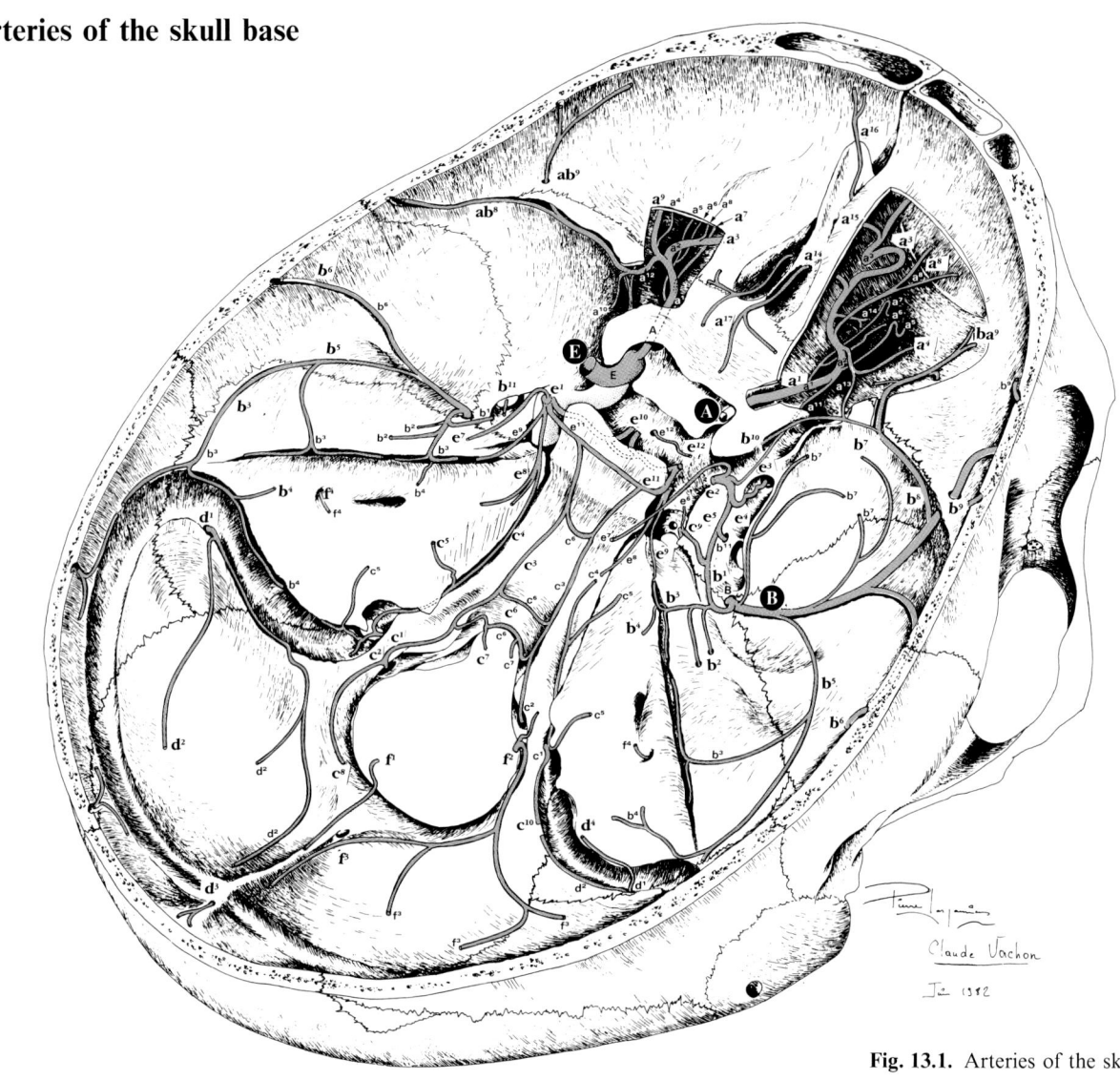

Fig. 13.1. Arteries of the skull base

A.	*Ophthalmic Artery*	*B.*	*Middle Meningeal Artery*

A. *Ophthalmic Artery*
- a^1 Intraorbital portion 1
- a^2 Intraorbital portion 2
- a^3 Intraorbital portion 3
- a^4 Lateral muscular artery
- a^5 Lateral ciliary artery
- a^6 Central retinal artery
- a^7 Medial ciliary artery
- a^8 Supra orbital artery
- a^9 Lacrymal artery
- a^{10} Recurrent tentorial artery
- a^{11} Deep recurrent ophthalmic artery
- a^{12} Recurrent meningeal artery
- a^{13} Meningo ophthalmic artery
- a^{14} Posterior ethmoidal artery
- a^{15} Anterior ethmoidal artery
- a^{16} Anterior falcine artery
- a^{17} Jugum sphenoidal branch
- ab^8 Meningeal branch for the sphenoid ridge
- ab^9 Anterior frontal meningeal branch

B. *Middle Meningeal Artery*
- b^1 Cavernous branch
- b^2 Petrous branch
- b^3 Basal tentorial branch
- b^4 Posterior fossa branch
- b^5 Petro squamosal branch
- b^6 Parieto occipital branch
- b^7 Middle cranial fossa branch
- b^8 Sphenoidal branch
- b^9 Frontal branch
- b^{10} Tentorial branch
- b^{11} Cavernous branch of the accessory meningeal artery
- ba^9 Meningo lacrymal artery

C. *Ascending Pharyngeal Artery*
- c^1 Jugular branch
- c^2 Hypoglossal branch
- c^3 Clival branch
- c^4 Inferior petrosal branch
- c^5 Cerebello pontine angle branch
- c^6 Midline anastomosis
- c^7 Odontoid arterial arch system
- c^8 Foramen magnum branch
- c^9 Carotid branch
- c^{10} Cerebellar fossa branch

D. *Occipital Artery*
- d^1 Mastoid branch
- d^2 Cerebellar fossa branch
- d^3 Torcular branch
- d^4 Cerebello pontine angle branch

E. *Internal Carotid Artery*
- e^1 Meningo hypophyseal trunk
- e^2 Infero lateral trunk (I.L.T.)
- e^3 Antero medial branch (I.L.T.)
- e^4 Antero lateral branch (I.L.T.)
- e^5 Posterior branch (I.L.T.)
- e^6 Recurrent artery of the foramen lacerum
- e^7 Marginal tentorial artery
- e^8 Lateral clival artery (medial branch)
- e^9 Lateral clival artery (lateral branch)
- e^{10} Postero inferior hypophyseal artery
- e^{11} Medial clival artery
- e^{12} Capsular artery

F. *Vertebral Artery*
- f^1 Artery of the falx cerebelli
- f^2 Posterior meningeal artery
- f^3 Cerebellar fossa branch
- f^4 Subarcuta artery

Craniofacial arteries, courses, and orifices of the skull base

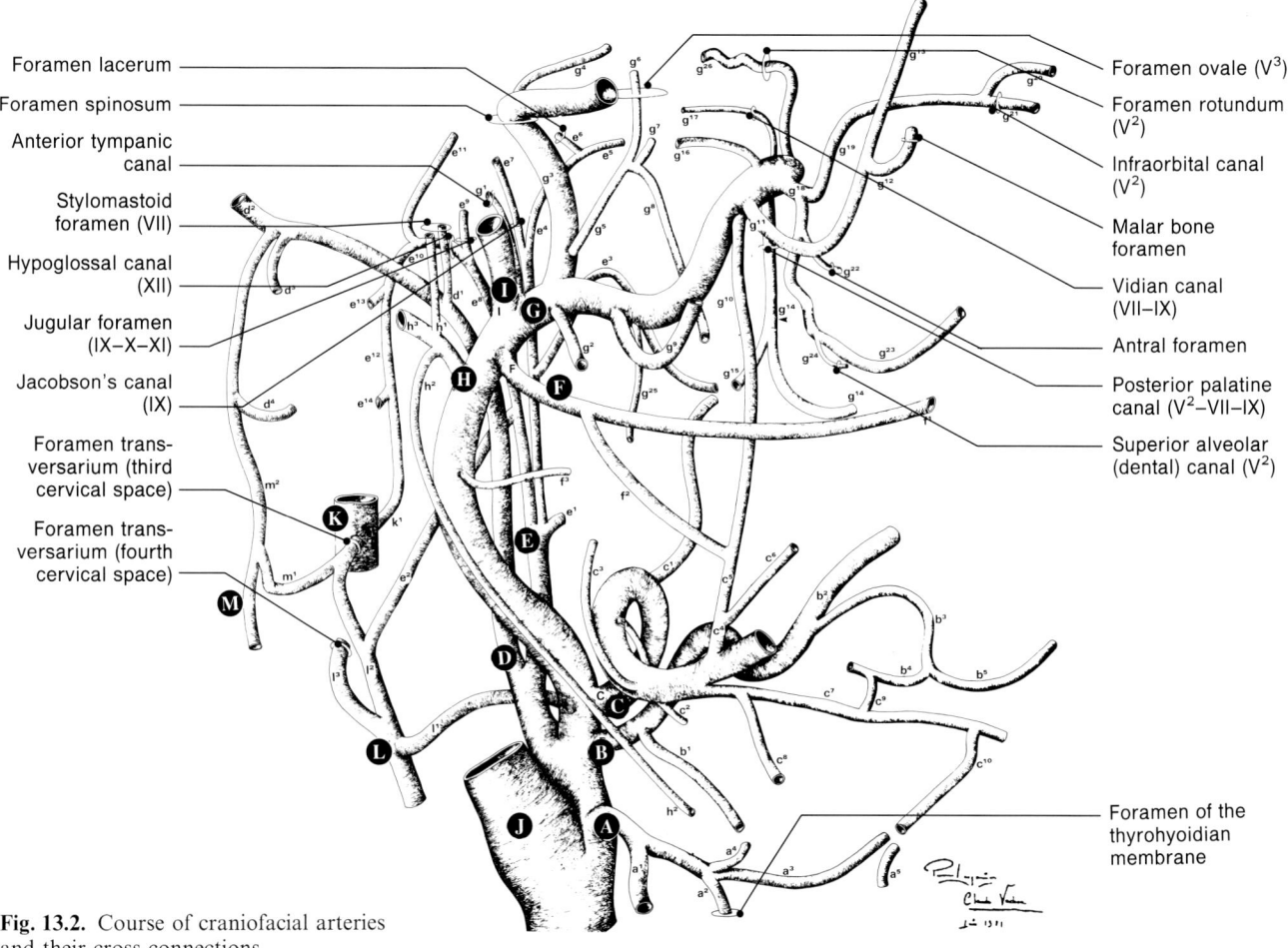

Fig. 13.2. Course of craniofacial arteries and their cross-connections

A. *Superior Thyroidal Artery*
a^1 Posterior branch (glandular)
a^2 Superior laryngeal artery
a^3 Anterior anastomotic branch
a^4 Hyoidian branch
a^5 Thyro-hyoidian branch

B. *Lingual Artery*
b^1 Hyoidian branch
b^2 Distal lingual artery
b^3 Sub-lingual artery
b^4 Sub-lingual anastomosis
b^5 Medial mandibular artery

C. *Facial Artery*
c^1 Ascending palatine artery
c^2 Sub-mandibular artery
c^3 Inferior masseteric artery
c^4 Bucco jugal trunk
c^5 Buccal artery
c^6 Posterior jugal artery
c^7 Sub-mental artery
c^8 Posterior hyoidian branch
c^9 Sub-lingual anastomosis
c^{10} Anterior hyoidian branch

D. *Occipital Artery*
d^1 Stylo-mastoid artery
d^2 Cutaneous branch
d^3 C1 occipito vertebral anastomosis
d^4 C2 occipito vertebral anastomosis

E. *Ascending Pharyngeal Artery*
e^1 Inferior pharyngeal branch
e^2 Musculo spinal branch
e^3 Middle pharyngeal branch
e^4 Superior pharyngeal branch
e^5 Inferior eustachian tube artery
e^6 Mandibular anastomosis
e^7 Inferior tympanic artery
e^8 Neuro-meningeal trunk
e^9 Jugular branch
e^{10} Hypoglossal branch
e^{11} Clival branch
e^{12} Odontoid arterial arch system
e^{13} Epidural branch (C1)
e^{14} Epidural branch (C2)

F. *Transverse Facial Artery*
f^1 Jugal branch
f^2 Superior masseteric artery
f^3 Middle masseteric artery

G. *Internal Maxillary Artery*
g^1 Anterior tympanic artery
g^2 Inferior dental artery
g^3 Middle meningeal artery
g^4 Cavernous branch
g^5 Accessory meningeal artery
g^6 Cavernous branch
g^7 Eustachian tube branch
g^8 Palatine branch
g^9 Middle deep temporal artery
g^{10} Buccal artery
g^{11} Anterior deep temporal artery
g^{12} Orbital branch
g^{13} Musculo-cutaneous branch
g^{14} Greater palatine artery
g^{15} Pterygoid branch
g^{16} Pterygo vaginal artery
g^{17} Vidian artery
g^{18} Infraorbital/superior alveolar trunk
g^{19} Infraorbital artery
g^{20} Orbital branch
g^{21} Jugal branch
g^{22} Antral branch
g^{23} Jugal branch
g^{24} Alveolar branch
g^{25} Deep masseteric artery
g^{26} Artery of the foramen rotundum

H. *Posterior Auricular Artery*
h^1 Stylo-mastoid artery
h^2 Stylo-muscular artery
h^3 Cutaneous branch

I. *Superficial Temporal Artery*

J. *Internal Carotid Artery*

K. *Vertebral Artery*
k^1 Odontoid arterial arch system

L. *Ascending Cervical Artery*
l^1 C4 collateral
l^2 Anterior anastomotic artery (C3)
l^3 Anterior anastomotic artery (C4)

M. *Deep Cervical Artery*
m^1 Posterior anastomotic artery (C3)
m^2 Posterior longitudinal anastomosis

Ophthalmic artery, anterior ethmoidal artery, nasal and frontal terminal branches of the ophthalmic artery, and anterior ciliary arteries

[See course of ophthalmic nerve (V^1), p. 81–93, (nasociliary frontal nerves (V^1)]

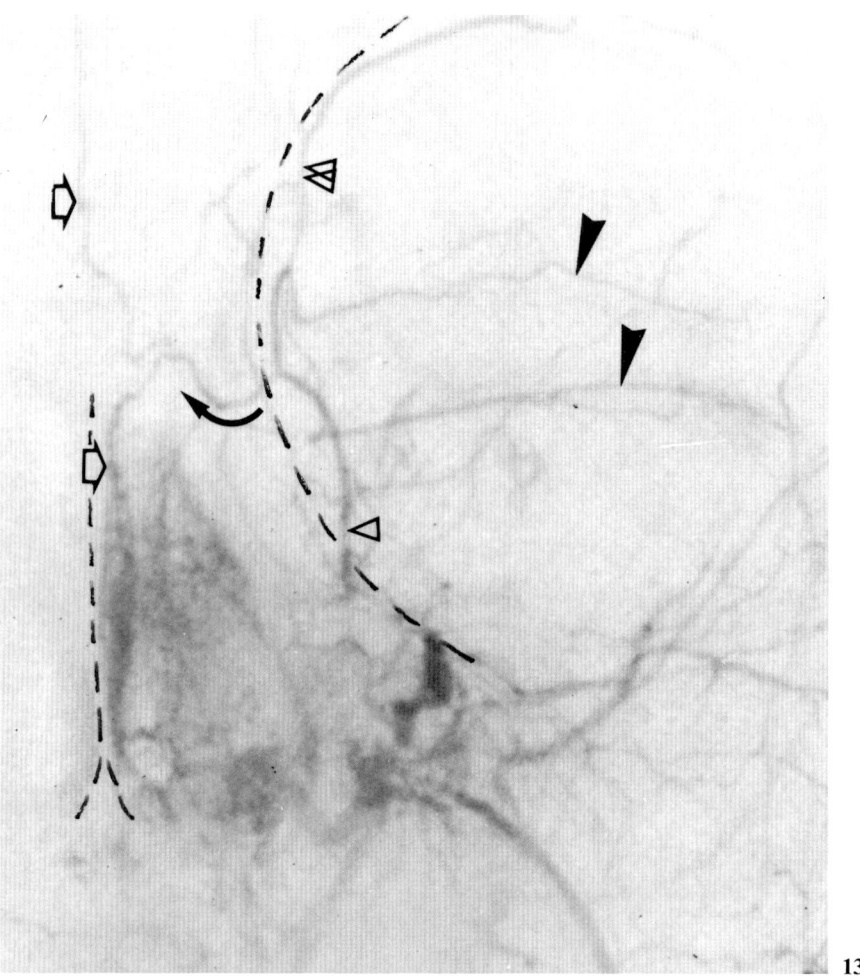

13.3

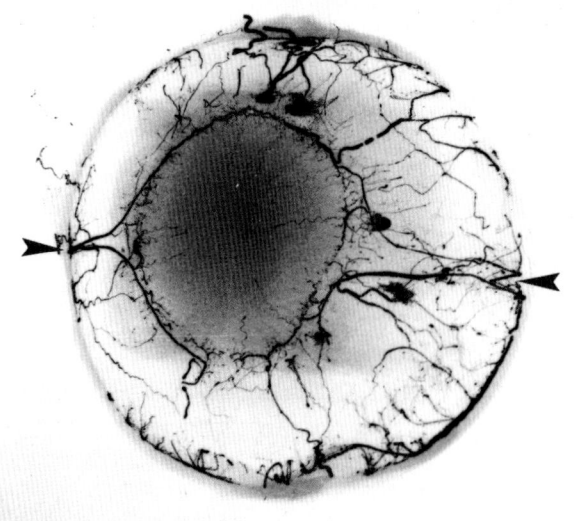

13.4

Fig. 13.3. Frontal subtraction distal maxillary angiogram. The *interrupted lines* represent the midline and the medial rim of the left orbit. Visualization of the anterior ethmoidal artery (*curved arrow*) and its septal and falcine branches (*open arrow*); opacification of both superior and inferior palpebral arteries (*arrowheads*), and of the nasal (*open arrowhead*) and frontal (*double open arrowhead*) terminal branches of the ophthalmic artery

Fig. 13.4. Microradiogram of an injected eyeball. Note the circle of the iris filled by the anterior ciliary arteries (*arrowheads*)

Artery of the foramen rotundum, infraorbital artery, vidian artery, pterygovaginal artery

[See ophthalmic nerve (V^1), pp. 83–93; maxillary nerve (V^2), pp. 95–109; infraorbital nerve (V^2), pp. 111–116; pterygoid nerve and canal (VII–IX), pp. 131, 194–197]

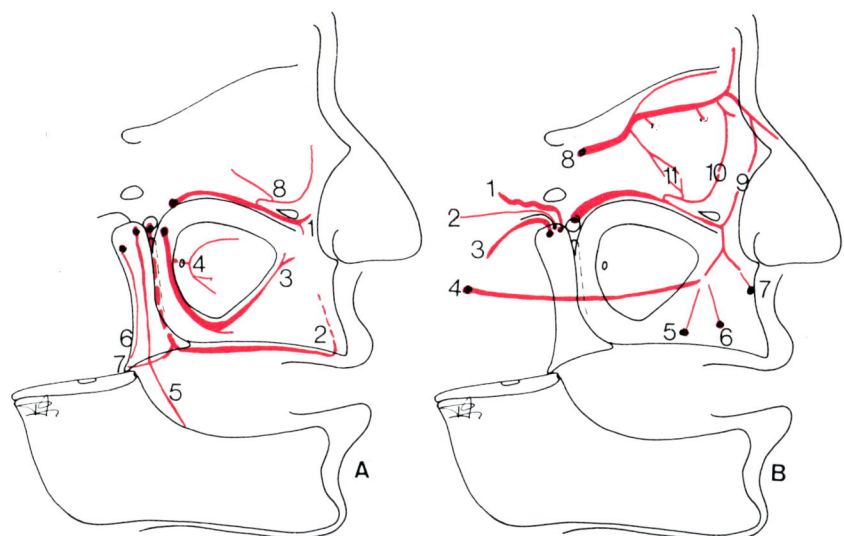

Fig. 13.5. Diagrammatic representation of the main arterial pedicles to the maxillary area. **A** Deep pedicles. *1*, infraorbital artery; *2*, greater palatine artery; *3*, superior alveolar artery; *4*, antral branch; *5*, buccal artery; *6*, pterygoidian artery; *7*, posterior branch of the descending palatine artery; *8*, orbital branch of the infraorbital artery. **B** Peripheral collaterals to the same area. *1*, artery of the foramen rotundum; *2*, Vidian artery; *3*, pterygovaginal artery; *4*, transverse facial artery; *5*, posterior jugal branch; *6*, middle jugal branch; *7*, anterior jugal branch; *8*, ophthalmic artery; *9*, naso-orbital artery; *10*, inferior palpebral artery; *11*, inferior muscular artery

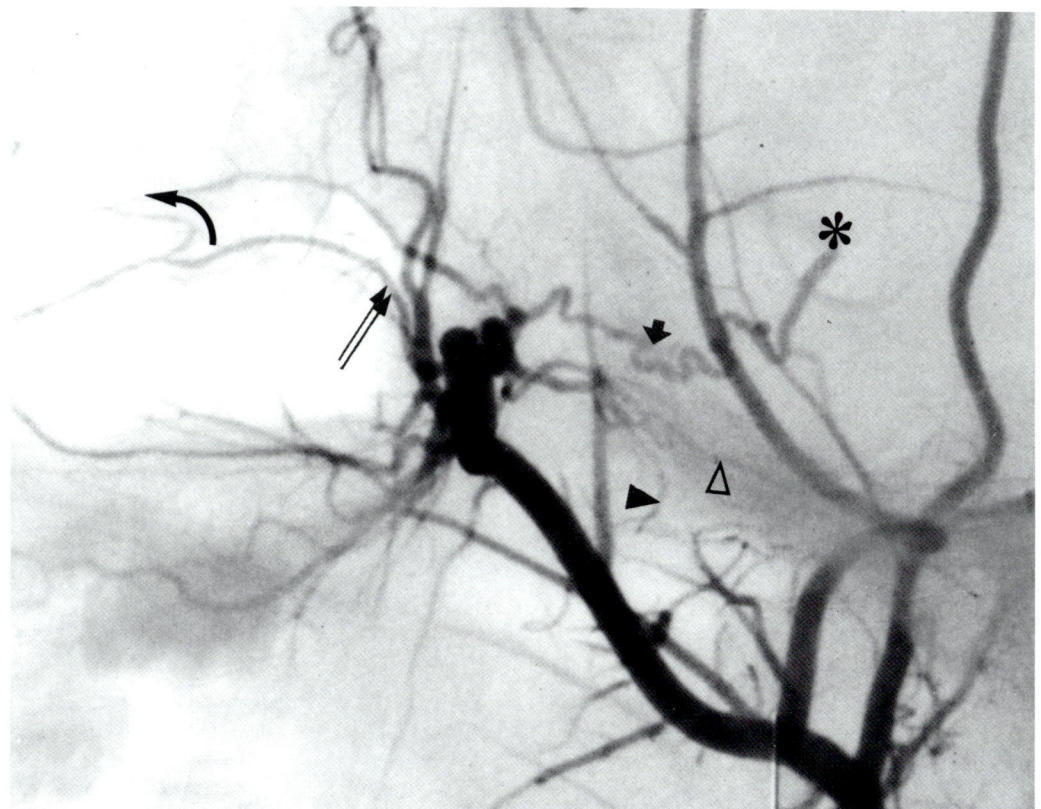

Fig. 13.6. Lateral subtraction angiogram of the distal external carotid artery. The distal collaterals of the internal maxillary artery are clearly visible: the infraorbital artery (*double arrow*) with its orbital branch (*curved arrow*), the pterygovaginal artery (*arrowhead*), the Vidian artery (*open arrowhead*); the artery of the foramen rotundum (*arrow*) opacify the inferolateral trunk (*asterisk*)

Superior alveolar and infraorbital arteries, greater palatine artery, arterial pedicles to the soft palate, and facial arteries

[See infraorbital nerve and superior alveolar branches (V^2), pp. 110–116; greater palatine nerve and foramen (V^2–VII–IX), p. 134; palatine nerves and incisive canal (hard palatine), p. 132]

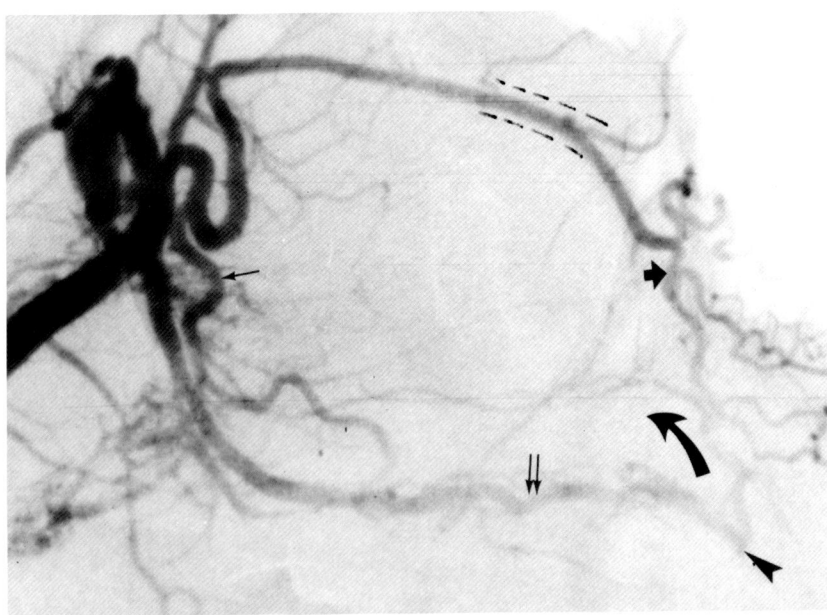

Fig. 13.7. Lateral subtraction angiogram of the internal maxillary artery (coned-down view). The *double interrupted line* indicates the infraorbital canal. The superior alveolar artery (*small arrow*) is clearly visible, as well as the greater palatine artery (*double, small arrows*) with the anterior palatine canal (*arrowhead*). At this point the descending palatine artery gives rise to its anastomotic channel with the septal system (*curved arrow*). The jugal supply from the infraorbital artery (*arrow*) in the nasolabial fold is seen

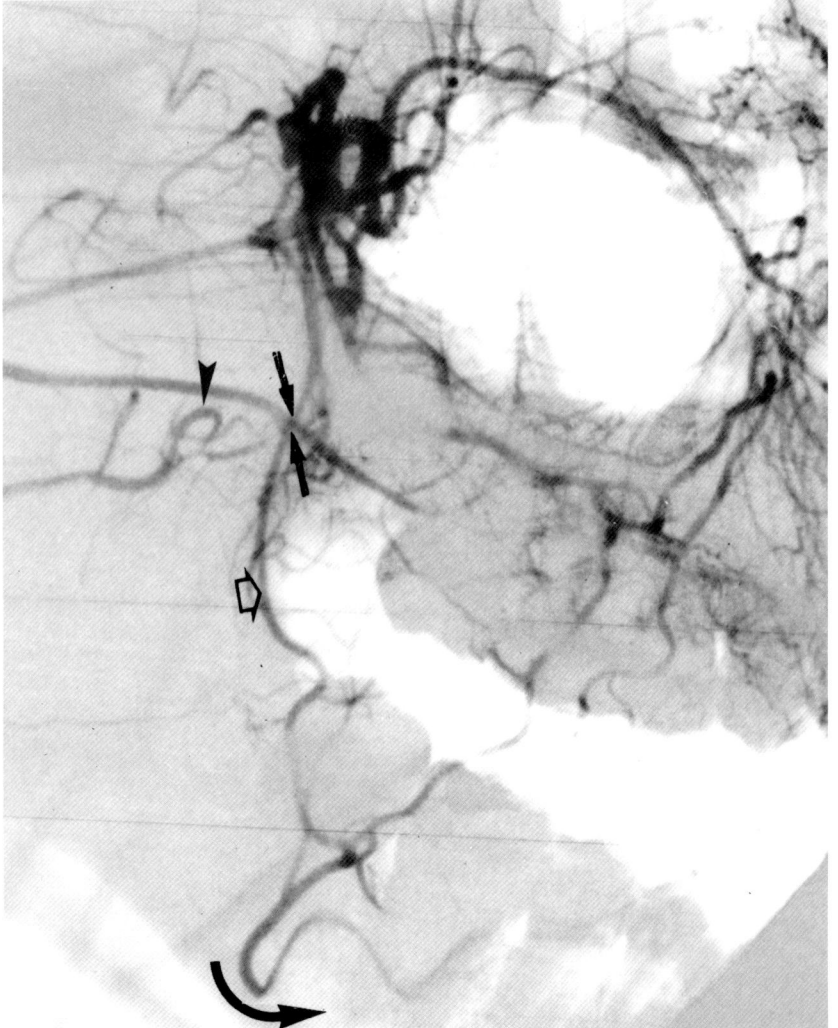

Fig. 13.8. Lateral subtraction angiogram of the distal internal maxillary artery. Note the crossing point of the buccal artery with the transverse facial artery (*arrows*). The facial artery (*curved arrow*) is opacified *via* the buccal system (*open arrow*). The pedicle to the soft palate (*arrowhead*) is filled *via* the greater palatine artery. Same case as in Fig. 2.60. Reprinted by permission from Lasjaunias, P. et al.: Bases radioanatomiques de l'embolisation artérielle au cours des épistaxes. Journal of Neuroradiology 6: 45–53, 1979

Infraorbital artery: labial, palpebral, and nasal branches

[See infraorbital canal and foramen (V^2), pp. 117–123]

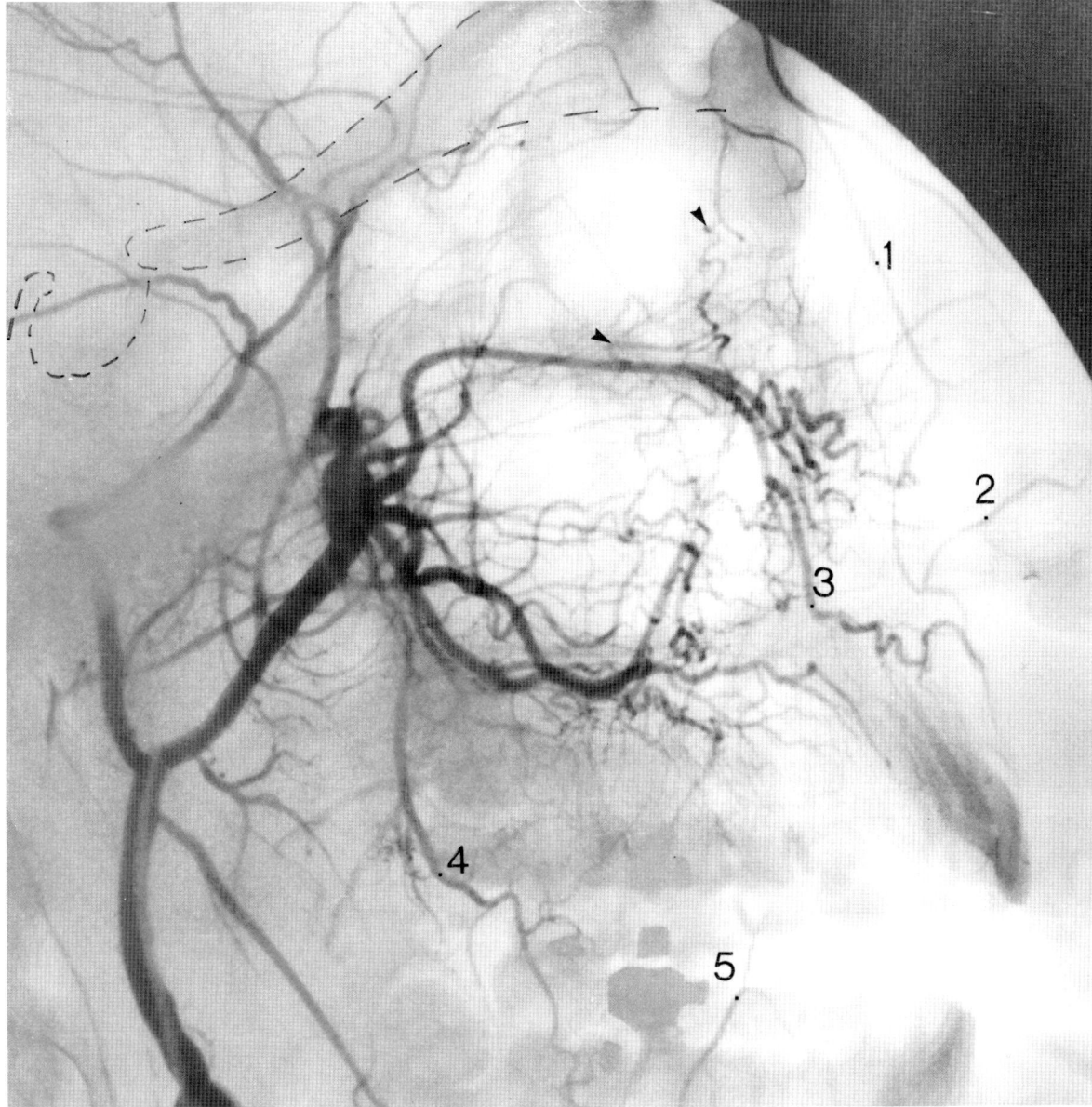

Fig. 13.9. Lateral subtraction angiogram of the internal maxillary artery. The infraorbital artery fills the inferior palpebral system through its orbital branch (*arrowheads*). Note the dominance of this system in the blood supply to the face: the nasoangular artery (*1*) supplies the alar pedicle (*2*); the anterior jugal system is supplied by the infraorbital artery (*3*); the buccal artery (*4*) fills the posterior jugal trunk (*5*)

Facial artery, and submental artery

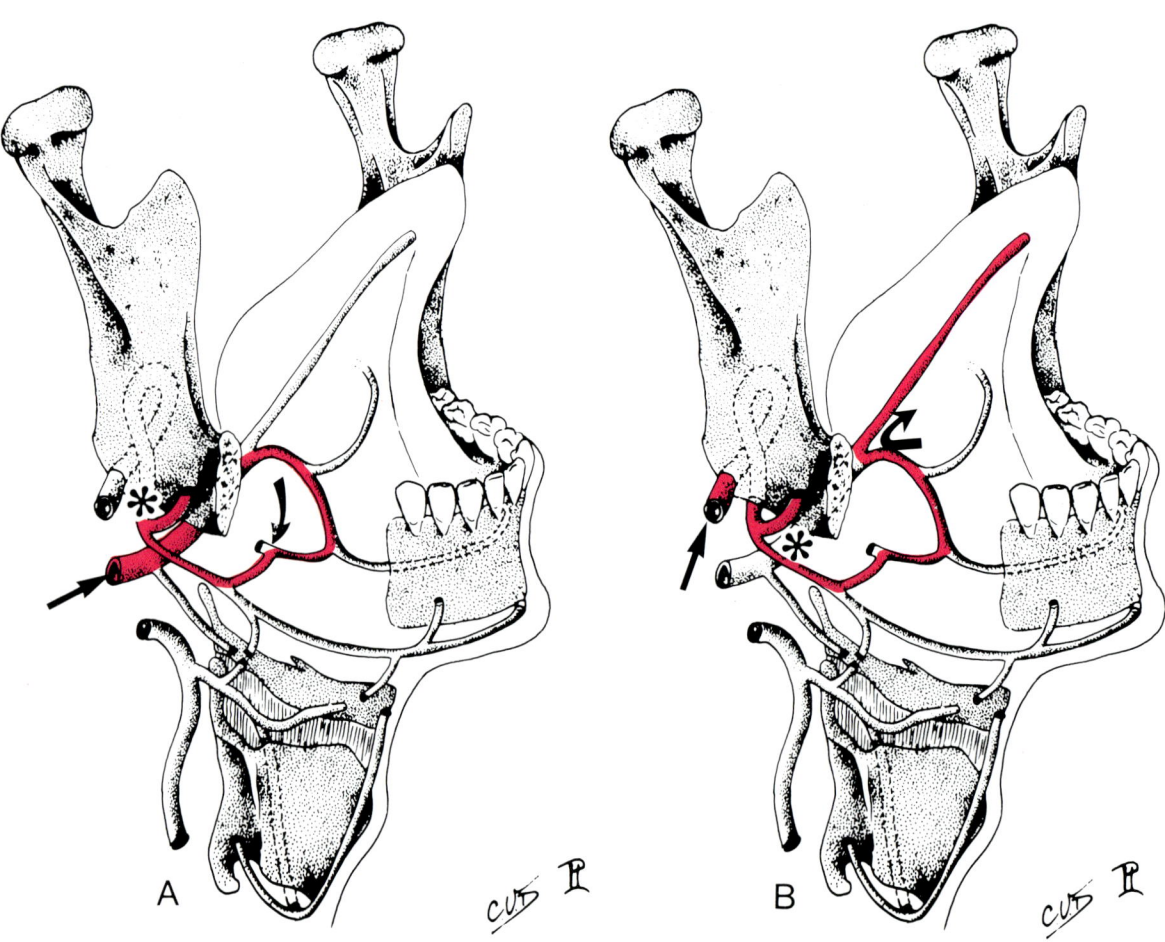

Fig. 13.10. Schematic representation of the linguofacial pattern viewed from the side and anteriorly. Two basic theoretical situations are illustrated. **A** The proximal facial occlusion (*asterisk*) induces the lingual (*arrow*) enlargement to supply the facial trunk through the sublingual anastomosis (*curved arrow*). **B** Proximal lingual occlusion (*asterisk*) induces facial (*arrow*) enlargement to supply the lingual trunk through the submental and sublingual anastomosis (*broken arrow*)

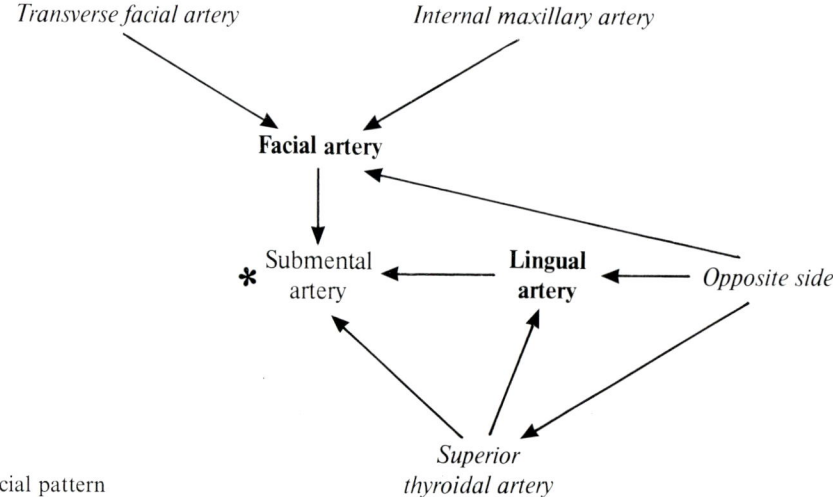

Fig. 13.10 C. Linguofacial pattern

Infraorbital artery: labial, palpebral, and nasal branches

[See infraorbital canal and foramen (V^2), pp. 117–123]

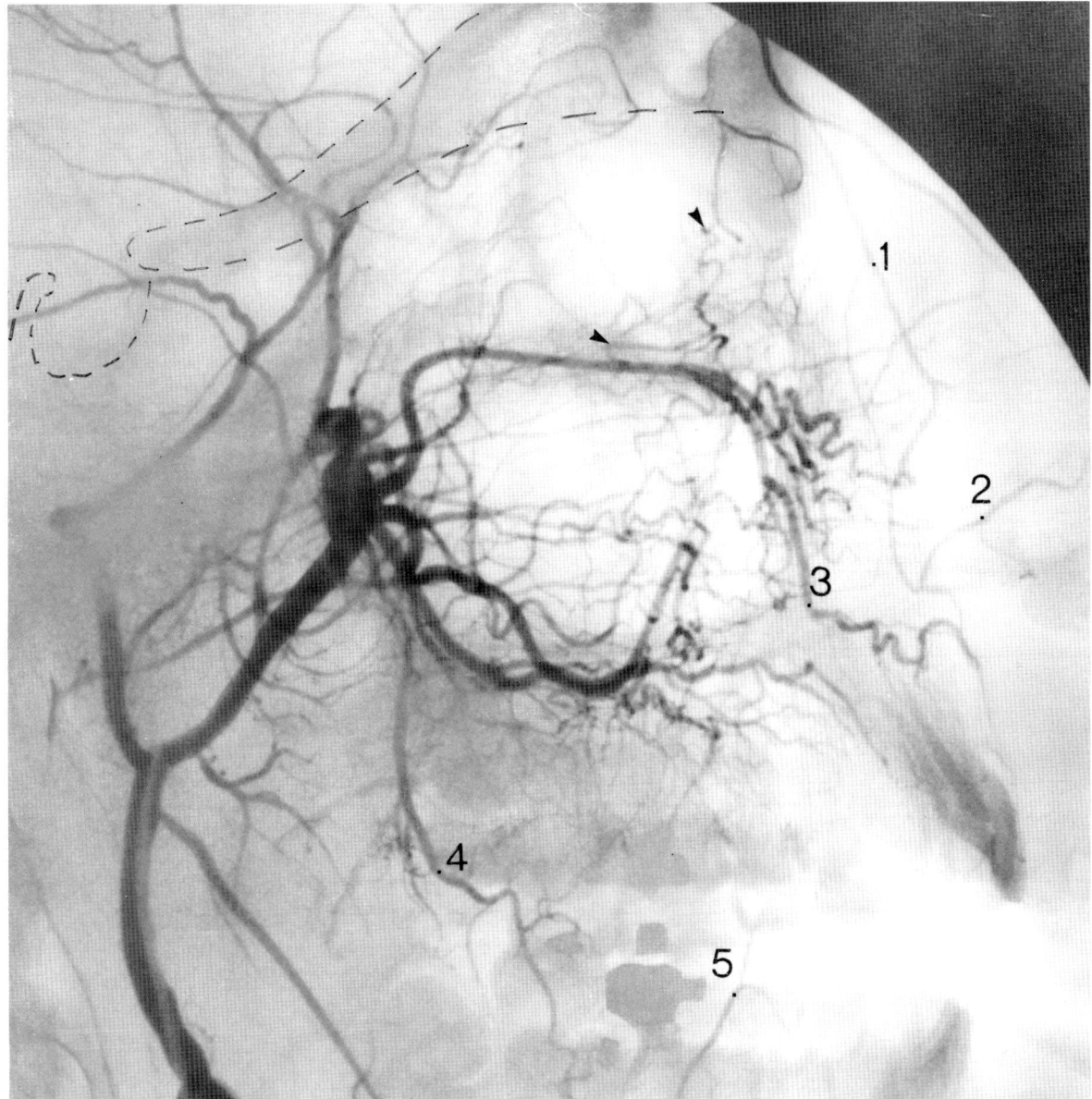

Fig. 13.9. Lateral subtraction angiogram of the internal maxillary artery. The infraorbital artery fills the inferior palpebral system through its orbital branch (*arrowheads*). Note the dominance of this system in the blood supply to the face: the nasoangular artery (*1*) supplies the alar pedicle (*2*); the anterior jugal system is supplied by the infraorbital artery (*3*); the buccal artery (*4*) fills the posterior jugal trunk (*5*)

Facial artery, and submental artery

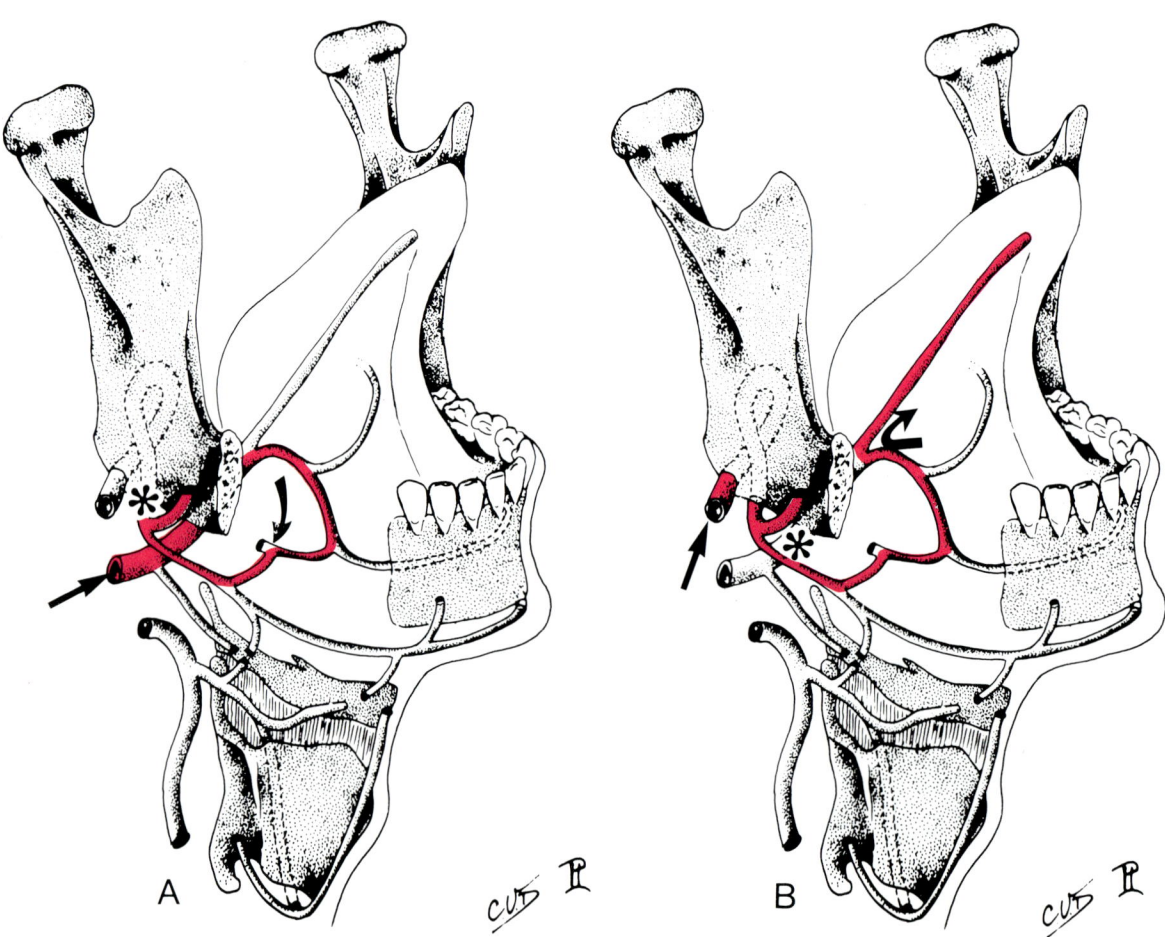

Fig. 13.10. Schematic representation of the linguofacial pattern viewed from the side and anteriorly. Two basic theoretical situations are illustrated. **A** The proximal facial occlusion (*asterisk*) induces the lingual (*arrow*) enlargement to supply the facial trunk through the sublingual anastomosis (*curved arrow*). **B** Proximal lingual occlusion (*asterisk*) induces facial (*arrow*) enlargement to supply the lingual trunk through the submental and sublingual anastomosis (*broken arrow*)

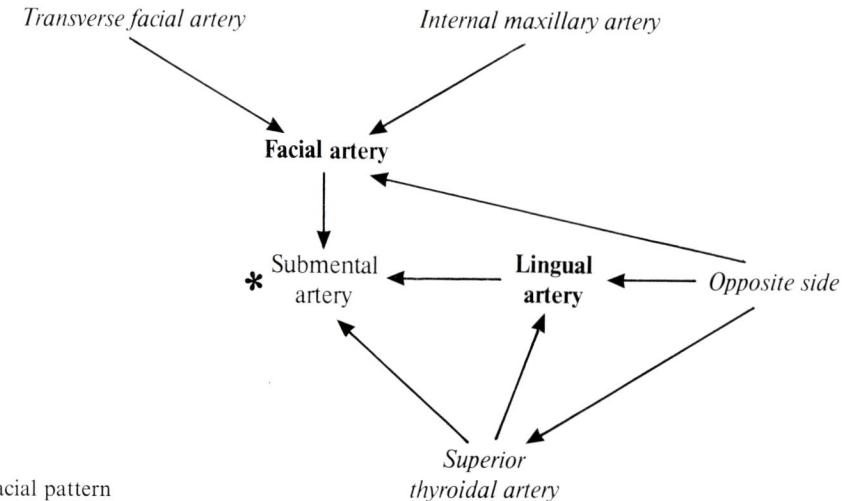

Fig. 13.10 C. Linguofacial pattern

Lingual branch, submental branch, submental artery, and medial mandibular branch

[See mandibular nerve (V³), pp. 202–203; inferior alveolar nerve (V³), pp. 147–152]

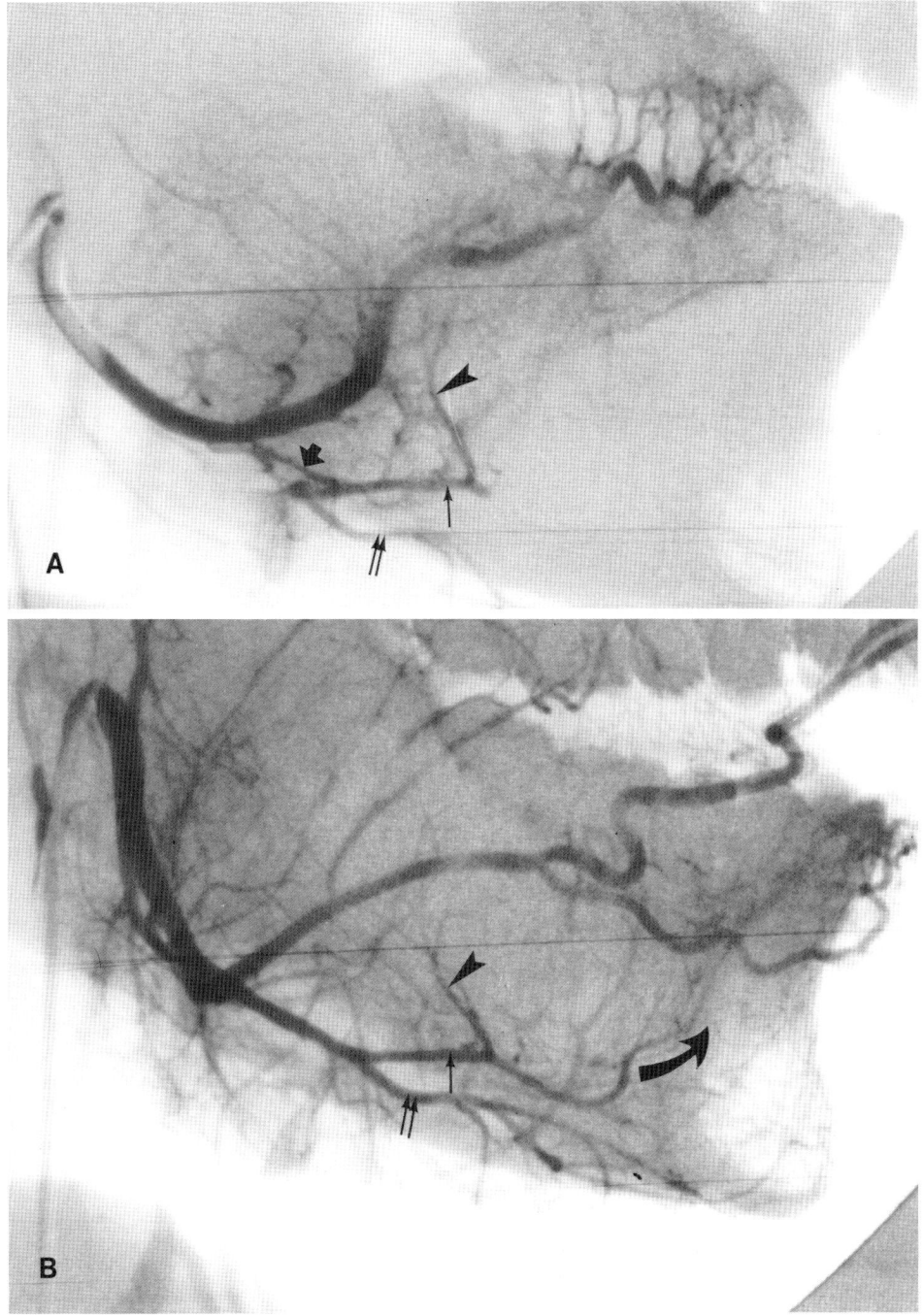

Fig. 13.11. Selective lingual (**A**) and facial (**B**) angiograms. Lateral projection, normal aspect. The vessels supplying the oral floor are seen. Submental dominance in the supply of that area. *Arrowhead:* periglandular ring; *solid arrow:* lingual branch; *small arrow:* submental branch; *double arrow:* submental artery; *curved arrow:* medial mandibular branch

Inferior labial artery, and facial artery

[See mental nerve and foramen (V^3), pp. 147–154]

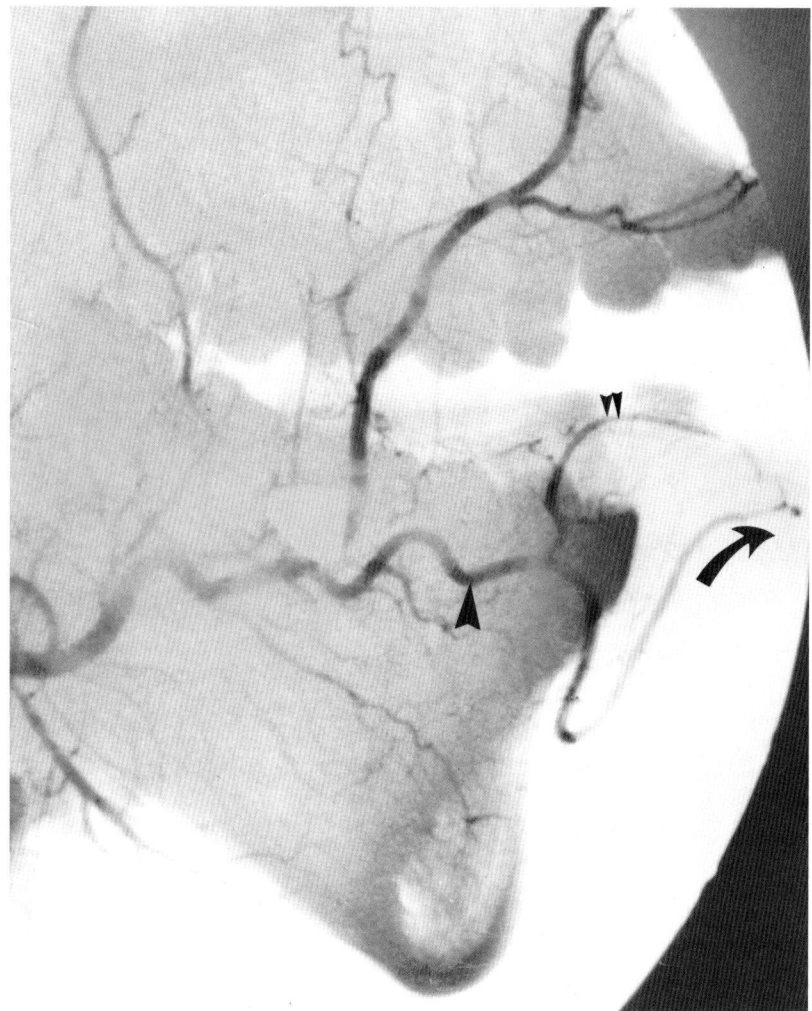

Fig. 13.12. Lateral subtraction angiogram of the facial artery. The inferior labial artery (*arrowhead*) demonstrates an arcade that reaches the limits of the face (*curved arrow*); also shown is the opposite inferior labial artery (*double, small arrowheads*)

Lingual branch, submental branch, submental artery, and medial mandibular branch

[See mandibular nerve (V³), pp. 202–203; inferior alveolar nerve (V³), pp. 147–152]

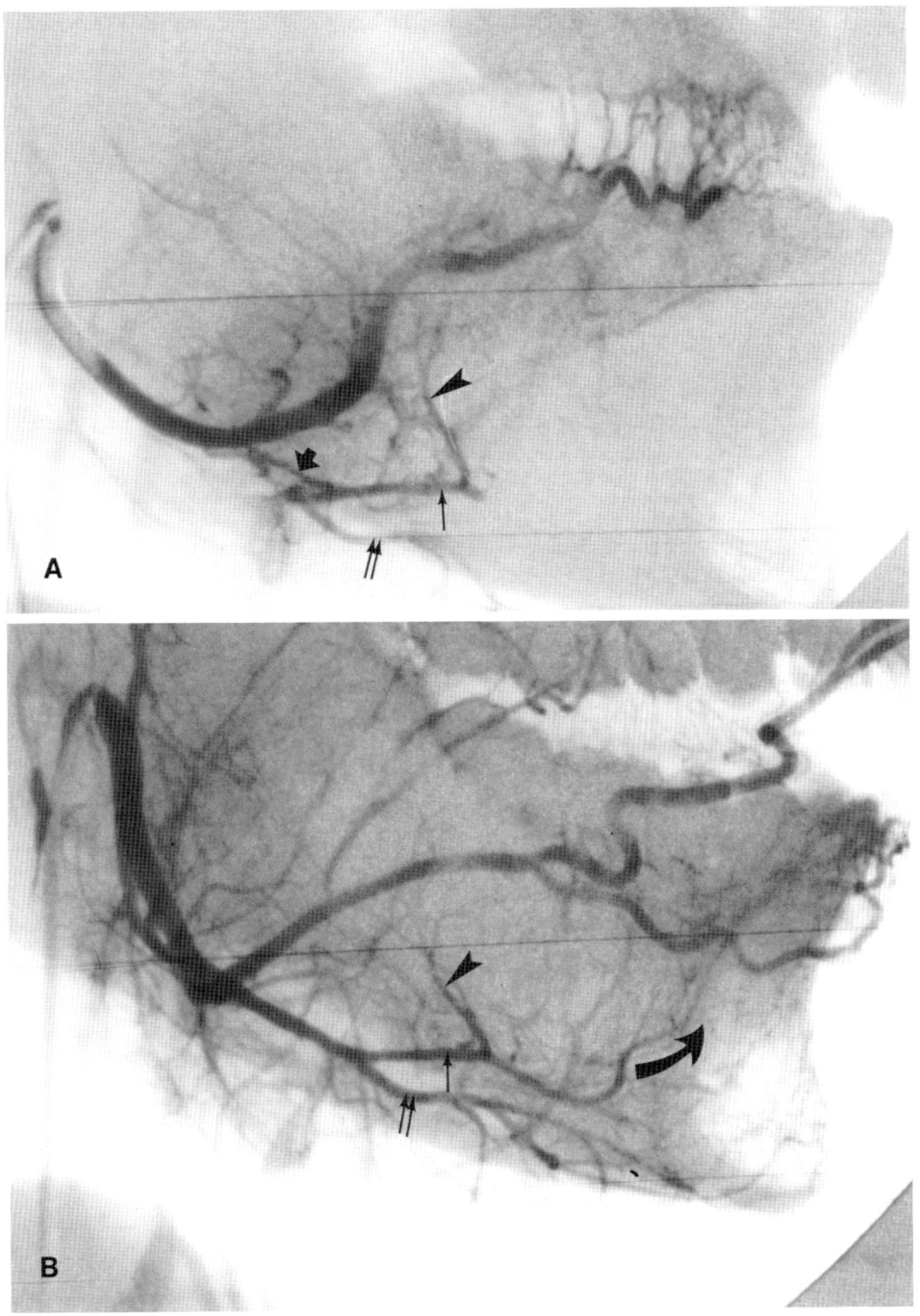

Fig. 13.11. Selective lingual (**A**) and facial (**B**) angiograms. Lateral projection, normal aspect. The vessels supplying the oral floor are seen. Submental dominance in the supply of that area. *Arrowhead:* periglandular ring; *solid arrow:* lingual branch; *small arrow:* submental branch; *double arrow:* submental artery; *curved arrow:* medial mandibular branch

Inferior labial artery, and facial artery

[See mental nerve and foramen (V^3), pp. 147–154]

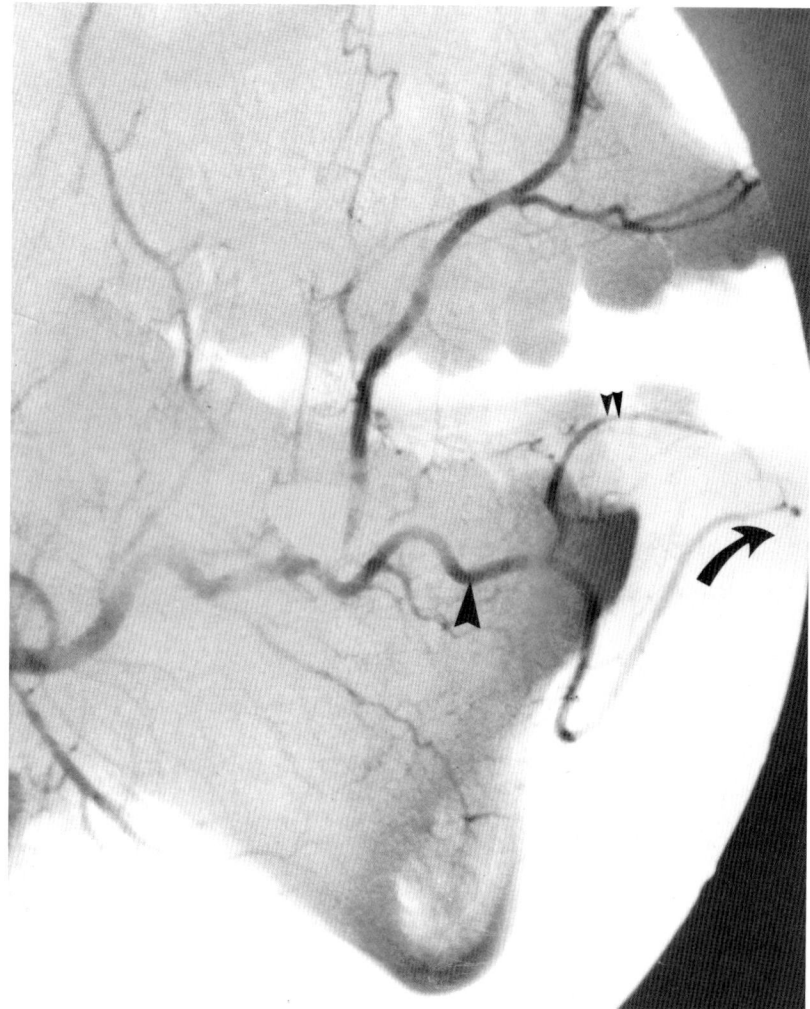

Fig. 13.12. Lateral subtraction angiogram of the facial artery. The inferior labial artery (*arrowhead*) demonstrates an arcade that reaches the limits of the face (*curved arrow*); also shown is the opposite inferior labial artery (*double, small arrowheads*)

Inferior alveolar artery, and mandibular canal

[See inferior alveolar nerve (V^3), mandibular canal, pp. 146–150]

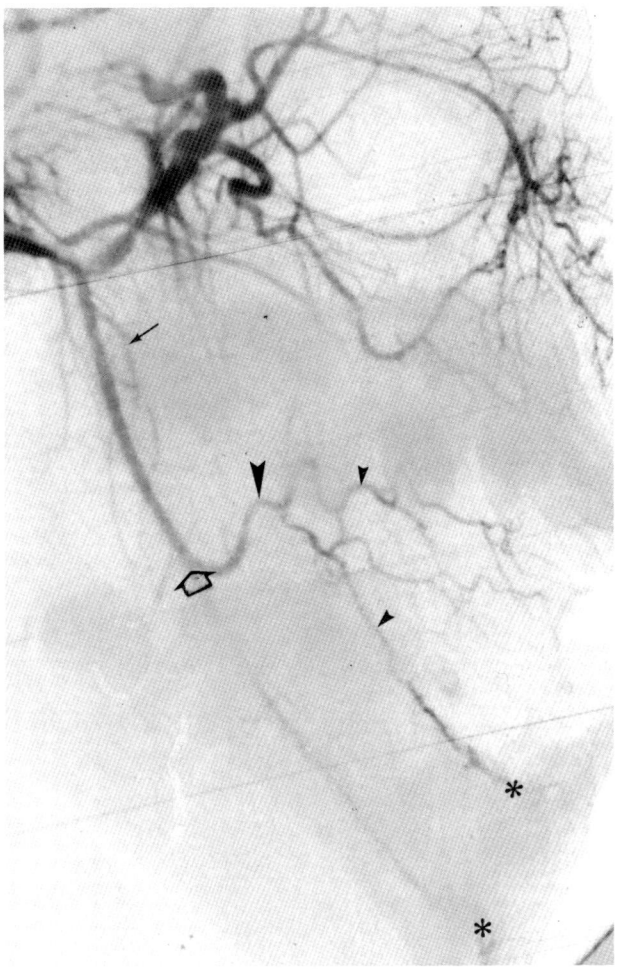

Fig. 13.13. Lateral subtraction angiogram of the internal maxillary artery. The inferior alveolar artery supplies a facial vascular malformation (*asterisks*); prior to entering the inferior dental canal (*open arrow*), the inferior dental artery gives a branch to the lingual nerve (*arrow*) and a jugal collateral to che cheek (*arrowheads*)

Arterial system of the facial nerve and the stylomastoid foramen, inferior tympanic artery, chorda tympani, and posterior auricular artery

[See intrapetrous and extrapetrous courses of the facial nerve (VII), pp. 171–210; tympanic nerve (IX) (Jacobson's nerve), pp. 235–239; petrotympanosquamous fissure, chorda tympani (VII), p. 202]

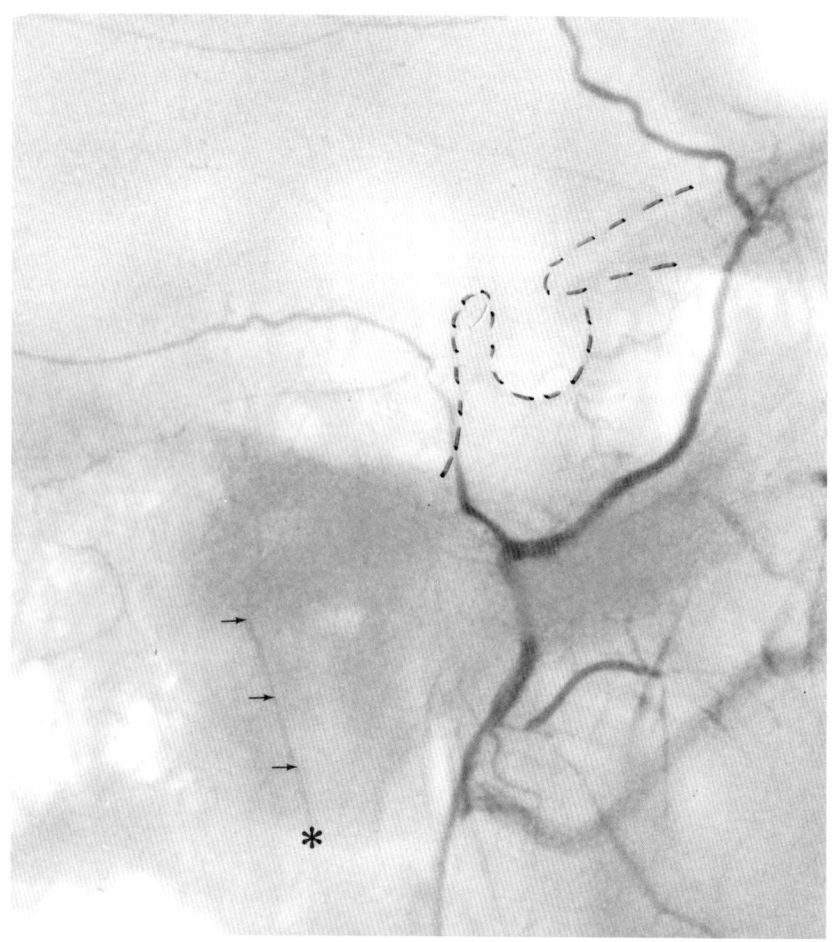

Fig. 13.14. Lateral subtraction angiogram of the middle meningeal artery. Visualization of the arterial system of the facial nerve (*small arrows*) and the stylomastoid foramen (*asterisk*)

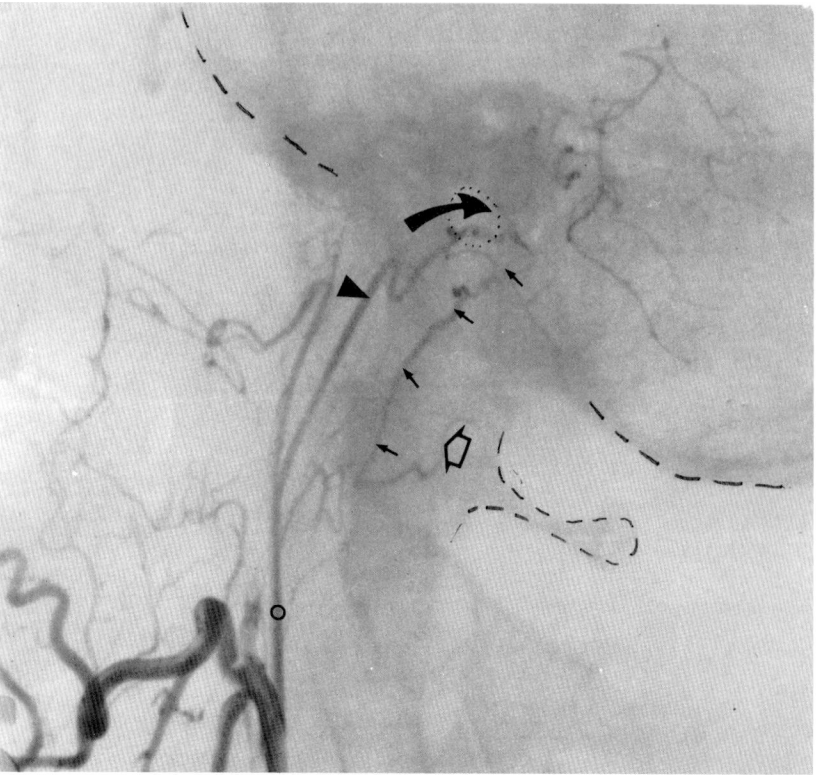

Fig. 13.15. Lateral subtraction angiogram of the ascending pharyngeal artery (○). The inferior tympanic artery (*arrowhead*) gives a branch coursing with the chorda tympani (*curved arrow*) with retrograde opacification of the stylomastoid artery (*small arrows*) arising from the posterior auricular artery (*open arrow*)

Artery of the submandibular gland, greater palatine artery, and pterygovaginal artery

[See greater palatine nerve (V^2–VII–IX), p. 134]

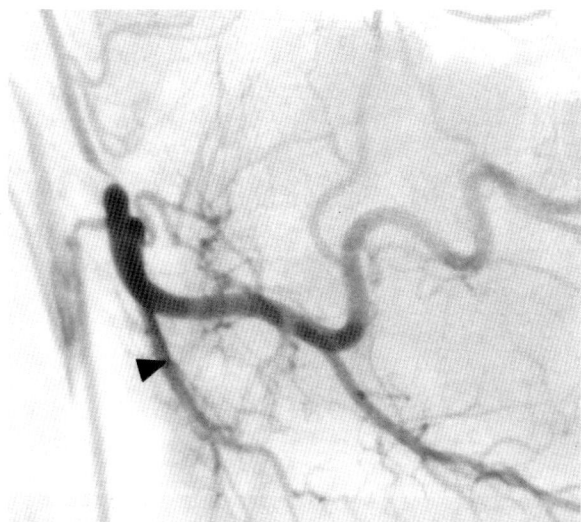

Fig. 13.16. Selective facial angiogram, lateral projection. The artery of the submandibular gland (*arrowhead*) is clearly seen. Note also its rapid branching in two

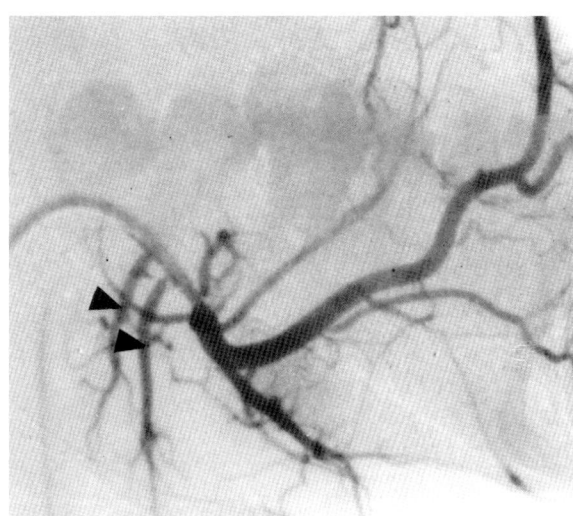

Fig. 13.17. Selective facial angiogram, lateral projection. Note the two pedicles for the submandibular gland (*arrowheads*)

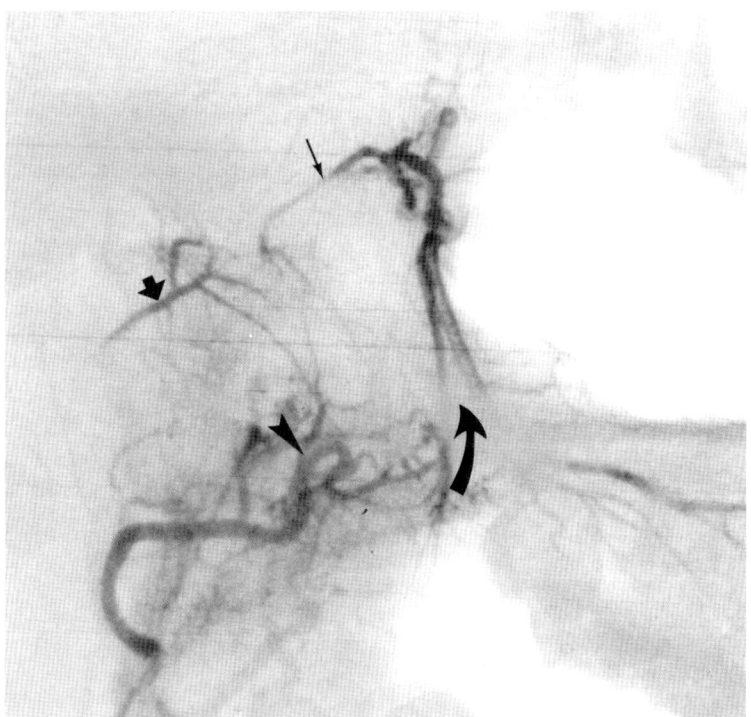

Fig. 13.18. Lateral subtraction angiogram of the ascending palatine artery (*arrowhead*) arising from the external carotid artery. Note retrograde opacification of the greater palatine artery (*curved arrow*) and the accessory meningeal artery (*arrow*) the pterygovaginal artery (*small arrow*)

Palatine branch of the accessory meningeal artery, and masseteric arteries

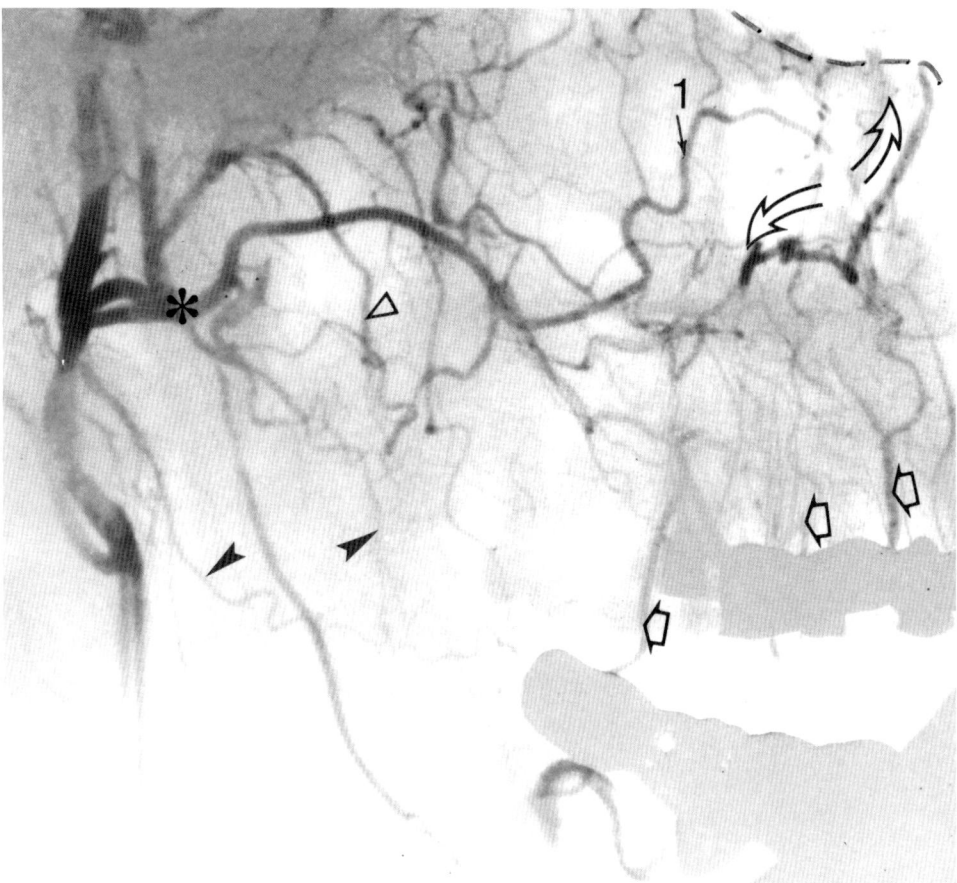

Fig. 13.19. Selective distal external carotid angiogram, lateral projection. Previous embolization of the maxillary artery distal to the middle meningeal origin (*asterisk*). The transverse facial artery (*1*) through its ascending and descending anastomoses (*open curved arrows*) reopacified the branches of the facial system (*open arrows*). The palatine branch of the accessory meningeal artery (*open arrowhead*) must be differentiated from the masseteric arteries (*arrowheads*)

Ascending pharyngeal artery, hypoglossal branch, accessory artery, mastoid branch of the occipital artery, and emissary vein of the inferior petrosal sinus

[See hypoglossal nerve and canal (XII), pp. 260–272; accessory nerve (XI), pp. 253–258; sinuses of skull base, afferent and emissary veins, p. 167]

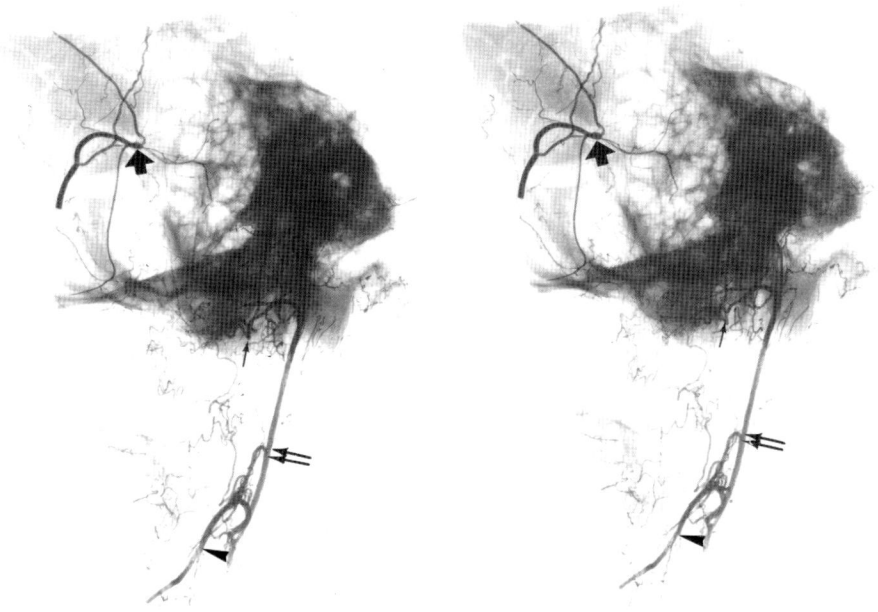

Fig. 13.20. Stereomicroradiogram of an injected base of the skull (lateral view). The neuromeningeal trunk (*double arrows*) of the ascending pharyngeal artery is preserved as well as the musculospinal artery (*arrowhead*). The trunk gives a large hypoglossal branch (*small arrow*). Note the mastoid branch of the occipital artery (*arrow*)

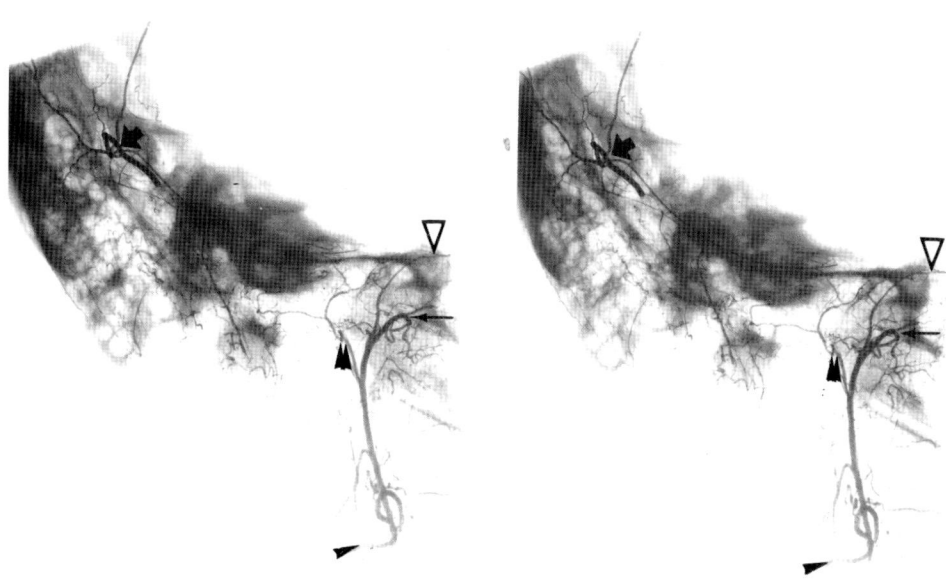

Fig. 13.21. Stereomicroradiogram of an injected base of the skull (anteroposterior view). The neuromeningeal trunk of the ascending pharyngeal artery is preserved (*arrowhead*). Its two branches, hypoglossal (*small arrow*) and jugular (*double arrowheads*), are visible. Note an accessory artery (*open arrowhead*) arising from the same trunk entering the skull through an emissary vein of the inferior petrosal sinus. Note also the mastoid branch of the occipital artery (*arrow*)

Cavernous sinus

Venous drainage at the skull base

[See cavernous sinus afferent and emissary veins, p. 167, optic canal (II), p. 22; superior orbital fissure (III–IV–V–VI), p. 82; foramen rotundum (V^2), p. 97; foramen ovale (V^3), p. 137; Arnold's foramen (VII–IX), p. 196; foramen lacerum, p. 80]

1. Anterior to the dorsum sellae course the anterior and posterior intercavernous or coronary sinuses, the capsular and the posteroinferior hypophyseal arteries.
2. Posterior to the dorsum sellae is the transverse occipital sinus and the medial artery of the clivus.

Thus, the two cavernous plexuses (Fig. 13.22) constitute an unexpansible extradural venous plexus.[1]

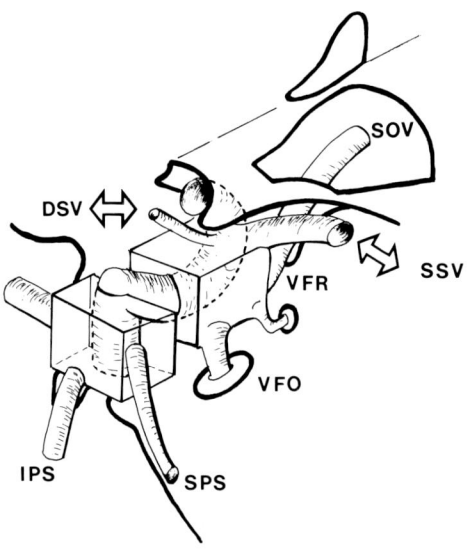

Fig. 13.22. Diagrammatic representation of the venous drainage of the base of the skull, seen from above and from the side. The cavernous sinus proper is clearly demonstrated with its tributaries and drainage. *SOV*, superior ophthalmic vein; *SSV*, superficial sylvian vein; *DSV*, deep sylvian vein; *VFO*, vein of the foramen ovale; *SPS*, superior petrosal sinus; *IPS*, inferior petrosal sinus to transverse occipital sinus; *VFR*, vein of the foramen rotundum

Foramen of the sellar and perisellar regions and their neurovascular contents

Pharyngohypophyseal canal (inconstant)	capsular branch (sinusal)
Optical canal	optic nerve
	ophthalmic artery
Superior orbital fissure	IIIrd
	IVth
	VIth
	Vth1
	autonomic nervous system
	deep recurrent ophthalmic artery
	ophthalmic vein
	recurrent meningeal or recurrent tentorial or meningo-ophthalmic artery depending on the variant
Foramen rotundum	Vth2
	emissary vein
	artery of the foramen rotundum
Foramen ovale	Vth3
	Vmth
	emissary vein
	cavernous branch of the accessory meningeal artery
Arnold's foramen (inconstant)	superficial and deep minor petrosal nerves, emissary vein
Vesalius foramen (inconstant)	emissary vein
	cavernous branch of the accessory meningeal artery (maxillary dominance)
Foramen lacerum	internal carotid artery
	pericarotid autonomic nervous system
	carotid branch of the ascending pharyngeal artery
	vidian nerve
Foramen spinosum (inconstant)	middle meningeal artery

---

[1] The venous plexus situated in the extradural space, lined with endothelium, is the counterpart of the vertebral epidural venous plexus, with which it communicates through the basilary plexus dorsal to the dorsum sellae.

Trigeminal artery, trunk in its lateral medullary portion

[See trigeminal nerve (V), p. 60; spinal roots of accessory nerve (XI), p. 255]

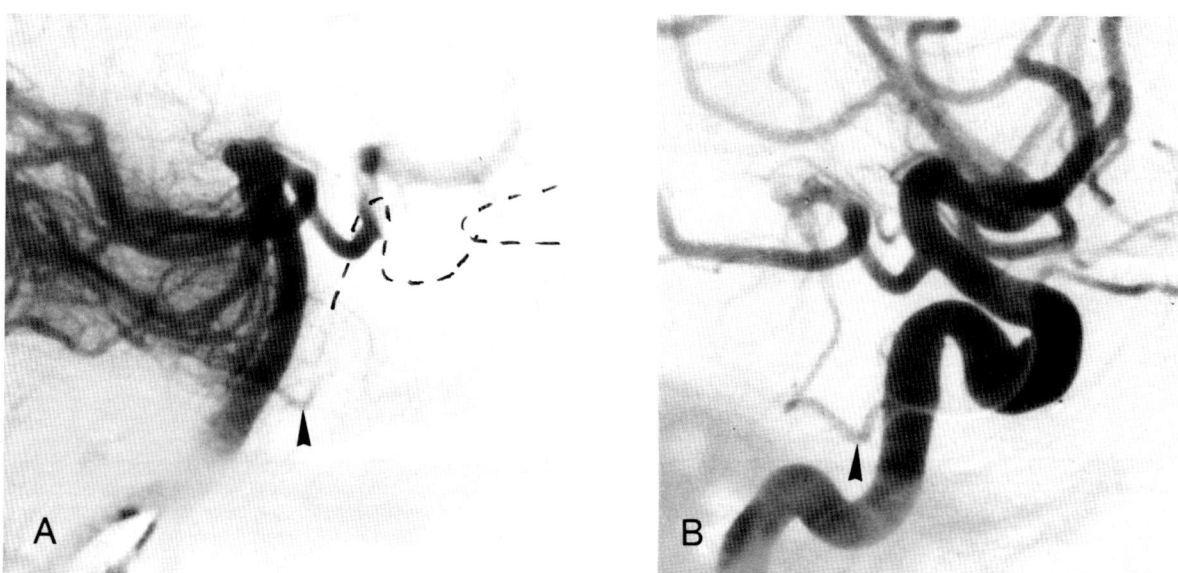

Fig. 13.23. **A** Selective injection of the vertebral artery, lateral view. **B** Internal carotid injection, lateral view, in a case of persistent trigeminal neuralgia. Note the partial trigeminal persistence (*arrowhead*)

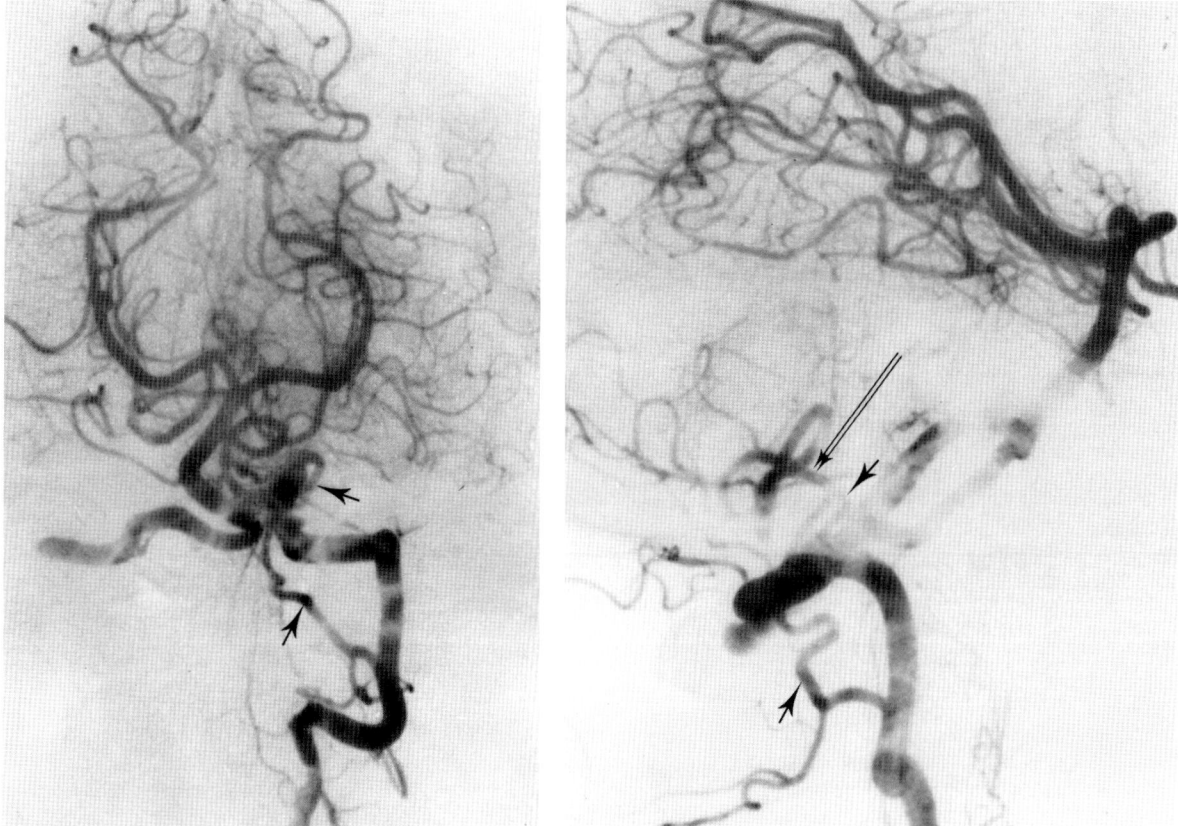

Fig. 13.24. Vertebral injection, (**A**) frontal and (**B**) lateral views. Double origin of the PICA at C1–C2 (*arrows*) which becomes a single trunk in its lateral medullary portion (*double arrow*)

Hypoglossal branch

[See hypoglossal nerve (XII), p. 260]

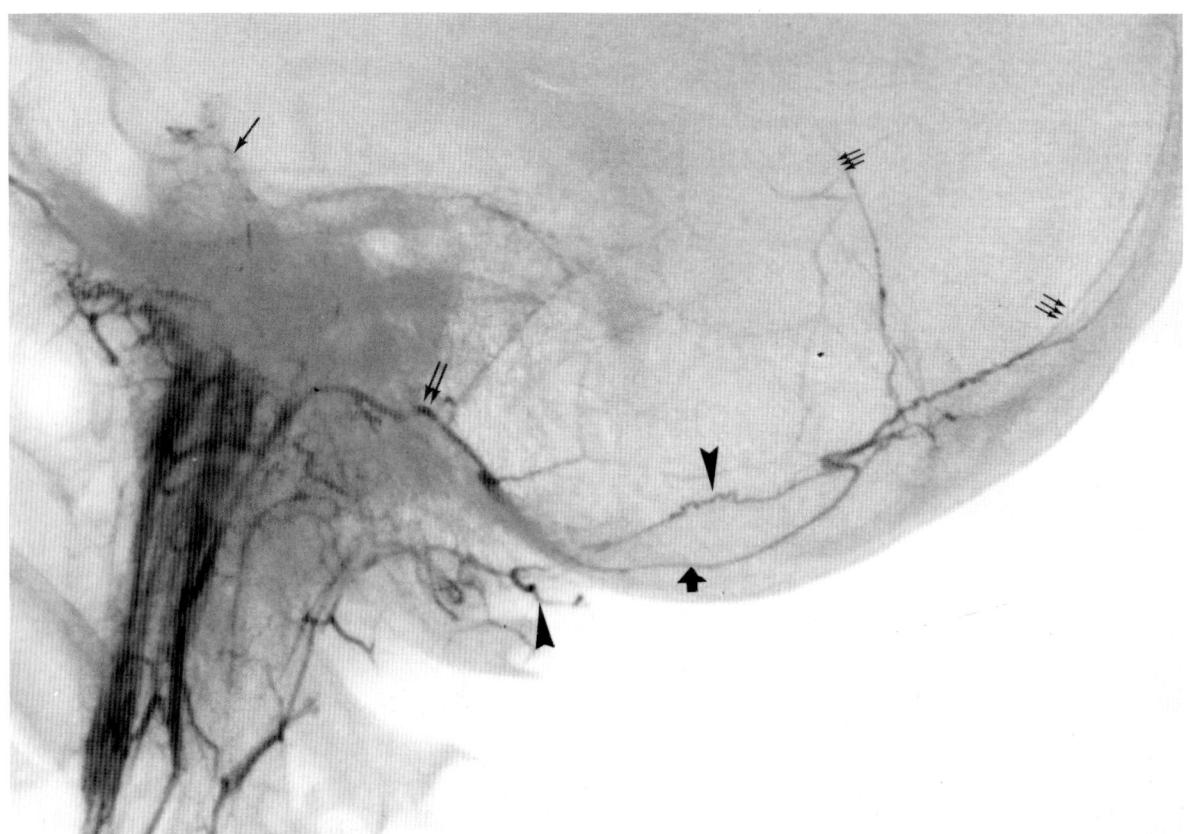

Fig. 13.25. Selective injection of the ascending pharyngeal artery. Lateral projection. The hypoglossal branch (*double arrow*) gives rise to the meningeal artery of the cerebellar fossa (*arrow*). Through this artery one can recognize the arterial system of the midline: the arteries of the falx cerebri, the straight sinus (*triple arrows*), and the falx cerebelli which originates here from the occipital artery (*arrowheads*). Note also the visualization of the posterior portion of the pituitary gland through the clival anastomotic channel (*small arrow*). Reprinted by permission from Lasjaunias, P. et al.: Vascularisation meningée de la fosse cérébrale moyenne. Journal of Neuroradiology 4: 361–384, 1977

Bibliography

Bouchet M, Dulac GL (1955) Anatomie radiographique du massif facial. Masson, Paris

Brant-Zawadzki M (1987) Magnetic resonance. Imaging of the central nervous system. Raven Press, New York

Brunner S, Pedersen CB (1970) Roentgen examination of the facial canal. Acta Radiol [Diagn] (Stockh) 10 (6):545

Cabanis EA, Tamraz J, Iba-Zizen MT (1986) IRM de la tête à 0,5 Tesla. Feuill Radiol 26:309–416

Chin FK (1970) Radiation dose to critical organs during petrous tomography. Radiology 94:623–627

Daniels DL, Haughton VM (1987) Cranial and spinal magnetic resonance imaging. An atlas and a guide. Raven Press, New York

Daniels DL, Herfkins R, Koehler PR, Millen SJ, Shaffer KA, Williams AL, Haughton VM (1984) Magnetic resonance imaging of the internal auditory canal. Radiology 151:105–108

Daniels DL, Pech P, Haughton VM (1984) Magnetic resonance imaging of the temporal bone. General Electric Medical Systems Group, Milwaukee

Daniels DL, Schenck JF, Foster T, Hart H Jr, Millent SJ, Meyer GA, Pech P, Haughton VM (1985) Magnetic resonance imaging of the jugular foramen. AJNR 6:699–703

Dolenc VV (1987) The cavernous sinus. Springer, Wien New York

Dulac GL (1955) Présentation du crâniographe. Application stéréoradiographique et aux incidences angulaires. J Radiol Electrol 36:11–12, 930–933

Dulac GL, Claus E, Barrois J (1973) Monographia otoradiologica. Bull Radiogr Agfa Gevaert, août 1973

Ericson S, Liliequist B (1973) Tomographic examination of the vertical segment of the facial canal. Acta Radiol [Diagn] (Stockh) 14:673

Fischgold H, David M, Bregeat P (1952) Tomographie de la base du crâne. Masson, Paris

Fischgold H, Metzger J, Korach G (1954) Tomographie de la région pétro-sphéno-occipitale. Incidence des quatre dernières paires crâniennes. Acta Radiol 42,1:56–64

Fischgold H, Salamon G, Guerinel G, Louis R, Metzger J, Legré J, Wackenheim A, Doyon D (1972) Traité de radiodiagnostic, tome XIII: Neuroradiologie. Fasc 1: Radioanatomie. Méthodes d'exploration. Masson, Paris

Fleury P, François J, Bourdon R (1964) Etude radio-tomo-anatomique des osselets. Ann Otolaryngol 81,1/2:45–52

Fowler EP (1961) Variations in the temporal bone course of the facial nerve. Laryngoscope 71 (8):937

Francke JP, Macke A, Clarisse J, Libersa JC, Dobbelaere P (1982) The internal carotid arteries. Anat Clin 3:243–261

Ge X, Spector G (1981) Labyrinthine segment and geniculate ganglion of facial nerve in fetal and adult human temporal bones. Ann Otol Rhinol Laryngol [Suppl 85]:2

Johnson DW (1984) Air cisternography of the cerebellopontine angle using high resolution computed tomography. Radiology 151 (2):401–404

Juster M, Fischgold H (1955) Etude radioanatomique de l'os temporal. Masson, Paris

Kodros A, Buckingham RA (1957) Anatomy of the descending portion of the facial nerve in the AMA. Arch Otolaryngol 66:735

Korach G, Vignaud J (1977) Manuel de techniques radiographiques du crâne. Masson, Paris

Kubik S, Oguz M (1983) Exploration of the facial nerve canal by high-resolution computed tomography. Anatomy and pathology. Neuroradiology 24:139

Kudo H, Nori S (1974) Topography of the facial nerve in the human temporal bone. Acta Anat (Basel) 90:467

Lang J (1981) Facial and vestibulocochlear nerve. Topographic anatomy and variations. In: Samii M, Jannetta PJ (eds) The cranial nerves. Springer, Berlin Heidelberg New York, p 363

Lang J (1981) Neuroanatomie der N. opticus, trigeminus, facialis, glossopharyngeus, vagus, accessorius und hypoglossus. Arch Otorhinolaryngol 231:1

Laudenbach P, Bonneau E, Korach G (1977) Radiographie panoramique dentaire et maxillo-faciale. Masson, Paris

Lazorthes G (1971) Le système nerveux périphérique. Masson, Paris

May M (1976) Anatomy of cross-section of facial nerve and temporal bone: clinical application. In: Fisch U (ed) Proceedings of the 3rd Symposium on Facial Nerve Surgery, August 1976, Zurich, Switzerland, p 40 (abstract)

Mündnich K, Frey K-W (1959) The tomogram of the ear. Das Röntgenschichtbild des Ohres. Thieme, Stuttgart

Nager G (1982) The facial canal. Normal anatomy, variations and anomalies. Ann Otol Rhinol Laryngol 91 [Suppl 97]:33

New PFJ, Bachow TB, Wismer GL, Rosen BR, Brady TJ (1985) MR imaging of the acoustic nerves and small acoustic neuromas at 0.6 T: prospective study. AJNR 6:165–170

Newton TH, Potts DG (1971) Radiology of the skull and train. Mosby, Saint Louis

Paturet G (1964) Traité d'anatomie humaine, tome IV: Système nerveux. Masson, Paris

Potter G (1964) Radiologic assessment of the facial nerve. Otolaryngol Clin North Am 7 (2):343

Proctor B, Nager G (1982) The facial canal. Normal anatomy, variations and anomalies. Ann Otol Rhinol Laryngol 91 [Suppl 97]:33

Rabischong P, Vignaud J, Paleirac R, Lamoth AP (1975) Tomographie et anatomie de l'oreille. Arts Graphiques A.P. Lamoth, Amsterdam

Rauschning W, Bergstrom K, Pech P (1983) Correlative craniospinal anatomy studies by computed tomography and cryomicrotomy. J Comput Assist Tomogr 7:9–13

Rhoton AL, Pulec JL, Hall GM, Boyd AS (1968) Absence of bone over the geniculate ganglion. J Neurosurg 28 (1):48–53

Ribet RM (1952) Les nerfs crâniens. Doin, Paris

Salamon G, Huang YP (1976) Radiologic anatomy of the brain. Springer, Berlin Heidelberg New York

Schubiger O (1983) High resolution CT of the normal and abnormal fallopian canal. Am J Neuroradiol 4:748

Swartz JD (1984) The facial nerve canal: CT analysis of the protruding tympanic segment. Radiology 153:443–447

Teresi LM, Kolin E, Lufkin RB, Hanafee WN (1987) MR imaging of the intraparotid facial nerve: normal anatomy and pathology. AJR 148:995–1000

Teresi LM, Lufkin RB, Wortham D, Flannigan B, Reicher M, Halbach V, Bentson J, Wilson G, Ward P, Hanafee WN (1987) MR imaging of the intratemporal facial nerve using surface coils. AJNR 8:49–54

Valavanis A, Kubik S, Oguz M (1983) Exploration of the facial nerve canal by high-resolution computed tomography. Anatomy and pathology. Neuroradiology 24:139

Valavanis A, Schubiger O (1983) High-resolution CT of the normal and abnormal fallopian canal. Am J Neuroradiol 4:748

Valvassori GE (1976) Radiography of the facial nerve canal. In: Fisch U (ed) Proceedings of the 3rd Symposium on Facial Nerve Surgery, August 1976, Zurich, Switzerland, p 174 (abstract)

Valvassori GE, Potter DG, Hanafee WN, Carter BL, Buckingham RA (1982) Radiology of the ear, nose and throat. Saunders, Philadelphia

Vignaud J (1974) Traité de radiodiagnostic, tome XVII.1: Temporal, fosses nasales, cavités accessoires. Masson, Paris

Vignaud J, Boulin A (1987) Tomodensitométrie crânio-encéphalique. Vigot, Paris

Vignaud J, Burlamaqui BJ, Augin ML (1970) Etude tomographique de l'aqueduc de Fallope. J Radiol Electrol 51:127–132

Vignaud J, Jardin C, Rosen L (1986) The ear – diagnostic imaging. Masson, New York

Vignaud J, Korach G (1969) Exploration radiologique du rocher normal. Feuill Electroradiol 51:52

Vignaud J, Sultan A, Leriche H (1969) Dislocations traumatiques de la chaîne des osselets. J Radiol Electrol 50,11:803–806

Wadin K, Wilbrand H (1987) The labyrinthine portion of the facial canal. A comparative radioanatomic investigation. Acta Radiol 28:17–32

Weill F (1975) Eléments programmés de radiologie oto-rhino-stomatologique. Masson, Paris

Wilbrand HF (1974) Multidirectional tomography of minor detail in the temporal bone. Acta Universitatis Upsaliensis, Upsala

Wilbrand HF (1975) Multidirectional tomography of the facial canal. Acta Radiol [Diagn] (Stockh) 16:654

Zacchi C, Vio S, Fiore D (1981) Anatomia radiologica dei neuri cranici. Piccin, Padova

Index

aditus ad antrum 223
angle, cerebellopontine 65, 66, 177, 178, 215, 231, 245
-, -, abducent nerve 64-67, 160-164, 176-179, 215, 231-233, 266
-, -, cistern of 66, 163, 177, 179, 189, 215, 232, 264
-, -, glossopharyngeal nerve 231, 232
antrum, mastoid 222
area striata 31
artery, basilar 215
-, cerebellar (superior) 40, 41
-, cerebral (posterior) 40, 41
-, ophthalmic 23, 24, 30

body, lateral geniculate 18, 31, 32
bulb, olfactory 2, 5, 9, 11, 13-15, 26
-, -, anatomy 12
-, -, imaging 12

canal, carotid 232
-, facial 190, 191, 195, 200, 201, 210
-, incisive 128, 132, 133
-, mandibular 147-150, 152
-, optic 11, 23
-, -, anatomy 21
-, -, computed tomography (CT) 23
-, -, imaging 21, 22
-, palatine 129
-, -, greater 129, 132, 133
-, -, -, sulcus 129, 134
-, -, lesser 129, 132
-, -, -, sulcus 129
-, pterygoid 194, 196-198
canaliculus, tympanic, imaging 237
cavities of the internal ear, anatomy 216
-, imaging 216
chiasm, optic 18, 20, 23, 24, 26-30, 32
chorda tympani 183, 202-204
cistern, of cerebellopontine angle 66, 163, 177, 179, 189, 215, 232, 264
-, chiasmatic 26, 28
-, of great cerebral vein 52, 53, 56
-, -, anatomy 51
-, -, imaging 51, 52
-, interpeduncular 38-41
-, -, anatomy 38
-, -, imaging 38, 39, 41
-, pontine 67, 164, 215
cochlea 215, 218, 219
colliculus, inferior 48, 52, 54, 56, 58
-, -, anatomy 51
-, -, imaging 51
concha, nasal, inferior 128
-, -, middle 128
-, -, superior 128
corpus callosum, genu 14
-, -, splenium 14
-, -, sulcus 13-15

ear, external 225
-, -, imaging 225
-, internal, anatomy 216-218
-, -, cavities, anatomy 216
-, -, -, imaging 216
-, middle, anatomy 219, 221-224
-, -, imaging 220-222
external ear see ear
eyeball muscle 45
eyelid, upper, levator muscle 44, 45

fissure, orbital, inferior 113
-, -, superior 43, 83, 164
-, -, -, imaging 55, 167
-, -, petrotympanosquamous 202, 203
foramen, ethmoidal 90, 91
-, -, anterior 89-93
-, -, imaging 90
-, -, posterior 89-93
-, incisive 133
-, infraorbital 117-122
-, jugular 232-235, 237, 245, 249, 257, 258
-, -, anatomy 233, 246
-, -, imaging 233, 246
-, mental 147-152
-, ovale 60, 137, 145
-, -, anatomy 138
-, -, imaging 138, 139
-, palatine 132-134
-, rotundum 97-109
-, sphenopalatine 128, 129, 134
-, stylomastoid 183, 205, 206
-, -, imaging 207
fossa, pterygopalatine 60, 65, 125, 127-131, 134, 194, 197
-, -, anatomy 126, 127, 132
-, -, imaging 126-131, 134
fossula, petrosal (sulcus of inferior ganglion) 228, 232, 234-237
-, -, anatomy 234
-, -, imaging 234

ganglion, ciliary 44, 46, 55, 105
-, geniculate 197, 200-202, 204, 209, 210
-, otic 143, 145, 197, 198
-, -, canal 198, 199
-, pterygopalatine 60, 124-131, 134, 194, 197, 209, 210
-, trigeminal 60, 65, 67, 70, 71, 73, 77-79
-, -, trigeminal impression, anatomy 72
-, -, -, imaging 72-78
-, -, trigeminal notch 71, 77, 80
-, vestibular 217
genu of corpus callosum 14
-, splenium 14
-, sulcus 13-15
gland, lacrimal 169, 209, 210
-, palatine 209
-, parotid 209
-, submandibular 209
gyrus, cingulate 14, 15
-, parahippocampal, anatomy 12
-, -, imaging 12

hammer see malleus

incus 219, 221, 222
internal ear see ear

lamina, spiral, bony 218
lingula of mandible 149, 150

malleus 219, 221, 222, 224
mandible, lingula 149, 150
meatus, acoustic, external, anatomy 215
-, -, -, imaging 202, 215, 216, 221, 224, 225
-, -, -, sensory ramus 181, 183, 200
-, -, internal 177-180, 188, 189, 215-218
middle ear see ear
muscle, dilator pupillae 46
-, -, sympathetic innervation 46
-, levator palpebrae superioris 44, 45
-, oblique, inferior 44, 45

–, –, superior 55–58
–, –, –, reflexion pulley (trochlea) 55–58
–, pterygoid, lateral 143
–, rectus, inferior 44, 55
–, –, lateral 163, 164, 168–170
–, –, medial 44, 45, 168
–, –, superior 44, 45
–, sphincter pupillae 46
–, –, parasympathetic innervation 46
–, styloglossus 235, 271
–, stylohyoid 235, 271
–, stylopharyngeus 235, 271
muscles, ocular 45

nerve, abducent 156–166, 168–170, 215
–, –, anatomy 157–159
–, –, cerebellopontine angle 64–67, 160–164, 176–179, 215, 231–233, 266
–, –, course 160–165, 169, 170
–, –, imaging 157–159
–, –, pathology 157–159
–, –, sulcus 164, 165, 168
–, –, sympathetic branch 169
–, accessory 128, 252, 255, 256, 258
–, –, anatomy 253, 255, 257
–, –, imaging 253, 255–258
–, –, roots 252, 255, 256
–, alveolar, inferior 137, 143, 145, 147, 149, 151
–, –, –, anatomy 148
–, –, –, imaging 148, 149
–, –, –, pathology 146
–, auriculotemporal 145, 209
–, buccal 145
–, ciliary 46
–, cochlear 212
–, ethmoidal, anatomy 89
–, –, anterior 88–92
–, –, –, imaging 89
–, –, posterior 88–92
–, –, –, imaging 89–91
–, –, sulcus 91, 93
–, facial 172–179, 185, 188, 189, 200, 205, 209, 210, 212, 217
–, –, anastomoses 182, 183, 204, 205
–, –, anatomy 173, 176
–, –, collaterals 175, 180, 183
–, –, extrapetrous course 184
–, –, imaging 173, 176, 185–187
–, –, intrapetrous course 180, 183, 188
–, –, pathology 173, 185–187
–, –, terminal branches 181, 210
–, frontal 37, 60, 83
–, glossopharyngeal 209, 228, 232, 238
–, –, anatomy 229, 231
–, –, branches 238, 239
–, –, cerebellopontine angle 231, 232
–, –, imaging 229, 231
–, –, parasympathetic nucleus 209
–, –, posterior lateral sulcus of medulla oblongata 228, 231, 232
–, hypoglossal 128, 160, 172, 260, 263–269, 271
–, –, anatomy 263, 267
–, –, branches 271
–, –, imaging 267, 268
–, infraorbital 110–116
–, –, anatomy 112, 118
–, –, imaging 112–114
–, –, labial, palpebral and nasal branches 117–123
–, –, pathology 110, 117
–, –, sulcus 111–116
–, intermedius 179, 183, 188, 200
–, lacrimal 57, 58, 60, 61, 71, 77, 83, 92
–, to levator labii superioris muscle 91, 92
–, –, sulcus 91, 93
–, mandibular 65, 71, 77, 79, 83, 136–138, 143–145
–, –, imaging 138–140, 143–150

–, –, pathology 136
–, masseteric 145
–, maxillary 60, 77, 83, 97–109
–, –, anatomy 98
–, –, imaging 98–100, 102, 103, 105–109
–, –, pathology 96
–, –, sulcus 101
–, mental, anatomy 148
–, –, imaging 148, 149, 151, 152
–, –, pathology 146
–, mylohyoid 61, 137
–, nasal, inferior 128
–, –, superior 127–129, 131
–, nasociliary 60, 61, 77, 92
–, –, nasopalatine 127–129, 131
–, –, anterior branch 132, 133
–, oculomotor 33–41, 44–46
–, –, anatomy 35, 38, 42, 44, 46
–, –, communicating branch with ciliary ganglion 46
–, –, extrinsic ocular movements 44, 45
–, –, imaging 35, 38–41
–, –, inferior branch 37, 44
–, –, parasympathetic innervation 46
–, –, pathology 35, 38, 42
–, –, sulcus 42, 43
–, –, superior branch 37, 44
–, ophthalmic 65–67, 71, 77, 79, 82, 83, 87, 101
–, –, meningeal branch 145
–, optic 18, 23, 24, 26–32
–, –, anatomy 19, 21, 25
–, –, imaging 19, 21–23, 25, 26
–, –, occipitotemporal fasciculus 31
–, –, pathology 19
–, palatine 129, 134
–, –, accessory 128, 132, 133
–, –, greater 124, 128, 132, 133
–, –, lesser 124, 128, 132, 133
–, petrosal 210
–, –, greater 183, 190, 192, 196–198, 200, 209
–, –, lesser 183, 190, 192, 196–198, 209, 210
–, pterygoid 129, 131, 134, 194, 195, 197
–, pterygopalatine 123, 125, 127, 129, 134, 194
–, to stapedius muscle 183, 201
–, temporal, deep 145
–, trigeminal 60, 61, 65–67
–, –, anatomy 63, 64
–, –, communicating branch with ciliary ganglion 60, 61, 123
–, –, imaging 63–65
–, –, impression 65–67, 71, 73–80
–, –, motor root 60, 65
–, –, nucleus 209
–, –, pathology 63
–, –, sensory root 60, 65
–, –, terminal branches 153
–, trochlear 48, 52, 54–56, 58
–, –, anatomy 49–51
–, –, imaging 49, 54
–, tympanic 236, 238, 239, 249
–, –, anatomy 236
–, –, branches 238
–, –, imaging 237
–, vagus 128, 242, 249, 252, 258, 260, 264, 266, 271
–, –, anatomy 243, 245, 246
–, –, auricular branch 183, 204, 249, 271
–, –, functions 250
–, –, imaging 245, 246, 248
–, –, pathology 243, 245, 246
–, vestibulocochlear 212, 215, 217, 224, 226
–, –, anatomy 213, 215, 216
nerves, olfactory 1–3, 5–7, 9, 11–15
–, –, anatomy 3, 6, 12
–, –, fibers 9, 15
–, –, imaging 3, 6–10, 12–15
–, –, pathology 3

–, to tensor tympani, tensor veli palatini and medial pterygoid muscles 145
notch, trigeminal 71, 77, 80

ossicles, chain of, imaging 220–222
ostium introitus 204, 205, 248, 249
–, anatomy 248, 249

pathways, olfactory, anatomy 12
–, –, imaging 2–16
–, optic 17–32
–, –, anatomy 21, 25
–, –, imaging 24, 29, 30
–, secretory, salivary and lacrimomuconasal 209
peduncle, cerebral 46, 58
–, –, anatomy 38
–, –, imaging 38
plate, cribriform 7–11, 13–15
–, –, of ethmoid, anatomy 6
–, –, –, imaging 6
plexus, internal carotid 46, 210, 239
pons 67
pulvinar 31, 32
pupil, dilator muscle 46
–, –, sympathetic innervation 46
–, sphincter muscle 46
–, –, parasympathetic innervation 46

radiations, optic 30, 31
recess, optic 23, 26

sinus, sphenoidal 91–93
stapes 219, 221, 222
stirrup *see* stapes
striae, longitudinal 15

substance, perforate, anterior 2, 15, 31
–, –, posterior 34, 40, 212
sulcus, calcarine 30–32
–, cavernous 54, 143, 162–164
–, –, anatomy 42, 162
–, –, imaging 42, 162–164
–, ethmoidal nerve 91, 93
–, infraorbital 112, 116
–, –, imaging 112, 113
–, medullopontine 160, 161, 172, 242

thalamus 23, 27, 30
tract, olfactory 2, 5, 9, 11, 15
–, –, intermediate 11
–, –, lateral 2, 11
–, –, medial 11
–, –, sulcus 13
–, optic 18, 20, 24, 29–32
–, –, computed tomography (CT) 29
trigone, olfactory 2, 9, 11, 15
tube, auditory 219, 222–225
–, –, anatomy 223
–, –, imaging 223, 224
tubercle, retrogasserian 80

uncus, hippocampal 16
–, –, anatomy 12
–, –, imaging 12

vein, great cerebral, cistern of 52, 53, 56
–, –, –, anatomy 51
–, –, –, imaging 51, 52
velum, medullary, superior 48, 52, 56
ventricle, lateral 31

window, vestibular 218, 219, 221, 222

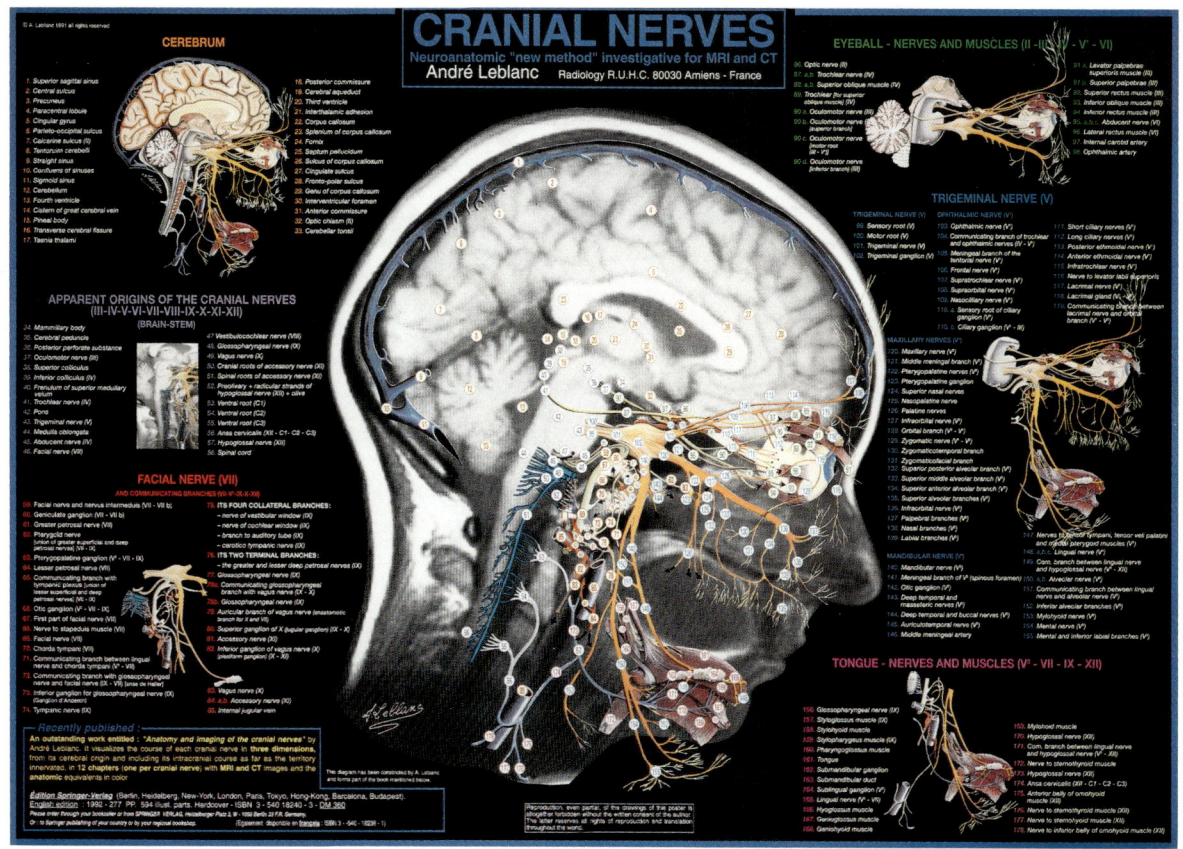
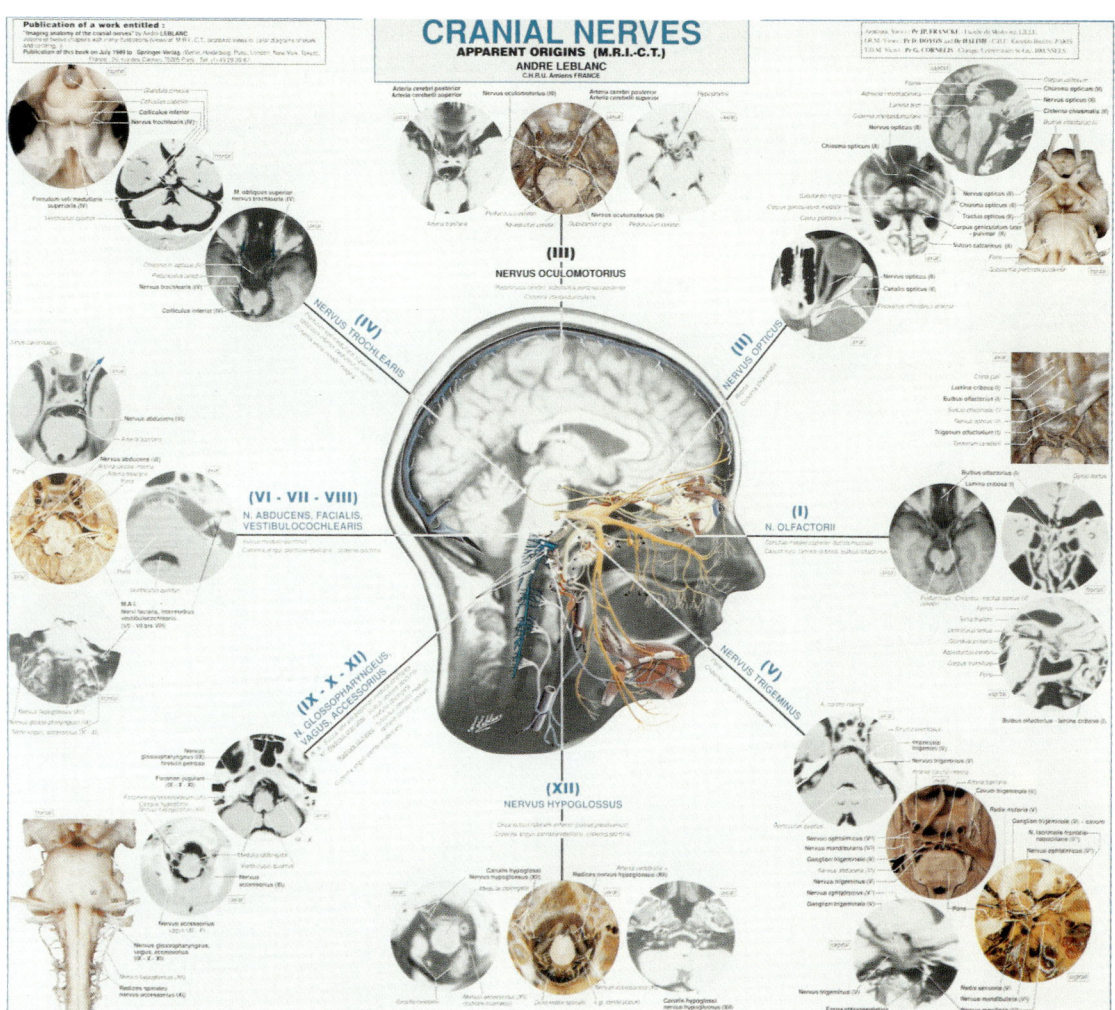

For all orders for these posters, please contact the author: Mr. André Leblanc, P.O. Box n° 2, 80800 Daours, France, [Fax: (+33) 22.48.31.23]

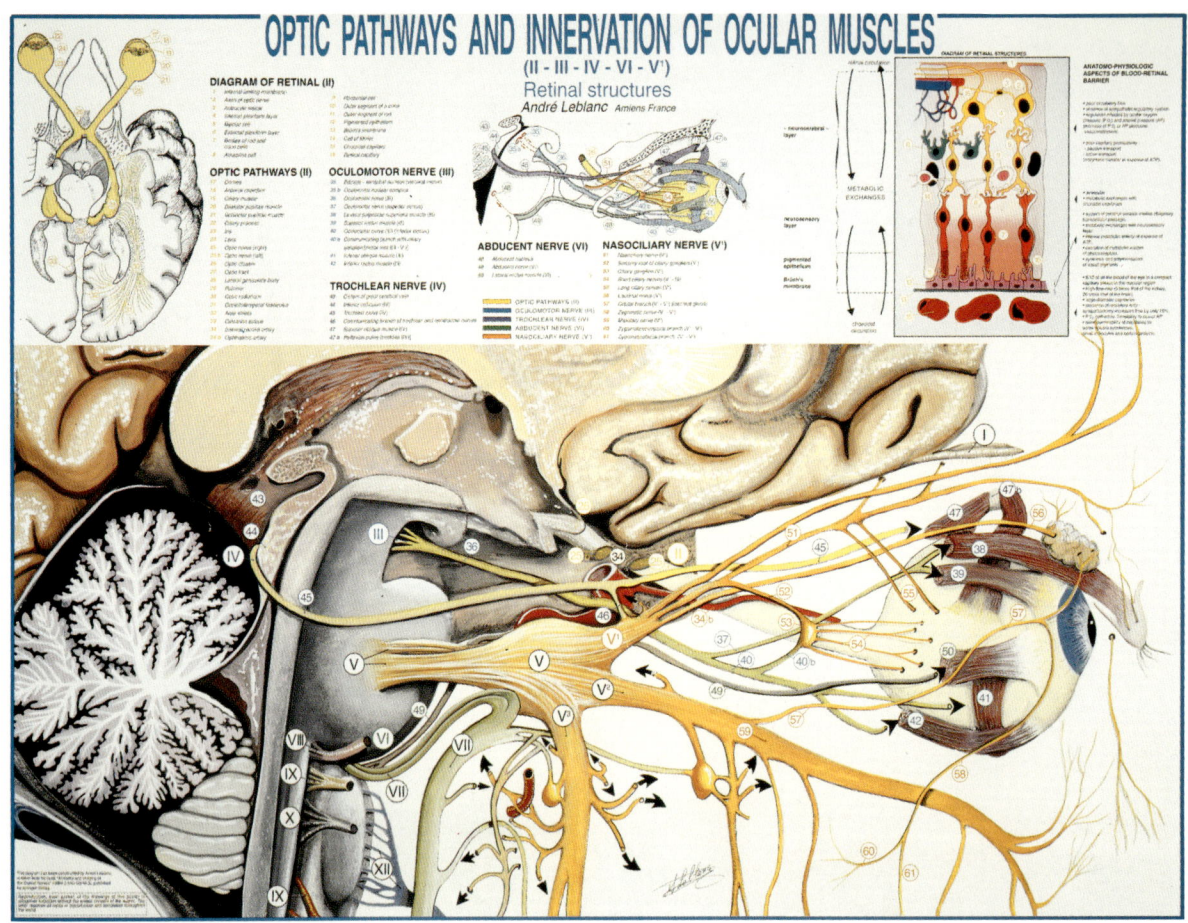
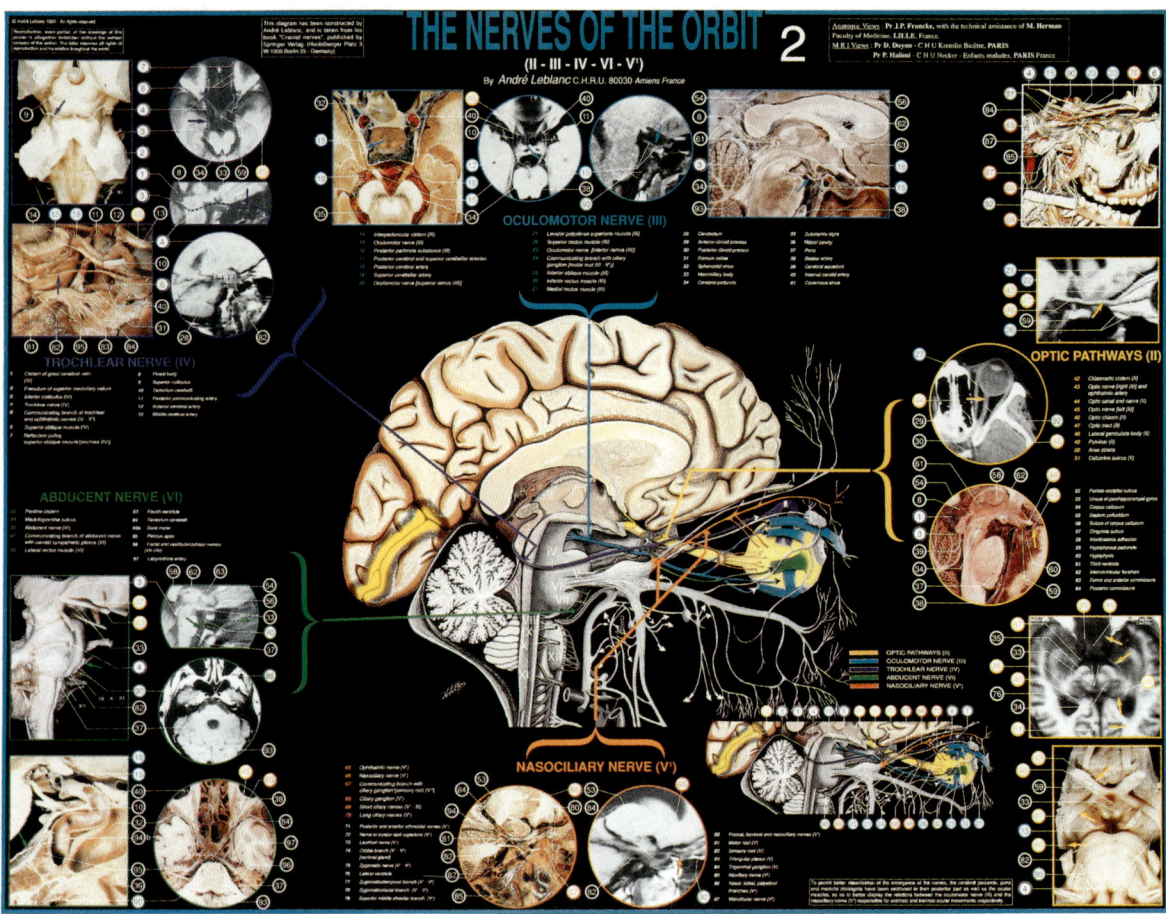

For all orders for these posters, please contact the author: Mr. André Leblanc, P.O. Box n° 2, 80800 Daours, France, [Fax: (+33) 22.48.31.23]